Sodium in Health and Disease

Sodium in Health and Disease

Edited by

Michel Burnier
University Hospital of Lausanne
CHUV, Switzerland

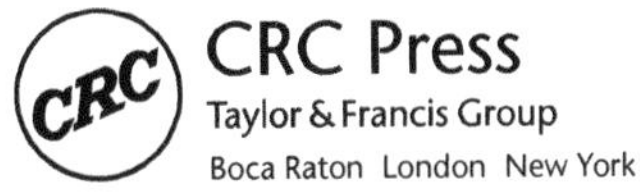

CRC Press is an imprint of the
Taylor & Francis Group, an **informa** business

CRC Press
Taylor & Francis Group
6000 Broken Sound Parkway NW, Suite 300
Boca Raton, FL 33487-2742

First issued in paperback 2019

ISBN-13: 978-0-8493-3978-3 (hbk)
ISBN-13: 978-0-367-38828-7 (pbk)

A CIP record for this book is available from the British Library.

Library of Congress Cataloging-in-Publication Data available on application

Visit the Taylor & Francis Web site at
http://www.taylorandfrancis.com

and the CRC Press Web site at
http://www.crcpress.com

To Marie France
and
Géraldine, Céline, and Pauline

One sees clearly only with the heart. Anything essential is invisible to the eyes.

Antoine de Saint Exupéry, in *Le Petit Prince*

Preface

Salt has long been recognized as the most determinant element of body fluid necessary to maintain the integrity of the *milieu intérieur*. Research on salt has always been intense, and has been characterized in the last ten years by major advances in our understanding of the mechanisms that contribute to the regulation of sodium balance in physiological and pathological conditions. Several renal transporters have been cloned and various monogenic forms of hypertension have been characterized in which specific alterations in renal tubular sodium handling have been described. The roles of many important regulators of sodium balance have been defined, such as that of 11-beta-hydroxysteroid dehydrogenase and the influence of renal structure proteins on sodium transport. Relevant information on the impact of sodium in diseases has also been gathered. Recent findings include the description of the link between sodium intake and pulse pressure and isolated systolic hypertension, and the surprising association between aldosterone and the metabolic syndrome.

The aim of *Sodium in Health and Disease* is to focus on the most recent developments that may be of interest for basic scientists as well as clinicians. It is addressed primarily to specialists in hypertension who are confronted with these salt issues almost every day, but also to cardiologists and nephrologists who have similar concerns regarding the role of salt in the development of cardiac and renal diseases. Interesting new information is provided for scientists working on the molecular biology of sodium transport. We hope to encourage new collaborations between scientists and clinicians.

The latest molecular and experimental mechanisms whereby body sodium homeostasis is maintained are described, followed by the clinical aspects of sodium and a review of the potential role of sodium in diseases such as hypertension, congestive heart failure, chronic renal failure, and cirrhosis. The basic science presented in this book provides exciting new data on renal sodium transporters. Eric Féraille, Olivier Bonny, and Peter A. Doris have written comprehensive reviews on the Na^+-K^+-ATPase, the epithelial sodium channel, and the renal handling of sodium by the proximal tubule. The authors give important insights into the biochemistry of renal sodium handling. In Chapter 4, Paolo Manunta presents an important new approach to the regulation of sodium excretion, i.e the impact of renal structure proteins on sodium transport. In recent years, considerable new information has been acquired regarding the role of mineralocorticoids and particularly aldosterone. These aspects are covered in Chapters 7 and 8 by Nicolette Farman and Paolo Ferrari in two excellent reviews on aldosterone and 11-beta-hydroxysteroid dehydrogenase. Sodium balance cannot be maintained without the crucial role of regulating hormones. Interestingly, new hormonal controls of sodium excretion are still being discovered. These hormonal systems are reviewed in light of the most recent data. Edward J. Johns discusses new aspects linked to the activity of the sympathetic nervous system in Chapter 6. Jean-Pierre Montani has risen to the challenge of providing an integrative approach to the multiple mechanisms involved in the regulation of sodium homeostasis.

In the future, even more research will be needed and new tools must be developed. In Chapter 10, Pierre Meneton presents the various animal models that have been generated and are now available for the study of the renal mechanisms of sodium excretion.

The chapters covering the clinical aspect of this topic include a discussion by Graham A. MacGregor on the controversial issue of the link between hypertension and sodium intake. Dr. McGregor handles this topic with conviction and presents several irrefutable arguments. Judith A. Miller provides interesting new data on gender differences in the way sodium balance is maintained, a topic that is rarely covered in textbooks.

Sodium in Health and Disease provides the most recent findings on the role of sodium in diseases such as hepatic cirrhosis, congestive heart failure, hypertension, and chronic renal failure. This research is presented by recognized leaders in the fields: Pere Ginès, William T. Abraham, Gerjan J. Navis, and Albert Mimran. Finally, Bernard Waeber and Nancy J. Brown address the role of diuretics in the management of hypertension and renal and cardiac diseases. In Chapter 23, Dr. Brown considers the escalating use of mineralocorticoid antagonists and the increasing evidence for clinical benefits of these agents beyond their capacity to enhance sodium excretion.

I have been fortunate that many distinguished authors, colleagues, and friends agreed to contribute to this exciting project. I would like to take this opportunity to thank them all very warmly. I would also like to thank Christine DeGunten for her excellent secretarial support and enthusiasm, and help in maintaining the deadlines. I have also appreciated the great help of the people at Informa Healthcare, who gave me the opportunity to edit this book and provided excellent professional support.

Michel Burnier

Contents

Contributors

William T. Abraham Division of Cardiovascular Medicine, Ohio State University, Columbus, Ohio, U.S.A.

Athanase Benetos Geriatric Center, Brabois Hospital, University of Nancy II, Nancy, France

Murielle Bochud Institute of Social and Preventive Medicine, University Hospital, University of Lausanne, Lausanne, Switzerland

Olivier Bonny Charles and Jane Pak Center for Mineral Metabolism and Division of Nephrology, Southwestern Medical Center, The University of Texas, Dallas, Texas, U.S.A.

Nancy J. Brown Division of Clinical Pharmacology, Departments of Medicine and Pharmacology, Vanderbilt University Medical Center, Nashville, Tennessee, U.S.A.

Michel Burnier Division of Nephrology and Hypertension Consultation, University Hospital, University of Lausanne, Lausanne, Switzerland

Mauro Bustamante Service of Nephrology, Fondation pour Recherches Médicales, University of Geneva, Geneva, Switzerland

Andrés Cárdenas Institute of Digestive Diseases and Metabolism, University of Barcelona, Barcelona, Spain

David Z. I. Cherney Division of Nephrology, Toronto General Hospital, University of Toronto, Toronto, Ontario, Canada

Lionel Coltamai Division of Nephrology and Hypertension Consultation, University Hospital, University of Lausanne, Lausanne, Switzerland

Robert Di Nicolantonio Department of Physiology, The University of Melbourne, Victoria, Australia

Peter A. Doris Center for Human Genetics, Institute of Molecular Medicine, University of Texas Health Science Center, Houston, Texas, U.S.A.

Nicolette Farman Faculté de Médecine, Xavier Bichat, Paris, France

Eric Féraille Service of Nephrology, Fondation pour Recherches Médicales, University of Geneva, Geneva, Switzerland

Paolo Ferrari Department of Nephrology, Fremantle Hospital and School of Medicine and Pharmacology, University of Western Australia, Perth, Australia

John W. Funder Prince Henry's Institute of Medical Research, Clayton, Victoria, Australia

Pere Ginès Institute of Digestive Diseases and Metabolism, University of Barcelona, Barcelona, Spain

Feng J. He Blood Pressure Unit, Cardiac and Vascular Sciences, St. George's University of London, London, U.K.

Srinivas Iyengar Division of Cardiovascular Medicine, Ohio State University, Columbus, Ohio, U.S.A.

Edward J. Johns Department of Physiology, University College Cork, Cork, Republic of Ireland

Graham A. MacGregor Blood Pressure Unit, Cardiac and Vascular Sciences, St. George's University of London, London, U.K.

Marc P. Maillard Division of Nephrology and Hypertension Consultation, University Hospital, University of Lausanne, Lausanne, Switzerland

Paolo Manunta Division of Nephrology, Dialysis, and Hypertension, San Raffaele University Hospital "Vita-Salute," Milan, Italy

Pierre Meneton Department of Public Health and Medical Information, Paris Descartes University, Paris, France

Judith A. Miller Division of Nephrology, Toronto General Hospital, University of Toronto, Toronto, Ontario, Canada

Albert Mimran Department of Medicine, Hospital Lapeyronie, Montpellier, France

Jean-Pierre Montani Division of Physiology, Department of Medicine, University of Fribourg, Fribourg, Switzerland

Trefor Owen Morgan Department of Physiology, The University of Melbourne, Victoria, Australia

Friso L. H. Muntinghe Department of Medicine, University Medical Center Groningen, Groningen, The Netherlands

Gerjan J. Navis Department of Medicine, University Medical Center Groningen, Groningen, The Netherlands

Jean Ribstein Department of Medicine, Hospital Lapeyronie, Montpellier, France

Michel E. Safar Department of Medicine, Paris Descartes University and AP-HP Hôtel-Dieu Hospital, Paris, France

Maria Teresa Sciarrone Division of Nephrology, Dialysis, and Hypertension, San Raffaele University Hospital "Vita-Salute," Milan, Italy

Bruce N. Van Vliet Division of Basic Medical Sciences, Faculty of Medicine, Memorial University of Newfoundland, St. John's, Newfoundland, Canada

Bruno Vogt Division of Nephrology and Hypertension Consultation, University Hospital, University of Lausanne, Lausanne, Switzerland

Bernard Waeber Division of Clinical Pathophysiology and Hypertension Consultation, Department of Medicine, University Hospital, University of Lausanne, Lausanne, Switzerland

Anne Zanchi Division of Nephrology, Department of Medicine, Centre Hospitalier Universitaire Vaudois and University of Lausanne, Lausanne, Switzerland

Introduction

Michel Burnier, the editor of *Sodium in Health and Disease*, was kind enough to select me, among many friends and many competent scientists, to write a preface to this promising book. This raised a question, "Should the introduction be written after or before reading the chapters?" I had no choice, knowing only the authors and the plan of the book. The readers, however should read the chapters and then return to this introduction.

The intention of the authors is to add a translation of scientific facts into social behavior and public health vision. Keep in mind two words that are more and more frequently used: *translational* (1) and *evidence-based* (2). These terms can be applied to the entire history of salt and health. Translational means the ability to integrate the basic knowledge recently acquired on the single nucleotide polymorphisms and mutations of the multiple genes coding for the many proteins involved in the control of sodium intake, and elimination within the analysis of both individual diseases characterized by a sodium excess or a sodium loss is linked to a high or a low blood pressure, and epidemiologic observations throughout the entire world (3). Translational means understanding the advantages and limitations of the information provided by multiple animal models—from the chimpanzees when they meet researchers like Denton and exposure to salt, or rats when they are bred by Dahl, Bianchi, Aoki, and Okamoto, and others—in relation to data collected in populations where either blood pressure levels or incidence of cardiovascular diseases, stomach cancer, osteoporosis, or asthma are most frequently found to be associated with salt intake or salt excretion or a decrease in these diseases are found to be in proportion to a reduction in sodium intake. Evidence-based refers to each of the studies, experimental or human, that should be planned, performed, and critically analyzed according to certain rules of internal and external validity. These studies have been progressively theorized, resulting in improvement in investigative technologies, statistical methodologies, and reasoning.

From genes to the environment, translation will inspire a health policy and its tools: periodic surveillance of population health parameters, professional training, consumer information, negotiations with or regimentations of salty-food manufacturers. It is not a unidirectional translation, going from active scientists to passive consumers and quiet tradesmen. Financial interests involved in pricing of salt and the volume of salt added to food react to the analysis of the health effects on their business, much like the reaction of those concerned with nicotine in cigarettes or calories in energy-dense diets rich in oils, fats, and simple sugars. Perhaps unconsciously at first, these businesses take advantage of the difficulties encountered by the translation of scientific results to health policy at the service of their own financial interests. Here begins "the (political) science of salt," as it was called by Gary Taubes in the journal *Science* (4). "Three decades (four now) of controversy over the putative benefits of salt reduction show how the demands of good science clash with the pressures of public health policy...."

The cartoon captions in Taubes's article get the point across: "The salt controversy is the number one perfect example of why science is a destabilizing force in public policy" (Sanford Miller). "You can say without any shadow of a doubt that the [NHLBI] has made a commitment to salt education that goes way beyond the scientific facts" (Drummond Rennie). "All I'm trying to do is save some lives" (Ed. Rocella). "The most slender piece of evidence in favor of a salt-blood pressure link is welcomed as further proof of the link, while failures to find such evidence is explained away" (Olaf Simpson). "Intersalt did not show blood pressure increases if you eat a lot of salt" (Lennart Hanson). "The position has been clarified: all the Intersalt analyses confirm salt as an important determinant of blood pressure" (Malcom Law). "As long as there are things in the media that say the salt controversy continues, the [salt interests] win" (Jeff Cutter). The last word in the article was given to Hennekens, "The problem with this field is that people have chosen sides. What we ought to do is let the science drive the system rather than the opinion." It is at this time that evidence-based medicine on politics of salt and blood pressure should intervene.

The information given to policy-makers to create a truly active policy on salt reduction in food is not the result of a vote among experts. This is true even if, among all those who did contribute by generating data and not opinions, a large majority is in favor of salt reduction. A structured process of risk assessment and risk management is necessary, as summarized in Figure 1. Neither the level of quality nor the level of evidence is the same for all published studies. However, there is already a proliferation of panel recommendations, constituted at the request of the World Health Organization (5), national food agencies, professional associations (6–8), and scientific collaborations (9), which finally conclude that attainment of lower sodium levels in the general population represents an important public health opportunity.

Most of the recommendations indicate that a minimum 50% reduction of sodium in processed foods, fast-food products, and restaurant meals should be achieved in the next decade. In each country, the main source of sodium in food should be known, since they are quite different between Japan, China, and the United States. Specific national efforts have to be targeted, such as the negotiations initiated in France for bakers to reduce the daily salt content of bread, which provides around 30% of the salt content of the French diet, to 18g/kg.

As to the individual advice given by health professionals to patients and families, they are unlikely to be successful in the absence of salt labeling in food (10). By contrast with the endless European negotiations, the United Kingdom has created a "front-of-product" traffic light-type labeling system that identifies products as high (red light), medium (orange) or low (green) in sodium (11). Consumer associations can also help the

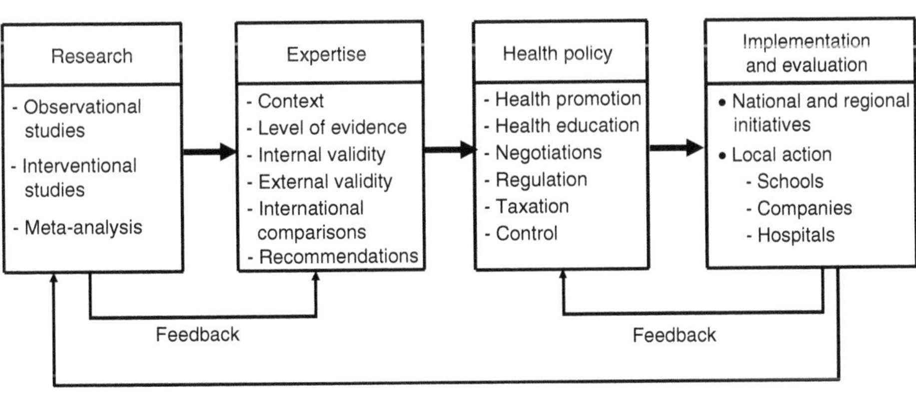

Figure 1 The independent and interrelated steps of risk assessment and risk management for salt intake and disease.

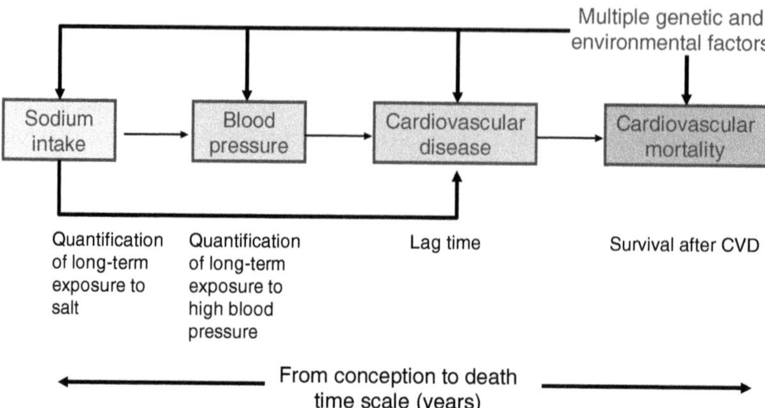

Figure 2 A conceptual framework for the relationship between salt consumption and cardiovascular mortality.

public and the authorities with periodic surveys that show, for instance, that the salt content of french fries ranges from 1.3 to 2.8 grams NaCl per 100 grams, when they bring 490 to 590 Kcalories/100gms.

The real issue today is not a lack of knowledge or an absence of objectives, but rather a deficit of public action. This failure is well demonstrated by the periodic measurements of sodium intake or sodium elimination in populations, which remains largely above 2.500 mg of sodium each day. This is even true for Finland, which was the most active in its nutritional health policy over the last 40 years. The 24-hour urinary sodium excretion for the Finnish population has decreased from 220 to 170 mmol/day in men, and from 180 to 130 mmol/day in women, remaining quite above the proposed target of 100 mmol/day value (12).

The majority of physicians and citizens are not aware of the major nutritional challenges of the twenty-first century. They only recognized the epidemic of obesity a few decades after it started, and some still look at sodium in the context of edemas. The lag time between salt exposure, rise in blood pressure, and cardiovascular and renal damage independent of blood pressure is not apparent (Figure 2). The public debate is dominated by the influence of the media and by different types of intervention from the food industry (13).

The most frequent type of lobbying promotes the potential risks to an individual's health from the extremely low salt diets studied in animals and humans (less than 2 grams of salt per day). These studies are not included in public health policies and push forward the salt-sensitivity paradigm to target salt intake limitation to a disputable "salt-sensitive" fraction of the population (14). This is similar to how the data about cancer sensitivity is used by the tobacco industry and gene-susceptibility for diabetes and obesity is applied by the food industry.

The salt industry also insists on the importance of the other risk factors of a low-salt diet, including caloric unbalance, taste of food, and liquid ingestion. Another more subtle lobbying tactic is the promotion of new "healthy" foods, in which the sodium content will be decreased, the potassium and calcium content will be increased, and the phytosterols will be introduced. The prices of these items will be increased in proportion to the magnitude of the advertisements designed to increase the market size. This leads to a curious society in which the young eat cheap fast foods and the old are fed a dream of immortality. Social inequalities in nutritional and health status will likely increase if what is considered healthy food becomes more and more expensive, as is already the case for fresh vegetables and fruits.

What will be the most complex and the most lengthy? The full understanding of gene functions, the description of genotype-phenotype correlations, and the discovery of a new pharmacology of the kidney, the heart, and the vessels? Or the implementation of the Consensus Action on Salt and Health (CASH: www.actiononsalt.org.uk) or the World Action on Salt and Health (WASH: wash@sgul.ac.uk), which promises that "if everyone achieved the 5g target of salt per day, 35,000 lives would be saved each year in the UK, and a further 35,000 people would be saved from the trauma and possible disability of a cardiovascular event which they survive?"

Developments in the understanding of sodium in health and disease will continue, so that the second edition of this book, five to ten years from now, may be even more interesting than this one.

Joel Ménard
Faculté de Médecine Paris-Descartes
Laboratoire de Santé Publique et d'Informatique Médicale
Paris, France

REFERENCES

1. Sung NS, Crowley WF, Jr., Genel M, Salber P, Sandy L, Sherwood LM, Johnson SB, Catanese V, Tilson H, Getz K, et al. Central challenges facing the national clinical research enterprise. J Am Med Assoc 2003; 289(10):1278–87.
2. Evidence-based medicine. A new approach to teaching the practice of medicine. Evidence-Based Medicine Working Group [see comments]. J Am Med Assoc 1992; 268(17):2420–5.
3. Meneton P, Jeunemaitre X, de Wardener HE, MacGregor GA. Links between dietary salt intake, renal salt handling, blood pressure, and cardiovascular diseases. Physiol Rev 2005; 85(2):679–715.
4. Taubes G. The (political) science of salt. Science 1998; 281:5379. 898–901, 903–7.
5. WHO. Reducing salt intake in populations. Report of a WHO Forum and Technical meeting. 5–7 October 2006. Paris (France).
6. Havas S, Roccella EJ, Lenfant C. Reducing the public health burden from elevated blood pressure levels in the United States by lowering intake of dietary sodium. Am J Public Health 2004; 94(1):19–22.
7. Dickinson BD, Havas S. Reducing the population burden of cardiovascular disease by reducing sodium intake: a report of the council on science and public health. Arch Intern Med 2007; 167(14):1460–8.
8. Lichtenstein AH, Appel LJ, Brands M, Carnethon M, Daniels S, Franch HA, Franklin B, Kris-Etherton P, Harris WS, Howard B, et al. Diet and lifestyle recommendations revision 2006: a scientific statement from the American Heart Association Nutrition Committee. Circulation 2006; 114(1):82–96.
9. He FJ, MacGregor GA. Effect of longer-term modest salt reduction on blood pressure. Cochrane Database Syst Rev 2004:3. CD004937. DOI: 10.1002/14651858.CD004937
10. Hooper L, Bartlett C, Davey SG, Ebrahim S. Advice to reduce dietary salt for prevention of cardiovascular disease. Cochrane Database Syst Rev 2004:Issue 1. Art. No.: CD003656. DOI: 10.1002/14651858.CD003656.pub2
11. Sharp D. Labelling salt in food: if yes, how? Lancet 2004; 364(9451):2079–81.

12. Laatikainen T, Pietinen P, Valsta L, Sundvall J, Reinivuo H, Tuomilehto J. Sodium in the Finnish diet: 20-year trends in urinary sodium excretion among the adult population. Eur J Clin Nutr 2006; 60(8):965–70.
13. Al-Awqati Q. Evidence-based politics of salt and blood pressure. Kidney Int 2006; 69(10):1707–8.
14. Luft FC, Weinberger MH. Heterogeneous responses to changes in dietary salt intake: the salt-sensitivity paradigm. Am J Clin Nutr 1997; 65(Suppl. 2):612S–7S.

1
Sodium-Potassium-ATPase

Mauro Bustamante and Eric Féraille
Service of Nephrology, Fondation pour Recherches Médicales, University of Geneva, Geneva, Switzerland

INTRODUCTION

The sodium-potassium-adenosinetriphosphatase (Na^+-K^+-ATPase), or sodium pump, belongs to the P-type ATPases family (also called E1,E2-ATPases). This family of ATPases comprises active transporters involved in unidirectional transport or exchange of monovalent (H^+, Na^+, K^+) or divalent (Ca^{2+}, Cu^{2+}, Mg^{2+}) ions. Transient phosphorylation during the catalytic cycle is the major characteristic of the P-type ATPase family. The Na^+-K^+-ATPase is a heteromeric integral membrane protein made of a main catalytic subunit, the α subunit, and a smaller glycosylated subunit, the β subunit. The Na^+-K^+-ATPase is present on the surface of every animal cell where its main function is to pump three intracellular sodium ions (Na^+) out of the cell and two extracellular potassium ions (K^+) within the cell. This ion transport performed against electrochemical Na^+ and K^+ gradients existing across the cell membrane requires energy provided by adenosine triphosphate (ATP) hydrolysis. The ion exchange performed by Na^+-K^+-ATPase maintains a high intracellular K^+ concentration and a low intracellular Na^+ concentration, and therefore participates in the resting potential of the cell. In specialized cells, Na^+-K^+-ATPase deserves additional major functions: (*i*) in excitable cells, Na^+-K^+-ATPase is essential for potassium ion re-uptake from the interstitial space during the repolarization phase (1) and (*ii*) in epithelial cells the polarized distribution of Na^+-K^+-ATPase energizes most reabsorption and secretion processes (2–6).

In sodium reabsorbing epithelia, including renal tubular cells, the Na^+-K^+-ATPase is exclusively located in the basolateral membrane (3,4). The Na^+ gradient generated by basolateral Na^+-K^+-ATPase is dissipated by passive Na^+ transport across the apical membrane. This organization results in a net transfer of Na^+ from the mucosal (luminal) to serosal (interstitial) compartment. Net sodium reabsorption is the major function of renal Na^+-K^+-ATPase and a close relationship is observed between Na^+-K^+-ATPase expression levels and the Na^+ reabsorption capacity of the successive renal tubule segments. In humans, the kidneys reabsorb about 600 g of Na^+ per day, which requires the consumption of about 2 kg of ATP by Na^+-K^+-ATPase.

In absorptive epithelia, Na^+-K^+-ATPase also energizes secondary active transport of a wide variety of charged (ions) or uncharged (glucose) solutes. Passive sodium entry into the cells is most often performed via cotransporters or antiporters coupled with the entry or exit of other solute(s). In addition, vectorial transport of charged solutes generates transepithelial potential differences that drive passive ion movements through the paracellular pathway.

FUNCTIONAL PROPERTIES OF THE Na^+-K^+-ATPase

The Na^+-K^+-ATPase can be considered either as an enzyme (ATPase) or as an ion transporter (the Na^+-pump). However, it is important to remember that ATPase activity and ion transport are intimately linked and are two aspects of the same function.

Enzymatic Properties of the Na^+-K^+-ATPase

The first experimental evidence revealing the fundamental properties of Na^+-K^+-ATPase, i.e., Na^+- and K^+-activated ATPase activity, was provided about 40 years ago by the 1997 Nobel Prize winner Jens Christian Skou (7). Na^+ and K^+ stimulate Na^+-K^+-ATPase activity from the cytoplasmic and extracellular side, respectively. The reported apparent mean Na^+ affinity constant of Na^+-K^+-ATPase ($K_{0.5Na}$) is comprised of between 5 and 15 mM in the presence of a low K^+ concentration (5–10 mM), and under these conditions the maximal velocity (V_{max}) is achieved in the presence of 60 to 100 mM Na^+. Since K^+ competes with Na^+ at the cytoplasmic site, $K_{0.5Na}$ is lower in the presence of the high K^+ concentration prevailing in intact cells (8). Intracellular Na^+ concentration is comprised of between 5 and 20 mM in intact cells, therefore, Na^+-K^+-ATPase works well below its V_{max} under basal conditions (9,10). Hence, any increase in intracellular Na^+ concentration stimulates Na^+-K^+-ATPase, which in turn extrudes more Na^+ out of the cell and tends to decrease intracellular Na^+ concentration. Reciprocally, a decrease in intracellular Na^+ concentration slows down Na^+-K^+-ATPase and thereby favors the return of intracellular Na^+ concentration to its initial levels. The Na^+ activation of Na^+-K^+-ATPase is a highly cooperative process, thus small variations of intracellular Na^+ concentration close to the $K_{0.5Na}$ produces larges variations in Na^+-K^+-ATPase activity. The reported apparent mean affinity constant for extracellular K^+ ($K_{0.5K}$) is comprised of between 0.5 and 1.5 mM. Therefore, except in the case of severe hypokalemia, extracellular K^+ is not rate-limiting for Na^+-K^+-ATPase activity.

The energy needed for ion transport is provided by ATP hydrolysis. The real substrate of the Na^+-K^+-ATPase is the Mg^{2+}-ATP complex, but magnesium is not particularly needed as it can be replaced by other divalent cations, such as manganese or cobalt. However, most divalent cations including calcium inhibit the Na^+-K^+-ATPase activity of the pump. The interaction of Mg^{2+}-ATP with Na^+-K^+-ATPase is complex and involves a high- and a low-affinity binding site. Since intracellular ATP concentration is maintained well above the $K_{0.5}$ of the low-affinity ATP binding site, ATP is not considered as a physiological modulator of Na^+-K^+-ATPase. ATP may become rate-limiting under pathologic conditions with decreased production such as ischemia. The Na^+-K^+-ATPase transports two Na^+ within the cell and three K^+ out of the cell for each molecule of ATP hydrolysed. Consequently Na–K-ATPase activity is electrogenic and directly participates to a part of the resting membrane potential (5–10 mV). The main part of the resting potential due to the flow of K^+ through K^+ channels is also dependent on Na^+-K^+-ATPase which maintains a high intracellular K^+ concentration.

As all P-type ATPases, the Na^+-K^+-ATPase cycles between two conformational states and is transiently phosphorylated. E_1 and E_2 conformations characterize the Na^+-K^+-ATPase according to its affinity for ions and substrate (sodium, potassium, and ATP) and to the availability of their intra- and extra-cellular docking sites. The E_1 conformation has a high affinity for Na^+ and ATP, a poor affinity for K^+, and the docking sites are accessible from the intracellular side of the cell. On the other hand, the E_2 conformation has a low affinity for Na^+ and ATP, a high affinity for K^+, and its docking sites are accessible from the extracellular side of the cell. The Na^+-K^+-ATPase is transiently phosphorylated when changing conformation. The pump cycles between E_1 and E_2 conformations according to the Albers–Post model (Fig. 1). When the Na^+-K^+-ATPase is in the E_1 conformation, ATP, Mg^{2+}, and Na^+ bind to their docking site on the intracellular side of the cell. This docking allows the phosphorylation of the Na^+-K^+-ATPase (E_1-P conformation) and the shutting of the sodium docking site, which prevents its release. After ADP release, the conformational change from E_1-P to E_2-P occurs. The E_2-P conformation allows the release of Na^+ outside the cell and the docking of extracellular K^+. Thereafter, the phosphate is released and a new conformation change from E_2-P to E_2 occurs. Lastly, the spontaneous conformation change from E_2 to E_1 releases K^+ inside the cell (11).

Pharmacology and Toxicology of the Na^+-K^+-ATPase

Digitalis glycosides that contain sugar and cyclic ester moieties are natural potent and specific inhibitors of Na^+-K^+-ATPase. Digitalis are mostly found in plants, although similar compounds have been identified in some animal species. Ouabain (or G-strophantidin) is generally used in vitro because it is the most water soluble, while digoxin is the most

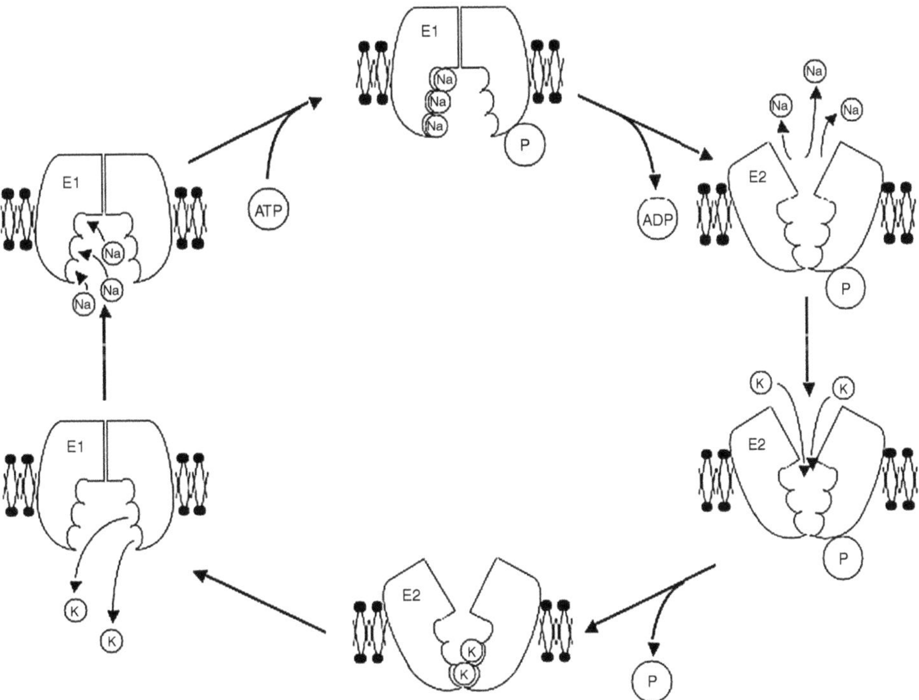

Figure 1 The Albers–Post model. This model shows the transitions between the main conformational states of the catalytic subunit of Na^+-K^+-ATPase (E_1, E_1-P, E_2-P, E_2).

widely used digitalic in therapy. The ouabain binding site is located on the Na^+-K^+-ATPase α subunit extracellular loops comprised between the transmembrane domains from M1 to M2 (12). Additional aminoacid residues that participate in ouabain binding were identified within M3-M4, M5-M6, and M7-M8 segments (13). The ouabain binding site is physically close to the K^+ docking site (14) and K^+ behaves as a competitive inhibitor of ouabain binding. Therefore, digitalis toxicity is greatly enhanced by hypokaliemia. Ouabain inhibits Na^+-K^+-ATPase activity through inhibition of dephosphorylation of the E_2-P conformation. The affinity of Na^+-K^+-ATPase for ouabain varies from the nM to the mM range between species. Rats, mice, and *Bufo marinus* exhibit ouabain-resistant enzymes (IC50 ~ 0.1 mM), while humans and rabbits exhibit ouabain-sensitive enzymes (IC50 ~ 0.1 μM). In addition, the affinity of Na^+-K^+-ATPase for ouabain differs from one organ to another. For instance the kidney Na^+-K^+-ATPase is less sensitive to ouabain than cardiac or brain enzyme. These differences are at least in part explained by the molecular heterogeneity of Na^+-K^+-ATPase (15,16).

Vanadate is an inhibitor of all ATPases that go through a phosphorylated state. Vandate acts as a phosphate analog and covalently binds to the phosphorylation site of P-type ATPases, blocking them in the E_2-P conformation.

STRUCTURE OF THE NA^+-K^+-ATPASE

The Na^+-K^+-ATPase is constituted of two subunits (α and β) associated in a 1:1 ratio. Theoretically, at least four α subunit isoforms can be associated with at least three β subunit isoforms to generate Na^+-K^+-ATPase isozymes with specific pharmacological and transport properties (17). The protomeric (one alpha and one beta subunit) or multimeric nature of Na^+-K^+-ATPase units located in plasma membranes is still debated since recent reports led to conflicting conclusions that in situ functional Na^+-K^+-ATPase units are monomeric (18) or multimeric (19).

Na^+-K^+-ATPase Subunits

The α Subunit

The α subunit, which contains about 1000 aminoacids and exhibits an apparent molecular weight close to 110 kDa, displays all the functional properties of the Na^+-pump and is therefore referred as the "catalytic" subunit. As schematized in Figure 2, it is an integral membrane protein that contains ten membrane-spanning domains from M1 to M10 with intracellular NH_2- and COOH-terminal domains (20). The docking site for ATP is located in a large intracellular loop between M4 and M5, which also contains the aspartic acid that becomes transiently phosphorylated during the catalytic cycle. The pore itself and the cation occlusion site are formed by the M4, M5, and M6 domains (13). Finally, the extracellular loop between domains M7 and M8 interacts with the β subunit. To date, four Na^+-K^+-ATPase α subunit isoforms, named α1 to α4, have been cloned (21,22). The α1 isoform is ubiquitous and is the only isoform identified in renal epithelial cells. The α2 isoform is expressed in heart, skeletal muscle, and brain (glial) cells, while the α3 isoform is expressed in nervous tissue (neurons) and ovaries (15,16). Finally, the α4 isoform is specifically expressed in testis (22).

Several aminoacid residues are phosphorylation sites for protein kinases. The first identified α subunit phosphorylation site was Ser-943, which is located within a typical protein kinase A (PKA) consensus site (23–25). However, the accessibility of this site under physiological conditions remains elusive (26). Serine Ser^{16} is a conserved site for

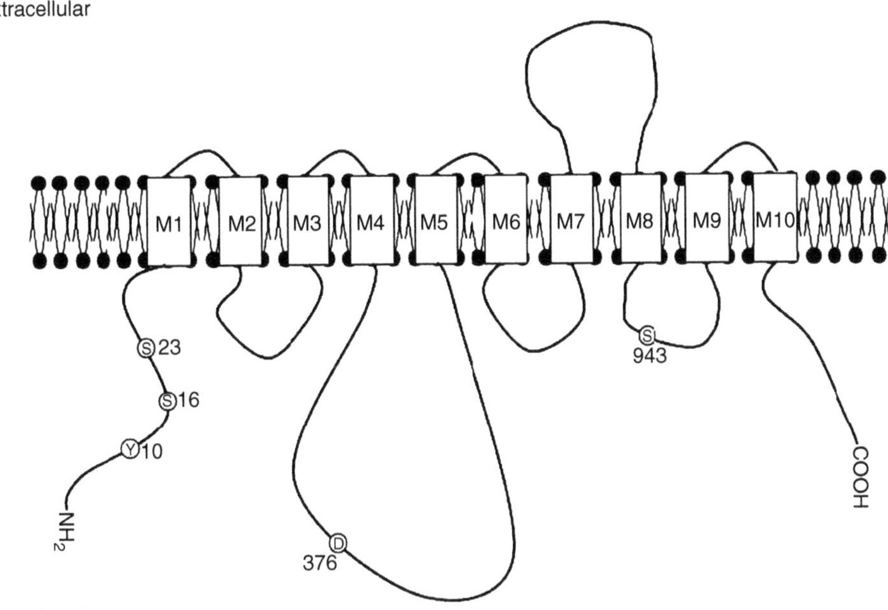

Figure 2 Schematic topology of the Na^+-K^+-ATPase α subunit. The Na^+-K^+-ATPase α subunit displays ten membrane-spanning domains with intracytoplasmic NH_2 and COOH termini. Phosphorylation sites for PKC (S16 and S23) and tyrosine kinases (Y10) are located in NH_2 terminus of the subunit. The PKA phosphorylation site (S943) is found into the M8-M9 intracellular loop. The aspartic acid (D376) residue located within the large M4-M5 intracellular loop is phosphorylated during the catalytic cycle of the pump.

protein kinase C (PKC) phosphorylation (25,27), while two additional PKC phosphorylation sites consisting of Thr^{15} and Ser^{23} are species specific. Indeed Thr^{15} is present only in *B. marinus* α1 subunit (25), and Ser^{23} is present only in rat α1 subunit (24,25,28). The Na^+-K^+-ATPase also exhibits phosphorylation sites for other protein kinases. For instance, the Na^+-K^+-ATPase α1 subunit can be phosphorylated by tyrosine kinases on Tyr^{10} (29,30) and by extracellular regulated kinases (31).

The β Subunit

The β subunit is only 300 aminoacids long, and displays a single membrane-spanning domain and a large extracellular end with several glycosylation sites (32,33). The extracellular domain interacts with the α subunit. The β subunit does not exhibit intrinsic enzymatic properties, but its association with the α subunit is necessary to the enzymatic activity of the Na^+-K^+-ATPase. It also allows an adequate folding of newly synthesized α subunits, a correct targeting to the membrane, and it stabilizes the Na^+-pump in the cellular membrane (34). The α subunit is not directed to the plasma membrane without being associated to the β subunit, and therefore Na^+-K^+-ATPase surface expression directly depends on the availability of β subunits. The β subunit may also modulate the apparent K^+ affinity of Na^+-K^+-ATPase (35).

The γ Subunit

Recently, a family of homologous small proteins ($\sim$10 kDa) sharing a conserved motif have been arranged in a group named the family of regulatory proteins (FXYD) proteins.

Currently, seven members of this family have been identified, and four of them (FXYD-1, -2, -4, and -7) can be associated with the Na^+-K^+-ATPase and modulate its function (36). The cloned γ subunit of the Na^+-K^+-ATPase (37), which was first co-purified with α and β subunits (38), is a member of this family and was renamed FXYD-2 (39). This small subunit is preferentially expressed in the kidney but is not necessary for routing or function of the Na^+-K^+-ATPase. The most noticeable effect of the association of FXYD-2 with Na^+-K^+-ATPase is decreased apparent Na^+ affinity of the enzyme (40,41). In contrast, association of Na^+-K^+-ATPase with FXYD-4 increases the apparent Na^+ affinity of Na^+-K^+-ATPase (41). It is worth noting that FXYD-2 is abundantly expressed in proximal tubule (PT) and loop of Henle, two segments with a Na^+-K^+-ATPase exhibiting a low apparent Na^+ affinity (8,42,43), while FXYD-4 is specifically expressed in collecting duct (CD) where the apparent affinity of Na^+-K^+-ATPase is high (8,44,45).

Functional Consequences of the Molecular Heterogeneity of Na^+-K^+-ATPase

Co-expression of specific α and β isoforms in heterologous expression systems indicates that any combination of αβ dimers studied is functional. However α subunit isoforms were shown to endow specific functional and pharmacological properties. It is well-established that rat α subunit isoforms display different affinities for cardiac glycosides. The rat α3β1 isozyme is the most ouabain-sensitive (IC50 ~ 2 nM), while α2β1 isozyme is intermediate (IC50 ~ 0.1 μM) and α1β1 isozyme is very ouabain-resistant (IC50 ~ 1 mM) (46). However, such differences in cardiac glycoside sensitivity are not observed in all species. Indeed, human α-isozymes display a similar affinity for ouabain (17). Differences in apparent Na^+ affinity of rat α-isozymes have been reported: α2β1 and α3β1 isozymes exhibit a high apparent Na^+ affinity while α1β1 isozyme exhibits a low Na^+ affinity (47). In contrast, the apparent Na^+ affinity human isozymes is α1β1 > α2β1 > α3β3 (17). Isozymes of Na^+-K^+-ATPase may also differ by their voltage dependence (17). Indeed, excitable cells which express α2 and α3 isoforms exhibit a voltage dependence of Na^+-K^+-ATPase within a wide range of membrane potentials from −100 to +50 mV, while Na^+-K^+-ATPase of renal epithelial cells which express the α1 isoform does not exhibit significant voltage dependence within the physiological range (−75 to −25 mV). The marked voltage dependence of Na^+-K^+-ATPase in excitable cells is physiologically sound since stimulation of Na^+-pump during depolarization facilitates the recovery of intracellular sodium. The absence of regulation of Na^+-pump by voltage is consistent with the absence of large variations of membrane potential in these cells.

REGULATION OF RENAL NA^+-K^+-ATPASE

Distribution and Properties of Renal Na^+-K^+-ATPase

In renal tubular epithelial cells, as in all Na^+-reabsorbing epithelia, the Na^+-K^+-ATPase is exclusively located in the basolateral membrane. Na^+-K^+-ATPase activity generates a Na^+ gradient that is dissipated by apical Na^+ entry through cell-specific transporters. This general organization of Na^+-reabsorbing epithelial cells generates an apical to basal vectorial Na^+ transport. In renal tubule epithelial, Na^+ reabsorption is the major function of Na^+-K^+-ATPase and a close relationship is observed between the Na^+ reabsorption capacity and the Na^+-K^+-ATPase activity of the different nephron segments (10,48,49).

Distribution of Na^+-K^+-ATPase along the renal tubule is highly heterogenous. In all animal species studied as yet, Na^+-K^+-ATPase activity is high in the thick ascending limb of Henle's loop (TAL) and in the distal convoluted tubule, intermediate in the PT and relatively low in the CD (10,48,49). A similar distribution profile was obtained by measurement of the number of active Na^+-pump by ^{3}[H]-ouabain binding (50).

The functional properties of Na^+-K^+-ATPase also varies along the nephron: in rat and rabbit, the CD exhibits a higher apparent Na^+ affinity as compared to the PT and the thick ascending limb (8,42,44). In addition, the rabbit CD displays a higher affinity for ouabain in comparison with the PT and the thick ascending limb of Henle (51). In the rat, two populations of Na^+-K^+-ATPase displaying different ouabain sensitivities are observed in each nephron segment studied (52). This functional heterogeneity of renal Na^+-K^+-ATPase is unlikely related on segment-specific expression of different isoforms of the α subunit since in situ hybridization and quantitative RT-PCR studies failed to demonstrate the presence of physiologically significant amounts of $\alpha 2$ and $\alpha 3$ subunit mRNA in the rat nephron (53,54). Therefore, the $\alpha 1\beta 1$ heterodimer is most likely the exclusive enzyme expressed in renal tubules and the functional heterogeneity of the enzyme may results from post translational modifications and/or association with regulatory molecules, i.e., γ subunit and/or corticosteroid hormone-induced factor (CHIF).

Regulation of the Na^+-K^+-ATPase in the PT

The PT reabsorbs over 70% of the filtered Na^+–K^+, Cl^-, bicarbonate, phosphate, and water. In this segment luminal Na^+ entry is mostly (80%) mediated via H^+ exchange via the isoform of Na^+/H^+ exchanger (NHE3). The remaining luminal Na^+ entry is mediated by various cotransporters including Na^+-glucose, Na^+-phosphate, Na^+-sulfate. Na^+ is extruded at the basolateral pole of the cell mostly by the Na^+-K^+-ATPase and accessorily by a Na^+–HCO_3^- cotransporter. In this part of nephron, sodium and fluid reabsorption is regulated by several hormones and neurotransmitters, including dopamine. As a general rule, Na^+ reabsorption is positively controlled by angiotensin II (ANG II), epinephrine and insulin, whereas the negative control is performed by dopamine and parathormone (55).

Positive Regulation by Angiotensin II

High concentrations of ANG II can be found in the lumen of PTs (56,57) suggesting that the major part of luminal ANG II derives from local synthesis. Indeed, PT cells express angiotensinogen (58), renin (59) and angiotensin I converting enzyme (60). Only a very small fraction of luminal ANG II is excreted in the urine, since it is almost entirely reabsorbed and degraded by PT (61). ANG II exerts a biphasic effect from both sides of PT: low ANG II concentrations (10^{-12}–10^{-10} M) stimulate while high ANG II concentrations (10^{-7}–10^{-6} M) inhibit fluid and solute reabsorption (62). Recent experiments revealed that ANG II also modulates Na^+-K^+-ATPase activity in a biphasic manner (63). At low concentrations, ANG II enhances Na^+-K^+-ATPase activity via increased apparent Na^+ affinity (64). However, the precise mechanism of Na^+-K^+-ATPase regulation by ANG II and its signaling pathway remain to be investigated. In addition to Na^+-K^+-ATPase, low concentrations of ANG II increase apical NHE3 exocytosis leading to stimulation of apical Na^+ influx (65) and also stimulates the activity of the basolateral Na^+–HCO_3^- cotransporter. Therefore, ANG II modulates PT Na^+ reabsorption via the coordinated control of both apical and basolateral Na^+ transporters.

Negative Regulation by Dopamine

Dopamine is locally produced by PT cells where it inhibits fluid and solute reabsorption (66,67). This local synthesis is increased by high Na^+ intake, and may therefore participate to the excretion of a Na^+ load (68).

Both locally synthesized and exogenous dopamine was repeatedly shown to inhibit the Na^+-K^+-ATPase via a decreased V_{max} of the enzyme (66,69,70). While dopamine increases the apparent Na^+ affinity of Na^+-K^+-ATPase in PT, the net resulting effect is inhibition of Na^+-K^+-ATPase activity (71). The inhibition of PT Na^+-K^+-ATPase activity by dopamine is PKC dependent (72,73). This effect also requires phospholipase A_2 (PLA_2) activation (74,75) and the synthesis of arachidonic acid metabolites via the cytochrome P-450 monooxygenase pathway (76). Studies performed in rat PT suspensions and in opossum kidney (OK) cells, a model of mammalian PT cell, showed that dopamine induces Na^+-K^+-ATPase redistribution from the basolateral membrane to cytoplasmic compartments. The number of Na^+-K^+-ATPase units found in a plasma membrane fraction is quickly reduced (within one minute), and associated with the sequential increase in amounts of Na^+-K^+-ATPase units found in isolated clathrin-coated pits (CCV) (after one minute), in a early endosomal fraction (after 2.5 minutes) and finally in a late endosomal fraction (after five minutes) (72,73).

The dopamine-induced redistribution of Na^+-K^+-ATPase is abolished in OK cells expressing a truncated rat $\alpha 1$ subunit lacking the 31 first aminoacids, suggesting that the extreme NH_2-terminus of the Na^+-K^+-ATPase α subunit plays a key role in this process (77). The NH_2-terminal portion of the rat $\alpha 1$ subunit contains two phosphorylation sites for PKC (Ser^{16} and Ser^{23}) (24,25,28) and a binding site for PI3-kinase (78). Expression of phosphorylation site and PI3-kinase binding site mutant rat $\alpha 1$ subunit in OK cells revealed that both phosphorylation of the $\alpha 1$ subunit on Ser^{23} and association of Na^+-K^+-ATPase with phosphatidyl-inositol 3′-kinase (PI3-kinase) (78) are required for dopamine-induced redistribution of Na^+-K^+-ATPase. Interestingly, despite its phosphorylation in response to dopamine, Ser^{16} does not participate to the dopamine-induced redistribution of Na^+-K^+-ATPase (77). The down regulation of Na^+-K^+-ATPase by dopamine is dependent on stimulation of PI3-kinase (74). Anchoring of PI3-kinase to the Na^+-K^+-ATPase via 14-3-3 protein which binds to phosphorylated Ser^{23} (79) would increase the local production of phosphatidylinositol 3-phosphate which increases the affinity of the adaptor protein-2 complex to its binding site centered by the α subunit Tyr^{542} (80). After endocytosis, the Na^+-K^+-ATPase is dephosphorylated in late endosomes (73) and it remains to be determined whether Na^+-K^+-ATPase units are degraded by lysosomes or recycle back to the plasma membrane. Figure 3 summarizes the mechanisms of regulation of Na^+-K^+-ATPase in response to dopamine.

In addition to Na^+-K^+-ATPase, dopamine induces internalization of apical NHE3 leading to inhibition of apical Na^+ influx (81). Therefore, dopamine modulates PT Na^+ reabsorption via the coordinated control of both apical and basolateral Na^+ transporters.

Regulation of Na^+-K^+-ATPase in the TAL

TAL reabsorbs close to 15% of the filtered Na^+ and also reabsorbs some bicarbonate and the divalent cations calcium and magnesium. The TAL is also called the diluting segment since it is impermeable to water and reabsorbs large amounts of solutes. Resulting from the transport process occurring along the TAL, the fluid delivered to the distal convoluted tubule is hypotonic and its NaCl concentration is close to 50 mM. This function of the TAL allows the build up of an osmotic corticopapillary gradient that is essential for water

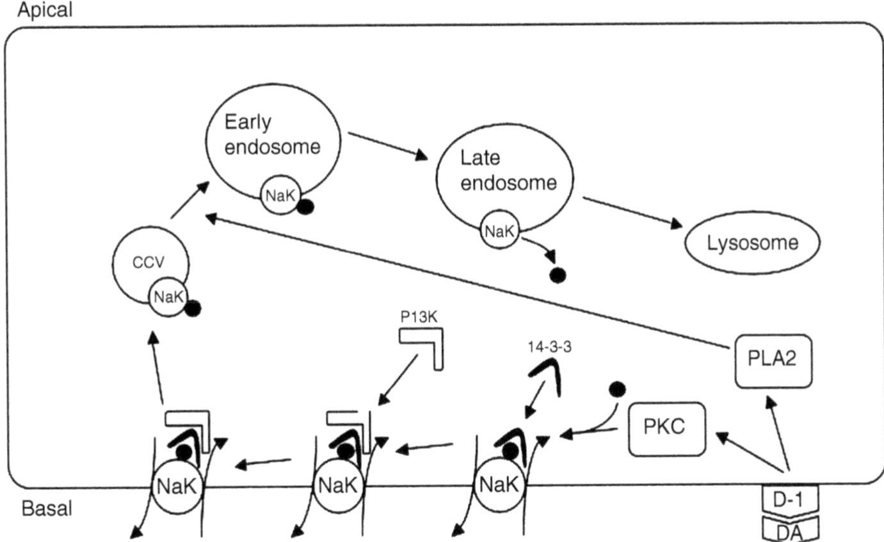

Figure 3 Regulation of Na^+-K^+-ATPase by dopamine in proximal tubule. Dopamine binding to D1-like receptors activates PKC and PLA_2 through yet undetermined mechanisms. PKC phosphorylates the Na^+-K^+-ATPase α subunit on Ser^{23}, which triggers the anchoring of PI3 kinase via 14-3-3 protein. The Na^+-K^+-ATPase then undergoes endocytosis through CCV and is targeted to early and late endosomes. The Na^+-K^+-ATPase is finally dephosphorylated in the late endosomal compartment by protein phosphatases.

reabsorption by the CD. Apical Na^+ entry is mediated by a furosemide-sensitive Na^+–K^+–$2Cl^-$ cotransporter (BSC1 or NKCC2) and is extruded by the basolateral Na^+-K^+-ATPase. On the other hand Cl^- leave the cell via Cl^-channels and a K^+–Cl^- cotransporter while K^+ is recycled back to the lumen via apical inwardly rectifying and voltage-insensitive K^+ channels rat outer medullary potassium channel, or KIR 1.1 (ROMK). Conductive diffusion of Cl^- and K^+ depolarizes the basolateral membrane and hyperpolarizes the apical membrane, respectively. These two diffusion potentials combine to generate a lumen positive transepithelial voltage which provides the driving force for paracellular cation reabsorption.

Micropuncture and in vitro microperfusion experiments showed that hormones coupled to adenylyl cyclase activation and cyclic-AMP (cAMP) analogs enhance NaCl reabsorption in the TAL (82–87). This stimulation of Na^+ reabsorption by the cAMP signaling pathway is at least in part mediated by stimulation of Na^+-K^+-ATPase activity (88). This stimulatory effect of cAMP on Na^+-K^+-ATPase activity was observed at V_{max} and required the presence of oxygen and metabolic substrates in sufficient amounts (88). Indeed, when metabolic supply is limiting, increasing cellular cAMP content inhibits Na^+-K^+-ATPase activity via generation of arachidonic acid metabolites through the cytochrome P450 pathway (88–91). The cAMP-induced Na^+-K^+-ATPase stimulation is correlated with increased phosphorylation levels of its α subunit (88). Whether this effect result from phosphorylation of the α subunit at Ser^{943} by PKA remains to be determined. In addition to Na^+-K^+-ATPase, cAMP increases apical NaCl influx via BSC1 (92) and basolateral Cl^- efflux via Cl^- channels (93) indicating that cAMP controls TAL NaCl reabsorption via the coordinated control of apical and basolateral transporters.

The stimulatory effect of the cAMP/PKA signaling pathway is subject to negative modulation by numerous signaling pathways including protein $G\alpha i$ activation by prostaglandins (94), cGMP generation in response to nitric oxide (95,96) and natriuretic peptides (97,98), and PKC stimulation in response to ANG II (92,99), bradykinin (100), and extracellular Ca^{2+} via activation of the extracellular Ca^{2+} receptor (101,102).

Regulation of the Na^+-K^+-ATPase in the CD

In mammals, the CD is the final site of regulation of Na^+–K^+, acid–base, and water excretion. The CD may accordingly reabsorb between 0% and 5% of the filtered Na^+. CD is made up of two different cell types: intercalated cells and principal cells. Intercalated cells are involved in acid/base regulation and their role is not discussed here. On the other hand, principal cells are responsible for water and Na^+ reabsorption as well as K^+ secretion. The function of principal cells requires the presence of specific membrane transporters to drive unidirectional Na^+–K^+ and H_2O fluxes. Figure 3 summarizes the functional organization of the CD principal cell: active electrogenic Na^+ transport generates a lumen-negative transepithelial voltage (0 to −60 mV), which is higher in the more cortical part of CD (−10 to −60 mV) and which decreases in the deeper medullary portions as a result of decreased Na^+ reabsorption by principal cells combined with increased electrogenic H^+ secretion by intercalated cells. Water enters the luminal (apical) side via aquaporin two water channels and leaves the cell through basolateral aquaporin three and four water channels. Although the driving force for water reabsorption is mainly provided by the countercurrent concentrating mechanism in the loop of Henle, Na^+ reabsorption along the CD, especially in the cortical part, dilutes the luminal fluid and contributes to the generation of an osmotic gradient favorable to water reabsorption. As depicted in Figure 4, Na^+ reabsorption in principal cells is linked to K^+ secretion through a two-step mechanism: pumping of K^+ within and Na^+ out of the cell by the basolateral Na^+-K^+-ATPase generates driving forces for apical Na^+ entry and K^+ exit. K^+ exit occurs through apical [belonging to the (ROMK) family] and basolateral K^+ channels, these latter being of several types of various conductance: their respective roles in K^+ transport is not clearly understood. Through this mechanism, K^+ secretion is primarily coupled to Na^+ reabsorption with the $2K^+$:$3Na^+$ stoichiometry of Na^+-K^+-ATPase. The apical Na^+ influx is mediated by amiloride-sensitive epithelial Na^+ channel (ENaC) and intracellular Na^+ is then extruded by basolateral Na^+-K^+-ATPase. The two major hormonal factors that positively control Na^+ reabsorption and Na^+-K^+-ATPase activity and expression are aldosterone and vasopressin. Moreover, recently an important role of intracellular Na^+ and extracellular osmolality in controlling Na^+-K^+-ATPase expression has been highlighted.

Regulation of Na^+-K^+-ATPase by Mineralocorticoids

The major physiological role of the mineralocorticoid hormone aldosterone is to increase extracellular volume in response to volume depletion. Aldosterone participates to the restoration of plasma volume mainly by stimulating the reabsorption of Na^+ from the lumen of the renal tubules and accessorily of other organs, such as the sweat glands and the distal colon. Aldosterone also plays an important role in the K^+ homeostasis: on the one hand, high extracellular K^+ is a stimulus for aldosterone secretion and, on the other hand, the secretion of K^+ into the kidney tubule is directly linked to the aldosterone-regulated Na^+ reabsorption that generates the electrical driving force for K^+ secretion (55). Aldosterone controls Na^+ reabsorption in CD principal cells by coordinated stimulation of the activities of apical ENaC and basolateral Na^+-K^+-ATPase. In renal epithelial cells, the Na^+-K^+-ATPase works at about 20% of its maximal rate (10), therefore,

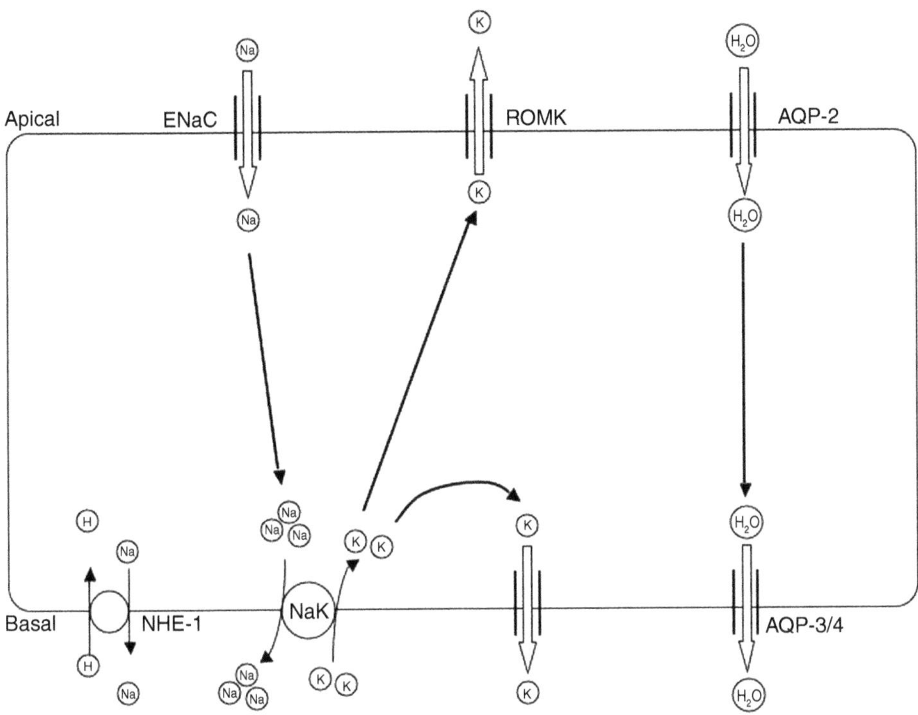

Figure 4 Sodium, potassium, and water transport in collecting duct principal cells. Sodium reabsorption occurs sequentially through apical Na-channels (ENaC) and basolateral Na^+, K^+-ATPase, and is linked to potassium secretion via luminal K-channels (ROMK). The Na-pump generates the driving forces for both Na^+ entry and K^+ exit at the apical side of the cell. Water permeability is mediated by sequential flow through apical aquaporin-2 water channel and basolateral aquaporin-3 and -4 water channels.

a large kinetic reserve allowing activation of Na^+-pump by intracellular Na^+ is available. However, a coordinated control of Na^+-K^+-ATPase that matches that of ENaC is necessary to maintain the constancy of intracellular [Na^+], and therefore ENaC function, over a broad range of reabsorption rates. Indeed, in the absence of simultaneous stimulation of ENaC and Na^+-K^+-ATPase, an increased Na^+ influx through ENaC would raise intracellular [Na^+] and subsequently decrease ENaC activity by feedback inhibition (103).

The physiological response to aldosterone action can be separated into short-term and long-term effect. The short-term (early) aldosterone effect on Na^+ reabsorption (and on K^+ secretion) can be observed after 30 minutes of aldosterone stimulation (104,105). The long-term (late) effect aldosterone induces a more sustained increase in the transport capacity of the target cells (106). In addition to these classical effects mediated by the corticosteroid receptor/DNA interaction, aldosterone has been shown to produce near-immediate effects whose physiological role of remains to be elucidated. These effects are mediated by a non-transcriptional mechanism (also denominated nongenomic or nonclassical) that must involve an as not yet identified receptor (107). Very recently, Le Moëllic et al. (108) have provided some experimental pieces of evidence indicating that aldosterone quickly stimulates transepithelial Na^+ transport through a nongenomic effect in cultured rat cortical collecting duct (CCD) cells.

Two decades ago, the long-term (days) treatment of adrenalectomized and adrenal-intact animals with aldosterone has been shown to increase the amount of Na^+-K^+-ATPase α subunit mRNA, protein, and activity in the CCD (55,106). This slow induction of Na^+-K^+-ATPase α_1 subunit protein synthesis (measurable after 6–18 hours) relies on a rapid transcriptional activation (measurable after 15 minutes) (109,110). This transcriptional control is most likely mediated by the several glucocorticoid response elements along the 5′-flanking region of Na^+-K^+-ATPase α_1 subunit gene (111). The long delay between the very early transcriptional response and the late accumulation of active Na^+-pumps is accounted for by the fact that the pumps are very numerous and represent a stable component of the transport machinery with a half-life of approximately one day.

The slow time course of cellular Na^+-K^+-ATPase accumulation is obviously not compatible with the short-term stimulation of Na^+-K^+-ATPase activity aldosterone. Indeed, early studies showed that the activity of the Na^+-K^+-ATPase, measured at V_{max} by hydrolytic activity after cell membrane permeabilization, slowly decreases after adrenalectomy (3–4 days) but rapidly returns (1–3 hours) to normal levels upon aldosterone infusion in the mammalian CCD (105,112). Similarly, ex vivo experiments performed in isolated CCDs from adrenalectomized rats showed that in the presence of 3,3′,5-triiodothyronine (T_3), three-hour incubation with aldosterone restored Na^+-K^+-ATPase activity (V_{max}) to normal levels (113). Subsequently, Barlet-Bas et al. (114) and Blot-Chabaud et al. (115) independently showed the presence of a mineralocorticoid-dependent pool of functionally silent Na^+-pumps. These observations raised the question whether aldosterone activates this latent pool of preexisting Na^+-K^+-ATPase units or whether it induces de novo synthesis of Na^+-K^+-ATPase. The mechanism of the short-term stimulation of Na^+-K^+-ATPase by aldosterone was studied in isolated rat CCDs and in mpkCCD$_{c14}$ cells (116), a model of mammalian CD principal cells. The mpkCCD$_{c14}$ cell model, derived from mouse CCD (117), develops a tight epithelium and retain expression of transporters specific for CD principal cells including ENaC and aquaporin two as well as controlled transepithelial Na^+ transport by aldosterone and vasopressin (117,118). Intravenous infusion of aldosterone in adrenalectomized rats induced a nearly threefold increase in Na^+-K^+-ATPase hydrolytic activity measured at V_{max}. This stimulation was associated with a severalfold increase in Na^+-K^+-ATPase cell surface expression measured by Western Blot performed after biotinylation and streptavidin precipitation of cell surface proteins. In contrast, the total cellular pool of Na^+-K^+-ATPase increased to a much lesser extent. Similar results were obtained in mpkCCD$_{c14}$ cells which displayed an increase in maximal Na^+-pump current and cell surface expression of Na^+-K^+-ATPase after short-term incubation (2–6 hour) with aldosterone. These results indicate that short-term aldosterone stimulates Na^+-K^+-ATPase activity through an increase in cell surface expression of active Na^+-K^+-ATPase units. Therefore, the short-term effect of aldosterone may rely on the translocation of an intracellular reservoir of Na^+-K^+-ATPase to the plasma membrane and is independent of increased abundance of total Na^+-K^+-ATPase subunits (Fig. 5). This aldosterone-recruitable pool of Na^+-K^+-ATPase remains to be identified by morphological studies.

The short-term stimulation of Na^+-K^+-ATPase activity and cell surface expression is independent of apical Na^+ entry trough ENaC and requires de novo transcription and translation (116). These results indicate that aldosterone-induced recruitment of Na^+-K^+-ATPase is not mediated by an increase in intracellular [Na^+] brought about by ENaC stimulation and it is most likely mediated by one of several short-term aldosterone-induced and/or repressed proteins. CHIF, the first identified aldosterone-induced protein (119), is expressed along the CD (120) and associates with the Na^+-K^+-ATPase to

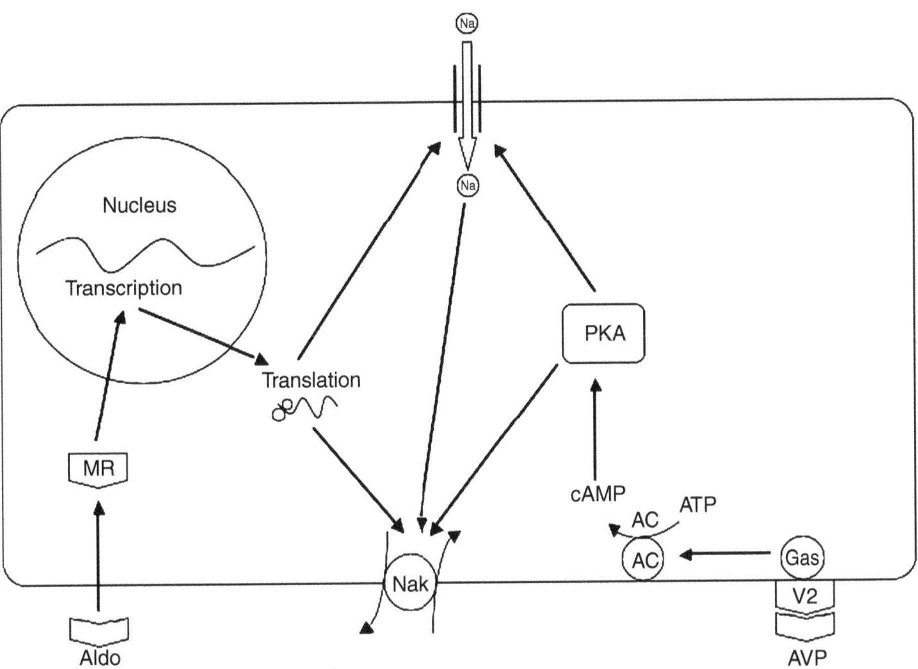

Figure 5 Regulation of Na^+-K^+-ATPase by aldosterone and vasopressin in collecting duct principal cells. Aldosterone (Aldo) binds to its intracellular receptor MR and induces transcription and translation of regulatory factors that stimulates Na^+-K^+-ATPase activity. Intracellular Na^+ directly activates Na^+-K^+-ATPase activity. Vasopressin (AVP) binding to V_2 receptor (V2) activates Gas protein, which in turn activates adenylate cyclase (AC). cAMP is synthesized from ATP and can therefore activate protein kinase cAMP-dependent PKA. Activated PKA phosphorylates Na^+-K^+-ATPase and stimulates its activity. Moreover, aldosterone and vasopressin also stimulate apical Na^+ channels (ENaC) and therefore Na^+ reabsorption.

increase its apparent Na^+ affinity (41). While CHIF expression is induced by aldosterone in the distal colon, this is not the case in the kidney (121). Therefore, CHIF is unlikely to play a major role in the early stimulation of CD Na^+-K^+-ATPase in response to aldosterone. Using a differential display strategy, the Verrey's group identified several aldosterone-induced transcripts in aldosterone-responsive epithelial A6 cells (122). Among them, K-ras, a small G-protein, was shown to stimulate ENaC current and surface expression in the *Xenopus laevis* oocyte expression system (123). However, K-ras mRNA is not induced by aldosterone in mammalian CD principal cells. Serial analysis of gene expression in cultured mouse $mpkCCD_{cl4}$ cells (124) and substractive hybridization on isolated rat CCD (125) identified several aldosterone-induced genes but their role in the modulation of transepithelial Na^+ transport remains to be established. Recently, the Serum- and Glucocorticoid-regulated Kinase 1 (SGK1) has received much attention as an aldosterone-induced protein. SGK1 is a serine/threonine kinase that was first identified in mammary tumor cells and subsequently in hepatoma cell line on the basis of its induction in response to high osmolarity (126). SGK1 is a component of the phosphoinositide 3-kinase signaling pathway and requires phosphorylation by PDK for activity and nuclear translocation (127). Experiments performed in adrenalectomized rats revealed that, in CD principal cells, SGK1 mRNA and protein are induced two hours after administration of aldosterone (128). Moreover, co-expression of SGK1 and ENaC subunits in the *Xenopus* oocyte expression system strongly stimulates ENaC activity and cell surface expression (129). However, induction of SGK1 per se is not sufficient to recruit ENaC to the cell surface: in aldosterone-infused adrenalectomized rats SGK1 was induced throughout the connecting tubule and CD while ENaC was translocated to the cell surface in connecting tubule and CCD only (128). In addition, expression of SGK1 in *Xenopus* oocyte was shown to stimulate the endogenous Na^+-pump current without variation of intracellular $[Na^+]$, suggesting that SGK1 primarily stimulates Na^+-K^+-ATPase activity (130). Another study revealed that co-expression of exogenous rat Na^+-K^+-ATPase and SGK1 in *Xenopus* oocyte increased both exogenous Na^+-pump current and Na^+-K^+-ATPase cell surface expression, as visualized by Western blotting of surface-biotinylated proteins (131). In contrast a kinase-dead mutant SGK1 had no effect on Na^+-K^+-ATPase activity and expression. The SGK1-dependent increase in Na^+-K^+-ATPase cell surface expression was independent of intracellular $[Na^+]$ and was specific since the cell surface expression of Na^+/phosphate cotransporter NaPi-IIa or heterodimeric aminoacid transporter LAT1-4F2hc were not altered by co-expression of SGK1. Taken together, these studies strongly suggest that SGK1 modulates ENaC and Na^+-K^+-ATPase cell surface expression in a coordinated manner. However, these findings require validation by further experiments performed in a reliable model of mammalian CD principal cells. The physiological control of renal Na^+ handling by SGK1 has been highlighted by the generation of SGK1-knockout mice which exhibit impaired ability to reduce urinary Na^+ excretion in response to dietetary Na^+ restriction (132). It should be mentioned that the relatively mild phenotype observed in SGK1-knockout mice might be explained by functional redundancy of SGK isoforms (133).

Finally, a recent study explored whether the short-term effect of aldosterone on Na^+-K^+-ATPase cell surface expression might depend on α subunit isoform-specific structures (134). Results obtained in mpkCCD$_{c14}$ cells expressing functional exogenous human $\alpha 1$ or $\alpha 2$ subunit showed that aldosterone stimulated only $\alpha 1$ subunit containing Na^+-K^+-ATPase isozymes, indicating that aldosterone responsiveness is dictated by $\alpha 1$ subunit-specific sequences.

Regulation of Na^+-K^+-ATPase by Vasopressin

Vasopressin (AVP) is coupled to adenylyl cyclase through its V_2 receptors and stimulates the cAMP/PKA signaling pathway in CD principal cells (Fig. 5). Stimulation of water reabsorption via increased water permeability of the apical membrane of principal cells in the major effect of AVP in CD. However, AVP also stimulates Na^+ reabsorption and K^+ secretion along the CD. In vitro microperfusion studies performed in rat CCD have shown that AVP, as well as cAMP analog, induce a rapid increase in Na^+ reabsorption (135,136). This effect of AVP on urinary Na^+ excretion has been recently confirmed by Bankir et al. who showed that in humans AVP decreases urinary Na^+ excretion via V_2 receptor activation (137). Recent experimental evidence indicate that AVP and cAMP stimulate Na^+ reabsorption by coordinated activation of ENaC and Na^+-K^+-ATPase. In isolated rat CCD stimulation of Na^+ transport in response to AVP/cAMP is associated with a sustained increase in the lumen-negative transepithelial voltage and in apical Na^+ conductance (138,139). The stimulatory effect of cAMP on ENaC was confirmed by patch-clamping experiments on the apical membrane of principal cells from isolated rat CCDs (140). In addition to these short-term (minutes) effect on apical Na^+ conductance, long-term (hours) AVP stimulation increases the translation rate of ENaC subunits in rat CCD cultured cells (141) and increased β and γENaC subunits expression in AVP-supplemented Bratlleboro rats (a rat strain exhibiting a spontaneous knockout of the AVP gene) (142). These reports demonstrate that AVP controls the synthesis and the activity of ENaC in mammalian CD principal cells.

Stimulation of Na^+-K^+-ATPase is a prerequisite for an increased Na^+ reabsorption, but initial studies reported an inhibitory effect of AVP and cAMP analogs on Na^+-K^+-ATPase activity in isolated rat CCD (90). However results from our laboratory indicated that this inhibitory pathway was promoted by metabolic stress related to the ex vivo experimental conditions (88): the inhibitory effect of cAMP is indirect and relied on the PLA_2/arachidonate/cytochrome P-450-monoxygenase pathway (90) and, indeed, in well-oxygenated isolated rat CCDs, cAMP analogs induced a twofold stimulation of both transport and hydrolytic Na^+-K^+-ATPase activity (143). The stimulation of Na^+-K^+-ATPase activity in response to cAMP analogs and AVP is rapid (5 minutes) and is associated with a proportional increase in Na^+-K^+-ATPase cell surface expression and without alteration of the total cellular pool of Na^+-K^+-ATPase (143,144). The identification of the cAMP-responsive pool of Na^+-K^+-ATPase and its relation to an aldosterone controlled reservoir remains also to be determined by morphological techniques.

Cyclic-AMP classically binds to the regulatory subunits of the PKA holoenzyme and release active catalytic PKA subunits (PKAc) by alleviating autoinhibitory contacts (145). In $mpkCCD_{cl4}$ cells, inhibition of PKA prevents the AVP-induced recruitment of Na^+-K^+-ATPase to the cell surface (144). However, the exact role of PKA in the short-term Na^+-K^+-ATPase upregulation, in CD principal cells remains to be elucidated. Transient expression of wild-type and mutant human $\alpha 1$ subunits in $mpkCCD_{c14}$ cells revealed that phosphorylation of the Na^+-K^+-ATPase α_1 subunit on Ser^{943}, the PKA phosphorylation site (23) is not involved in the recruitment of Na^+-K^+-ATPase to the cell surface in response to PKA activation (144). Therefore, the effect of PKA may rely on phosphorylation of intermediate target(s) that ultimately leads to increased cell surface expression of Na^+-K^+-ATPase.

Control of Na–K-ATPase by Na^+ and Osmolality

Na^+-K^+-ATPase in CD exhibits an apparent affinity for Na^+ that is twice higher than in the PT and TAL (8,44). Therefore the kinetic reserve for activation of Na^+-K^+-ATPase by intracellular [Na^+] is much lower in the CD than in the more proximal nephron segments. Thus principal cells must face the challenge to maintain intracellular [Na^+] within a narrow range, a priority with respect to many cellular functions and ENaC activity, despite a lower Na^+ affinity of the Na^+-K^+-ATPase and a lower extracellular [Na^+] (about 95% of the filtered Na^+ is reabsorbed by the more proximal renal tubule segments).

In mammalian CCD a rise in intracellular [Na^+] was shown to rapidly and proportionally increase the Na^+-K^+-ATPase activity and the number of functional Na^+-K^+-ATPase units independently of transcriptional activation and/or de novo protein synthesis (114). These reports raised the possibility that silent Na^+-K^+-ATPase units already located at the cell membrane are activated or alternatively, that preexisting intracellular Na^+-K^+-ATPase units are shuttled to the cell surface. We recently demonstrated that, in microdissected rat CCDs and in $mpkCCD_{c14}$ cells, a rise in intracellular [Na^+] increases Na^+-K^+-ATPase activity and recruits Na^+-K^+-ATPase units to the cell surface (146), similarly to the regulation of the Na^+-K^+-ATPase by cAMP (147) and aldosterone (116), discussed above. The Na^+-induced increase in Na^+-K^+-ATPase cell surface expression is aldosterone-dependent (114,115,146), suggesting the requirement of an aldosterone-dependent expression of regulatory protein(s) exerting a permissive effect. Conversely, the early stimulation of Na^+-K^+-ATPase activity by aldosterone is independent of an increment of the intracellular [Na^+] brought about by increased apical Na^+ conductance (116). As summarized in Figure 6, we showed that the cellular mechanism leading to the recruitment of active Na^+-K^+-ATPase units in CD principal cells, relies at least in part on cAMP-independent and proteasomal-dependent PKA activation (146). Recently, a cAMP-independent mechanism of PKA activation has been demonstrated in response to cytokines and vasoactive peptides. In this setting, free active PKAc is released upon dissociation of a multi-protein complex containing PKAc, IκBα and NF-κBp65, and subsequent proteasomal degradation of IκBα (148,149). Recent results from our laboratory show that in $mpkCCD_{cl4}$ cells, increasing intracellular [Na^+]i induces the dissociation of an endogenous PKAc/IκBα/NF-κBp65 complex resulting in stimulation of PKA activity and recruitment of active Na^+-K^+-ATPase units to the cell surface (150).

Since CD cells are physiologically exposed to variations of interstitial and tubular fluid osmolarities, we studied the effects of extracellular anisotonicity on Na^+-K^+-ATPase cell surface expression. Results obtained in $mpkCCD_{cl4}$ cells indicate that extracellular hypotonocity increases both cell volume and Na^+-K^+-ATPase cell surface expression. In contrast, extracellular hypertonicity which induces cell shrinkage did not alter the subcellular Na^+-K^+-ATPase localization. The effect of hypotonicity is not

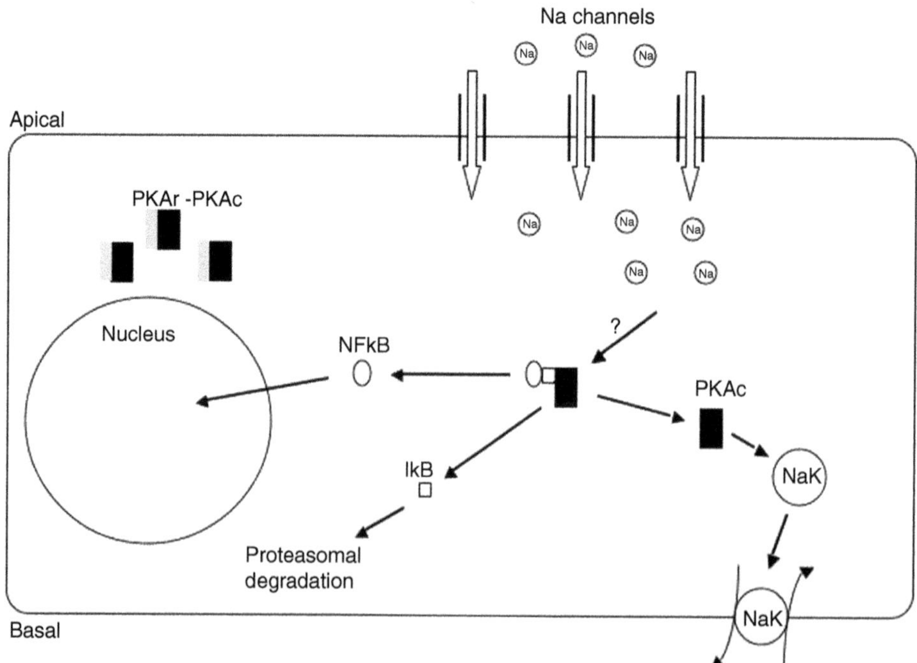

Figure 6 Regulation of Na^+-K^+-ATPase by sodium in collecting duct principal cells. An increase in intracellular Na^+ concentration stimulates Na^+-K^+-ATPase activity and recruits Na^+-K^+-ATPase units to the cell surface via dissociation of a protein complex containing PKAc/IκBα/NF-κBp65. Release of free PKAc results in stimulation of PKA activity and recruitment of active Na^+-K^+-ATPase units to the cell surface.

directly related to cell volume variations while it relies on stimulation of ENaC-mediated apical Na^+ influx leading to PKA activation (151).

Therefore, increased apical Na^+ influx brought about by ENaC activation or by incubation of cells with a Na^+ ionophore induces a coordinated increase in basolateral Na^+-K^+-ATPase activity that may rely on the activity of an intracellular [Na^+] sensor which remains to be identified. Activation of this putative [Na^+] sensor leads to the dissociation of a cytosolic PKAc/IκBα/NF-κBp65 complex leading to PKA activation and recruitment of active Na^+-K^+-ATPase units to the plasma membrane of CD principal cells.

Dysregulation of Na^+-K^+-ATPase in Nephrotic Syndrome

Nephrotic syndrome is characterized by massive albuminuria associated with hypoalbuminemia. In humans, nephrotic syndrome is either a primary disease without glomerular morphologic alterations or a consequence of inflammatory or deposit glomerular diseases. Nephrotic syndrome is associated with avid renal Na^+ retention leading to extracellular fluid expansion and edema. Early in vivo micropuncture experiments performed in the unilateral model of puromycin aminonucleoside (PAN)-induced nephrotic syndrome in rats have shown that the CD is a major site of Na retention (152). This observation was recently confirmed by in vitro microperfusion experiments on isolated CCDs from PAN nephrotic rats (153). Na retention in nephrotic syndrome is at least in part explained by increased Na^+-K^+-ATPase activity, which provides the driving force for tubular Na^+ reabsorption. Indeed, Na^+-K^+-ATPase activity was specifically increased in CCD of several rat models of nephrotic syndrome, such as PAN and adriamycin nephrosis, Heyman nephritis or mercury chloride-induced glomerulonephritis and correlated closely to decreased urinary Na^+ excretion (153). Moreover, experiments performed in adrenalectomized rats and in Brattleboro rats, which exhibit spontaneous knockout of the vasopressin gene, have established that increased Na^+-K^+-ATPase expression and Na^+ retention are independent of aldosterone and vasopressin in PAN nephrotic rats (154,155).

We have recently investigated the mechanism of increased Na^+-K^+-ATPase activity in CCD of PAN nephrotic rats (143). The twofold increase in maximal Na^+-K^+-ATPase hydrolytic activity was associated with a proportional increase of cell surface and total Na^+-K^+-ATPase. Indirect immunofluorescence imaging showed that increased Na^+-K^+-ATPase expression was restricted to CCD principal cells and that the enzyme was properly located at the basolateral pole of principal cells. These results suggest that increased Na^+-K^+-ATPase activity results from an increase in Na^+-K^+-ATPase subunits synthesis and delivery of newly synthesized Na^+-pumps to the plasma membrane in PAN nephrotic rat CCD. This interpretation was further supported by the observed increase of the number of mRNA encoding Na^+-K^+-ATPase α1 and β1 subunits.

REFERENCES

1. Clausen T. Na^+–K^+ pump regulation and skeletal muscle contractility. Physiol Rev 2003; 83(4):1269–324.
2. Amerongen HM, Mack JA, Wilson JM, et al. Membrane domains of intestinal epithelial cells: distribution of Na^+-K^+-ATPase and the membrane skeleton in adult rat intestine during fetal development and after epithelial isolation. J Cell Biol 1989; 109(5):2129–38.

3. Kyte J. Immunoferritin determination of the distribution of ($Na^+ + K^+$) ATPase over the plasma membranes of renal convoluted tubules. II. Proximal segment. J Cell Biol 1976; 68(2):304–18.
4. Kyte J. Immunoferritin determination of the distribution of ($Na^+ + K^+$) ATPase over the plasma membranes of renal convoluted tubules. I. Distal segment. J Cell Biol 1976; 68(2):287–303.
5. Smith ZD, Caplan MJ, Forbush B, et al. Monoclonal antibody localization of Na^+-K^+-ATPase in the exocrine pancreas and parotid of the dog. Am J Physiol Gastrointest Liver Physiol 1987; 253(2):G99–109.
6. Gundersen D, Orlowski J, Rodriguez-Boulan E. Apical polarity of Na,K-ATPase in retinal pigment epithelium is linked to a reversal of the ankyrin–fodrin submembrane cytoskeleton. J Cell Biol 1991; 112(5):863–72.
7. Skou JC. The influence of some cations on adenosine triphosphatase from peripheral nerves. Biochim Biophys Acta 1957; 18(2):394–401.
8. Barlet-Bas C, Cheval L, Khadouri C, et al. Difference in the Na affinity of Na–K-ATPase along the rabbit nephron: modulation by K. Am J Physiol Renal Physiol 1990; 259(2): F246–50.
9. Blot-Chabaud M, Jaisser F, Gingold M, et al. Na^+-K^+-ATPase-dependent sodium flux in cortical collecting duct. Am J Physiol Renal Fluid Electrolyte Physiol 1988; 255(24): F605–13.
10. Cheval L, Doucet A. Measurement of Na–K-ATPase-mediated rubidium influx in single segments of rat nephron. Am J Physiol Renal Physiol 1990; 259(1):F111–21.
11. Kaplan JH. Ion movements through the sodium pump. Annu Rev Physiol 1985; 47: 535–44.
12. Lingrel JB, Van Huysse J, O'Brien W, Jewell-Motz E, Askew R, Schultheis P. Structure–function studies of the Na,K-ATPase. Kidney Int 1994; 44:S32–9.
13. Lingrel JB, Arguello JM, Van Huysse J, et al. Cation and cardiac glycoside binding sites of the Na,K-ATPase. Ann NY Acad Sci 1997; 834:194–206.
14. Palasis M, Kuntzweiler TA, Arguello JM, et al. Ouabain interactions with the H5-H6 hairpin of the Na,K-ATPase reveal a possible inhibition mechanism via the cation binding domain. J Biol Chem 1996; 271(40):14176–82.
15. Sweadner KJ. Isozymes of the Na^+/K^+-ATPase. Biochim Biophys Acta 1989; 988(2): 185–220.
16. Levenson R. Isoforms of the Na–K-ATPase: family members in search of function. Rev Physiol Biochem Pharmacol 1994; 123:1–45.
17. Crambert G, Hasler U, Beggah AT, et al. Transport and pharmacological properties of nine different human Na,K-ATPase isozymes. J Biol Chem 2000; 275(3):1976–86.
18. Martin DW, Marecek J, Scarlata S, et al. $\alpha\beta$ protomers of Na^+-K^+-ATPase from microsomes of duck salt gland are mostly monomeric: formation of higher oligomers does not modify molecular activity. Proc Natl Acad Sci USA 2000; 97(7):3195–200.
19. Laughery M, Todd M, Kaplan JH. Oligomerization of the Na,K-ATPase in cell membranes. J Biol Chem 2004; 279(37):36339–48.
20. Shull GE, Schwartz A, Lingrel JB. Amino-acid sequence of the catalytic subunit of the ($Na^+ + K^+$)ATPase deduced from a complementary DNA. Nature 1985; 316(6030):691–5.
21. Shull GE, Greeb J, Lingrel JB. Molecular cloning of three distinct forms of the Na^+-K^+-ATPase α-subunit from rat brain. Biochemistry 1986; 25(25):8125–32.
22. Shamraj OI, Lingrel JB. A putative fourth Na^+-K^+-ATPase α-subunit gene is expressed in testis. Proc Natl Acad Sci USA 1994; 91(26):12952–6.
23. Fisone G, Cheng SXJ, Nairn AC, et al. Identification of the phosphorylation site for cAMP-dependent protein kinase on Na^+-K^+-ATPase and effects of site-directed mutagenesis. J Biol Chem 1994; 269(12):9368–73.
24. Feschenko MS, Sweadner KJ. Conformation-dependent phosphorylation of Na,K-ATPase by protein kinase A and protein kinase C. J Biol Chem 1994; 269(48):30436–44.

25. Béguin P, Beggah AT, Chibalin AV, et al. Phosphorylation of the Na,K-ATPase α-subunit by protein kinase A and C in vitro and in intact cells. Identification of a novel motif for PKC-mediated phosphorylation. J Biol Chem 1994; 269(39):24437–45.
26. Sweadner KJ, Feschenko MS. Predicted location and limited accessibility of protein kinase A phosphorylation site on Na–K-ATPase. Am J Physiol Cell Physiol 2001; 280(4):C1017–26.
27. Béguin P, Peitsch MC, Geering K. $\alpha1$ but not $\alpha2$ or $\alpha3$ isoforms of Na,K-ATPase are efficiently phosphorylated in a novel protein kinase C motif. Biochemistry 1996; 35(45): 14098–108.
28. Belusa R, Wang Z-M, Matsubara T, et al. Mutation of the protein kinase C phosphorylation site on rat $\alpha1$ Na^+-K^+-ATPase alters regulation of intracellular Na^+ and pH and influences cell shape and adhesiveness. J Biol Chem 1997; 272(32):20179–84.
29. Féraille E, Carranza ML, Gonin S, et al. Insulin-induced stimulation of Na^+-K^+-ATPase activity in kidney proximal tubule cells depends on phosphorylation of the α-subunit at Tyr-10. Mol Biol Cell 1999; 10(9):2847–59.
30. Chibalin AV, Kovalenko MV, Ryder JW, et al. Insulin- and glucose-induced phosphorylation of the Na^+–K^+-adenosine triphosphatase α-subunits in rat skeletal muscle. Endocrinology 2001; 142(8):3474–82.
31. Al-Khalili L, Kotova O, Tsuchida H, et al. ERK1/2 mediates insulin stimulation of Na,K-ATPase by phosphorylation of the α-subunit in human skeletal muscle cells. J Biol Chem 2004; 279(6):25211–8.
32. Kawakami K, Nojima H, Ohta T, et al. Molecular cloning and sequence analysis of human Na,K-ATPase β-subunit. Nucleic Acids Res 1986; 14(7):2833–44.
33. Shull GE, Lane LK, Lingrel JB. Amino-acid sequence of the β-subunit of the $(Na^+ + K^+)$-ATPase deduced from a cDNA. Nature 1986; 321(6068):429–31.
34. Hasler U, Wang X, Crambert G, et al. Role of beta-subunit domains in the assembly, stable expression intracelluar routing, and functional properties of Na, K-ATPase. J Biol Chem 1998 Nov 13; 273(46):30826–35.
35. Jaisser F, Jaunin P, Geering K, et al. Modulation of the Na,K-pump function by β-subunit isoforms. J Gen Physiol 1994; 103(4):605–23.
36. Sweadner KJ, Arystarkhova E, Donnet C. FXYD proteins as regulators of the Na,K-ATPase in the kidney. Ann NY Acad Sci 2003; 986:382–7.
37. Mercer RW, Biemesderfer D, Bliss DP, et al. Molecular cloning and immunological characterization of the γ polypeptide, a small protein associated with the Na,K-ATPase. J Cell Biol 1993; 121(3):579–86.
38. Forbush B, Kaplan JH, Hoffman JF. Characterization of a new photoaffinity derivative of ouabain: labeling of the large polypeptide and of a proteolipid component of the Na, K-ATPase. Biochemistry 1978; 17(17):3667–76.
39. Sweadner K, Rael E. The FXYD gene family of small ion transport regulators or channels: cDNA sequence, protein signature sequence, and expression. Genomics 2000; 68(1):41–56.
40. Arystarkhova E, Wetzel RK, Asinovski NK, et al. The γ subunit modulates Na^+ and K^+ affinity of the renal Na,K-ATPase. J Biol Chem 1999; 274(47):33183–5.
41. Béguin P, Crambert G, Guennoun S, et al. CHIF, a member of the FXYD protein family, is a regulator of Na,K-ATPase distinct from the γ-subunit. EMBO J 2001; 20(15):3993–4002.
42. Féraille E, Carranza ML, Rousselot M, et al. Insulin enhances sodium sensivity of Na–K-ATPase in isolated rat proximal convoluted tubule. Am J Physiol Renal Physiol 1994; 267(1):F55–62.
43. Wetzel RK, Sweadner KJ. Immunocytochemical localization of Na–K-ATPase α and γ subunits in rat kidney. Am J Physiol Renal Physiol 2001; 281(3):531–45.
44. Féraille E, Rousselot M, Rajerison R, et al. Insulin primarily stimulates Na^+-K^+-ATPase in rat collecting duct. J Physiol 1995; 488(1):171–80.
45. Shi H, Levy-Holzman R, Cluzeaud F, et al. Membrane topology and immunolocalization of CHIF in kidney and intestine. Am J Physiol Renal Physiol 2001; 280(3):F505–12.
46. Munzer JS, Daly SE, Jewell-Motz EA, et al. Tissue- and isoform-specific kinetic behavior of the Na,K-ATPase. J Biol Chem 1994; 269(24):16668–76.

47. Jewell EA, Lingrel JB. Comparison of the substrate dependence properties of the rat Na,K-ATPase $\alpha 1$, $\alpha 2$, and $\alpha 3$ isoforms expressed in HeLa cells. J Biol Chem 1991; 266(25): 16925–30.
48. Doucet A, Katz AI, Morel F. Determination of Na–K-ATPase activity in single segments of the mammalian nephron. Am J Physiol Renal Fluid Electrolyte Physiol 1979; 237(2): F105–13.
49. Katz AI, Doucet A, Morel F. Na–K-ATPase activity along the rabbit, rat, and mouse nephron. Am J Physiol Renal Fluid Electrolyte Physiol 1979; 237(2):F114–20.
50. El Mernissi G, Doucet A. Quantitation of [^{3}H]ouabain binding and turnover of Na–K-ATPase along the rabbit nephron. Am J Physiol Renal Fluid Electrolyte Physiol 1984; 247(1): F158–67.
51. Doucet A, Barlet C. Evidence for differences in the sensitivity to ouabain of NaK-ATPase along the nephrons of rabbit kidney. J Biol Chem 1986; 261(3):993–5.
52. Féraille E, Barlet-Bas C, Cheval L, et al. Presence of two isoforms of Na,K-ATPase with different pharmacological and immunological properties in the rat kidney. Pflugers Arch 1995; 430(2):205–12.
53. Farman N, Corthesy-Theulaz I, Bonvalet J-P, et al. Localization of α-isoforms of Na–K-AtPase in rat kidney by in situ hybridization. Am J Physiol Cell Physiol 1991; 260(3): C468–74.
54. Lücking K, Nielsen JM, Pedersen PA, et al. Na–K-ATPase isoform ($\alpha 3$, $\alpha 2$, $\alpha 1$) abundance in rat kidney estimated by competitive RT-PCR and ouabain binding. Am J Physiol Renal Physiol 1996; 271(2):F253–60.
55. Féraille E, Doucet A. Sodium–potassium-adenosinetriphosphatase-dependent sodium transport in the kidney: hormonal control. Physiol Rev 2001; 81(1):345–418.
56. Boer WH, Braam B, Fransen R, et al. Effects of reduced renal perfusion pressure and acute volume expansion on proximal tubule and whole kidney angiotensin II content in the rat. Kidney Int 1997; 51(1):44–9.
57. Navar LG, Harrison-Bernard LM, Imig JD, et al. Intrarenal angiotensin II generation and renal effects of AT1 receptor blockade. J Am Soc Nephrol 1999; 10(S12):S266–72.
58. Ingelfinger JR, Zuo WM, Fon EA, et al. In situ hybridization evidence for angiotensinogen messenger RNA in the rat proximal tubule. An hypothesis for the intrarenal renin angiotensin system. J Clin Invest 1990; 85(2):417–23.
59. Moe OW, Ujiie K, Star RA, et al. Renin expression in renal proximal tubule. J Clin Invest 1993; 91(3):774–9.
60. Bruneval P, Hinglais N, Alhenc-Gelas F, et al. Angiotensin I converting enzyme in human intestine and kidney. Ultrastructural immunohistochemical localization. Histochemistry 1986; 85(1):73–80.
61. Peterson DR, Oparil S, Flouret G, et al. Handling of angiotensin II and oxytocin by renal tubular segments perfused in vitro. Am J Physiol Renal Fluid Electrolyte Physiol 1977; 232(4):F319–24.
62. Harris PJ, Young JA. Dose-dependent stimulation and inhibition of proximal tubular sodium reabsorption by angiotensin II in the rat kidney. Pflugers Arch 1977; 367(3):295–7.
63. Bharatula M, Hussain T, Lokhandwala MF. Angiotensin II AT1 receptor/signaling mechanisms in the biphasic effect of the peptide on proximal tubular Na^+-K^+-ATPase. Clin Exp Hypertens 1998; 20(4):465–80.
64. Aperia A, Holtbäck U, Syrén M-L, et al. Activation/deactivation of renal Na^+-K^+-ATPase: a final common pathway for regulation of natriuresis. FASEB J 1994; 8(6):336–439.
65. Du Cheyron D, Chalumeau C, Defontaine N, et al. Angiotensin II stimulates NHE3 activity by exocytic insertion of the transporter: role of PI 3-kinase. Kidney Int 2003; 64(3): 939–49.
66. Seri I, Kone BC, Gulans SR, et al. Locally formed dopamine inhibits Na–K-ATPase activity in rat renal cortical tubule cells. Am J Physiol Renal Fluid Electrolyte Physiol 1988; 255(4):F666–73.

67. Eklöf A-C, Holtbäck U, Sundelöf M, et al. Inhibition of COMT induces dopamine-dependent natriuresis and inhibition of proximal tubular Na^+-K^+-ATPase. Kidney Int 1997; 52(3): 742–7.
68. Seri I, Kone BC, Gulans SR, et al. Influence of Na intake on dopamine-induced inhibition of renal cortical Na–K-ATPase. Am J Physiol Renal Physiol 1990; 258(1):F52–60.
69. Aperia A, Bertorello A, Seri I. Dopamine causes inhibition of Na^+-K^+-ATPase activity in rat proximal convoluted tubule segments. Am J Physiol Renal Fluid Electrolyte Physiol 1987; 252(1):F39–45.
70. Bertorello A, Aperia A. Inhibition of proximal tubule Na–K-ATPase activity requires simultaneous activation of DA1 and DA2 receptors. Am J Physiol Renal Physiol 1990; 259(6):F924–8.
71. Ibarra F, Aperia A, Svensson L-B, et al. Bidirectional regulation of Na,K-ATPase activity by dopamine and an α-adrenergic agonist. Proc Natl Acad Sci USA 1993; 90(1):21–4.
72. Chibalin AV, Katz AI, Berggren P-O, et al. Receptor-mediated inhibition of renal Na^+-K^+-ATPase is associated with endocytosis of its α- and β-subunits. Am J Physiol Renal Physiol 1997; 273(5):C1458–65.
73. Chibalin AV, Pedemonte CH, Katz AI, et al. Phosphorylation of the catalytic α-subunit constitutes a triggering signal for Na^+-K^+-ATPase endocytosis. J Biol Chem 1998; 273(15):8814–9.
74. Chibalin AV, Zierath JR, Katz AI, et al. Phosphatidylinositol 3-kinase-mediated endocytosis of renal Na^+-K^+-ATPase α subunit in response to dopamine. Mol Biol Cell 1998; 9(5):1209–20.
75. Satoh T, Ominato M, Katz AI. Different mechanisms of renal Na–K-ATPase regulation by dopamine in the proximal and distal nephron. Hypertens Res 1995; 18(S11):S137–40.
76. Ominato M, Satoh T, Katz AI. Regulation of Na–K-ATPase activity in the proximal tubule: role of the protein kinase C pathway and ecosanoids. J Membrane Biol 1996; 152(3):235–43.
77. Chibalin AV, Ogimoto G, Pedemonte CH, et al. Dopamine-induced endocytosis of Na^+-K^+-ATPase is initiated by phosphorylation of Ser^{18} in the rat α-subunit and is responsible for the decreased activity in epithelial cells. J Biol Chem 1999; 274(4):1920–7.
78. Yudowski GA, Efendiev R, Pedemonte CH, et al. Phosphoinositide-3 kinase binds to a proline-rich motif in the Na^+-K^+-ATPase α-subunit and regulates its trafficking. Proc Natl Acad Sci USA 2000; 97(12):6556–61.
79. Efendiev R, Chen Z, Krmar RT, et al. The 14-3-3 protein translates the Na^+-K^+-ATPase $\alpha 1$-subunit phosphorylation signal into binding and activation of phosphoinositide 3-kinase during endocytosis. J Biol Chem 2005; 280(16):16272–7.
80. Doné SC, Leibiger IB, Efendiev R, et al. Tyrosine 537 within the Na^+-K^+-ATPase α-subunit is essential for AP-2 binding and clathrin-dependent endocytosis. J Biol Chem 2002; 277(19):17108–11.
81. Hu MC, Fan L, Crowder LA, et al. Dopamine acutely stimulates Na^+/H^+ exchanger (NHE3) endocytosis via clathrin-coated vesicles dependence on protein kinase A-mediated NHE3 phosphorylation. J Biol Chem 2001; 276(29):26906–15.
82. Bailly C, Imbert-teboul M, Roinel N, et al. Isoproterenol increases Ca, Mg, and NaCl reabsorption in mous thick ascending limb. Am J Physiol Renal Physiol 1990; 258(5): F1224–31.
83. Di Stefano A, Wittner M, Nitschke R, et al. Effects of parathyroid hormone and calcitonin on Na^+-Cl^-, K^+, Mg^{2+} and Ca^{2+} transport in cortical and medullary thick ascending limbs of mouse kidney. Pflugers Arch 1990; 417(2):161–7.
84. Wittner M, Di Stefano A, Mandon B, et al. Stimulation of NaCl reabsorption by antidiuretic hormone in the cortical thick ascending limb of Henle's loop of the mouse. Pflugers Arch 1991; 419(2):212–4.
85. Wittner M, Mandon B, Roinel N, et al. Hormonal stimulation of Ca^{++} and Mg^{++} transport in the cortical thick ascending limb of Henle's loop of the mouse: evidence for a change in the paracellular pathway permeability. Pflugers Arch 1993; 423(5–6):387–96.

86. Di Stefano A, Wittner M, Nitschke R, et al. Effects of glucagon on Na^+, Cl^-, K^+, Mg^{2+} and Ca^{2+} transports in cortical and medullary thick ascending limbs of mouse kidney. Pflugers Arch 1989; 414(6):640–6.
87. Elalouf J-M, Roinel N, De Rouffignac C. Effects of dDAVP on rat juxtamedullary nephrons: stimulation of medullary K recycling. Am J Physiol Renal Fluid Electrolyte Physiol 1985; 249(2):F291–8.
88. Kiroytcheva M, Cheval L, Carranza ML, et al. Effect of cAMP on the activity and the phosphorylation of Na^+-K^+-ATPase in rat thick ascending limb of Henle. Kidney Int 1999; 55(5):1819–31.
89. Satoh T, Cohen HT, Katz AI. Different mechanisms of renal Na–K-ATPase regulation by protein kinases in proximal and distal nephron. Am J Physiol Renal Physiol 1993; 265(3):F399–405.
90. Satoh T, Cohen HT, Katz AI. Intracellular signaling in the regulation of renal Na–K-ATPase. J Clin Invest 1992; 89(2):1496–500.
91. Satoh T, Cohen HT, Katz AI. Intracellular signaling in the regulation of renal Na–K-ATPase. J Clin Invest 1993; 91(2):409–15.
92. Amlal H, Legoff C, Vernimmen C, et al. ANG II controls Na–K^+(NH_4^+)–2Cl^- cotransport via 20-HETE and PKC in medullary thick ascending limb. Am J Physiol Cell Physiol 1998; 274(4):C1047–56.
93. Schlatter E, Greger R. cAMP increases the basolateral Cl^- conductance in the isolated perfused medullary thick ascending limb of Henle's loop of the mouse. Pflugers Arch 1985; 405(4):367–76.
94. Stokes JB. Effect of prostaglandin E2 on chloride transport across the rabbit thick ascending limb of Henle. Selective inhibition of the medullary portion. J Clin Invest 1979; 64(2): 495–502.
95. Plato CF, Stoos BA, Wang D, et al. Endogenous nitric oxide inhibits chloride transport in the thick ascending limb. Am J Physiol Renal Physiol 1999; 276(2):F159–63.
96. Ortiz PA, Hong NJ, Garvin JL. NO decreases thick ascending limb chloride absorption by reducing Na^+–K^+–2Cl^- cotransporter activity. Am J Physiol Renal Physiol 2001; 281(5): F819–25.
97. Nonoguchi H, Tomita K, Marumo F. Effects of atrial natriuretic peptide and vasopressin on chloride transport in long- and short-looped medullary thick ascending limbs. J Clin Invest 1992; 90(2):349–57.
98. Bailly C. Effect of luminal atrial natriuretic peptide on chloride reabsorption in mouse cortical thick ascending limb: inhibition by endothelin. J Am Soc Nephrol 2000; 11(10):1791–7.
99. Lerolle N, Bourgeois S, Leviel F, et al. Angiotensin II inhibits NaCl absorption in the rat medullary thick ascending limb. Am J Physiol Renal Physiol 2004; 287(3):F404–10.
100. Grider JS, Falcone JC, Kilpatrick EL, et al. P450 arachidonate metabolites mediate bradykinin-dependent inhibition of NaCl transport in the rat thick ascending limb. Can J Physiol Pharmacol 1997; 75(2):91–6.
101. De Jesus Ferreira MC, Bailly C. Extracellular Ca^{2+} decreases chloride reabsorption in rat CTAL by inhibiting cAMP pathway. Am J Physiol Renal Physiol 1998; 275(2):F198–203.
102. Riccardi D, Hall AE, Chattopadhyay N, et al. Localization of the extracellular Ca^{2+}/polyvalent cation-sensing protein in rat kidney. Am J Physiol Renal Physiol 1998; 274(3): F611–22.
103. Kellenberger S, Gautschi I, Rossier BC, et al. Mutations causing Liddle syndrome reduce sodium-dependent downregulation of the epithelial sodium channel. J Clin Invest 1998; 101(12):2741–50.
104. Horisberger JD, Diezi J. Effects of mineralocorticoids on Na and K excretion in the adrenalectomized rat. Am J Physiol Renal Fluid Electrolyte Physiol 1983; 246(1):F89–99.
105. ElMernissi G, Doucet A. Specific activity of Na,K-ATPase after adrenalectomy and hormone replacement along the rabbit nephron. Pflugers Arch 1984; 402(3):258–63.
106. Verrey F. Transcriptional control of sodium transport in tight epithelia by adrenal steroids. J Membrane Biol 1995; 144:93–110.

107. Losel RM, Feuring M, Falkenstein E, et al. Nongenomic effects of aldosterone: cellular aspects and clinical implications. Steroids 2002; 67(6):493–8.
108. Le Moëllic C, Ouvrard-Pascaud A, Capurro C, et al. Early nongenomic events in aldosterone action in renal collecting duct cells: PKC activation, mineralocorticoid receptor phosphorylation, and cross-talk with the genomic response. J Am Soc Nephrol 2004; 15(5):1145–60.
109. Johnson JP, Jones D, Wiesmann WP. Hormonal regulation of Na,K-ATPase in cultured epithelial cells. Am J Physiol Cell Physiol 1986; 251(2):C186–90.
110. Leal T, Crabbé J. Effect of aldosterone on ($Na^+ + K^+$)-ATPase of amphibian sodium-transporting epithelial cells (A6) in culture. J Steroid Biochem 1989; 34(1–6):581–4.
111. Yagawa Y, Kawakami K, Nagano K. Cloning and analysis of the 5′-flanking region of rat Na,K-ATPase α_1 subunit gene. Biochim Biophys Acta 1990; 1049(3):286–92.
112. Horster M, Schmid H, Schmidt U. Aldosterone in vitro restores nephron Na,K-ATPase of distal segments from adrenalectomized rabbits. Pflugers Arch 1980; 384(3):203–6.
113. Barlet-Bas C, Khadouri C, Marsy S, et al. Sodium-independent in vitro induction of Na^+-K^+-ATPase by aldosterone in renal target cells: permissive effect of triiodothyronine. Proc Natl Acad Sci USA 1988; 85(5):1707–11.
114. Barlet-Bas C, Khadouri C, Marsy S, et al. Enhanced intracellular sodium concentration in kidney cells recruits a latent pool of Na–K-ATPase whose size is modulated by corticosteroids. J Biol Chem 1990; 265(14):7799–803.
115. Blot-Chabaud M, Wanstok F, Bonvalet J-P, et al. Cell sodium-induced recruitment of Na–K-AtPase pumps in rabbit cortical collecting tubules is aldosterone-dependent. J Biol Chem 1990; 265(20):11676–81.
116. Summa V, Mordasini D, Roger F, et al. Short-term effect of aldosterone on Na,K-ATPase cell surface expression in kidney collecting duct cells. J Biol Chem 2001; 276(50):47087–93.
117. Bens M, Vallet V, Cluzeaud F, et al. Corticosteroid-dependent sodium transport in a novel immortalized mouse collecting duct principal cell line. J Am Soc Nephrol 1999; 10:923–34.
118. Vandewalle A, Bens M. Duong Van Huyen J-P. Immortalized kidney epithelial cells as tools for hormonally regulated ion transport studies. Curr Opin Nephrol Hypertens 1999; 8(5):581–7.
119. Attali B, Latter H, Rachamim N, et al. A corticosteroid-induced gene expressing an "IsK-Like" K^+ channel activity in *Xenopus* oocytes. Proc Natl Acad Sci USA 1995; 92(13): 6092–6.
120. Capurro C, Coutry N, Bonvalet J-P, et al. Cellular localization and regulation of CHIF in kidney and colon. Am J Physiol Cell Physiol 1996; 271(3):C753–62.
121. Wald H, Goldstein O, Asher C, et al. Aldosterone induction and epithelial distribution of CHIF. Am J Physiol Renal Physiol 1996; 271:F322–6.
122. Spindler B, Mastroberardino L, Custer M, et al. Characterization of early aldosterone-induced RNAs identified in A6 kidney epithelia. Pflugers Arch 1997; 434(3):323–31.
123. Mastroberardino L, Spindler B, Forster I, et al. Ras pathway activates epithelial Na^+ channel and decreases its surface expression in *Xenopus* oocytes. Mol Biol Cell 1998; 9(12): 3417–27.
124. Robert-Nicoud M, Flahaut M, Elalouf J-M, et al. Transcriptome of a mouse kidney cortical collecting duct cell line: effects of aldosterone and vasopressin. Proc Natl Acad Sci USA 2001; 98(5):2712–6.
125. Boulkroun S, Fay M, Zennaro MC, et al. Characterization of rat NDRG2 (N-Myc Downstream Regulated Gene 2), a novel early mineralocorticoid-specific induced gene. J Biol Chem 2002; 277(35):31506–15.
126. Waldegger S, Barth P, Raber G, et al. Cloning and characterization of a putative human serine/threonine protein kinase transcriptionally modified during anisotonic and isotonic alterations of cell volume. Proc Natl Acad Sci USA 1997; 94(9):4440–5.
127. Park J, Leong ML, Buse P, et al. Serum and glucocorticoid-inducible kinase (SGK) is a target of the PI 3-kinase-stimulated signaling pathway. EMBO J 1999; 18(11):3024–33.

128. Loffing J, Zecevic M, Féraille E, et al. Aldosterone induces rapid apical translocation of ENaC in early portion of enal collecting system: possible role of SGK. Am J Physiol Renal Physiol 2001; 280(4):F675–82.
129. Chen S-Y, Bhargava A, Mastroberardino L, et al. Epithelial sodium channel regulated by aldosterone-induced protein sgk. Proc Natl Acad Sci USA 1999; 96(5):2514–9.
130. Setiawan I, Henke G, Feng Y, et al. Stimulation of *Xenopus* oocyte Na^+–K^+ATPase by the serum and glucocorticoid-dependent kinase sgk1.Pflugers Arch 2002; 444:426–31.
131. Zecevic M, Heitzmann D, Camargo SM, et al. SGK1 increases Na,K-ATPase cell-surface expression and function in *Xenopus laevis* oocytes. Pflugers Arch 2004; 448(1):29–35.
132. Wulff P, Vallon V, Huang DY, et al. Impaired renal Na^+ retention in the sgk1-knockout mouse. J Clin Invest 2002; 110(9):1263–8.
133. Friedrich B, Feng Y, Cohen P. The serine/threonine kinases SGK2 and SGK3 are potent stimulators of the epithelial Na^+ channel α,β,γ-ENaC. Pflugers Arch 2003; 445(6):693–6.
134. Summa V, Camargo SM, Bauch C, et al. Isoform specificity of human Na^+-K^+-ATPase localization and aldosterone regulation in mouse kidney cells. J Physiol 2004; 555(2):355–64.
135. Hawk CT, Kudo LH, Rouch AJ, et al. Inhibition by epinephrine of AVP- and cAMP-stimulated Na and water transport in Dahl rat CCD. Am J Physiol Renal Physiol 1993; 265(3):F449–60.
136. Hawk CT, Li L, Schafer JA. AVP and aldosterone at physiological concentrations have synergistic effects on Na^+ transport in rat CCD. Kidney Int 1996; 50(12):S35–41.
137. Bankir L, Fernandes S, Bardoux P, et al. Vasopressin-V2 receptor stimulation reduces sodium excretion in healthy humans. J Am Soc Nephrol 2005; 16(7):1920–8.
138. Reif MC, Troutman SL, Schafer JA. Sodium transport by rat cortical collecting tubule. Effects of vasopressin and desoxycorticosterone. J Clin Invest 1986; 77(4):1291–8.
139. Schafer JA, Troutman SL. cAMP mediates the increase in apical membrane Na^+ conductance produced in rat CCD by vasopressin. Am J Physiol Renal Fluid Electrolyte Physiol 1990; 259(5):F823–31.
140. Frindt G, Silver RB, Windhager EE, et al. Feedback regulation of Na channels in rat CCT III. Response to cAMP. Am J Physiol Renal Physiol 1995; 268(3):F480–9.
141. Djelidi S, Fay M, Cluzeaud F, et al. Transcriptional regulation of sodium transport by vasopressin in renal cells. J Biol Chem 1997; 272(52):32919–24.
142. Ecelbarger CA, Kim G-H, Terris J, et al. Vasopressin-mediated regulation of epithelial sodium channel abundance in rat kidney. Am J Physiol Renal Physiol 2000; 279(1):F46–53.
143. Deschênes G, Gonin S, Zolty E, et al. Increased synthesis and AVP unresponsiveness of Na,K-ATPase in collecting duct from nephrotic rats. J Am Soc Nephrol 2001; 12(11):2241–52.
144. Mordasini D, Bustamante M, Rousselot M, et al. Stimulation of Na^+ transport by arginine-vasopressin is independent of PKA phosphorylation of the Na,K-ATPase α-subunit in collecting duct principal cells. Am J Physiol Renal Physiol 2005; 289(5):F1031–9.
145. Taylor SS. cAMP-dependent protein kinase. J Biol Chem 1989; 264(15):8443–6.
146. Vinciguerra M, Deschênes G, Hasler U, et al. Intracellular Na^+ controls cell surface expression of Na,K-ATPase via a cAMP-independent PKA pathway in mammalian kidney collecting duct cells. Mol Biol Cell 2003; 14(7):2677–88.
147. Gonin S, Deschênes G, Roger F, et al. Cyclic AMP increases cell surface expression of functional Na,K-ATPase units in mammalian cortical collecting duct principal cells. Mol Biol Cell 2001; 12(2):255–64.
148. Dulin NO, Niu J, Browning DD, et al. Cyclic AMP-independent activation of protein kinase A by vasoactive peptides. J Biol Chem 2001; 276(24):20827–30.
149. Zhong H, SuYang H, Erdjument-Bromage H, et al. The transcriptional activity of NF-κB is regulated by the IκB-associated PKAc subunit through cyclic-AMP-independent mechanism. Cell 1997; 89(3):413–24.
150. Vinciguerra M, Hasler H, Mordasini D, et al. Cytokines and sodium induce PKA-dependent cell-surface Na,K-ATPase recruitment via dissociation of NFκB/IκB/PKAc complex in collecting duct principal cells. J Am Soc Nephrol 2005; 16(9):2576–85.

151. Vinciguerra M, Arnaudeau S, Mordasini D, et al. Extracellular hypotonicity increases Na,K-ATPase cell surface expression via enhanced Na^+ influx in cultured renal collecting duct cells. J Am Soc Nephrol 2004; 15(10):2537–47.
152. Ichikawa I, Rennke HG, Hoyer JR, et al. Role for intrarenal mechanisms in the impaired salt excretion of experimental nephrotic syndrome. J Clin Invest 1983; 71(1):91–103.
153. Deschênes G, Wittner M, Di Stefano A, et al. Collecting duct is a site of sodium retention in PAN nephrosis: a rationale for amiloride therapy. J Am Soc Nephrol 2001; 12(3):598–601.
154. Vogt B, Favre H. Na^+-K^+-ATPase activity and hormones in single nephron segments from nephrotic rats. Clin Sci 1991; 80(6):599–604.
155. Deschênes G, Doucet A. Collecting duct Na^+/K^+-ATPase activity is correlated with urinary sodium excretion in nephrotic syndromes. J Am Soc Nephrol 2000; 11(4):604–15.

2
The Epithelial Sodium Channel

Olivier Bonny
Charles and Jane Pak Center for Mineral Metabolism and Division of Nephrology, Southwestern Medical Center, The University of Texas, Dallas, Texas, U.S.A.

INTRODUCTION

As sodium is the most abundant cation of the extracellular fluid (ECF) and sodium salts account for the most important part of the osmotically active solutes in the plasma and interstitial fluids, the amount of sodium in the body is a prime determinant of the ECF volume. Therefore, multiple regulatory mechanisms have evolved in terrestrial animals to tightly control its concentration in the body. Through the operation of these regulatory mechanisms, the amount of sodium excreted is adjusted to equal the amount ingested over a wide range of dietary intakes, allowing individuals to stay in sodium and volume balance.

Such a regulatory system requires sensors that detect changes in ECF volume and/or sodium concentration and effectors that eventually modify the rate of sodium excretion/reabsorption to maintain sodium homeostasis. This chapter focuses on the effector pathway controlling salt balance, with emphasis on the special role played by the epithelial sodium channel (ENaC) in dealing with this issue.

EFFECTORS OF SALT HOMEOSTASIS: THE ROLE OF THE KIDNEY

Effectors of sodium homeostasis should be located in tissues where sodium is excreted and reabsorbed in a controlled manner. Feces, urine, and secretions of exocrine glands (sweat, salivary, lachrymal and mammary glands) contain sodium. Thus, colon, kidneys, and principal ducts of the sweat and salivary glands control salt and water excretion and/or reabsorption, mainly under the control of the hormone aldosterone (1,2). The kidney is however the only organ able to vary sodium excretion in urine over many orders of magnitude and thus plays a special role in salt homeostasis and in the control of the ECF volume (3). Moreover, the kidney has a quantitative advantage over other salt-excreting organs, due to its filtrating capacities: with a glomerular filtration rate of 125 mL/min and a plasma sodium concentration of 145 mmol/L, the kidney is filtrating more than 26 moles of sodium a day (or about 1.5 kg of NaCl). More than 99% of the filtered sodium must be reabsorbed along the nephron to keep sodium in balance.

In the kidney, sodium is filtered from the blood through the glomerulus and then sequentially reabsorbed along the different segments of the nephron. Quantitative measurements of sodium reabsorption along the nephron were performed using micropuncture experiments. In the proximal tubule, between 50% and 75% of the filtered sodium is reabsorbed via secondary active cotransporters, together with amino acids, glucose, and phosphate, or in exchange for protons extruded via the apical sodium/hydrogen exchanger, type 3 (NHE3 or SLC9A3) or, possibly, type 8 (NHE8 or SLC9A8). The thin descending loop of Henle does not reabsorb sodium. By contrast, the thick ascending loop of Henle accounts for 20% to 25% of total sodium reabsorption in the nephron. In this segment, sodium enters the apical side of the cells through the Na^+–K^+–$2Cl^-$ cotransporter (NKCC2 or SLC12A1), which is inhibited by the diuretic furosemide. In the early distal tubule, about 5% to 10% of the filtered sodium is reabsorbed through the sodium chloride cotransporter (NCC or SLC12A3), targeted by the thiazide diuretics. Only a small percentage (2–5%) of the filtered sodium enters the late distal tubule where the fine regulation takes place mainly under the control of aldosterone and where the diuretics spironolactone and amiloride block its reabsorption. By definition, this segment includes the late distal convoluted tubule, the connecting tubule and the CCT and is often referred to as the aldosterone-sensitive distal nephron (ASDN). Throughout this segment, two cell types are present which account for the transport of different ions. Principal cells are responsible for sodium reabsorption and potassium secretion and intercalated cells are involved in potassium reabsorption, and proton or bicarbonate secretion. Due to the presence of tight junctions, all these cells form a tight epithelia resulting in high transepithelial resistances, forcing transcellular sodium reabsorption. Although the sodium reaching the late ASDN represents quantitatively only a small fraction of the filtered sodium, this segment is the place where the final decision is made on how much sodium will be excreted.

SODIUM REABSORPTION ACROSS ASDN: THE APICAL SODIUM CONDUCTANCE

Active transport of sodium through epithelia was first studied in frog skin and toad urinary bladder. In 1958, Koefoed-Johnsen and Ussing proposed a general model of sodium transport through frog skin (Fig. 1A) (4). They emphasized the role of the basolateral Na^+–K^+-ATPase at the origin of the skin potential and concluded that the active transport of sodium is, in reality, a forced exchange of sodium against potassium. The ASDN is a very close representation of the Koefoed-Johnsen and Ussing model and micropuncture experiments have allowed a better understanding of the apical conductance for sodium (Fig. 1B). In 1968, Bentley identified the inhibitory effect of amiloride on sodium transport across toad bladder and its potential role as a diuretic (5). This drug proved to be a valuable tool to study apical epithelial sodium transport, as it turned out to be a specific blocker of the apical sodium conductance at micromolar concentrations. Lindemann and Van Driessche first reported that specific sodium pores allowed high throughput of sodium ions through frog skin (6). In 1980, Palmer et al. performed a current–voltage analysis of apical sodium transport of the toad urinary bladder after depolarization of the basolateral surface by exposure to 85 mM KCl and 50 mM sucrose. Noise analysis established that the single channel conductance was as low as about 5 pS and that the selectivity of the channel for sodium over potassium was greater than 100:1 (7). Later on, the patch-clamp technique of single channels allowed a finer characterization of the amiloride-sensitive apical sodium conductance. However, the first patch-clamp results obtained from purified

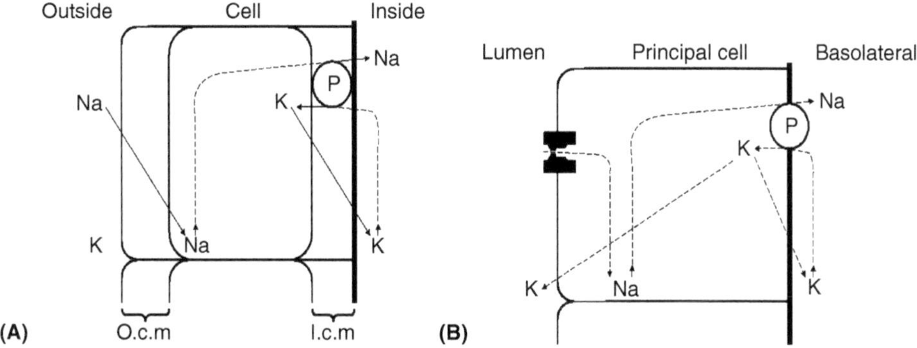

Figure 1 General mechanism of sodium reabsorption through tight epithelia. (**A**) The Valborg Koefoed-Johnsen and Hans H. Ussing model of sodium reabsorption through the frog skin. The Na^+–K^+-ATPase is represented by P. (**B**) An adaptation of the Koefoed-Johnsen/Ussing model for the principal cell in the aldosterone-sensitive distal nephron. The apical epithelial sodium channel is depicted in black. The Na^+–K^+-ATPase is represented by a P. *Source*: From Ref. 4.

amiloride-sensitive ENaC reconstituted into planar lipid bilayer (8) or from A6 cells (9) did not fit the characteristics of the native channel described at that point. In 1986, Palmer and Frindt published the first data obtained by patch-clamping apical membranes of rat CCT that matched the characteristics of the ENaC (10). This work established the fundamental references of the native ENaC in mammalian kidney.

From electrophysiological studies, basic characteristics of the epithelial channel are defined in terms of biophysical properties (low single channel conductance, sodium selectivity, slow gating) and pharmacological properties (sensitivity to amiloride or analogs). The single channel conductance of the ENaC is about 5 pS at room temperature with sodium as the conducted ion and 9 pS at room temperature in the presence of lithium. The channel is highly selective for sodium over potassium, with a ratio described up to 1000:1. The only other known permeable ions are H^+ and Li^+. The apparent K_m for sodium is about 40 mM as defined by single channel measurements. The gating of the channel is very slow, with open and closed time in the magnitude of the second, and with highly variable open probability (p_o). These kinetics are only slightly affected by voltage. Amiloride sensitivity is high, with a K_i for amiloride of about 0.1 μM. The block conferred by amiloride is slightly voltage dependent and is competitively inhibited by sodium ions, suggesting that amiloride might be plugged in the outer mouth of the channel pore.

CLONING OF THE ENAC

With molecular tools being developed and with the first cloning of genes coding for ion transporters, cloning of amiloride-sensitive apical sodium channel genes was highly anticipated in the early 1990s. Functionally expressing a rat colon cDNA library in *Xenopus laevis* oocytes, Canessa et al. isolated a clone able to induce tiny but characteristic amiloride-sensitive sodium currents (11). By complementing the found α subunit in the same assay, they published one year later that the ENaC is made of three subunits, called α, β and γ (12). When all three subunits were expressed in *Xenopus* oocytes, they reproduced the known features of the native channel. Noteworthy, Linguelia et al. were able to clone the rat ENaC at almost the same time, using the same functional cloning assay (13).

A fourth ENaC subunit, δ, which is actually an α-like subunit has been cloned by homology in humans (14). It shares 37% homology with α and 25% to 30% with β and γ subunits. When expressed in oocytes, it can assemble with β and γ subunits and give rise to sodium currents with slight biophysical differences when compared with the wild-type (αβγ) channel. The amiloride sensitivity is lower and the lithium over sodium selectivity ratio is decreased. δ is mainly expressed in nonepithelial tissues like testis, ovary, pancreas, brain and heart. δ was first found in human and chimpanzee, but Brockway et al. identified it in rabbit retina (15) and nucleotide databases show sequences homologs of δ ENaC in *Bos taurus*, *Canis familiaris* and even *Mus musculus*. Expression of δ ENaC in other species than human will allow a better evaluation of its function, but remains speculative so far. Another peculiarity of δ ENaC is its pH sensitivity, with activation at low pH values [half-maximal pH for activation is 5.0 (16) or 6.0 (17)]. One way of regulating ENaC surface expression is through the interaction of a PPXY domain present in the intracellular C-terminus of all three subunits with the WW domain of NEDD4-2, an ubiquitin ligase. Once the binding occurs, ENaC is retrieved from the cell surface and directed for degradation. In δ ENaC the PPXY motif is not conserved, suggesting that δ-containing channels could be regulated in another way. Indeed, Biasio et al. reported about the regulation of δ ENaC by Murr1, an intracellular ubiquitous protein that could be involved in copper transport (18). Murr1 was identified by yeast-two-hybrid screen of a human brain library using δ ENaC C-terminus as bait. When δβγ and even αβγ are coexpressed in *X. laevis* oocytes, amiloride-sensitive sodium currents are inhibited by Murr1 in a dose-dependent manner. Some reports have disclosed pharmacological activation of δβγ channels by capsazepine, a competitive antagonist for transient receptor potential vanilloid subfamily 1 (19) and by icilin (20) and inhibition by Evan's blue (21).

Babini et al. have reported on the cloning of ε ENaC, an α/δ-like ENaC subunit found in *X. laevis* (22). It is mainly expressed in the kidney and the bladder of *X. laevis* and to a lesser extent in the brain and skeletal muscle. It can form functional channel on its own, but produces only tiny currents. Associated with β and γ subunits, currents have the same amplitude as αβγ-formed channels, but display a lower amiloride sensitivity compared with αβγ and a strong inhibition by extracellular sodium. Like δ, ε is lacking the PPXY motif involved in the regulation of surface expression of the channel.

Cloning of the ENaC allowed the elucidation of two rare genetic traits linked to gain-of-function (Liddle's syndrome) or to decreased function [systemic type I pseudohypoaldosteronism (PHA-1)] of ENaC in humans, highlighting the central role of ENaC in sodium homeostasis. Moreover, ENaC cloning has facilitated the dissection of intracellular signaling pathways regulating ENaC and has linked known hormonal effects with sodium reabsorption in the distal nephron. ENaC cloning was the starting point for the identification of several homologous genes grouped in the degenerin (DEG)/ENaC family.

ENAC: A MEMBER OF THE LARGE HETEROGENEOUS DEG/ENAC FAMILY

Sequence alignment showed that ENaC has substantial homology with genes previously identified by genetic screen of the mechanosensitive pathway of *Caenorhabditis elegans*, called degenerins (11). These proteins were named after the discovery that mutations of the genes deg-1 and mec-4 induced a swelling and degeneration of sensory neurons of the worm *C. elegans* (23). The DEG/ENaC family consists of channels found in nematodes, insects, mollusks and mammals and covers a large variety of functions and a wide tissue distribution. The *C. elegans* genome contains several genes sharing homology with the

DEG/ENaC family, which are mainly involved in mechanosensation. In the fly *Drosophila melanogaster*, two gene families are related to the DEG/ENaC family (24) and seem to be important for different functions such as locomotion (25), lung liquid clearance (26) or even salt taste (27). In the snail *Helix aspersa*, an amiloride-sensitive sodium channel is expressed in the nervous tissue and is activated by the neuropeptide FMRF (28).

By extension, genes related to the DEG/ENaC family were found in other species including mammals. For instance, Sakai et al. cloned a rat homolog (BLINaC), which is expressed mainly in the small intestine, brain and liver (29). Schaefer et al. cloned hINaC from human small intestine (30). The function of these genes has not been reported yet.

Channels of the DEG/ENaC family can be constitutively active (ENaC) or activated by small peptide (FaNaC), proton (ASIC) or mechanical stimuli, as showed for the *C. elegans* degenerins.

The newly described genes have broadened the heterogeneity of the family and may explain the diversity of channels with biophysical differences described by electrophysiologists previous to the cloning era (31). With the completion of the human genome sequencing, it seems unlikely that other new human clones will join the family.

ENAC: SUBUNIT TOPOLOGY AND STOICHIOMETRY

ENaC is a heteromultimeric complex made of the assembly of three proteins α, β and γ ENaC. These three subunits share about 35% homology and have presumably the same secondary structure, with two transmembrane domains and intracellular amino and carboxy ends, exposing a large extracellular loop that constitutes about two-third of the protein mass (32–34).

Quantitative assessment of cell surface abundance of ENaC showed that α, β and γ subunits assemble according to a fixed stoichiometry to constitute the channel pore (35). If everyone adheres to this assertion, the question of how many subunits and which subunits are forming the functional channel complex is still under debate. Several approaches have been used to address this issue. Biophysical and biochemical methods, concatameric construct expression, freeze-fracture electron microscopy and, more recently, fluorescence resonance energy transfer (FRET) were used (Table 1). Even if the biophysical method developed by MacKinnon was successful in assessing subunit stoichiometry of several channels (46), it seems that the data obtained for more complex and heteromultimeric channels like ENaC may be more conflicting. The results obtained for ENaC so far by this method and others can be separated in two groups (Table 1): (*i*) ENaC is either a heterotetrameric complex consisting in 2α:1β:1γ (36–39,45) or (*ii*) is an equimolar complex of higher order, type 3α:3β:3γ (40–44). These contradictory results have led laboratories to search for alternative methods to solve this issue (freeze-fracture electron microscopy or FRET), but no consensus has been reached so far, even if one can argue that octameric or nonameric complexes described in some studies might reflect dimers of a basic unit consisting in a heterotetramer. Emphasis on tetramer assembly of ENaC subunits comes from the fact that homologous channels like ASICs, FaNaC and potassium two-transmembrane spanning channels are homotetramers. The visualization of the crystal structure of ENaC is expected to give a definitive answer to this question, but is still awaited.

If all three subunits are homologous and participate in the pore structure, they do not have the same relative function. The α subunit plays a special role. When injected alone in the *Xenopus* oocyte, the α subunit produces small but significant amiloride-sensitive sodium currents (11), which allowed its cloning. By contrast, neither β nor γ could do the same. δ ENaC can produce tiny currents when injected alone in oocytes (14). However,

Table 1 Reported Studies on ENaC Subunit Stoichiometry

Species and channel	Expression system	Method	Proposed subunit stoichiometry	Reference
Rat ENaC	Oocyte	Biophysical quantitative cell-surface binding assay concatameric constructs	$2\alpha:1\beta:1\gamma$	36
Rat ENaC	Lipid bilayer	Biophysical	$2\alpha:1\beta:1\gamma$	37
Mouse ENaC	Oocyte	Biophysical	$2\alpha:1\beta:1\gamma$	38
Rat ENaC	Oocyte	Biochemical	Heterotetramer	39
Human ENaC	Oocyte	Freeze-fracture EM biophysical	Eight or nine total subunits with at least 2γ	40
Human ENaC (FaNac+BNC1)	Oocyte COS cells	Biophysical biochemical	Nine subunit: $3\alpha:3\beta:3\gamma$	41,42
Mouse ENaC	COS and CHO cells	FRET biochemical	$1\alpha:1\beta:1\gamma$ or higher equimolar ratio (3:3:3)	43,44
Helix aspersa FaNac	HEK cells	Biochemical	Homotetrameric	45

whether α or δ alone could form a channel by themselves or whether endogenous subunits present in *Xenopus* oocytes contribute to the expression of heteromultimeric ENaC at the cell surface is still unclear. In particular, the ε ENaC subunit, PCR cloned from *X. laevis*, could associate with β and γ and form functional channels (22).

Surface binding experiments demonstrated the close correlation between the number of channel molecules present at the oocyte surface and the current measured in individual oocytes (35). One study has suggested that the α subunit could play a role in the trafficking of the channel to the cell surface (47). Indeed, in the surface binding assay, all complexes comprising α subunits reached the cell surface, though less efficiently for αβ, αγ and α alone compared with αβγ-injected oocytes, while no signal could be detected on oocytes injected only with β and/or γ subunits after two days of incubation (35). Using the same quantitative surface binding assay, Firsov et al. showed that oocytes injected with α, β, and γ ENaC present twice more α at the cell surface compared with βγ-injected oocytes (36). The central role of α ENaC subunit is further illustrated by the fact that most of ENaC loss-of-function mutations found in humans affected by systemic PHA-1 are located in the gene coding for α ENaC (48).

If all three ENaC subunits are present in the same cell, they preferentially assemble in heteromeric complexes instead of homomeric. The mechanism for this heteromeric preferential assembly is not known. In certain tissues, however, only one or two of the three subunits have been found, leading to speculation about the functional relevance of possible monomer, homo- or heterodimers. However, one should be aware that a missing subunit in a specific organ could result either from a downregulation of this subunit in certain circumstances or from technical difficulties to efficiently demonstrate the presence of a given subunit in this organ. Characteristics of heterodimers were assessed electrophysiologically. Canessa and collaborators have shown that channel activity recorded after injection of oocytes with rat αβ have different sensitivity to amiloride and a different Li^+/Na^+ ratio selectivity compared with αβγ or αγ (49,50). We confirmed these results for the rat $\alpha\beta$ heterodimers and, in addition, found that when $\beta\gamma$ or an α truncated mutant ($\alpha_{L535stop}\beta\gamma$) are injected in oocytes, they behave the same way as $\alpha\beta$, with decreased amiloride sensitivity and decreased Li^+/Na^+ ratio selectivity (51). Interestingly, these differences were not encountered when human $\alpha\beta$, $\alpha\gamma$ or the corresponding α truncated mutant ($\alpha_{R508stop}\beta\gamma$) ENaC subunits were injected in oocytes. This species difference in the selectivity and amiloride sensitivity of currents recorded from oocytes injected with $\alpha\beta$, $\alpha\gamma$ or mutant $\alpha_{R508stop}\beta\gamma$ ENaC has not been explained so far.

TISSUE EXPRESSION OF ENAC

All three subunits are expressed in sodium reabsorbing organs in humans: from the late distal convoluted tubule to outer medullary collecting duct of the kidney, the distal colon, and the ducts of salivary and sweat glands (52). This expression pattern coincides with the expression of the mineralocorticoid receptor (MR) and the 11β-hydroxysteroid dehydrogenase type 2, two required proteins for an adequate and regulated response to aldosterone.

In the kidney, the three ENaC subunits were found by immunochemistry in the late distal convoluted tubule, the connecting tubule, the CCT and the outer medullary collecting tubule (52–55). The presence of ENaC subunit in the inner medullary collecting duct is unclear. Duc did not detect it by immunochemistry, but Volk et al. showed the presence of the transcripts along this segment of the tubule (56). Electrophysiological data suggest that the sodium channel present in this part of the nephron could be different from ENaC (56,57).

The three ENaC subunits were identified along the respiratory system, starting from the nose down to type II pneumocytes in alveoli (55,58–62). The role of ENaC in the respiratory system is different in the sense that it is not involved in overall salt balance but rather in maintaining a local and appropriate level of hydration of the fluid layer lining the surface of the epithelium (63).

ENaC has been described in the colon (52,55,64,65), but has been poorly studied at the functional level. Wang et al. measured amiloride-sensitive transepithelial potential difference (PD) in the colon and showed its regulation by the diet and circadian rhythm (66). ENaC may also be involved in the pathogenesis of diarrhea in patients with ulcerative colitis (67).

In the skin, all three ENaC subunits are expressed in keratinocytes and in hair follicles (68), but their role still remain elusive. Brouard et al. failed to show sodium transport through cultured human keratinocytes (69). These authors and others (70) suggest that ENaC might be involved in cell differentiation in the skin. Indeed, α ENaC inactivation in the mouse leads to a skin phenotype with epithelial hyperplasia, abnormal nuclei, premature secretion of lipids, and abnormal keratohyaline granules (71,72). Moreover, skin-specific inactivation of the channel activating protease (CAP), known to upregulate ENaC activity in epithelia, leads to a drastic phenotype, with death intervening before 60 hours of life (73). These mice die of dehydration and present a lower body weight and abnormal skin permeability, with severe malformation of the stratum corneum and absence of the tight-junction protein occludin. As CAP could act not only on ENaC but also on several transporters present in the keratinocytes, its specific relationship with ENaC in the skin is not established yet.

An amiloride-sensitive Na^+ conductance has been described in a human lymphocyte cell line as well as in freshly isolated rat and human lymphocytes, using the whole-cell patch-clamp technique (74) and the three ENaC subunits have been localized in lymphocytes. However, the function of the channels in the lymphocyte is unknown.

ENaC was identified in several sense organs, such as taste buds, inner ear and eye. Taste buds on the surface of the tongue express ENaC and the perception of salty taste in humans can be attenuated by amiloride (see Ref. 75 for review). Gründer et al. found expression of all three ENaC subunits in the inner ear (76), where ENaC or its regulating proteins [for instance, TMPRSS3, a serine protease which activates ENaC and, when mutated in human, leads to deafness (77)] might play a role in the endolymphatic sodium homeostasis or in transducing mechanosensitive signals. However, Peters et al. found no evidence of hearing loss in two patients suffering from systemic PHA-1 (78). In the eye, ENaC was found in the corpus ciliary and in the retina (79), but its function remains elusive. Fricke described the presence of all three subunits in mechanosensitive neurons of the trigeminal ganglia and hypothesized a role in mechanosensation (80). Drummond and his group found β and γ subunits in vascular smooth muscle cells of kidney and speculate about the possible involvement of these subunits in mechanosensation (81), though without functional data.

STRUCTURE/FUNCTION

In the absence of a crystal structure for DEG/ENaC proteins, studies of ENaC mutants (naturally occurring or generated) were the chosen route for exploring the structure/function of the channel. Using this approach, functional domains have been identified on intracellular N- and C-termini and on the large extracellular loop of the three ENaC subunits. A model of the external mouth of the channel pore has been proposed and the site for amiloride block was identified (82). Starting from the N-terminus, a review of the significant functional domains follows.

In the cytoplasmic N-terminal domain, a highly conserved region preceding the first transmembrane domain is involved in the gating of the channel, as illustrated by a homozygous mutation found in human and leading to systemic PHA-1 (83,84). Another important feature of the amino-terminal region is the presence of numerous lysine residues. Staub et al. have shown that these residues are involved in the ubiquitination process of ENaC subunits, especially of α and γ subunits, and thus could be key elements in determining the half-life of the channel (85). Others have identified a motif present on the rat α subunit (KGDK) that could play a role in regulating the endocytosis of the channel (86). Finally, the N-terminal domain was reported to be involved in channel assembly as demonstrated for the γ subunit (87).

The extracellular loop is the largest domain of the protein, encoded by 10 different exons, in comparison with N- and the C-intracellular termini, which are both encoded by only one exon. It contains several putative glycosylation sites (32,34). Two cysteine-rich boxes (CRBs) are present in the loop. CRB1 contains 6 cysteines and CRB2 10 cysteines. Firsov et al. have demonstrated interactions between cysteines 1 and 6 in CRB1, and cysteines 11 and 12 in CRB2, both of which are critical for channel function, especially in the trafficking of the channel to the cell surface (88). Using anti-amiloride antibodies, Ismailov et al. identified an amiloride binding site in the extracellular loop (89), but no functional significance of this site could be demonstrated. Waldmann et al. and Schild et al. have highlighted the importance of a specific segment localized upstream of the second transmembrane domain, called pre-M2, for the amiloride block and for filter selectivity (90,91). Schild et al. found point mutations that affect substantially the amiloride sensitivity on the three subunits (90). In the same lab, Kellenberger et al. have studied the molecular aspects of the selectivity filter and have proposed a model of the external pore of the channel based on electrophysiological data (92,93). Regulation of ENaC activity intervenes in the same pre-M2 segment, as point mutations in this segment lead to cell swelling and neurodegeneration in the worm *C. elegans* (94,95) or to a twofold increase in ENaC activity in a patient with Liddle's syndrome (96).

The intracellular carboxy terminus contains several functional domains involved in the regulation of the number of channels present at the cell surface. A PPxY motif (or PY motif) is present on all ENaC subunits, except δ and ε. Its deletion on the β and γ subunits in patients affected by Liddle's syndrome underscores its importance in ENaC regulation (97–100). In Liddle's syndrome, channels are hyperactive due to two factors: an increased number of channels present at the cell surface and an increased activity of ENaC. Staub et al. demonstrated that the PY motif is the target of Nedd4-2, an ubiquitin protein ligase, which binds to the PY motif through its WW domains (101). The binding allows the ubiquitination of ENaC and its retrieval from the cell surface. In Liddle's syndrome, the interaction between Nedd4-2 and the PY motif of β and γ subunits is disrupted by the absence of the PY motif and results in an increased number of hyperactive channels at the cell surface. An alternative explanation for the regulation of the number of channels present at the cell surface was pointed out by Shimkets et al. (102). They put forward that the PY motif could play a role as an endocytic signal, deleted in Liddle's patients. These two hypotheses are not mutually exclusive and identified the PY motif as essential in regulating the number of channels present at the cell surface. The intracellular C-terminus contains several putative phosphorylation sites. Serines and threonines, but not tyrosines, were found to be phosphorylated in the C-termini of β and γ subunits at basal state when channel subunits were stably expressed in Madin Darby canine kidney (MDCK) cells (103). In these cells, aldosterone and insulin increased the basal phosphorylation, but did not phosphorylate the α subunit. However, the phosphorylated residues have not yet been identified and their functional relevance not yet established. A more detailed description of phosphorylation events is given later. Finally, a proline-rich domain in the C-terminus of the α subunit that resembles a SH3 protein–protein interaction domain was involved in the interaction with an element of the cytoskeleton, α-spectrin (47). This interaction could play a role in the localization of the channel at the cell surface.

ENAC REGULATION

ENaC regulation is complex and may intervene at each processing step in the cell, transcriptional and posttranslational, such as heteromerization, trafficking, retrieval from the cell membrane, recycling and degradation. With a cell surface half-life of about one hour, retrieval of ENaC from the cell surface plays a critical role in regulating overall channel activity. This was emphasized by the finding that in Liddle's syndrome, ENaC retrieval from the cell surface is decreased and thus more channels are present at the surface, leading to excessive salt reabsorption and volume expansion.

Control by Ions and pH

Once inserted at the cell surface, ENaC is subjected to regulation by several ions and particularly by the main carried ion, sodium. High extracellular sodium concentrations inhibit ENaC by a mechanism known as self-inhibition that involves a decrease in ENaC p_o (104,105). Interestingly, mutations of histidine residues in the extracellular loop of α and γ ENaC modulate self-inhibition of ENaC by extracellular sodium, suggesting that the extracellular loop may be involved in luminal salt sensing (106). High intracellular sodium concentration has an inhibitory effect on ENaC, which is called feedback inhibition (107,108) and preserves cell volume homeostasis and cell survival. This mechanism is lacking in Liddle's syndrome, thus contributing to the increase in salt reabsorption in this syndrome (109). It is not known whether feedback inhibition is the result of a direct action of intracellular sodium on ENaC (110)] or results from indirect mechanisms, such as activation of G-protein or from a rise in intracellular calcium resulting from a cross talk with the basolateral membrane and activation of the sodium–calcium exchanger. According to the latter hypothesis, an elevation of intracellular sodium drives calcium influx through the sodium–calcium exchanger and the resulting intracellular rise of calcium inhibits ENaC activity.

Cytoplasmic calcium concentration is involved in the regulation of ENaC activity. The first indication that calcium may influence transepithelial transport came from studies done in the toad bladder exposed to quinidine, known to increase intracellular calcium. Quinidine was shown to inhibit the net transport of sodium in isolated toad bladder (111). Similar phenomena have been observed in the rabbit (112) or rat CCT (107). Since sodium transport was inhibited (*i*) when intracellular sodium was raised by ouabain, (*ii*) when basolateral sodium concentration was lowered or (*iii*) when ionophore was used apically, it has been postulated that basolateral extrusion of sodium by the Na–Ca exchanger could be involved in this inhibition. However, other mechanisms have been advanced for this inhibition. Ishikawa et al. found that when ENaC was stably expressed in MDCK cells, the single channel activity in excised inside-out patches was inhibited by increasing cytosolic Ca^{2+} concentration from 1 nM to 1 μM without changing the single channel conductance (110). By contrast, this direct effect has not been observed by Abriel and Horisberger in the cut-open oocyte system (113) or by Palmer (114). In the latter elegant study, Palmer measured the effect of changing intracellular calcium concentration in excised inside-out patches from rat CCT and found no direct effect of calcium on sodium current. However, in cell-attached patches obtained from rat CCT cells previously treated with the Ca^{2+}-ionophore ionomycin, a decrease in channel activity was observed. Thus, calcium-dependent inhibition of sodium current could arise by three different mechanisms: (*i*) A direct effect of calcium on ENaC (115), but this issue is highly debatable as reported by Abriel et al. and Palmer et al. (*ii*) An indirect effect through activation of intracellular calcium-dependent transducers, such as protein kinase C (PKC), calmodulin, phospholipases or phosphatidylinositol-4,5-bisphosphate (PIP2). (*iii*) An effect of calcium on ENaC trafficking, for instance through Nedd4, as Nedd4 trafficking is known to be calcium dependent. This issue is not yet resolved and will need further studies.

Chloride has been shown to be a regulator of ENaC activity either directly (116–118) or in the context of the complex ENaC regulation/interaction by cystic fibrosis transmembrane conductance regulator (CFTR) (119,120).

Intracellular pH has been shown to regulate ENaC. A low pHi directly inhibits ENaC, as shown in rat CCT (114,121), frog skin epithelium (122) or oocytes (113,123). Inhibition of ENaC by low intracellular pH may contribute to the activation of the Na^+–H^+ exchanger and thus to the restoration of normal intracellular pH.

Control by the Membrane Context

The membrane context surrounding ENaC complexes has been shown to play a role in modulating ENaC activity. If stretch activation of ENaC is still under debate (124,125), it seems that at least in some expression systems or specific tissues, this kind of ENaC regulation may be relevant (81,126). Membrane hyperpolarization has been shown to increase ENaC activity (124), but its physiological relevance remains elusive.

Cholesterol content of the plasma membrane may play a role in ENaC regulation, as shown in A6 cells by two different groups (127,128), but its physiological relevance is still unknown.

PIP2 and phosphatidylinositol 3,4,5-trisphosphate (PIP3) have been shown to increase ENaC activity in A6 cells (129) and in the *Xenopus* oocyte expression system (130). Regulation of ENaC activity by anionic lipids of the cell membrane may account for the inhibitory effect of extracellular adenosine tri-phosphate (ATP) on ENaC function via P2Y (131,132) and P2X receptors (133) or for a direct nongenomic stimulatory effect of aldosterone on ENaC via PI3 kinase (134). Even if the definitive ENaC domains interacting with PIPs have not been identified yet, evidence that the intracellular N-termini of both β and γ ENaC subunits (132,135) or the region immediately distal to the second transmembrane domain of the γ subunit (136) may modulate ENaC activity has recently been put forward.

Cytoskeleton elements have been associated with regulation of ENaC function. α-Spectrin (47) or actin (137) were reported to influence ENaC function. ENaC trafficking has been shown to be regulated by syntaxins and by the Rab pathway (138–140). Syntaxin 1a was shown to inhibit ENaC and syntaxin 3 to activate ENaC expressed in the *X. laevis* oocyte (141–143).

Hormonal Control

Hormones like aldosterone, glucocorticoids, vasopressin (82), insulin (144–149), angiotensin II (150,151), progesterone (152,153), estrogen (154) or prolonged treatment with atrial natriuretic peptide (ANP) (155) have been shown to regulate ENaC expression and/or activity from the basolateral compartment in the ASDN or in cell models. By contrast, adenosine (156,157) and prostaglandins E2 (158,159) are hormones regulating ENaC activity from the luminal side. Historically and from a physiological point of view, aldosterone plays by far the most recognized role.

Aldosterone action defines the ASDN, where ENaC, the 11-β hydroxysteroid dehydrogenase type 2, the MR and the Na^{+}–K^{+}-ATPase are coexpressed as effectors of its action. The aldosterone effect results in sodium absorption from the urinary compartment toward the interstitial compartment, as well as potassium and proton secretion. As studied in amphibian epithelial models, the aldosterone effect on sodium reabsorption is typically divided into three periods related to different cellular events (160). First, a period of latency is characterized by de novo synthesis of aldosterone-induced transcripts (AITs) and aldosterone-repressed transcripts (ARTs) without effect on sodium reabsorption. Then follows an early response period, during which transepithelial sodium transport increases rapidly, concomitant to a drop in transepithelial resistance. Finally, a late response period is characterized by a slower but continuous rise in transepithelial sodium reabsorption without further change in transepithelial resistance. Eventually, morphological and long-term changes may occur upon chronic exposure to increased aldosterone levels. The time course of these periods varies from one experimental system to the other (161,162) and is probably less clear cut in vivo (163). The cascade of cellular and molecular events leading to ENaC activation upon aldosterone stimulation still remains to be elucidated, but significant progress has been made in recent years. In particular, several different approaches were successfully used to identify early AITs or ARTs. Chen et al. used a subtracted cDNA library built from A6 cells and functionally coexpressed with ENaC in the oocyte expression system to identify the serum and glucocorticoid-regulated kinase 1 (sgk1) as a sevenfold inducer of ENaC activity (164). Others used a combination of PCR-based subtractive hybridization and differential display techniques and identified the same transcript among several clones induced by aldosterone treatment (10 nM for one hour) of rabbit cortical collecting duct (CCD) cells (165). Alvarez de la Rosa et al. confirmed a significant increase of ENaC activity by coexpression of ENaC with sgk1 and showed that it was due to an increased number of channels present at the cell surface, but that this effect was not mediated through the carboxy termini of any ENaC subunits (166). The targets of sgk1 were quickly identified. The interaction of sgk1 with Nedd4-2 was put forward by the group of Staub et al. They found that sgk1 phosphorylates Nedd4-2 in the *Xenopus* oocyte (167) and in a CCD cell line (168) and thus decreases the chance for Nedd4-2 to retrieve ENaC from the cell surface leading to increased sodium reabsorption. A negative feedback loop allows tight control of this process, as phosphorylated Nedd4-2 appears to ubiquitinate and eventually to enable sgk1 degradation (169). An alternative pathway by which sgk1 may regulate ENaC activity was proposed based on electrophysiological studies. Diakov and Kormacher showed a two- to threefold increase in ENaC current in outside-out patches obtained from oocytes injected with ENaC subunits and exposed to recombinant constitutively active sgk1 (170). This effect was lost when a C-terminus α mutant or even only an α S621A mutant was injected, but not when β or γ C-terminus truncations were injected. Taken together, these data indicate that sgk1 may interact directly with ENaC and modulate its activity by phosphorylation. However, these data are in contradiction with those from Alvarez de la Rosa et al. showing that none of the C-terminus truncated subunits were able to abrogate the induction of ENaC activity by sgk (166).

A major advance in the field of regulation of ENaC activity by sgk1 was made when a cofactor of the sgk/Nedd4-2 phospho-interaction was found by a Japanese group working on proteins 14-3-3. Proteins 14-3-3 recognize phosphopeptide consensus sequence motifs and regulate the activity, localization or function of the targeted phosphoprotein. In an attempt to search for new targets of 14-3-3, Ichimura et al. identified Nedd4-2 and showed that proteins 14-3-3 bind to phosphorylated Nedd4-2 and protect it from dephosphorylation (171). This interaction resulted in a decrease of ENaC ubiquitination and, thus, in a lower retrieval of ENaC from the cell surface. Bhalla et al. confirmed this important modulation in an epithelial cell line (172). Which of the 14-3-3 proteins is involved in this interaction in vivo and whether these isoforms are regulated by aldosterone were important questions addressed by the group of Frizzel and colleagues (173). Working with the mpkCCD_{c14} cell line, they identified 14-3-3 β as the isoform regulating the Nedd4-2/sgk1 interaction. Moreover, they showed that 14-3-3 β is upregulated by 10 nM aldosterone in this cell line.

If sgk1 plays a central and integrative role in the signaling pathway from aldosterone to ENaC and if the downstream partners are known (sgk1, 14-3-3, Nedd4-2 and finally ENaC), the upstream pathway was less explored. However, two groups identified WNK1, a serine–threonine protein kinase in which intronic deletion in humans leads to familial hyperkalemic hypertension (174), as an upstream regulator of sgk1. First, Naray-Fejes-Toth et al. showed that the expression of a kidney-specific WNK1 isoform, but not the long ubiquitous WNK1, was rapidly induced by aldosterone in a MR overexpressing cell line (175). When the kidney-specific isoform was overexpressed in cells, they noted an increase of the transepithelial sodium transport. Another group, seeking partners interacting with WNK1 by performing a yeast-two-hybrid screen, identified sgk1 as interacting with WNK1 (176). They further demonstrated that WNK1 activates ENaC through sgk1.

Several groups tried to identify other aldosterone-induced or -repressed proteins, using different approaches. Using a differential display PCR method to compare cDNA fragments generated from RNA of control and aldosterone treated A6 cells, Spindler et al. showed that only a small proportion of RNA ($<0.5\%$) was significantly regulated during the latent period of aldosterone action (177). They identified two aldosterone-induced RNA (adrenal steroid upregulated RNA) encoding (*i*) the *Xenopus* homolog of E16/TA1, a permease-related gene product of unknown function and (*ii*) the *Xenopus* A splice variant of the small G-protein K-Ras2. K-Ras2 mRNA was rapidly induced by aldosterone, even before any sodium transport response (178). Coexpression of K-Ras2 in *Xenopus* oocytes led to stimulation of ENaC activity at the cell surface suggesting a regulatory role of K-Ras2 transcriptionally controlled by aldosterone. Using the serial analysis of gene expression method, Robert-Nicoud et al. compared mRNA libraries of the $mpkCCD_{c14}$ cell line treated or not with aldosterone for four hours (179). They found 34 AITs and 29 ARTs, from which they validated two AITs and one ART by northern blot or by RT-PCR. Among the validated AITs, the glucocorticoid-induced leucine zipper (GILZ) mRNA was induced as early as 30 minutes after aldosterone stimulation, reaching an 11-fold induction four hours after stimulation. In vivo, GILZ was induced together with sgk1 in adrenalectomized rat substituted with 1 nM aldosterone for 2.5 hours (180). Pearce's group performed a microarray analysis of aldosterone-induced $mpkCCD_{c14}$ cells (1 μM, one or six hours) and found 49 AITs and 179 ARTs (181). GILZ was found again among the AITs and they showed that it was activating transepithelial sodium transport via the extracellular signal-regulated kinase (ERK) pathway (181).

Gumz et al. used the mouse IMCD3 cell line to perform an oligonucleotide array on 12,000 genes after aldosterone stimulation for one hour (182). They obtained several AITs and confirmed four of them by northern blot or RT-PCR. Confirmed AITs included sgk1, the connective tissue growth factor, the period homolog and preproendothelin. Except for sgk1, already shown to play an important physiological role in ENaC regulation, further studies are needed to establish the importance of these AITs.

Taken together, the results of these screens trying to identify new AITs showed a large diversity of putative ENaC regulators and highlighted the importance of phosphorylation and in particular the central role of sgk1 in the aldosterone signaling pathway. A brief summary of some regulation pathways discussed here are shown in Figure 2.

Control by Phosphorylation

In general, regulation of ENaC by protein kinases has been well established. The effect of protein kinase A (PKA) on ENaC has been reported (31). Permeable cyclic adenosine monophosphate (cAMP) analogs, inhibitors of phosphodiesterase and activators of adenylate cyclase can fully mimic the antidiuretic hormone (ADH)/vasopressin-induced activation of the channel. Thus, it is highly likely that this hormonal action is mediated by cell cAMP. It is generally assumed that the increase in channel activity results from the activation of PKA and a specific phosphorylation event. Not clear is the nature of protein whose phosphorylation affects the Na^+ channel activity. In general, two schemes have been proposed. One is a direct phosphorylation of the channel protein that increases its p_o. However, no conserved intracellular PKA site is contained in the amino acid sequence of the three subunits of ENaC and most of the data for a direct phosphorylation came from studies using a 730-kDa complex reconstituted in lipid bilayers, or from a guinea pig α subunit (183,184). The other is an insertion of new channels into the apical membrane resulting from the phosphorylation of other proteins, such as proteins of the cytoskeleton or regulating proteins. Most evidence favors this latter interpretation. Butterworth et al. have put forward an interesting model of how ENaC activity might be upregulated by cAMP (185,186). They showed in mpkCCD14 cells that cAMP stimulates ENaC via an exocytic pathway, ENaC being recycled from an intracellular pool. Others showed that PKA could phosphorylate Nedd4-2 directly on the same serines targeted by sgk1 (187).

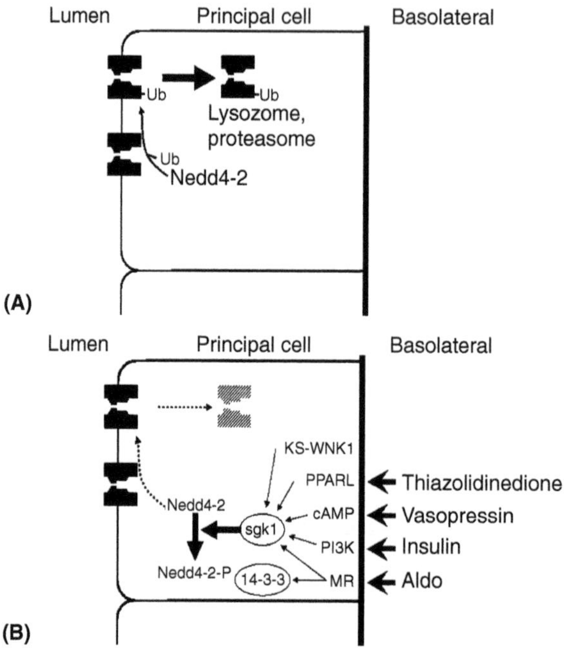

Figure 2 ENaC regulation by Nedd4-2 and sgk1. (**A**) Nedd4-2 comes in close contact with the PY motifs of ENaC, and ENaC ubiquitination takes place and leads to the retrieval of the channel from the cell surface. (**B**) When activated, sgkl interacts and phosphorylates Nedd4-2, the conformation of which is then stabilized by proteins 14-3-3. Nedd4-2 action on ENaC retrieval is thus prevented and the cell reabsorbs more sodium from the apical to the basolateral side.

Activation of PKC reduces sodium transport in A6 cells [Isc (188), cell-attached patches (189)], rat CCT [cell-attached patches (190)], rabbit cortical tubules [microperfusion (191)], LLC-PK1 renal epithelial cell line [$^{22}Na^+$ uptake (192)] and oocytes [whole cell (193), impedance analysis (194)]. It is unknown whether PKC regulation is due to direct ENaC phosphorylation or phosphorylation of regulators. Five putative regulation sites for PKC are conserved among human, rat, and *Xenopus* ENaC. Shimkets et al. showed that β and γ ENaC subunits but not α are phosphorylated at basal state (103). Their data suggest that aldosterone, insulin and PKA and C modulate the activity of ENaC by phosphorylation of the carboxy termini of the β and γ subunits. Others have shown that activation of PKC decreased β and γ subunits expression in A6 cells (195). And Yan et al. have shown in the oocyte expression system that the specific δ isoform of PKC may regulate ENaC activity by controlling cell surface expression of α ENaC (196).

Other kinases/phosphorylation processes might be involved in ENaC regulation. Shi et al. performed an in vitro phosphorylation assay and found three protein kinases involved in the phosphorylation of the carboxy termini of β and γ ENaC (197). They identified casein kinase 2 as one of these kinases and showed that it binds and phosphorylates the carboxy termini of β and, to a lesser extent, γ ENaC subunits (198). Its relevance in vivo has not yet been determined. Performing a yeast-two-hybrid screen with the mouse β ENaC carboxy termini as bait, Lebowitz et al. found a direct interaction of IkB-kinase β with β and γ ENaC subunits (199). The MAP kinase pathway has been involved in ENaC regulation by vasopressin (200) and by cross talking to the PIP3 kinase pathway (201).

Control by PPAR γ

Observations that treatment of patients with PPAR γ agonists thiazolidinediones (TZDs) has been associated with side effects such as fluid retention and edema led to the discovery of a new ENaC regulating pathway. Even though a small study did not find any effect of rosiglitazone (a TZD) on ENaC subunits of rat treated for three days (202), and even though Nofziger et al. found a downregulation of ENaC by the same compound in three ENaC expressing cell lines (203), there is strong in vivo evidence that ENaC is involved in this drug side effect. Zhang et al. (204) and Guan et al. (205) have shown that knockout of PPAR γ in mouse CCT prevents TZD-induced fluid retention and edema formation, similar to amiloride treatment. Moreover, Guan showed that ENaC γ subunit was upregulated in mice carrying the CCD-specific knockout of PPAR γ, identifying ENaC γ as a target of PPAR γ. It has been suggested that sgk1 could play a role in mediating PPAR γ effect (206); however, the exact sequence of events remains to be elucidated.

Control by Serine Proteases

Activation of epithelial sodium transport by luminal proteases such as kallikrein and urokinase has been described (207,208) and, conversely, inhibition of short-circuit current in toad urinary bladder by protease inhibitors such as aprotinin (209) has raised the possibility of ENaC regulation by proteases. Chraibi et al. have shown that trypsin activates short-circuit current of A6 cells previously treated by aprotinin (210). Their results indicated that ENaC activity might be regulated by an endogenous protease, whose effect can be mimicked by trypsin. Using functional complementation of a cDNA library made from A6 cells and expressed in *Xenopus* oocytes, Vallet et al. identified a clone coding for a GPI-anchored serine protease, named CAP1, for channel activating protein 1 (211). Two other CAP proteins were identified in the mouse and were shown to increase ENaC activity by several times, essentially by increasing the p_o without changing the cell surface expression (212,213). In the lung, near-silent ENaCs are activated upon exposure to trypsin or more specifically to neutrophil elastase (214,215). In humans, the mCAP1 ortholog prostasin and the mCAP2 ortholog TMPRSS4 are serine proteases that have been showed to regulate ENaC activity in vitro. In vivo, nafamostat mesilate, a synthetic protease inhibitor, decreases sodium excretion in the rat kidney and leads occasionally to hyponatremia and/or hyperkalemia in patients given this medication for pancreatitis and disseminated intravascular coagulation (216). In 18 human subjects (8 hypertensive and 10 normal), prostasin levels were detected in urine and seemed to be affected by the fluid replenishment of the subjects (217). The mechanisms by which CAPs activate ENaC are not yet understood. Some evidence indicates that CAPs could directly activate α and γ subunits by proteolytic processing (218). It has been shown that CAP binding to the cell surface is required for its function: when the GPI anchor is specifically deleted, *Xenopus* CAP1 is secreted, but is no longer able to activate ENaC (219). The degree of ENaC activation by proteases is highly variable between different cell lines and expression systems. In A6 cells, ENaC seems to be constitutively activated, as addition of trypsin to the cell does not induce any increase in transepithelial sodium transport. The basal sodium current is however totally abrogated by the addition of aprotinin (220). Conversely, the transepithelial sodium current in the CCD cell line mpkCCD$_{C14}$ is only 50% sensitive to aprotinin. These differences could be accounted for by differences in intracellular protease activity. Hughey et al. have shown that furin, a pro-protein processing endoprotease shuttling between the trans-Golgi network and the plasma membrane cleaves and activates ENaC and may be a major posttranslational ENaC regulator (221).

ENAC AND MOUSE MODELS

Manipulating ENaC genes in the mouse turned out to be an essential tool for the understanding of ENaC function in vivo and revealed an unexpected role of ENaC in the lung and a less important than expected role of ENaC in the CCD (Table 2). Moreover these mouse models provide us with the opportunity to compare the phenotypes observed in patients carrying alterations of ENaC function with those obtained in mice manipulated on one unique ENaC gene. These mouse models might be contributive to the elaboration of therapeutical approach in ENaC diseases.

Inactivation of the genes coding for α, β or γ ENaC have clearly demonstrated that all three ENaC subunits are independently essential for survival, as all the pups carrying an homozygous deleted allele died within 48 hours after birth (222,225,229). Mice deficient in the α ENaC gene locus [α(−/−) mice] presented with costal retractions and cyanosis within a few hours postpartum (222). They died 40 hours after birth with their lungs filled with fluid, demonstrating the importance of the α ENaC subunit in perinatal lung liquid clearance. Measurements of the amiloride-sensitive transepithelial PDs in α(−/−) mice revealed that ENaC activity was completely abolished, thus showing the insufficiency of β and γ subunits to form an efficient channel. An incomplete rescue of these mice was

Table 2 ENaC Genes Manipulation in Mice

Gene targeted	Construct	Phenotype	Reference
α ENaC	Knockout	Perinatal death. Inability to clear the lung of fluid. Metabolic acidosis and hyperkalemia	222
α ENaC	Transgenic α ENaC expression under control of CMV promoter in the α−/− background	50% survival to adulthood, with high postnatal lethality. Salt wasting, hyperkalemia, metabolic acidosis	223
α ENaC	CCD-specific knockout (Cre recombinase under the control of HoxB7 promoter)	No phenotype. Mice are salt and volume compensated	224
β ENaC	Knockout	Perinatal death. Salt wasting, hyperkalemia, metabolic acidosis	225
β ENaC	Partial destabilization of β ENaC RNA	Salt wasting under salt restriction. Viable	226
β ENaC	Knock-in of a Liddle's mutation	Under normal diet, slightly decreased aldosterone level and increased amiloride-sensitive transepithelial voltage difference in the colon. Under high salt diet, metabolic alkalosis, hypokalemia, and hypertension	227
β ENaC	Pulmonary overexpression under the control of the Clara cell secretory protein promoter	Airway surface liquid depletion, increased mucus concentration leading to severe lung disease mimicking cystic fibrosis	228
γ ENaC	Knockout	Perinatal death. Salt wasting, hyperkalemia, metabolic acidosis	229

Abbreviation: CMV, cytomegalovirus.

performed by introducing a transgenic rat α ENaC cDNA expressed under the control of the ubiquitous cytomegalovirus (CMV) promoter [α(−/−)Tg mice] (223). The resulting phenotype is a renal PHA-1 with about 50% neonatal lethality which is not due to pulmonary problems, but the result of the renal phenotype. This mouse model showed us that a partial rescue of ENaC activity in the α(−/−) background does not lead to neonatal respiratory failure, but is still insufficient to cope with the renal defect. These mice encountered more difficulties with fluid clearance from their lungs when challenged with thiourea or hyperoxia (230). Mice deficient in either β ENaC [β(−/−)] or γ ENaC [γ(−/−)] showed increased lung water contents measured as lung wet/dry ratio after birth, but otherwise did not exhibit the same lethal respiratory distress symptoms as α(−/−) mice (225,229).

Mice having only one allele of the gene coding for the α subunit of ENaC [α(+/−)] appear to have a phenotype comparable to that of wild-type mice. However, looking at regulation by plasma renin, angiotensin II and aldosterone under low, regular or high salt diet, Wang et al. have shown that these mice have developed a compensation mechanism leading to an activation of the renin–angiotensin system and to an upregulation of angiotensin II type 1 (AT1) receptor (151).

In contrast to α(−/−) mice which die mainly from pulmonary problems, β(−/−) and γ(−/−) mice exhibit a significant defect in renal function appearing a few hours after birth and leading to death within 48 hours. Lethargy and failure to thrive were associated with urinary Na^+ wasting, K^+ retention and increased plasma aldosterone concentrations, reflecting the same renal phenotype found in PHA-1 patients. The transgenic rescued mice α(−/−)Tg present a renal phenotype evoking the human PHA-1, but with some differences compared with β(−/−) and γ(−/−) mice (223). The symptoms appear later (about five days after birth) and are less dramatic compared with β(−/−) and γ(−/−) mice (50% survival to adulthood). A partial β knockout mouse model [β(m/m)] showed reduced ENaC activity and elevated plasma aldosterone levels (226). These mice develop a renal phenotype with weight loss, hyperkalemia, and salt wasting under salt restriction only. The phenotype difference observed between β(m/m) and β(−/−) mice is due to the strategy used to prepare these models. β(m/m) mice were obtained in the course of generating a mouse model for Liddle's syndrome. In these mice, β ENaC mRNA expression is very low (about 1% in lung and kidney) probably due to a destabilization by the inserted loxP site. This transcript level, however, is sufficient to rescue both lung and kidney phenotypes under normal salt conditions. Therefore, a very low level of β subunit mRNA seems to confer enough ENaC activity to maintain salt and water homeostasis under normal salt conditions, but is pathogenic if salt restriction is imposed.

Using the Cre-loxP–mediated recombination and a knock-in strategy, a mouse model for Liddle's syndrome was generated by introducing a stop codon (corresponding to residue R566 in human) into the mouse Scnn1b (β ENaC) gene locus (227). This animal model reproduces to a large extent a human form of salt-sensitive hypertension. Under regular salt diet, mice heterozygous and homozygous for the Liddle's mutation develop normally during the first three months of life. In these mice, blood pressure is not different from wild-type despite evidence for increased sodium reabsorption in the distal colon as well as low plasma aldosterone suggesting chronic increased extracellular volume. Under high salt intake, mice homozygous for Liddle's mutation develop high blood pressure, metabolic alkalosis and hypokalemia, together with cardiac and renal hypertrophy. This mouse model clearly established a causal relationship between dietary salt, ENaC and hypertension. A caveat of this model is that the mice have to be homozygous and challenged with a high salt diet to reproduce the human phenotype that occurs in heterozygous Liddle's patients under normal diet. Mouse peculiarities of the renin–angiotensin–aldosterone system could account for these species differences. It has been shown that these mice have a conserved aldosterone regulation and thus that the Liddle's mutation does not impair aldosterone response (231).

Rubera et al. have created a CCD-specific α ENaC knockout mouse, using the Cre recombinase driven by the HoxB7 promoter (224). Surprisingly, these mice are able to maintain sodium and volume homeostasis, suggesting that ENaC expression in the CCT is not critical for salt balance. One possible explanation is that α ENaC present in DCT2 and the connecting tubule, which is not deleted by the Cre recombinase in this mouse model, are sufficient to compensate for the deletion of α ENaC in the CCD. Indeed, as measured and calculated by Frindt and Palmer in the rat, ENaC activity in the CNT is probably sufficient to cope with the knockout of α ENaC in the CCD (232).

Overexpressing the β subunit in mouse lung under the control of the Clara cell secretory protein promoter, Mall et al. were able to show that ENaC overactivity in the lung leads to a cystic fibrosis like syndrome (228). These mice present an increased amiloride-sensitive short-circuit current across tracheal epithelia, a depletion of airway surface liquid volume, increased mucus concentration, delayed mucus transport and mucus adhesion to airway surfaces. Over time, these mice develop a severe lung disease mimicking cystic fibrosis, including mucus obstruction, goblet cell metaplasia, neutrophilic inflammation and bacterial superinfection. This mouse phenotype was confirmed in human patients suffering from nonclassic cystic fibrosis in which novel mutations in ENaC β subunit were identified, noteworthy in the absence of overt renal disease (233).

ENAC AND HUMAN DISEASES

Cloning of ENaC subunits revealed that a hereditary monogenic form of hypertension, namely Liddle's syndrome, is due to mutations deleting the PY motif present in the C-terminus of the β or γ ENaC subunits (97,98,100). Soon after, a salt-wasting syndrome in infancy, the systemic form of PHA-1, was also demonstrated to be caused by genetic defects in the three genes coding for ENaC (234,235). This emphasized the importance of ENaC in salt homeostasis and demonstrated that either gain-of-function or loss-of-function mutations could arise on the same genes and lead to mirror phenotypes. Implication of ENaC in tight regulation of salt homeostasis, control of extracellular volume and blood pressure has opened a new field of investigation and revealed ENaC and all its regulating factors as candidate proteins potentially involved in essential hypertension.

Liddle's Syndrome

Liddle's syndrome is a rare autosomal dominant Mendelian form of severe hypertension with early onset. It was first described by Liddle and coworkers in 1963 in a family in which multiple siblings had hypertension associated with hypokalemic alkalosis, suppressed plasma renin activity and low levels of aldosterone (236). No effect of spironolactone on blood pressure could be demonstrated. However, administration of the sodium channel blocker triamterene together with restriction of salt intake tended to normalized blood pressure. This suggested to Dr Liddle that hypertension was due to excessive sodium reabsorption in the distal nephron. Indeed, when the index case described by Dr Liddle was kidney transplanted, correction of all the abnormalities was obtained (237).

Using a candidate gene approach, mutations in the C-termini of the genes coding for β and γ ENaC subunits were identified (97,98,100). The mutations were either frameshifts or premature stop codons deleting part of the intracellular C-termini or missense mutations pointing out a proline-rich segment in the C-termini of β and γ ENaC, PPXY. When expressed in the oocyte system, the Liddle's variants revealed a significant increase in ENaC activity, resulting from an increased number of channels at the cell surface and an increase in p_o (35). Two hypotheses have been suggested for the prolonged half-life of mutant channels at the cell surface. (*i*) Nedd4-2 is a cytosolic protein–containing WW domains that specifically interact with the PPXY sequence of ENaC subunits (238). These proteins have ubiquitin ligase domains, suggesting that interaction with ENaC subunits leads to their ubiquitination, targeting them for degradation. Indeed, ENaC α and γ subunits were demonstrated to be ubiquitinated in the lysine residues of their intracellular N-termini (85). In Liddle's syndrome, the interaction between Nedd4-2 and ENaC through the deleted or mutated PPXY domain is lost so that channels are less efficiently cleared from the cell surface and accumulate. (*ii*) Inhibition of endocytosis via clathrin-coated pits by dominant-negative dynamin induces the same electrophysiological phenotype as seen with Liddle's syndrome (102). This suggests that clearance of ENaC from the cell surface could occur via this pathway which is deficient in Liddle's syndrome. Of note, Kellenberger et al. have shown that feedback inhibition is deficient in Liddle's mutants expressed in the *Xenopus* oocyte system, thus facilitating salt reabsorption through ENaC (109).

Hiltunen et al. have published the only mutation conferring Liddle's syndrome without interfering with the retrieval of channels from the cell surface (96). This γ ENaC N530S mutant is located in the outer mouth of the channel pore, close to the amiloride-binding site. Expression of the mutant in *Xenopus* oocytes demonstrated a twofold increase in ENaC activity compared with wild-type channel, without a change in cell surface expression.

Pseudohypoaldosteronism

Pseudohypoaldosteronism is a syndrome grouping different diseases resulting from the inability of aldosterone to produce its effects. It has been commonly classified into three types (239), all characterized by hyperkalemia, metabolic acidosis and abnormally elevated plasma aldosterone concentrations.

PHA-1 is characterized by an early and severe manifestation of salt wasting, life-threatening hyperkalemia, metabolic acidosis and dehydration. Treatment with fludrocortisone is ineffective, but salt supplementation alone may be sufficient to decrease the sodium wasting and stabilize the patient. Plasma aldosterone concentrations and plasma renin activity are elevated, further demonstrating peripheral resistance of target organs to these hormones and showing an adequate adrenal function. Type I PHA is heterogeneous and has been subdivided clinically into at least two entities, based on inheritance and phenotype of the disease (240). The identification of two distinct molecular defects has strengthened this subdivision. Type I PHA is caused by mutations present in the gene coding for the MR in the kidney-limited autosomal dominant form, and in the genes coding for the three subunits of ENaC in the systemic autosomal recessive form.

Renal type I PHA

An autosomal dominant pattern of inheritance is associated with a renal phenotype characterized by salt wasting, hyperkalemia, and metabolic acidosis. It has a milder course compared with the autosomal recessive systemic type I PHA and spontaneous remissions are often observed over time. Geller et al. studied five kindreds fulfilling the criteria for renal type I PHA and found four mutations in the gene coding for the MR, introducing frameshift, premature stop codon or splice donor site deletion (241). Another group found a missense mutation in a Japanese family with autosomal dominant PHA-1 (242). This heterozygous L924P mutation leads to a complete abolition of MR function. Out of three studied kindreds, Viemann et al. found an insertion (Ins2871C, codon 958) in a sporadic form of renal PHA-1, leading to a frameshift (243). Interestingly, one mutation described by Geller and the mutation found by Viemann are de novo mutations, suggesting that sporadic cases could be present in the trait. Sartorato et al. reported on 14 families and found six new mutations leading to frameshift, nonsense and three missense mutations (244). Other nonsense mutations have been published (245–247). Geller et al. have extended some published kindreds and described six new mutations (four de novo), reaching a total of 22 disease-causing mutations in this syndrome (248). They presented some evidence that haploinsufficiency might be sufficient to cause the trait. Interestingly, they showed that adults carrying the mutations are clinically undistinguishable from wild-type individuals except that they have high aldosterone and renin levels.

How one mutated allele of the MR can lead to a renal phenotype is striking, and whether this is due to haploinsufficiency or to a dominant negative effect remains to be demonstrated. By contrast, heterozygous knockout mice for the MR+/− grew and bred normally (249). Only homozygous knockout mice (MR−/−) display the same renal phenotype as patients affected by the renal PHA-1, with severe salt wasting, dehydration and a rapid death, about 10 days after birth. These MR−/− mice could be rescued by subcutaneous salt injection until the animals had reached a body mass of 8.5 g (250). Most of these animals survive with this regimen and cope with their defect. This indicates that, as in humans, survival is possible after the critical neonatal period, where the kidney is too immature to handle sodium and where sodium chloride supply in milk feeding is insufficient to compensate for renal losses. In that respect, differences in maturation of the kidney in the neonatal period between human and mice could explain the observed species differences. In adult carrying MR mutations, only higher levels of aldosterone are found, without any electrolytes or blood pressure abnormalities (248).

Systemic type I PHA

Type I PHA inherited as an autosomal recessive mode is characterized by a renal phenotype similar to the one described in the renal autosomal dominant form. However, no spontaneous remission is observed over time. This so-called systemic form exhibits defects in salt reabsorption in organs other than the kidney. Lung abnormalities were described, manifesting as recurrent respiratory infections within weeks or months after birth, characterized by cough, tachypnea, fever and wheezing (251–256). Cultures are sometimes negative, but CMV, RSV and *Staphylococcus aureus*, *Haemophilus influenzae*, *Streptococcus pneumonia*, *Moraxella catarrhalis* and even *Pseudomonas aeruginosa* were isolated in others. Kerem et al. measured the volume of the airway surface liquid in PHA-1 patients and found an increased volume of more than twice the normal (253). They hypothesized that the liquid could narrow airway lumen and/or dilute surface-active materials that stabilize small airways. The excess liquid in the airways of these patients results from an absence of electrogenic sodium transport, as demonstrated by the assessment of the nasal transepithelial voltage difference. The lung phenotype identified in mice deficient for α ENaC and reports of a lung phenotype in children and young adults have prompted pediatricians to search for implications of ENaC in neonatal respiratory distress syndrome (RDS), and especially in surfactant-resistant RDS. Malagon-Rogers first associated a case of RDS with pseudohypoaldosteronism (257). However, some features of this case are incompatible with an ENaC-related PHA-1. First, the patient was premature and it is established that premature infants have less nasal transepithelial amiloride-sensitive PD and are more susceptible to developing RDS (258). Second, the patient responded quickly to a mineralocorticoid treatment, which is an exclusion criterion for PHA-1. And finally, systemic phenotype, putative consanguinity of the parents, and genotype were not reported or not tested respectively. Akcay et al. have described a premature newborn with RDS, increased sweat electrolytes and pseudohypoaldosteronism, but no genotyping was performed, so that a direct association with ENaC cannot be made (259). Prince et al. measured the nasal transepithelial voltage PD in a neonate affected by PHA-1, but without any RDS (260). They found a basal value of zero and absence of an amiloride-sensitive voltage. No mutation was found on genes coding for ENaC, but the patient is clearly affected by the systemic form of PHA-1.

Other phenotypes described in systemic PHA may result from the impairment of ENaC expression in other tissues. These include gallbladder, where cholelithiasis has been described (261,262), Meibomian glands (239), skin (263–267) and placenta with some association with polyhydramnios (268–272). Only cases reported with skin or Meibomian glands phenotypes were clearly associated with the systemic form of PHA-1. The relevance of other findings and their link with the syndrome are less clear.

Systemic type I PHA was linked to chromosome 12p and 16p in humans (273). At the same time, Chang et al. identified three homozygous mutations in five kindreds originating from the Near East (234). All probants were products of consanguineous unions and all of them have the typical characteristics of systemic PHA-1. Deletion of 2 bp on the α subunit leads to a frameshift at position I68 (αI68fs). A premature stop codon in the extracellular loop of the α subunit predicts, if the mRNA is processed, a truncated α ENaC lacking the second transmembrane domain and the intracellular C-terminus (αR508stop). A missense mutation in a highly conserved domain in the intracellular N-terminus of the β subunit (βG37S) reveals genetic heterogeneity of systemic PHA-1. Heterogeneity was reinforced by the report of a splice-site mutation on the γ subunit leading to abnormal splicing that resulted either in a truncated γ protein or in the replacement of three conserved amino acid residues by a novel one (235). Numerous mutations have been described since (253,256,274–280). The majority of them are on the α ENaC subunit, thus illustrating the importance of this subunit in the function of ENaC. By contrast, activating mutations of the Liddle's syndrome were found only in the genes coding for β and γ subunits. Of note is the description of a patient suffering from type I PHA carrying a homozygous deletion of the upstream regulatory region of β ENaC, leading to near-total absence of β ENaC expression (279).

Compound heterozygous mutations on the genes coding for the ENaC subunits were reported in PHA-1 patients, adding more complexity in the analysis of the trait (253,256). In particular, these PHA-1 patients may not have any consanguineous familial history and may appear as sporadic cases.

Other groups also reported polymorphisms on the genes coding for ENaC and suggested that they could be related to type I PHA (281–283), especially if associated with polymorphisms present in the gene coding for the MR. Polymorphisms on ENaC that do not lead to a loss-of-function per se, but only when associated with polymorphisms on other genes could be of high relevance. They may confer a protection against excessive salt consumption and salt-sensitive hypertension, but remain purely speculative.

Iwai et al. found a polymorphism on the promoter region of the γ subunit [G(−173)A] which was linked to hypotension in a large Japanese population (284). The adenosine (AA) genotype was associated with an 11 mmHg decrease in systolic blood pressure and with a higher prevalence of hypotension. In a luciferase assay in MDCK and HRE cells, they showed that the allele A was associated with a drop of the promoter activity of about 50% compared with the G allele activity. This highlights the importance of potential polymorphisms in the promoter region of ENaC genes to influence blood pressure. However the clinical characteristics of the patients bearing the polymorphism were not detailed and we are not aware whether or not they have a salt-loosing nephropathy, a higher aldosterone concentration or other features of PHA-1.

Even though many of the PHA-1 patients reported in the literature have not been genotyped, it seems that not all cases of systemic PHA-1 are due to mutations of ENaC genes. In the series of Chang et al. and Kerem et al., no ENaC mutations were found in two of seven kindreds (234) and three of nine kindreds (253), respectively. This 30% of unknown causes of PHA-1 could be the result of a low sensitivity of the method used for the screening or could arise from mutations of the promoter (279) or of regulatory proteins that were missed by the screening. Moreover, we could imagine loss-of-function mutations on genes upregulating ENaC (CAP-1) or transducing the mineralocorticoid response from the MR to ENaC (the aldosterone-induced protein, sgk1, for instance). Conversely, genes involved in the repression of ENaC could be hyperactivated and become candidate genes for PHA-1 (Nedd4 or other). Further studies will help in resolving this issue. Using a candidate gene approach, Ludwig et al. did not find any association with prostasin, α-spectrin or Nedd4 (285). A similar attempt with claudin-8 was negative as well (286).

ENaC and Essential Hypertension

The physiology of blood pressure is determined by Ohm's law: blood pressure is proportional to cardiac output and to vascular resistance to blood flow. Thus, a wide variety of physiological systems that have pleiotropic effects and interact with vast complexity have been found to influence blood pressure (baroreceptors, natriuretic peptides, the renin angiotensin aldosterone system (RAAS), the kinin–kallikrein system, the adrenergic system, NO, endothelin, etc.). The contribution of some of these systems to short-term blood pressure control is well established. However, the determination of which of these pathways contributes to long-term blood pressure control has proved more problematic. The key role of the kidney in the long-term determination of blood pressure was put forward by Guyton (3). As studies of blood pressure variation in the general population are complicated by multifactorial determination, with a variety of demographic, environmental and genetic factors contributing to the trait, one alternative approach has been the investigation of rare Mendelian forms of blood pressure variation. Molecular genetic studies have identified a number of mutations that cause Mendelian forms of hypertension or hypotension. Interestingly, all of the mutated gene products act in the same physiological pathway in the kidney, altering net renal salt reabsorption and thus reinforcing Guyton's theory (287). Moreover, the pathophysiological link between salt and blood pressure is predictable from the relationship between salt and vascular volume homeostasis.

For ENaC and the MR genes, gain-of-function (leading to Liddle's syndrome) and loss-of-function (leading to PHA-1) mutations intervening in the same genes with opposite effects have established the importance of these genes in the setting of blood pressure. Although these traits have quantitatively large effects in affected individuals, they likely account for a very small fraction of the variation in blood pressure in the general population. Efforts to identify genes predisposing to hypertension in the general population have lead to the performance of genome-wide scans (288,289), searches for genetic linkage between candidate loci (previously identified by the Mendelian form of hypertension) and hypertension, and investigation into single nucleotide polymorphisms associated with hypertension (290).

Numerous loci are under investigation on chromosomes 17q, 15q, 2p25-p24 and 12p to mention only the more significant. Numerous genes have been proposed as candidate genes for essential hypertension in recent years: angiotensin-converting enzyme, angiotensinogen [especially the angiotensinogen gene variant M235T that increases the transcription of the gene (291)], α-adducin, the β_2-adrenergic receptor, the G-protein β_3-subunit, the endothelin-converting enzyme, the TNF receptor, the CYP3A5 and the prostacyclin synthase gene. Due to their special role in salt balance and their implication in hypo- or hypertension in Mendelian and rare diseases, the genes coding for the ENaC have received special attention and were screened by several groups in several different populations. No linkage was found between ENaC genes and hypertensive patients investigated in the Caribbeans (West African origin) (292), Sweden (293), China (294), Japan (295,296), France (297,298) or South Africa (299). However, a significant linkage between systolic blood pressure and polymorphic microsatellite markers of chromosome 16p12 (where genes coding for β and γ ENaC subunits are localized) was established by screening 286 white families from Australia (300). Nagy et al. found a quantitative trait locus for systolic blood pressure near the SCNN1b gene coding for β ENaC (301). Iwai et al. found a polymorphism in the promoter of the α subunit (A2139G) which is associated with both hypertension and proteinuria (284). The odds ratio for hypertension with the guanosine (GA) and the GG genotype was 1.3 in the large cohort they examined (3898 Japanese people) and 1.8 among subjects <60 years of age.

A special note concerns the T594M variant of β ENaC subunit, which has been associated with hypertension in a black population living in London (302–304). This polymorphism is notable, because so much emphasis has been given to it. Su et al. first described a heterozygous polymorphism at position 594 (T594M) in the β ENaC subunit present in 6.1% of subjects of African-American origin, but not in Caucasian people (305). However, no significant difference in blood pressure was found between people having the βT594M polymorphism or not. Persu et al. found also 6% βT594M polymorphism in people of Afro-Caribbean origin with essential hypertension (297). Tiago et al. found a 7% frequency of the βT594M variant in a population of 59 South African black subjects with mild-to-moderate hypertension (299). Another study performed on patients of African origin in South Africa found 4.2% frequency of the βT594M variant in hypertensive participants compared with 4.5% in normotensive subjects (306). In a study by Ambrosius et al., the allele frequencies of the βT594M variant determined in a cohort of normotensive children and adolescents in Indiana was 3% for blacks and 0.6% for whites (307). No correlation with hypertension was found in this study despite a sufficient power. A study assessed the incidence of the βT594M polymorphism in a hypertensive population in Japan and found no βT594M variant on 803 people screened (308). By contrast, a case–control study of black people who lived in London demonstrated a significant association between the βT594M variant and hypertension (302): 8.3% of the hypertensive patients carried the βT594M variant compared with 2.1% carriers of the βT594M in normotensive people (odds ratio 4.17, $p=0.029$). This was the first study demonstrating a statistical correlation between the βT594M polymorphism and the hypertension. A population-based study performed by the same group of authors in a population living in the same region (black people living in London who are the first-generation immigrants of African origin) confirmed that the βT594M variant is associated with hypertension (304). Indeed, a significant trend of increasing prevalence of the variant across increasing blood pressure categories was found. The frequency of the βT594M variant (hetero- and homozygous) was 4.6% in that study. In an attempt to identify factors explaining divergences between positive studies performed on a black population in London and negative studies performed in Africa, Dong et al. compared the frequency of βT594M variant in a small normotensive population from Ghana with a population of Ghanaian emigrants in London. They found a high frequency of the T594M variant in the young normotensive population of Ghana (13.7%), compared with 4.4% in the Ghanaian population of London, all hypertensive, but older (303). As most of the studies aiming at reporting T594M variant association with hypertension are limited by their sample size, Hollier et al. probed two random and well-characterized populations: one from Dallas County (Dallas Heart Study, $n=3137$) and the other from Jamaica (International Collaborative Study of Hypertension in Blacks, $n=1666$) (309). The incidence of T594M in African-American subjects living in Dallas and Jamaica was about 6%, but no association with hypertension was found in both populations. Moreover, six hypertensive patients carrying the T594M polymorphism and treated with amiloride did show a similar decrease of their blood pressure condition during the treatment period when compared with a 22 control population.

In the study of Su et al., the aldosterone profile of people carrying the T594M variant was significantly higher than that in T594T people, but there was no statistical difference when the urine aldosterone level was normalized for potassium excretion (which is a better indicator of RAAS activity) (305). The plasma renin activity was similar in both groups. In the study of Baker et al., the plasma renin activity was significantly lower in patients carrying the βT594M variant than in individuals without the variant, but the plasma aldosterone concentrations were similar in both groups (302).

To understand the molecular mechanisms underlying the T594M polymorphism, Persu et al. tested the T594M variant in the oocyte expression system. They found a nonsignificant increase of the amiloride-sensitive Na^+ current with αβT594Mγ compared with the wild-type αβγ and a nonsignificant decrease of the $^{22}Na^+$ flux compared with the wild-type channel (297). Su et al. examined an amiloride-sensitive sodium activity in freshly isolated human B lymphocytes by measuring the membrane slope conductance with the whole-cell patch-clamp method (305). The basal slope conductance values were similar for B lymphocytes from people with or without the βT594M. But in the presence of 8-CPT-cAMP, slope conductance of the responsive cells was more increased in cells carrying the βT594M than in wild-type cells. As inferred by the authors, the βT594M variant seems to be more responsive to 8-CPT-cAMP. When amiloride was co-applied with 8-CPT-cAMP, it blocked the response to cAMP, suggesting that the enhancement in slope conductance by 8-CPT-cAMP occurs via an amiloride-sensitive conductance. Cui et al. performed the same experiments on Epstein Barr virus (EBV)-transformed B lymphocytes and found the same activation of the slope conductance by 8-CPT-cAMP in lymphocytes from people carrying the βT594M variant (310). Moreover, they found that the 8-CPT-cAMP-induced activation of the slope conductance can be blocked by PMA, a phorbol ester that stimulates PKC. The block is partial (and highly variable) in B lymphocytes from people heterozygous for the βT594M variant, but is complete in B lymphocytes from people homozygous for the variant. This block is prevented by the application of chelerythrin, an inhibitor of the PKC, further suggesting the implication of the PKC in the blocking effect. The threonine at position 594 has been proposed to be a consensus site for PKC, and mutation of this residue to a methionine in the variant could lead to a loss of inhibition to PKC. However, the interpretation of these data is limited by at least two important caveats. First, the B lymphocytes are not epithelial in nature and the amiloride-sensitive sodium channel of the B lymphocyte is not well characterized. Second, the concentration of cAMP used in these studies is very high (300 μM 8-CPT-cAMP) and is at least 30-fold greater than the concentration needed to activate the B-cell sodium channel. In summary, βT594M polymorphism has been associated with hypertension in some specific populations (mainly a population of immigrants of African origin living in London), but not in several other populations, and so far the molecular determinants leading to a putative ENaC hyperactivity has proved to be difficult to identify and needs further studies.

In conclusion, the role of ENaC in salt homeostasis and blood pressure determination is well established, with its direct implication in Liddle's syndrome and PHA-1, but remains confined to very few individuals. Its participation in blood pressure variation among the general population remains to be demonstrated, though evidence from some linkage studies is growing. In particular, some ENaC polymorphisms were associated with hypertension in linkage studies. Functional studies of ENaC variants are lacking so far and would add more evidence for the implication of ENaC in blood pressure control. Moreover, ENaC regulating proteins are de facto candidates for essential hypertension. Some emerging data attempted to address this issue with a spontaneous variant of Nedd4-2 (311) or sgk1 (312), though without sufficient power to be conclusive.

CONCLUSION

The ENaC has proven to be a key and determinant player in salt balance. Cloning of the genes coding for its three subunits has allowed invaluable progress in the comprehension of its structure, of the pathways regulating its activity, and of its role in other organs. In the future, insights are expected from high-resolution solving of its crystal structure and from a more detailed characterization of its regulating pathways. Moreover, the relative role of variants of the ENaC in essential hypertension definitely warrants further investigation.

ACKNOWLEDGMENTS

I am thankful to Drs. Alexandru Bobulescu and David Sas for a careful review of the manuscript. The work of the author has been supported by the Swiss Foundation for Medical-Biological Grants, the Swiss National Science Foundation and the National Kidney Foundation.

REFERENCES

1. Kenouch S, Lombes M, Delahaye F, et al. Human skin as target for aldosterone: coexpression of mineralocorticoid receptors and 11 beta-hydroxysteroid dehydrogenase. J Clin Endocrinol Metab 1994; 79(5):1334–41.
2. Zennaro MC, Farman N, Bonvalet JP, et al. Tissue-specific expression of alpha and beta messenger ribonucleic acid isoforms of the human mineralocorticoid receptor in normal and pathological states. J Clin Endocrinol Metab 1997; 82(5):1345–52.
3. Guyton AC. Blood pressure control-special role of the kidneys and body fluids. Science 1991; 252(5014):1813–6.
4. Koefoed-Johnsen V, Ussing HH. The nature of the frog skin potential. Acta Physiol Scand 1958; 42(3–4):298–308.
5. Bentley PJ. Amiloride: a potent inhibitor of sodium transport across the toad bladder. J Physiol 1968; 195(2):317–30.
6. Lindemann B, Van Driessche W. Sodium-specific membrane channels of frog skin are pores: current fluctuations reveal high turnover. Science 1977; 195(4275):292–4.
7. Palmer LG, Edelman IS, Lindemann B. Current–voltage analysis of apical sodium transport in toad urinary bladder: effects of inhibitors of transport and metabolism. J Membr Biol 1980; 57(1):59–71.

8. Sariban-Sohraby S, Latorre R, Burg M, et al. Amiloride-sensitive epithelial Na+ channels reconstituted into planar lipid bilayer membranes. Nature 1984; 308(5954):80–2.
9. Hamilton KL, Eaton DC. Single-channel recordings from amiloride-sensitive epithelial sodium channel. Am J Physiol 1985; 249(3 Pt 1):C200–7.
10. Palmer LG, Frindt G. Amiloride-sensitive Na channels from the apical membrane of the rat cortical collecting tubule. Proc Natl Acad Sci USA 1986; 83(8):2767–70.
11. Canessa CM, Horisberger JD, Rossier BC. Epithelial sodium channel related to proteins involved in neurodegeneration. Nature 1993; 361(6411):467–70.
12. Canessa CM, Schild L, Buell G, et al. Amiloride-sensitive epithelial Na+ channel is made of three homologous subunits. Nature 1994; 367(6462):463–7.
13. Lingueglia E, Voilley N, Waldmann R, et al. Expression cloning of an epithelial amiloride-sensitive Na+ channel. A new channel type with homologies to *Caenorhabditis elegans* degenerins. FEBS Lett 1993; 318(1):95–9.
14. Waldmann R, Champigny G, Bassilana F, et al. Molecular cloning and functional expression of a novel amiloride-sensitive Na+ channel. J Biol Chem 1995; 270(46):27411–4.
15. Brockway LM, Zhou ZH, Bubien JK, et al. Rabbit retinal neurons and glia express a variety of ENaC/DEG subunits. Am J Physiol Cell Physiol 2002; 283(1):C126–34.
16. Yamamura H, Ugawa S, Ueda T, et al. Protons activate the delta-subunit of the epithelial Na+ channel in humans. J Biol Chem 2004; 279(13):12529–34.
17. Ji HL, Bishop LR, Anderson SJ, et al. The role of Pre-H2 domains of alpha- and delta-epithelial Na+ channels in ion permeation, conductance, and amiloride sensitivity. J Biol Chem 2004; 279(9):8428–40.
18. Biasio W, Chang T, McIntosh CJ, et al. Identification of Murr1 as a regulator of the human delta epithelial sodium channel. J Biol Chem 2004; 279(7):5429–34.
19. Yamamura H, Ugawa S, Ueda T, et al. Capsazepine is a novel activator of the delta subunit of the human epithelial Na+ channel. J Biol Chem 2004; 279(43):44483–9.
20. Yamamura H, Ugawa S, Ueda T, et al. Icilin activates the delta-subunit of the human epithelial Na+ channel. Mol Pharmacol 2005; 68(4):1142–7.
21. Yamamura H, Ugawa S, Ueda T, et al. Evans blue is a specific antagonist of the human epithelial Na+ channel delta-subunit. J Pharmacol Exp Ther 2005; 315(2):965–9.
22. Babini E, Geisler HS, Siba M, et al. A new subunit of the epithelial Na+ channel identifies regions involved in Na+ self-inhibition. J Biol Chem 2003; 278(31):28418–26.
23. Mano I, Driscoll M. DEG/ENaC channels: a touchy superfamily that watches its salt. Bioessays 1999; 21(7):568–78.
24. Adams CM, Anderson MG, Motto DG, et al. Ripped pocket and pickpocket, novel Drosophila DEG/ENaC subunits expressed in early development and in mechanosensory neurons. J Cell Biol 1998; 140(1):143–52.
25. Ainsley JA, Pettus JM, Bosenko D, et al. Enhanced locomotion caused by loss of the Drosophila DEG/ENaC protein Pickpocket1. Curr Biol 2003; 13(17):1557–63.
26. Liu L, Johnson WA, Welsh MJ. Drosophila DEG/ENaC pickpocket genes are expressed in the tracheal system, where they may be involved in liquid clearance. Proc Natl Acad Sci USA 2003; 100(4):2128–33.
27. Liu L, Leonard AS, Motto DG, et al. Contribution of Drosophila DEG/ENaC genes to salt taste. Neuron 2003; 39(1):133–46.
28. Lingueglia E, Champigny G, Lazdunski M, et al. Cloning of the amiloride-sensitive FMRFamide peptide-gated sodium channel. Nature 1995; 378(6558):730–3.
29. Sakai H, Lingueglia E, Champigny G, et al. Cloning and functional expression of a novel degenerin-like Na+ channel gene in mammals. J Physiol 1999; 519(Pt 2):323–33.
30. Schaefer L, Sakai H, Mattei M, et al. Molecular cloning, functional expression and chromosomal localization of an amiloride-sensitive Na(+) channel from human small intestine. FEBS Lett 2000; 471(2–3):205–10.
31. Garty H, Palmer LG. Epithelial sodium channels: function, structure, and regulation. Physiol Rev 1997; 77(2):359–96.

32. Canessa CM, Merillat AM, Rossier BC. Membrane topology of the epithelial sodium channel in intact cells. Am J Physiol 1994; 267(6 Pt 1):C1682–90.
33. Renard S, Lingueglia E, Voilley N, et al. Biochemical analysis of the membrane topology of the amiloride-sensitive Na+ channel. J Biol Chem 1994; 269(17):12981–6.
34. Snyder PM, McDonald FJ, Stokes JB, et al. Membrane topology of the amiloride-sensitive epithelial sodium channel. J Biol Chem 1994; 269(39):24379–83.
35. Firsov D, Schild L, Gautschi I, et al. Cell surface expression of the epithelial Na channel and a mutant causing Liddle syndrome: a quantitative approach. Proc Natl Acad Sci USA 1996; 93(26):15370–5.
36. Firsov D, Gautschi I, Merillat AM, et al. The heterotetrameric architecture of the epithelial sodium channel (ENaC). Embo J 1998; 17(2):344–52.
37. Berdiev BK, Karlson KH, Jovov B, et al. Subunit stoichiometry of a core conduction element in a cloned epithelial amiloride-sensitive Na+ channel. Biophys J 1998; 75(5): 2292–301.
38. Kosari F, Sheng S, Li J, et al. Subunit stoichiometry of the epithelial sodium channel. J Biol Chem 1998; 273(22):13469–74.
39. Dijkink L, Hartog A, van Os CH, et al. The epithelial sodium channel (ENaC) is intracellularly located as a tetramer. Pflugers Arch 2002; 444(4):549–55.
40. Eskandari S, Snyder PM, Kreman M, et al. Number of subunits comprising the epithelial sodium channel. J Biol Chem 1999; 274(38):27281–6.
41. Cheng C, Prince LS, Snyder PM, et al. Assembly of the epithelial Na+ channel evaluated using sucrose gradient sedimentation analysis. J Biol Chem 1998; 273(35):22693–700.
42. Snyder PM, Cheng C, Prince LS, et al. Electrophysiological and biochemical evidence that DEG/ENaC cation channels are composed of nine subunits. J Biol Chem 1998; 273(2):681–4.
43. Staruschenko A, Adams E, Booth RE, et al. Epithelial Na+ channel subunit stoichiometry. Biophys J 2005; 88(6):3966–75.
44. Staruschenko A, Medina JL, Patel P, et al. Fluorescence resonance energy transfer analysis of subunit stoichiometry of the epithelial Na+ channel. J Biol Chem 2004; 279(26):27729–34.
45. Coscoy S, Lingueglia E, Lazdunski M, et al. The Phe-Met-Arg-Phe-amide-activated sodium channel is a tetramer. J Biol Chem 1998; 273(14):8317–22.
46. MacKinnon R. Determination of the subunit stoichiometry of a voltage-activated potassium channel. Nature 1991; 350(6315):232–5.
47. Rotin D, Bar-Sagi D, O'Brodovich H, et al. An SH3 binding region in the epithelial Na+ channel (alpha rENaC) mediates its localization at the apical membrane. Embo J 1994; 13(19):4440–50.
48. Bonny O, Rossier BC. Disturbances of Na/K balance: pseudohypoaldosteronism revisited. J Am Soc Nephrol 2002; 13(9):2399–414.
49. Fyfe GK, Canessa CM. Subunit composition determines the single channel kinetics of the epithelial sodium channel. J Gen Physiol 1998; 112(4):423–32.
50. McNicholas CM, Canessa CM. Diversity of channels generated by different combinations of epithelial sodium channel subunits. J Gen Physiol 1997; 109(6):681–92.
51. Bonny O, Chraibi A, Loffing J, et al. Functional expression of a pseudohypoaldosteronism type I mutated epithelial Na+ channel lacking the pore-forming region of its alpha subunit. J Clin Invest 1999; 104(7):967–74.
52. Duc C, Farman N, Canessa CM, et al. Cell-specific expression of epithelial sodium channel alpha, beta, and gamma subunits in aldosterone-responsive epithelia from the rat: localization by in situ hybridization and immunocytochemistry. J Cell Biol 1994; 127(6 Pt 2):1907–21.
53. Loffing J, Loffing-Cueni D, Valderrabano V, et al. Distribution of transcellular calcium and sodium transport pathways along mouse distal nephron. Am J Physiol Renal Physiol 2001; 281(6):F1021–7.
54. Loffing J, Pietri L, Aregger F, et al. Differential subcellular localization of ENaC subunits in mouse kidney in response to high- and low-Na diets. Am J Physiol Renal Physiol 2000; 279(2):F252–8.

55. Renard S, Voilley N, Bassilana F, et al. Localization and regulation by steroids of the alpha, beta and gamma subunits of the amiloride-sensitive Na+ channel in colon, lung and kidney. Pflugers Arch 1995; 430(3):299–307.
56. Volk KA, Sigmund RD, Snyder PM, et al. rENaC is the predominant Na+ channel in the apical membrane of the rat renal inner medullary collecting duct. J Clin Invest 1995; 96(6):2748–57.
57. Light DB, McCann FV, Keller TM, et al. Amiloride-sensitive cation channel in apical membrane of inner medullary collecting duct. Am J Physiol 1988; 255(2 Pt 2):F278–86.
58. Farman N, Talbot CR, Boucher R, et al. Noncoordinated expression of alpha-, beta-, and gamma-subunit mRNAs of epithelial Na+ channel along rat respiratory tract. Am J Physiol 1997; 272(1 Pt 1):C131–41.
59. Matsushita K, McCray PB, Jr., Sigmund RD, et al. Localization of epithelial sodium channel subunit mRNAs in adult rat lung by in situ hybridization. Am J Physiol 1996; 271(2 Pt 1):L332–9.
60. Talbot CL, Bosworth DG, Briley EL, et al. Quantitation and localization of ENaC subunit expression in fetal, newborn, and adult mouse lung. Am J Respir Cell Mol Biol 1999; 20(3):398–406.
61. Watanabe S, Matsushita K, Stokes JB, et al. Developmental regulation of epithelial sodium channel subunit mRNA expression in rat colon and lung. Am J Physiol 1998; 275(6 Pt 1): G1227–35.
62. Rochelle LG, Li DC, Ye H, et al. Distribution of ion transport mRNAs throughout murine nose and lung. Am J Physiol Lung Cell Mol Physiol 2000; 279(1):L14–24.
63. Matthay MA, Folkesson HG, Clerici C. Lung epithelial fluid transport and the resolution of pulmonary edema. Physiol Rev 2002; 82(3):569–600.
64. Lingueglia E, Renard S, Waldmann R, et al. Different homologous subunits of the amiloride-sensitive Na+ channel are differently regulated by aldosterone. J Biol Chem 1994; 269(19):13736–9.
65. Carey HV, Hayden UL, Spicer SS, et al. Localization of amiloride-sensitive Na+ channels in intestinal epithelia. Am J Physiol 1994; 266(3 Pt 1):G504–10.
66. Wang Q, Horisberger JD, Maillard M, et al. Salt- and angiotensin II-dependent variations in amiloride-sensitive rectal potential difference in mice. Clin Exp Pharmacol Physiol 2000; 27(1–2):60–6.
67. Greig ER, Boot-Handford RP, Mani V, et al. Decreased expression of apical Na+ channels and basolateral Na+, K+-ATPase in ulcerative colitis. J Pathol 2004; 204(1): 84–92.
68. Roudier-Pujol C, Rochat A, Escoubet B, et al. Differential expression of epithelial sodium channel subunit mRNAs in rat skin. J Cell Sci 1996; 109(Pt 2):379–85.
69. Brouard M, Casado M, Djelidi S, et al. Epithelial sodium channel in human epidermal keratinocytes: expression of its subunits and relation to sodium transport and differentiation. J Cell Sci 1999; 112(Pt 19):3343–52.
70. Oda Y, Imanzahrai A, Kwong A, et al. Epithelial sodium channels are upregulated during epidermal differentiation. J Invest Dermatol 1999; 113(5):796–801.
71. Guitard M, Leyvraz C, Hummler E. A nonconventional look at ionic fluxes in the skin: lessons from genetically modified mice. News Physiol Sci 2004; 19:75–9.
72. Mauro T, Guitard M, Behne M, et al. The ENaC channel is required for normal epidermal differentiation. J Invest Dermatol 2002; 118(4):589–94.
73. Leyvraz C, Charles RP, Rubera I, et al. The epidermal barrier function is dependent on the serine protease CAP1/Prss8. J Cell Biol 2005; 170(3):487–96.
74. Oh Y, Warnock DG. Expression of the amiloride-sensitive sodium channel beta subunit gene in human B lymphocytes. J Am Soc Nephrol 1997; 8(1):126–9.
75. Lindemann B. Receptors and transduction in taste. Nature 2001; 413(6852):219–25.
76. Grunder S, Muller A, Ruppersberg JP. Developmental and cellular expression pattern of epithelial sodium channel alpha, beta and gamma subunits in the inner ear of the rat. Eur J Neurosci 2001; 13(4):641–8.

77. Guipponi M, Vuagniaux G, Wattenhofer M, et al. The transmembrane serine protease (TMPRSS3) mutated in deafness DFNB8/10 activates the epithelial sodium channel (ENaC) in vitro. Hum Mol Genet 2002; 11(23):2829–36.
78. Peters TA, Levtchenko E, Cremers CW, et al. No evidence of hearing loss in pseudohypoaldosteronism type 1 patients. Acta Otolaryngol 2006; 126(3):237–9.
79. Dyka FM, May CA, Enz R. Subunits of the epithelial sodium channel family are differentially expressed in the retina of mice with ocular hypertension. J Neurochem 2005; 94(1):120–8.
80. Fricke B, Lints R, Stewart G, et al. Epithelial Na+ channels and stomatin are expressed in rat trigeminal mechanosensory neurons. Cell Tissue Res 2000; 299(3):327–34.
81. Jernigan NL, Drummond HA. Vascular ENaC proteins are required for renal myogenic constriction. Am J Physiol Renal Physiol 2005; 289(4):F891–901.
82. Kellenberger S, Schild L. Epithelial sodium channel/degenerin family of ion channels: a variety of functions for a shared structure. Physiol Rev 2002; 82(3):735–67.
83. Grunder S, Firsov D, Chang SS, et al. A mutation causing pseudohypoaldosteronism type 1 identifies a conserved glycine that is involved in the gating of the epithelial sodium channel. Embo J 1997; 16(5):899–907.
84. Grunder S, Jaeger NF, Gautschi I, et al. Identification of a highly conserved sequence at the N-terminus of the epithelial Na+ channel alpha subunit involved in gating. Pflugers Arch 1999; 438(5):709–15.
85. Staub O, Gautschi I, Ishikawa T, et al. Regulation of stability and function of the epithelial Na+ channel (ENaC) by ubiquitination. Embo J 1997; 16(21):6325–36.
86. Chalfant ML, Denton JS, Langloh AL, et al. The NH(2) terminus of the epithelial sodium channel contains an endocytic motif. J Biol Chem 1999; 274(46):32889–96.
87. Adams CM, Snyder PM, Welsh MJ. Interactions between subunits of the human epithelial sodium channel. J Biol Chem 1997; 272(43):27295–300.
88. Firsov D, Robert-Nicoud M, Gruender S, et al. Mutational analysis of cysteine-rich domains of the epithelium sodium channel (ENaC). Identification of cysteines essential for channel expression at the cell surface. J Biol Chem 1999; 274(5):2743–9.
89. Ismailov, II, Kieber-Emmons T, Lin C, et al. Identification of an amiloride binding domain within the alpha-subunit of the epithelial Na+ channel. J Biol Chem 1997; 272(34): 21075–83.
90. Schild L, Schneeberger E, Gautschi I, et al. Identification of amino acid residues in the alpha, beta, and gamma subunits of the epithelial sodium channel (ENaC) involved in amiloride block and ion permeation. J Gen Physiol 1997; 109(1):15–26.
91. Waldmann R, Champigny G, Lazdunski M. Functional degenerin-containing chimeras identify residues essential for amiloride-sensitive Na+ channel function. J Biol Chem 1995; 270(20):11735–7.
92. Kellenberger S, Gautschi I, Schild L. A single point mutation in the pore region of the epithelial Na+ channel changes ion selectivity by modifying molecular sieving. Proc Natl Acad Sci USA 1999; 96(7):4170–5.
93. Kellenberger S, Hoffmann-Pochon N, Gautschi I, et al. On the molecular basis of ion permeation in the epithelial Na+ channel. J Gen Physiol 1999; 114(1):13–30.
94. Driscoll M, Chalfie M. The mec-4 gene is a member of a family of *Caenorhabditis elegans* genes that can mutate to induce neuronal degeneration. Nature 1991; 349(6310): 588–93.
95. Champigny G, Voilley N, Waldmann R, et al. Mutations causing neurodegeneration in *Caenorhabditis elegans* drastically alter the pH sensitivity and inactivation of the mammalian H+-gated Na+ channel MDEG1. J Biol Chem 1998; 273(25):15418–22.
96. Hiltunen TP, Hannila-Handelberg T, Petajaniemi N, et al. Liddle's syndrome associated with a point mutation in the extracellular domain of the epithelial sodium channel gamma subunit. J Hypertens 2002; 20(12):2383–90.
97. Hansson JH, Nelson-Williams C, Suzuki H, et al. Hypertension caused by a truncated epithelial sodium channel gamma subunit: genetic heterogeneity of Liddle syndrome. Nat Genet 1995; 11(1):76–82.

98. Hansson JH, Schild L, Lu Y, et al. A de novo missense mutation of the beta subunit of the epithelial sodium channel causes hypertension and Liddle syndrome, identifying a proline-rich segment critical for regulation of channel activity. Proc Natl Acad Sci USA 1995; 92(25):11495–9.
99. Schild L, Lu Y, Gautschi I, et al. Identification of a PY motif in the epithelial Na channel subunits as a target sequence for mutations causing channel activation found in Liddle syndrome. Embo J 1996; 15(10):2381–7.
100. Shimkets RA, Warnock DG, Bositis CM, et al. Liddle's syndrome: heritable human hypertension caused by mutations in the beta subunit of the epithelial sodium channel. Cell 1994; 79(3):407–14.
101. Staub O, Verrey F. Impact of Nedd4 proteins and serum and glucocorticoid-induced kinases on epithelial Na+ transport in the distal nephron. J Am Soc Nephrol 2005; 16(11):3167–74.
102. Shimkets RA, Lifton RP, Canessa CM. The activity of the epithelial sodium channel is regulated by clathrin-mediated endocytosis. J Biol Chem 1997; 272(41):25537–41.
103. Shimkets RA, Lifton R, Canessa CM. In vivo phosphorylation of the epithelial sodium channel. Proc Natl Acad Sci USA 1998; 95(6):3301–5.
104. Fuchs W, Larsen EH, Lindemann B. Current-voltage curve of sodium channels and concentration dependence of sodium permeability in frog skin. J Physiol 1977; 267(1): 137–66.
105. Palmer LG, Sackin H, Frindt G. Regulation of Na+ channels by luminal Na+ in rat cortical collecting tubule. J Physiol 1998; 509(Pt 1):151–62.
106. Sheng S, Bruns JB, Kleyman TR. Extracellular histidine residues crucial for Na+ self-inhibition of epithelial Na+ channels. J Biol Chem 2004; 279(11):9743–9.
107. Silver RB, Frindt G, Windhager EE, et al. Feedback regulation of Na channels in rat CCT. I. Effects of inhibition of Na pump. Am J Physiol 1993; 264(3 Pt 2):F557–64.
108. Komwatana P, Dinudom A, Young JA, et al. Cytosolic Na+ controls and epithelial Na+ channel via the Go guanine nucleotide-binding regulatory protein. Proc Natl Acad Sci USA 1996; 93(15):8107–11.
109. Kellenberger S, Gautschi I, Rossier BC, et al. Mutations causing Liddle syndrome reduce sodium-dependent downregulation of the epithelial sodium channel in the *Xenopus* oocyte expression system. J Clin Invest 1998; 101(12):2741–50.
110. Ishikawa T, Marunaka Y, Rotin D. Electrophysiological characterization of the rat epithelial Na+ channel (rENaC) expressed in MDCK cells. Effects of Na+ and Ca2+. J Gen Physiol 1998; 111(6):825–46.
111. Taylor A. Effect of quinidine on the action of vasopressin. Fed Proc 1975; 34:385.
112. Frindt G, Windhager EE. Ca2(+)-dependent inhibition of sodium transport in rabbit cortical collecting tubules. Am J Physiol 1990; 258(3 Pt 2):F568–82.
113. Abriel H, Horisberger JD. Feedback inhibition of rat amiloride-sensitive epithelial sodium channels expressed in *Xenopus laevis* oocytes. J Physiol 1999; 516(Pt 1):31–43.
114. Palmer LG, Frindt G. Effects of cell Ca and pH on Na channels from rat cortical collecting tubule. Am J Physiol 1987; 253(2 Pt 2):F333–9.
115. Rao US, Baker JM, Pluznick JL, et al. Role of intracellular Ca2+ in the expression of the amiloride-sensitive epithelial sodium channel. Cell Calcium 2004; 35(1):21–8.
116. Bachhuber T, Konig J, Voelcker T, et al. Cl− interference with the epithelial Na+ channel ENaC. J Biol Chem 2005; 280(36):31587–94.
117. Niisato N, Eaton DC, Marunaka Y. Involvement of cytosolic Cl− in osmoregulation of alpha-ENaC gene expression. Am J Physiol Renal Physiol 2004; 287(5):F932–9.
118. Kunzelmann K. ENaC is inhibited by an increase in the intracellular Cl(−) concentration mediated through activation of Cl(−) channels. Pflugers Arch 2003; 445(4):504–12.
119. Stutts MJ, Canessa CM, Olsen JC, et al. CFTR as a cAMP-dependent regulator of sodium channels. Science 1995; 269(5225):847–50.
120. Briel M, Greger R, Kunzelmann K. Cl− transport by cystic fibrosis transmembrane conductance regulator (CFTR) contributes to the inhibition of epithelial Na+ channels (ENaCs) in *Xenopus* oocytes co-expressing CFTR and ENaC. J Physiol 1998; 508(Pt 3): 825–36.

121. Silver RB, Frindt G, Palmer LG. Regulation of principal cell pH by Na/H exchange in rabbit cortical collecting tubule. J Membr Biol 1992; 125(1):13–24.
122. Harvey BJ, Thomas SR, Ehrenfeld J. Intracellular pH controls cell membrane Na+ and K+ conductances and transport in frog skin epithelium. J Gen Physiol 1988; 92(6):767–91.
123. Chalfant ML, Denton JS, Berdiev BK, et al. Intracellular H+ regulates the alpha-subunit of ENaC, the epithelial Na+ channel. Am J Physiol 1999; 276(2 Pt 1):C477–86.
124. Palmer LG, Frindt G. Gating of Na channels in the rat cortical collecting tubule: effects of voltage and membrane stretch. J Gen Physiol 1996; 107(1):35–45.
125. Benos DJ. Sensing tension: recognizing ENaC as a stretch sensor. Hypertension 2004; 44(5):616–7.
126. Drummond HA, Gebremedhin D, Harder DR. Degenerin/epithelial Na+ channel proteins: components of a vascular mechanosensor. Hypertension 2004; 44(5):643–8.
127. Balut C, Steels P, Radu M, et al. Membrane cholesterol extraction decreases Na+ transport in A6 renal epithelia. Am J Physiol Cell Physiol 2006; 290(1):C87–94.
128. West A, Blazer-Yost B. Modulation of basal and peptide hormone-stimulated Na+ transport by membrane cholesterol content in the A6 epithelial cell line. Cell Physiol Biochem 2005; 16(4–6):263–70.
129. Yue G, Malik B, Yue G, et al. Phosphatidylinositol 4,5-bisphosphate (PIP2) stimulates epithelial sodium channel activity in A6 cells. J Biol Chem 2002; 277(14):11965–9.
130. Ma HP, Saxena S, Warnock DG. Anionic phospholipids regulate native and expressed epithelial sodium channel (ENaC). J Biol Chem 2002; 277(10):7641–4.
131. Lehrmann H, Thomas J, Kim SJ, et al. Luminal P2Y2 receptor-mediated inhibition of Na+ absorption in isolated perfused mouse CCD. J Am Soc Nephrol 2002; 13(1):10–8.
132. Kunzelmann K, Bachhuber T, Regeer R, et al. Purinergic inhibition of the epithelial Na+ transport via hydrolysis of PIP2. Faseb J 2005; 19(1):142–3.
133. Wildman SS, Marks J, Churchill LJ, et al. Regulatory interdependence of cloned epithelial Na+ channels and P2X receptors. J Am Soc Nephrol 2005; 16(9):2586–97.
134. Ma HP, Eaton DC. Acute regulation of epithelial sodium channel by anionic phospholipids. J Am Soc Nephrol 2005; 16(11):3182–7.
135. Helms MN, Liu L, Liang YY, et al. Phosphatidylinositol 3,4,5-trisphosphate mediates aldosterone stimulation of epithelial sodium channel (ENaC) and interacts with gamma-ENaC. J Biol Chem 2005; 280(49):40885–91.
136. Pochynyuk O, Staruschenko A, Tong Q, et al. Identification of a functional phosphatidylinositol 3,4,5-trisphosphate binding site in the epithelial Na+ channel. J Biol Chem 2005; 280(45):37565–71.
137. Berdiev BK, Prat AG, Cantiello HF, et al. Regulation of epithelial sodium channels by short actin filaments. J Biol Chem 1996; 271(30):17704–10.
138. Saxena S, Quick MW, Warnock DG. Interaction of syntaxins with epithelial ion channels. Curr Opin Nephrol Hypertens 2000; 9(5):523–7.
139. Saxena S, Singh M, Engisch K, et al. Rab proteins regulate epithelial sodium channel activity in colonic epithelial HT-29 cells. Biochem Biophys Res Commun 2005; 337(4): 1219–23.
140. Saxena SK, Singh M, Shibata H, et al. Rab4 GTP/GDP modulates amiloride-sensitive sodium channel (ENaC) function in colonic epithelia. Biochem Biophys Res Commun 2006; 340(2):726–33.
141. Berdiev BK, Jovov B, Tucker WC, et al. ENaC subunit-subunit interactions and inhibition by syntaxin 1A. Am J Physiol Renal Physiol 2004; 286(6):F1100–6.
142. Qi J, Peters KW, Liu C, et al. Regulation of the amiloride-sensitive epithelial sodium channel by syntaxin 1A. J Biol Chem 1999; 274(43):30345–8.
143. Saxena S, Quick MW, Tousson A, et al. Interaction of syntaxins with the amiloride-sensitive epithelial sodium channel. J Biol Chem 1999; 274(30):20812–7.
144. Song J, Hu X, Riazi S, et al. Regulation of blood pressure, the epithelial sodium channel (ENaC), and other key renal sodium transporters by chronic insulin infusion in rats. Am J Physiol Renal Physiol 2005; 22:22.

145. Blazer-Yost BL, Record RD, Oberleithner H. Characterization of hormone-stimulated Na+ transport in a high-resistance clone of the MDCK cell line. Pflugers Arch 1996; 432(4):685–91.
146. Blazer-Yost BL, Liu X, Helman SI. Hormonal regulation of ENaCs: insulin and aldosterone. Am J Physiol 1998; 274(5 Pt 1):C1373–9.
147. Baxendale-Cox LM, Duncan RL. Insulin increases sodium (Na+) channel density in A6 epithelia: implications for expression of hypertension. Biol Res Nurs 1999; 1(1):20–9.
148. Blazer-Yost BL, Esterman MA, Vlahos CJ. Insulin-stimulated trafficking of ENaC in renal cells requires PI3-kinase activity. Am J Physiol Cell Physiol 2003; 284(6):C1645–53.
149. Zhang YH, Alvarez de la Rosa D, Canessa CM, et al. Insulin-induced phosphorylation of ENaC correlates with increased sodium channel function in A6 cells. Am J Physiol Cell Physiol 2005; 288(1):C141–7.
150. Peti-Peterdi J, Warnock DG, Bell PD. Angiotensin II directly stimulates ENaC activity in the cortical collecting duct via AT(1) receptors. J Am Soc Nephrol 2002; 13(5):1131–5.
151. Wang Q, Hummler E, Maillard M, et al. Compensatory up-regulation of angiotensin II subtype 1 receptors in alpha ENaC knockout heterozygous mice. Kidney Int 2001; 59(6):2216–21.
152. Michlig S, Harris M, Loffing J, et al. Progesterone down-regulates the open probability of the amiloride-sensitive epithelial sodium channel via a Nedd4-2-dependent mechanism. J Biol Chem 2005; 280(46):38264–70.
153. Thomas CP, Liu KZ, Vats HS. Medroxyprogesterone acetate binds the glucocorticoid receptor to stimulate {alpha}-ENaC and sgk1 expression in renal collecting duct epithelia. Am J Physiol Renal Physiol 2006; 290(2):F306–12.
154. Gambling L, Dunford S, Wilson CA, et al. Estrogen and progesterone regulate alpha, beta, and gammaENaC subunit mRNA levels in female rat kidney. Kidney Int 2004; 65(5): 1774–81.
155. Wang W, Li C, Nejsum LN, et al. Biphasic effects of ANP infusion in conscious, euvolumic rats: roles of AQP2 and ENaC trafficking. Am J Physiol Renal Physiol 2006; 290(2):F530–41.
156. Ma H, Ling BN. Luminal adenosine receptors regulate amiloride-sensitive Na+ channels in A6 distal nephron cells. Am J Physiol 1996; 270(5 Pt 2):F798–805.
157. Wei Y, Sun P, Wang Z, et al. Adenosine inhibits ENaC via cytochrome P-450 epoxygenase-dependent metabolites of arachidonic acid. Am J Physiol Renal Physiol 2006; 290(5): F1163–8.
158. Guan Y, Zhang Y, Breyer RM, et al. Prostaglandin E2 inhibits renal collecting duct Na+ absorption by activating the EP1 receptor. J Clin Invest 1998; 102(1):194–201.
159. Wegmann M, Nusing RM. Prostaglandin E2 stimulates sodium reabsorption in MDCK C7 cells, a renal collecting duct principal cell model. Prostaglandins Leukot Essent Fatty Acids 2003; 69(5):315–22.
160. Verrey F, Hummler E, Schild L, et al. Control of sodium transport by aldosterone. In: Giebisch DWSaG et al, ed. The Kidney, Physiology and Physiopathology. 3rd ed., Vol. I. Philadelphia, PA: Lippincott Williams & Wilkins, 2000:1441–71.
161. Bens M, Vallet V, Cluzeaud F, et al. Corticosteroid-dependent sodium transport in a novel immortalized mouse collecting duct principal cell line. J Am Soc Nephrol 1999; 10(5): 923–34.
162. May A, Puoti A, Gaeggeler HP, et al. Early effect of aldosterone on the rate of synthesis of the epithelial sodium channel alpha subunit in A6 renal cells. J Am Soc Nephrol 1997; 8(12):1813–22.
163. Loffing J, Zecevic M, Feraille E, et al. Aldosterone induces rapid apical translocation of ENaC in early portion of renal collecting system: possible role of SGK. Am J Physiol Renal Physiol 2001; 280(4):F675–82.
164. Chen SY, Bhargava A, Mastroberardino L, et al. Epithelial sodium channel regulated by aldosterone-induced protein sgk. Proc Natl Acad Sci USA 1999; 96(5):2514–9.
165. Naray-Fejes-Toth A, Canessa C, Cleaveland ES, et al. Sgk is an aldosterone-induced kinase in the renal collecting duct. Effects on epithelial Na+ channels. J Biol Chem 1999; 274(24):16973–8.

166. Alvarez de la Rosa D, Zhang P, Naray-Fejes-Toth A, et al. The serum and glucocorticoid kinase sgk increases the abundance of epithelial sodium channels in the plasma membrane of *Xenopus* oocytes. J Biol Chem 1999; 274(53):37834–9.
167. Debonneville C, Flores SY, Kamynina E, et al. Phosphorylation of Nedd4-2 by Sgk1 regulates epithelial Na(+) channel cell surface expression. Embo J 2001; 20(24):7052–9.
168. Flores SY, Loffing-Cueni D, Kamynina E, et al. Aldosterone-induced serum and glucocorticoid-induced kinase 1 expression is accompanied by Nedd4-2 phosphorylation and increased Na+ transport in cortical collecting duct cells. J Am Soc Nephrol 2005; 16(8):2279–87.
169. Zhou R, Snyder PM. Nedd4-2 phosphorylation induces serum and glucocorticoid-regulated kinase (SGK) ubiquitination and degradation. J Biol Chem 2005; 280(6):4518–23.
170. Diakov A, Korbmacher C. A novel pathway of epithelial sodium channel activation involves a serum- and glucocorticoid-inducible kinase consensus motif in the C terminus of the channel's alpha-subunit. J Biol Chem 2004; 279(37):38134–42.
171. Ichimura T, Yamamura H, Sasamoto K, et al. 14-3-3 proteins modulate the expression of epithelial Na+ channels by phosphorylation-dependent interaction with Nedd4-2 ubiquitin ligase. J Biol Chem 2005; 280(13):13187–94.
172. Bhalla V, Daidie D, Li H, et al. Serum- and glucocorticoid-regulated kinase 1 regulates ubiquitin ligase neural precursor cell-expressed, developmentally down-regulated protein 4-2 by inducing interaction with 14-3-3. Mol Endocrinol 2005; 19(12):3073–84.
173. Liang X, Peters KW, Butterworth MB, et al. 14-3-3 isoforms are induced by aldosterone and participate in its regulation of epithelial sodium channels. J Biol Chem 2006; 12:12.
174. Wilson FH, Disse-Nicodeme S, Choate KA, et al. Human hypertension caused by mutations in WNK kinases. Science 2001; 293(5532):1107–12.
175. Naray-Fejes-Toth A, Snyder PM, Fejes-Toth G. The kidney-specific WNK1 isoform is induced by aldosterone and stimulates epithelial sodium channel-mediated Na+ transport. Proc Natl Acad Sci USA 2004; 101(50):17434–9.
176. Xu BE, Stippec S, Chu PY, et al. WNK1 activates SGK1 to regulate the epithelial sodium channel. Proc Natl Acad Sci USA 2005; 102(29):10315–20.
177. Spindler B, Mastroberardino L, Custer M, et al. Characterization of early aldosterone-induced RNAs identified in A6 kidney epithelia. Pflugers Arch 1997; 434(3):323–31.
178. Mastroberardino L, Spindler B, Forster I, et al. Ras pathway activates epithelial Na+ channel and decreases its surface expression in *Xenopus* oocytes. Mol Biol Cell 1998; 9(12):3417–27.
179. Robert-Nicoud M, Flahaut M, Elalouf JM, et al. Transcriptome of a mouse kidney cortical collecting duct cell line: effects of aldosterone and vasopressin. Proc Natl Acad Sci USA 2001; 98(5):2712–6.
180. Muller OG, Parnova RG, Centeno G, et al. Mineralocorticoid effects in the kidney: correlation between alphaENaC, GILZ, and Sgk-1 mRNA expression and urinary excretion of Na+ and K+. J Am Soc Nephrol 2003; 14(5):1107–15.
181. Soundararajan R, Zhang TT, Wang J, et al. A novel role for glucocorticoid-induced leucine zipper protein in epithelial sodium channel-mediated sodium transport. J Biol Chem 2005; 280(48):39970–81.
182. Gumz ML, Popp MP, Wingo CS, et al. Early transcriptional effects of aldosterone in a mouse inner medullary collecting duct cell line. Am J Physiol Renal Physiol 2003; 285(4):F664–73.
183. Schnizler M, Mastroberardino L, Reifarth F, et al. cAMP sensitivity conferred to the epithelial Na+ channel by alpha-subunit cloned from guinea-pig colon. Pflugers Arch 2000; 439(5):579–87.
184. Chraibi A, Schnizler M, Clauss W, et al. Effects of 8-cpt-cAMP on the epithelial sodium channel expressed in *Xenopus* oocytes. J Membr Biol 2001; 183(1):15–23.
185. Butterworth MB, Edinger RS, Johnson JP, et al. Acute ENaC stimulation by cAMP in a kidney cell line is mediated by exocytic insertion from a recycling channel pool. J Gen Physiol 2005; 125(1):81–101.
186. Butterworth MB, Frizzell RA, Johnson JP, et al. PKA-dependent ENaC trafficking requires the SNARE-binding protein complexin. Am J Physiol Renal Physiol 2005; 289(5):F969–77.

187. Snyder PM, Olson DR, Kabra R, et al. cAMP and serum and glucocorticoid-inducible kinase (SGK) regulate the epithelial Na(+) channel through convergent phosphorylation of Nedd4-2. J Biol Chem 2004; 279(44):45753–8.
188. Yanase M, Handler JS. Activators of protein kinase C inhibit sodium transport in A6 epithelia. Am J Physiol 1986; 250(3 Pt 1):C517–22.
189. Ling BN, Eaton DC. Effects of luminal Na+ on single Na+ channels in A6 cells, a regulatory role for protein kinase C. Am J Physiol 1989; 256(6 Pt 2):F1094–103.
190. Frindt G, Palmer LG, Windhager EE. Feedback regulation of Na channels in rat CCT. IV. Mediation by activation of protein kinase C. Am J Physiol 1996; 270(2 Pt 2):F371–6.
191. Hays SR, Baum M, Kokko JP. ***Effects of protein kinase C activation on sodium, potassium, chloride, and total CO2 transport in the rabbit cortical collecting tubule. J Clin Invest 1987; 80(6):1561–70.
192. Mohrmann M, Cantiello HF, Ausiello DA. Inhibition of epithelial Na+ transport by atriopeptin, protein kinase C, and pertussis toxin. Am J Physiol 1987; 253(2 Pt 2):F372–6.
193. Awayda MS, Ismailov I,I, Berdiev BK, et al. Protein kinase regulation of a cloned epithelial Na+ channel. J Gen Physiol 1996; 108(1):49–65.
194. Awayda MS. Specific and nonspecific effects of protein kinase C on the epithelial Na (+) channel. J Gen Physiol 2000; 115(5):559–70.
195. Stockand JD, Bao HF, Schenck J, et al. Differential effects of protein kinase C on the levels of epithelial Na+ channel subunit proteins. J Biol Chem 2000; 275(33):25760–5.
196. Yan W, Suaud L, Kleyman TR, et al. Differential modulation of a polymorphism in the COOH terminus of the {alpha}-subunit of the human epithelial sodium channel by protein kinase C{delta}. Am J Physiol Renal Physiol 2006; 290(2):F279–88.
197. Shi H, Asher C, Chigaev A, et al. Interactions of beta and gamma ENaC with Nedd4 can be facilitated by an ERK-mediated phosphorylation. J Biol Chem 2002; 277(16):13539–47.
198. Shi H, Asher C, Yung Y, et al. Casein kinase 2 specifically binds to and phosphorylates the carboxy termini of ENaC subunits. Eur J Biochem 2002; 269(18):4551–8.
199. Lebowitz J, Edinger RS, An B, et al. Ikappab kinase-beta (ikkbeta) modulation of epithelial sodium channel activity. J Biol Chem 2004; 279(40):41985–90.
200. Nicod M, Michlig S, Flahaut M, et al. A novel vasopressin-induced transcript promotes MAP kinase activation and ENaC downregulation. Embo J 2002; 21(19):5109–17.
201. Tong Q, Booth RE, Worrell RT, et al. Regulation of Na+ transport by aldosterone: signaling convergence and cross talk between the PI3-K and MAPK1/2 cascades. Am J Physiol Renal Physiol 2004; 286(6):F1232–8.
202. Song J, Knepper MA, Hu X, et al. Rosiglitazone activates renal sodium- and water-reabsorptive pathways and lowers blood pressure in normal rats. J Pharmacol Exp Ther 2004; 308(2):426–33.
203. Nofziger C, Chen L, Shane MA, et al. PPARgamma agonists do not directly enhance basal or insulin-stimulated Na(+) transport via the epithelial Na(+) channel. Pflugers Arch 2005; 451(3):445–53.
204. Zhang H, Zhang A, Kohan DE, et al. Collecting duct-specific deletion of peroxisome proliferator-activated receptor gamma blocks thiazolidinedione-induced fluid retention. Proc Natl Acad Sci USA 2005; 102(26):9406–11.
205. Guan Y, Hao C, Cha DR, et al. Thiazolidinediones expand body fluid volume through PPARgamma stimulation of ENaC-mediated renal salt absorption. Nat Med 2005; 11(8):861–6.
206. Hong G, Lockhart A, Davis B, et al. PPARgamma activation enhances cell surface ENaCalpha via up-regulation of SGK1 in human collecting duct cells. Faseb J 2003; 17(13):1966–8.
207. Lewis SA, Alles WP. Urinary kallikrein: a physiological regulator of epithelial Na+ absorption. Proc Natl Acad Sci USA 1986; 83(14):5345–8.
208. Lewis SA, Clausen C. Urinary proteases degrade epithelial sodium channels. J Membr Biol 1991; 122(1):77–88.
209. Orce GG, Castillo GA, Margolius HS. Inhibition of short-circuit current in toad urinary bladder by inhibitors of glandular kallikrein. Am J Physiol 1980; 239(5):F459–65.

210. Chraibi A, Vallet V, Firsov D, et al. Protease modulation of the activity of the epithelial sodium channel expressed in *Xenopus* oocytes. J Gen Physiol 1998; 111(1):127–38.
211. Vallet V, Chraibi A, Gaeggeler HP, et al. An epithelial serine protease activates the amiloride-sensitive sodium channel. Nature 1997; 389(6651):607–10.
212. Vuagniaux G, Vallet V, Jaeger NF, et al. Synergistic activation of ENaC by three membrane-bound channel-activating serine proteases (mCAP1, mCAP2, and mCAP3) and serum- and glucocorticoid-regulated kinase (Sgk1) in *Xenopus* oocytes. J Gen Physiol 2002; 120(2):191–201.
213. Vuagniaux G, Vallet V, Jaeger NF, et al. Activation of the amiloride-sensitive epithelial sodium channel by the serine protease mCAP1 expressed in a mouse cortical collecting duct cell line. J Am Soc Nephrol 2000; 11(5):828–34.
214. Caldwell RA, Boucher RC, Stutts MJ. Serine protease activation of near-silent epithelial Na+ channels. Am J Physiol Cell Physiol 2004; 286(1):C190–4.
215. Caldwell RA, Boucher RC, Stutts MJ. Neutrophil elastase activates near-silent epithelial Na+ channels and increases airway epithelial Na+ transport. Am J Physiol Lung Cell Mol Physiol 2005; 288(5):L813–9.
216. Iwashita K, Kitamura K, Narikiyo T, et al. Inhibition of prostasin secretion by serine protease inhibitors in the kidney. J Am Soc Nephrol 2003; 14(1):11–6.
217. Olivieri O, Castagna A, Guarini P, et al. Urinary prostasin: a candidate marker of epithelial sodium channel activation in humans. Hypertension 2005; 46(4):683–8.
218. Hughey RP, Mueller GM, Bruns JB, et al. Maturation of the epithelial Na+ channel involves proteolytic processing of the alpha- and gamma-subunits. J Biol Chem 2003; 278(39):37073–82.
219. Vallet V, Pfister C, Loffing J, et al. Cell-surface expression of the channel activating protease xCAP-1 is required for activation of ENaC in the *Xenopus* oocyte. J Am Soc Nephrol 2002; 13(3): 588–94.
220. Adebamiro A, Cheng Y, Johnson JP, et al. Endogenous protease activation of ENaC: effect of serine protease inhibition on ENaC single channel properties. J Gen Physiol 2005; 126(4):339–52.
221. Hughey RP, Bruns JB, Kinlough CL, et al. Epithelial sodium channels are activated by furin-dependent proteolysis. J Biol Chem 2004; 279(18):18111–4.
222. Hummler E, Barker P, Gatzy J, et al. Early death due to defective neonatal lung liquid clearance in alpha-ENaC-deficient mice. Nat Genet 1996; 12(3):325–8.
223. Hummler E, Barker P, Talbot C, et al. A mouse model for the renal salt-wasting syndrome pseudohypoaldosteronism. Proc Natl Acad Sci USA 1997; 94(21):11710–5.
224. Rubera I, Loffing J, Palmer LG, et al. Collecting duct-specific gene inactivation of alphaENaC in the mouse kidney does not impair sodium and potassium balance. J Clin Invest 2003; 112(4):554–65.
225. McDonald FJ, Yang B, Hrstka RF, et al. Disruption of the beta subunit of the epithelial Na+ channel in mice: hyperkalemia and neonatal death associated with a pseudohypoaldosteronism phenotype. Proc Natl Acad Sci USA 1999; 96(4):1727–31.
226. Pradervand S, Barker PM, Wang Q, et al. Salt restriction induces pseudohypoaldosteronism type 1 in mice expressing low levels of the beta-subunit of the amiloride-sensitive epithelial sodium channel. Proc Natl Acad Sci USA 1999; 96(4):1732–7.
227. Pradervand S, Wang Q, Burnier M, et al. A mouse model for Liddle's syndrome. J Am Soc Nephrol 1999; 10(12):2527–33.
228. Mall M, Grubb BR, Harkema JR, et al. Increased airway epithelial Na+ absorption produces cystic fibrosis-like lung disease in mice. Nat Med 2004; 10(5):487–93.
229. Barker PM, Nguyen MS, Gatzy JT, et al. Role of gammaENaC subunit in lung liquid clearance and electrolyte balance in newborn mice. Insights into perinatal adaptation and pseudohypoaldosteronism. J Clin Invest 1998; 102(8):1634–40.
230. Egli M, Duplain H, Lepori M, et al. Defective respiratory amiloride-sensitive sodium transport predisposes to pulmonary oedema and delays its resolution in mice. J Physiol 2004; 560(Pt 3):857–65.

231. Dahlmann A, Pradervand S, Hummler E, et al. Mineralocorticoid regulation of epithelial Na+ channels is maintained in a mouse model of Liddle's syndrome. Am J Physiol Renal Physiol 2003; 285(2):F310–8.
232. Frindt G, Palmer LG. Na channels in the rat connecting tubule. Am J Physiol Renal Physiol 2004; 286(4):F669–74.
233. Sheridan MB, Fong P, Groman JD, et al. Mutations in the beta-subunit of the epithelial Na+ channel in patients with a cystic fibrosis-like syndrome. Hum Mol Genet 2005; 14(22): 3493–8.
234. Chang SS, Grunder S, Hanukoglu A, et al. Mutations in subunits of the epithelial sodium channel cause salt wasting with hyperkalaemic acidosis, pseudohypoaldosteronism type 1. Nat Genet 1996; 12(3):248–53.
235. Strautnieks SS, Thompson RJ, Gardiner RM, et al. A novel splice-site mutation in the gamma subunit of the epithelial sodium channel gene in three pseudohypoaldosteronism type 1 families. Nat Genet 1996; 13(2):248–50.
236. Liddle GW, Bledsoe T, Coppage WS. A familial renal disorder simulating primary aldosteronism but with negligible aldosterone secretion. Trans Assoc Am Physicians 1963; 76:199–213.
237. Botero-Velez M, Curtis JJ, Warnock DG. Brief report: Liddle's syndrome revisited—a disorder of sodium reabsorption in the distal tubule. N Engl J Med 1994; 330(3):178–81.
238. Staub O, Dho S, Henry P, et al. WW domains of Nedd4 bind to the proline-rich PY motifs in the epithelial Na+ channel deleted in Liddle's syndrome. Embo J 1996; 15(10):2371–80.
239. Kuhnle U. Pseudohypoaldosteronism: mutation found, problem solved? Mol Cell Endocrinol 1997; 133(2):77–80.
240. Hanukoglu A. Type I pseudohypoaldosteronism includes two clinically and genetically distinct entities with either renal or multiple target organ defects. J Clin Endocrinol Metab 1991; 73(5):936–44.
241. Geller DS, Rodriguez-Soriano J, Vallo Boado A, et al. Mutations in the mineralocorticoid receptor gene cause autosomal dominant pseudohypoaldosteronism type I. Nat Genet 1998; 19(3):279–81.
242. Tajima T, Kitagawa H, Yokoya S, et al. A novel missense mutation of mineralocorticoid receptor gene in one Japanese family with a renal form of pseudohypoaldosteronism type 1. J Clin Endocrinol Metab 2000; 85(12):4690–4.
243. Viemann M, Peter M, Lopez-Siguero JP, et al. Evidence for genetic heterogeneity of pseudo-hypoaldosteronism type 1: identification of a novel mutation in the human mineralocorticoid receptor in one sporadic case and no mutations in two autosomal dominant kindreds. J Clin Endocrinol Metab 2001; 86(5):2056–9.
244. Sartorato P, Lapeyraque AL, Armanini D, et al. Different inactivating mutations of the mineralocorticoid receptor in fourteen families affected by type I pseudohypoaldosteronism. J Clin Endocrinol Metab 2003; 88(6):2508–17.
245. Nystrom AM, Bondeson ML, Skanke N, et al. A novel nonsense mutation of the mineralocorticoid receptor gene in a Swedish family with pseudohypoaldosteronism type I (PHA1). J Clin Endocrinol Metab 2004; 89(1):227–31.
246. Riepe FG, Krone N, Morlot M, et al. Identification of a novel mutation in the human mineralocorticoid receptor gene in a German family with autosomal-dominant pseudohypoaldosteronism type 1: further evidence for marked interindividual clinical heterogeneity. J Clin Endocrinol Metab 2003; 88(4):1683–6.
247. Riepe FG, Krone N, Morlot M, et al. Autosomal-dominant pseudohypoaldosteronism type 1 in a Turkish family is associated with a novel nonsense mutation in the human mineralocorticoid receptor gene. J Clin Endocrinol Metab 2004; 89(5):2150–2.
248. Geller DS, Zhang J, Zennaro MC, et al. Autosomal dominant pseudohypoaldosteronism type 1: mechanisms, evidence for neonatal lethality, and phenotypic expression in adults. J Am Soc Nephrol 2006; 17(5):1429–36.
249. Berger S, Bleich M, Schmid W, et al. Mineralocorticoid receptor knockout mice: pathophysiology of Na+ metabolism. Proc Natl Acad Sci USA 1998; 95(16):9424–9.

250. Bleich M, Warth R, Schmidt-Hieber M, et al. Rescue of the mineralocorticoid receptor knock-out mouse. Pflugers Arch 1999; 438(3):245–54.
251. Hanukoglu A, Bistritzer T, Rakover Y, et al. Pseudohypoaldosteronism with increased sweat and saliva electrolyte values and frequent lower respiratory tract infections mimicking cystic fibrosis. J Pediatr 1994; 125(5 Pt 1):752–5.
252. Hogg RJ, Marks JF, Marver D, et al. Long term observations in a patient with pseudohypoaldosteronism. Pediatr Nephrol 1991; 5(2):205–10.
253. Kerem E, Bistritzer T, Hanukoglu A, et al. Pulmonary epithelial sodium-channel dysfunction and excess airway liquid in pseudohypoaldosteronism. N Engl J Med 1999; 341(3):156–62.
254. MacLaughlin EF. Pseudohypoaldosteronism and sodium transport. Pediatr Pulmonol 1996; 13:181–2.
255. Marthinsen L, Kornfalt R, Aili M, et al. Recurrent *Pseudomonas* bronchopneumonia and other symptoms as in cystic fibrosis in a child with type I pseudohypoaldosteronism. Acta Paediatr 1998; 87(4):472–4.
256. Schaedel C, Marthinsen L, Kristoffersson AC, et al. Lung symptoms in pseudohypoaldosteronism type 1 are associated with deficiency of the alpha-subunit of the epithelial sodium channel. J Pediatr 1999; 135(6):739–45.
257. Malagon-Rogers M. A patient with pseudohypoaldosteronism type 1 and respiratory distress syndrome. Pediatr Nephrol 1999; 13(6):484–6.
258. Barker PM, Gowen CW, Lawson EE, et al. Decreased sodium ion absorption across nasal epithelium of very premature infants with respiratory distress syndrome. J Pediatr 1997; 130(3):373–7.
259. Akcay A, Yavuz T, Semiz S, et al. Pseudohypoaldosteronism type 1 and respiratory distress syndrome. J Pediatr Endocrinol Metab 2002; 15(9):1557–61.
260. Prince LS, Launspach JL, Geller DS, et al. Absence of amiloride-sensitive sodium absorption in the airway of an infant with pseudohypoaldosteronism. J Pediatr 1999; 135(6):786–9.
261. Akkurt I, Kuhnle U, Ringenberg C. Pseudohypo-aldosteronism and cholelithiasis: coincisdence or pathogenetic correlation? Eur J Pediatr 1997; 156(5):363–6.
262. Hanaki K, Ohzeki T, Iitsuka T, et al. An infant with pseudohypoaldosteronism accompanied by cholelithiasis. Biol Neonate 1994; 65(2):85–8.
263. Reddy MM, Wang XF, Gottschalk M, et al. Normal CFTR activity and reversed skin potentials in pseudohypoaldosteronism. J Membr Biol 2005; 203(3):151–9.
264. Martin JM, Calduch L, Monteagudo C, et al. Clinico-pathological analysis of the cutaneous lesions of a patient with type I pseudohypoaldosteronism. J Eur Acad Dermatol Venereol 2005; 19(3):377–9.
265. Garty BZ. Chronic *Pseudomonas* colonization of the skin, ear and eyes in a child with type I pseudohypoaldosteronism. Acta Paediatr 1999; 88(4):472–3.
266. Aberer E, Gebhart W, Mainitz M, et al. Sweat glands in pseudohypoaldosteronism. Hautarzt 1987; 38(8):484–7.
267. Urbatsch A, Paller AS. Pustular miliaria rubra: a specific cutaneous finding of type I pseudohypoaldosteronism. Pediatr Dermatol 2002; 19(4):317–9.
268. Liotta A, Maggio MC, Iachininoto R, et al. Fetal pseudohypoaldosteronism: a rare cause of hydramnios. Pediatr Med Chir 2003; 25(5):375–7.
269. Narchi H, Santos M, Kulaylat N. Polyhydramnios as a sign of fetal pseudohypoaldosteronism. Int J Gynaecol Obstet 2000; 69(1):53–4.
270. Wong GP, Levine D. Congenital pseudohypoaldosteronism presenting in utero with acute polyhydramnios. J Matern Fetal Med 1998; 7(2):76–8.
271. Greenberg D, Abramson O, Phillip M. Fetal pseudohypoaldosteronism: another cause of hydramnios. Acta Paediatr 1995; 84(5):582–4.
272. Abramson O, Zmora E, Mazor M, et al. Pseudohypoaldosteronism in a preterm infant: intrauterine presentation as hydramnios. J Pediatr 1992; 120(1):129–32.
273. Strautnieks SS, Thompson RJ, Hanukoglu A, et al. Localisation of pseudohypoaldosteronism genes to chromosome 16p12.2-13.11 and 12p13.1-pter by homozygosity mapping. Hum Mol Genet 1996; 5(2):293–9.

274. Adachi M, Tachibana K, Asakura Y, et al. Compound heterozygous mutations in the gamma subunit gene of ENaC (1627delG and 1570-1G→A) in one sporadic Japanese patient with a systemic form of pseudohypoaldosteronism type 1. J Clin Endocrinol Metab 2001; 86(1):9–12.
275. Bonny O, Knoers N, Monnens L, et al. A novel mutation of the epithelial Na+ channel causes type 1 pseudohypoaldosteronism. Pediatr Nephrol 2002; 17(10):804–8.
276. Edelheit O, Hanukoglu I, Gizewska M, et al. Novel mutations in epithelial sodium channel (ENaC) subunit genes and phenotypic expression of multisystem pseudohypoaldosteronism. Clin Endocrinol (Oxf) 2005; 62(5):547–53.
277. Grunder S, Chang SS, Lifton R, et al. PHA-1: a novel thermosensitive mutation in the ectodomain of alpha ENaC. J Am Soc Nephrol 1998; 9:S069 (Abstract).
278. Saxena A, Hanukoglu I, Saxena D, et al. Novel mutations responsible for autosomal recessive multisystem pseudohypoaldosteronism and sequence variants in epithelial sodium channel alpha-, beta-, and gamma-subunit genes. J Clin Endocrinol Metab 2002; 87(7):3344–50.
279. Thomas CP, Zhou J, Liu KZ, et al. Systemic pseudohypoaldosteronism from deletion of the promoter region of the human beta epithelial Na(+) channel subunit. Am J Respir Cell Mol Biol 2002; 27(3):314–9.
280. Thomas CP, Zhou J, Liu KZ, et al. Gene symbol: SCNN1B. Disease: pseudohypoaldosteronism, type 1. Hum Genet 2004; 114(4):402.
281. Arai K, Nakagomi Y, Iketani M, et al. Functional polymorphisms in the mineralocorticoid receptor and amirolide-sensitive sodium channel genes in a patient with sporadic pseudohypoaldosteronism. Hum Genet 2003; 112(1):91–7.
282. Arai K, Zachman K, Shibasaki T, et al. Polymorphisms of amiloride-sensitive sodium channel subunits in five sporadic cases of pseudohypoaldosteronism: do they have pathologic potential? J Clin Endocrinol Metab 1999; 84(7):2434–7.
283. Ludwig M, Bolkenius U, Wickert L, et al. Common polymorphisms in genes encoding the human mineralocorticoid receptor and the human amiloride-sensitive sodium channel. J Steroid Biochem Mol Biol 1998; 64(5-6):227–30.
284. Iwai N, Baba S, Mannami T, et al. Association of sodium channel gamma-subunit promoter variant with blood pressure. Hypertension 2001; 38(1):86–9.
285. Ludwig M, Bidlingmaier F, Reissinger A. Pseudohypoaldosteronism type 1 and the genes encoding prostasin, alpha-spectrin, and Nedd4. Int J Mol Med 2004; 14(6):1101–4.
286. Huey CL, Riepe FG, Sippell WG, et al. Genetic heterogeneity in autosomal dominant pseudohypoaldosteronism type I: exclusion of claudin-8 as a candidate gene. Am J Nephrol 2004; 24(5):483–7.
287. Lifton RP, Gharavi AG, Geller DS. Molecular mechanisms of human hypertension. Cell 2001; 104(4):545–56.
288. Levy D, DeStefano AL, Larson MG, et al. Evidence for a gene influencing blood pressure on chromosome 17. Genome scan linkage results for longitudinal blood pressure phenotypes in subjects from the framingham heart study. Hypertension 2000; 36(4):477–83.
289. Xu X, Rogus JJ, Terwedow HA, et al. An extreme-sib-pair genome scan for genes regulating blood pressure. Am J Hum Genet 1999; 64(6):1694–701.
290. Halushka M, Fan J-B, Bentley K, et al. Patterns of single-nucleotide polymorphisms in candidate genes for blood pressure homeostasis. Nat Genet 1999; 22:239–47.
291. Jeunemaitre X, Soubrier F, Kotelevtsev YV, et al. Molecular basis of human hypertension: role of angiotensinogen. Cell 1992; 71(1):169–80.
292. Munroe PB, Strautnieks SS, Farrall M, et al. Absence of linkage of the epithelial sodium channel to hypertension in black Caribbeans. Am J Hypertens 1998; 11(8 Pt 1):942–5.
293. Melander O, Orho M, Fagerudd J, et al. Mutations and variants of the epithelial sodium channel gene in Liddle's syndrome and primary hypertension. Hypertension 1998; 31(5):1118–24.
294. Niu T, Xu X, Cordell HJ, et al. Linkage analysis of candidate genes and gene-gene interactions in chinese hypertensive sib pairs. Hypertension 1999; 33(6):1332–7.
295. Chang H, Fujita T. Lack of mutations in epithelial sodium channel beta-subunit gene in human subjects with hypertension. J Hypertens 1996; 14(12):1417–9.

296. Matsubara M, Metoki H, Suzuki M, et al. Genotypes of the betaENaC gene have little influence on blood pressure level in the Japanese population. Am J Hypertens 2002; 15(2 Pt 1):189–92.
297. Persu A, Barbry P, Bassilana F, et al. Genetic analysis of the beta subunit of the epithelial Na+ channel in essential hypertension. Hypertension 1998; 32(1):129–37.
298. Persu A, Coscoy S, Houot AM, et al. Polymorphisms of the gamma subunit of the epithelial Na+ channel in essential hypertension. J Hypertens 1999; 17(5):639–45.
299. Tiago AD, Nkeh B, Candy GP, et al. Association study of eight candidate genes with renin status in mild-to-moderate hypertension in patients of African ancestry. Cardiovasc J S Afr 2001; 12(2):75–80.
300. Wong ZY, Stebbing M, Ellis JA, et al. Genetic linkage of beta and gamma subunits of epithelial sodium channel to systolic blood pressure. Lancet 1999; 353(9160):1222–5.
301. Nagy Z, Busjahn A, Bahring S, et al. Quantitative trait loci for blood pressure exist near the IGF-1, the Liddle syndrome, the angiotensin II-receptor gene and the renin loci in man. J Am Soc Nephrol 1999; 10(8):1709–16.
302. Baker EH, Dong YB, Sagnella GA, et al. Association of hypertension with T594M mutation in beta subunit of epithelial sodium channels in black people resident in London. Lancet 1998; 351(9113):1388–92.
303. Dong YB, Plange-Rhule J, Owusu I, et al. T594M mutation of the beta-subunit of the epithelial sodium channel in Ghanaian populations from Kumasi and London and a possible association with hypertension. Genet Test 2002; 6(1):63–5.
304. Dong YB, Zhu HD, Baker EH, et al. T594M and G442V polymorphisms of the sodium channel beta subunit and hypertension in a black population. J Hum Hypertens 2001; 15(6):425–30.
305. Su YR, Rutkowski MP, Klanke CA, et al. A novel variant of the beta-subunit of the amiloride-sensitive sodium channel in African Americans. J Am Soc Nephrol 1996; 7(12):2543–9.
306. Nkeh B, Samani NJ, Badenhorst D, et al. T594M variant of the epithelial sodium channel beta-subunit gene and hypertension in individuals of African ancestry in South Africa. Am J Hypertens 2003; 16(10):847–52.
307. Ambrosius WT, Bloem LJ, Zhou L, et al. Genetic variants in the epithelial sodium channel in relation to aldosterone and potassium excretion and risk for hypertension. Hypertension 1999; 34(4 Pt 1):631–7.
308. Matsubara M, Ohkubo T, Michimata M, et al. Japanese individuals do not harbor the T594M mutation but do have the P592S mutation in the C-terminus of the beta-subunit of the epithelial sodium channel: the Ohasama study. J Hypertens 2000; 18(7):861–6.
309. Hollier JM, Martin DF, Bell DM, et al. Epithelial sodium channel allele T594M is not associated with blood pressure or blood pressure response to amiloride. Hypertension 2006; 47(3):428–33.
310. Cui Y, Su YR, Rutkowski M, et al. Loss of protein kinase C inhibition in the beta-T594M variant of the amiloride-sensitive Na+ channel. Proc Natl Acad Sci USA 1997; 94(18): 9962–6.
311. Fouladkou F, Alikhani-Koopaei R, Vogt B, et al. A naturally occurring human Nedd4-2 variant displays impaired ENaC regulation in *Xenopus laevis* oocytes. Am J Physiol Renal Physiol 2004; 287(3):F550–61.
312. Busjahn A, Aydin A, Uhlmann R, et al. Serum- and glucocorticoid-regulated kinase (SGK1) gene and blood pressure. Hypertension 2002; 40(3):256–60.

3
The Sodium-Hydrogen Exchange System

Peter A. Doris
Center for Human Genetics, Institute of Molecular Medicine, University of Texas Health Science Center, Houston, Texas, U.S.A.

INTRODUCTION

Eukaryotic cells are separated from their surrounding aqueous environment by a lipid bilayer membrane. This cell membrane encloses the soluble cell proteins and is largely impermeable to them. These proteins are predominantly negatively charged at normal cellular pH and are neutralized by potassium ions, which are much more abundant in the intracellular fluid (~150 meq/L) than the extracellular fluid (~4 meq/L). The cell membrane is permeable to potassium ions, allowing these ions to enter and neutralize negatively charged proteins. However, the proteins generate an osmotic effect that tends to draw water into the cells across the relatively water-permeable membrane. Swelling of cells is prevented by opposing the osmotic pressure generated by intracellular proteins with a high concentration of sodium ions outside the cell (~140 meq/L), while maintaining a low intracellular sodium content (~15 meq/L). This distribution of ions is essential to protect the cell from bursting as a result of osmotic swelling.

Identification of the mechanism responsible for generating asymmetric distribution of ions across the cell membrane engaged fundamental cell physiology research for several decades in the last century. Ultimately it was proven that the transmembrane (TM) gradient of sodium is sustained by an energy-dependent secretory process to remove sodium from inside the cell, which in turn lead to the identification of a membrane ATPase that transports sodium ions asymmetrically from inside the cell in exchange for potassium ions outside the cell (1,2). The electrochemical gradient provided by this energy-driven distribution of sodium ions provides the driving force that animates the biological roles played by a large family of sodium–proton exchangers that have become specialized to permit intestinal absorption of dietary sodium, to maintain cell volume in the face of osmotic shrinkage, to remove excess protons resulting from metabolism, to maintain the pH and sodium ion content of intracellular organelles, to contribute to renal tubular mechanisms involved in bulk reabsorption of sodium by the proximal tubule, and to support acid secretion by the stomach and the distal renal tubule.

FUNDAMENTAL ASPECTS

Studies of the sodium–proton exchanger have their origins in the work of Peter Mitchell, whose chemiosmotic hypothesis of mitochondrial coupling of electron transport and ATP synthesis to proton gradients envisioned the necessity of facilitated cation/proton exchange across an otherwise impermeable mitochondrial membrane (3,4). The biological activity of the transporter was first demonstrated in a prokaryote, *Streptococcus faecalis*, in 1972 (5). Murer and colleagues demonstrated the activity of the sodium–proton exchanger in mammalian cells in 1976 (6) and the fundamental facets of the function of the exchanger came clearly into focus. The mammalian sodium–proton exchanger is a tightly coupled, electroneutral exchanger with a stoichiometry of 1 proton:1 sodium ion. The exchange reaction is bi-directional with TM chemical gradients of sodium and protons providing the proximal driving force. Normally, the inward diffusional gradient for sodium ions is created by active transport of sodium out of the cell by sodium–potassium-ATPase (Na^+–K^+-ATPase) this allows sodium to enter the cell via the sodium–proton exchanger which, in turn, drives cellular proton extrusion from the cytoplasm. Internal pH (pH_i) is a major factor regulating activity of the exchanger with increasing intracellular proton concentration providing a powerful stimulus to activity. These advances in functional insight were soon followed by the emergence of molecular genetic techniques that have laid the foundation for understanding the structural and functional diversity of the many isoforms of the sodium–proton exchanger encoded in the mammalian genome.

Cloning of the first sodium–proton exchanger, NHE-1, was accomplished by Pouysségur and colleagues who used an expression strategy to identify a cDNA that, when expressed in antiporter-deficient fibroblast cells (7), was able to protect the cells from an otherwise lethal intracellular acidification challenge (8). The availability of a single NHE cDNA sequence provided important leverage to the search for other NHE genes whose existence was anticipated because of differences in the pharmacological responsiveness and hormonal regulation observed in in vitro studies. Homology cloning using low stringency hybridization to the NHE-1 cDNA probe rapidly resulted in the cloning of NHE-2, -3, and -4 (9–12) and allowed comparison of the inferred amino acid sequences. Secondary structures predicted from the sequences were examined to illuminate structural homologies and differences among NHE family members and tissue distribution patterns were also established. A fifth member of the NHE family was soon recognized and four additional members have now been identified which appear to serve specific intracellular organelle functions. In addition, a sperm-specific isoform necessary for flagellar activity and fertility has been identified (13). The NHE family is outlined in Table 1.

THE NHE GENE FAMILY: EVOLUTIONARY ORIGINS AND HOMOLOGIES

A number of schema have been developed to define NHE-specific protein motifs and have been subsequently applied to the rapidly-growing number of genome sequence databases for a wide range of organisms to identify and classify evolutionary relationships among NHE proteins. Collectively, these proteins belong to the cation proton antiporter (CPA) family as defined in the Transport Protein Database (14–16). CPA1 and CPA2 proteins are eukaryotic, having evolved from prokaryotic precursors. All known, characterized mammalian NHE's, except the sperm-specific NHE protein, belong to the CPA1 group. The sperm NHE shows greatest homology to ancestral prokaryotic progenitors of CPA1 and CPA2 proteins. CPA2 proteins, generally referred to as NhaA proteins in prokaryotes, exist in the genomes of higher eukaryotes, but are presently functionally uncharacterized. The eukaryotic CPA1 genes share ancestry with NhaP genes in prokaryotes that transport

Table 1 The NHE Protein Family in Mammals

Isoform	Tissues expressing	Subcellular distribution	Gene name	Evolutionary emergence
NHE1	Widespread	Cell membrane, basolateral surface of polarized epithelia	Slc9a1	Vertebrates
NHE2	Intestine, muscle, kidney, brain	Cell membrane, apical surface of polarized epithelia	Slc9a2	Vertebrates
NHE3	Intestine, kidney	Cell membrane, apical surface and recycling endosomes or polarized epithelia	Slc9a3	Invertebrates
NHE4	Stomach, kidney, brain	Cell membrane, basolateral surface of polarized epithelia	Slc9a4	Vertebrates
NHE5	Brain	Cell membrane, synaptic vesicles	Slc9a5	Invertebrates
NHE6	Widespread	Recycling endosomes (early)	Slc9a6	Fungi
NHE7	Widespread	trans-Golgi	Slc9a7	Fungi
NHE8	Widespread	trans-Golgi	Slc9a8	Slime mold
NHE9	Widespread	Recycling endosomes (late)	Slc9a9	Fungi
Sperm NHE	Spermatozoa	Flagella	Slc9a10	—

Na^+ or Li^+ in exchange for H^+. In prokaryotes the coupling stoichiometry of the NhaP transporters is $1Na^+{:}2H^+$. The prokaryotic carriers are energized by proton gradients created by H^+-ATPases (in contrast to the Na^+–K^+-ATPases that generate the sodium gradient exploited by NHE in higher eukaryotes) and their action to extrude sodium and facilitate proton entry allows prokaryote survival and growth in high sodium and alkaline environments.

The comprehensive analysis provided by Brett and colleagues offers a rigorous and broad assessment of the evolutionary origins and relationships of the NHE family members (17). Brett and colleagues divide these transporters into two clades: plasma membrane and intracellular NHE's, with the plasma membrane clade further subdivisible into resident and recycling clusters (17). In the plasma membrane clade, the membrane resident cluster appears to be a relatively recent evolutionary occurrence and emerges first in early vertebrates (18), while lacking orthologs in plants and yeast. The recycling cluster appears to be older with early orthologs emerging in nematodes and insects (19,20). Among the intracellular clade, the endosomal cluster is quite ancient with early representatives in yeast (21) where their role as endosomal contributors to salt sequestration, regulation of vacuolar pH and vesicle trafficking are established (22–24). The vacuolar NHE cluster are represented strongly among plant species where they play important roles in adaptation to salt and osmotic stresses (25,26). The plant members of this group appear to transport both Na^+ and K^+ in exchange for H^+(27) and some forms at least have been shown to regulate vacuolar pH (25,26). Finally the NHE-8-like intracellular cluster has its earliest ortholog in slime molds (28) and representatives are also present in invertebrates and vertebrates, though not in plants (17). This group is not fully functionally characterized.

STRUCTURE–FUNCTION RELATIONSHIPS

Hydropathy analysis of the NHE amino acid sequences from mammals predicts a 12 trans-membrane-spanning domain topology with intracytoplasmic N- and C-terminal sequences. The fundamental TM topology seems to have emerged early as electron cryomicroscopy studies of the NhaP from *Escherichia coli* indicate a similar topography (29). A wide range of additional experimental data lends support to and extends insight into the organization of the TM domains in mammals. These include studies that have attempted to localize immunological epitopes to the interior or exterior of the cells (30), studies to examine glycosylation sites (31), studies of protease cleavage (32) and of intra- versus extracellular accessibility of cysteine-binding sulfhydryl reagents to cysteine substitutions (33). The latter studies have been particularly thoroughly exploited and have suggested additional subtlety to the membrane insertion in which the intracellular loops between segments TM4 and TM5 as well as TM8 and TM9 and the extracellular loop between TM9 and TM10 re-enter the membrane bilayer, but do not penetrate it (Fig. 1). These segments may face into and line a membrane pore that contains an aqueous milieu and that is accessible from both sides of the cell membrane (33). Some evidence suggests that NHE-1 and NHE-3 form stable, functional homodimers in the cell membrane (34).

NHE-1 and NHE-2 appear to be glycosylated, while NHE-3 is not (31). NHE-1 is N-glycosylated at the Asn-75 residue of the N-terminal chain (31), while NHE-2 has only O-glycosylation sites (35). The functional significance of this post-translational modification, if any, has not emerged. Sequence conservation among the human isoforms of NHE is highest in the region of TM6 and TM7 with approximately 95% amino acid

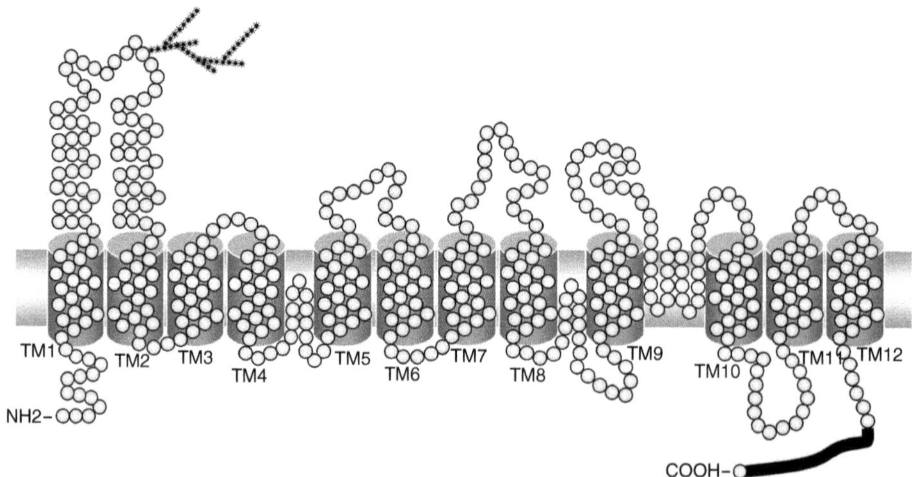

Figure 1 Topology model of human NHE-1.The 12 transmembrane (TM) domain structure is a common feature of NHE proteins that emerges early in the evolution of these proteins. This model has recently been extended particularly through studies in which targeted mutation of residues to cysteine has been used to create sites that can be tagged by thiol-reactive compounds applied either at the extra- or intracellular surface. This work has somewhat revised previous models and now incorporates two intracellular loops that enter, but do not completely penetrate the cell membrane. These loops appear to be accessible from the extracellular surface and may participate in the formation and lining of the TM pore. *Source*: From Ref. 33.

identity, implying conservation of critical functions within this region. This implication is borne out by amino acid substitution experiments that show that E^{262} in TM7 is critical for proton translocation (34). Ion transport activity of NHE isoforms resident in the plasma membrane display $[H^+]$ relationship greater than first order, indicating a possible co-operative allosteric mechanism in which an internal site may be subject to $[H^+]$-dependent modification that amplifies the effect of increasing $[H^+]$ at the proton transport site (36). Some insight into this mechanism has emerged from mutation studies of residues in and around the TM11 of the human NHE-1 that have implicated residues R^{440}, G^{445}, and G^{446} in modifying sensitivity of the transport mechanism to pH_i (37). It is also possible that the formation of exchanger homodimers provides another means by which cooperative proton binding may occur. Only one residue in the human NHE-1, F^{162}, has been shown to be critical for Na^+ binding (38). In contrast to high conservation pressures on these core functional elements of the transporter, conservation in the N- and C-terminals is weak. The C-terminal region appears to function as an important location to which isoform-specific regulatory mechanisms are targeted and is discussed further below.

ISOFORM-SPECIFICITY OF TRANSPORT INHIBITORS

Two major classes of NHE inhibitory drugs are recognized and contain either a pyrazinylcarbonylguanidine (such as amiloride and its derivatives) or a benzoylguanidine nucleus (e.g., HOE642, cariporide) (Fig. 2). The guanidine moiety is protonated at physiological pH. Development of inhibitors of NHE has been advanced by studies showing that sodium and guanidine function as simple competitors that appear to act at the same extracellular sodium binding site (39), presumably this competition occurs between the protonated guanidinium group in the inhibitor and sodium ions. Amiloride lacks specificity and shows cross-inhibition of epithelial sodium channels as well as the sodium–calcium exchanger (40). Drug development using amiloride as a lead compound involved further substitution of the 5-amino group of the pyrazine ring and has yielded a number of derivatives, such as ethylisopropylamiloride, and 5-*N*-methylpropylamiloride that show greater specificity as selective NHE inhibitors. However, isoform specificity remains relatively weak with greatest potency towards NHE-1 > NHE-2 > NHE-5 > NHE-3.

Further pharmacological development lead to the emergence of the benzoylguanidines including cariporide (HOE642) and related compounds (HOE694, eniporide), which show much greater isoform selectivity to NHE-1 and have become useful tools to evaluate the clinical opportunities provided by selective NHE-1 inhibition. As competitive inhibitors of the sodium ion, these drugs are active in their protonated form. While amiloride and closely related derivatives are fully protonated at physiological pH, some of these drugs (e.g., cariporide, $pK_a = 6.2$) demonstrate the particularly useful property of having pK_a's that result in the formation of active protonated forms of the drug under ischemic conditions, while under normoxic conditions at physiological pH they are present as uncharged forms of lower activity. Selective NHE-3 inhibitors, notably S3226, have now also emerged (41).

Pharmacological inhibitors of NHE have provided a further tool to investigate the structure–function relationships within the protein. Amiloride appears to act, as would be expected on the basis of its competition with sodium ions, from the extracellular surface (42). A single point mutation in NHE-1 (L^{167} to F^{167}) that lies in the middle of the TM4 domain, along with gene amplification of this allele, provided the basis for amiloride resistance (43). This insight provides some understanding of the isoform specificity of

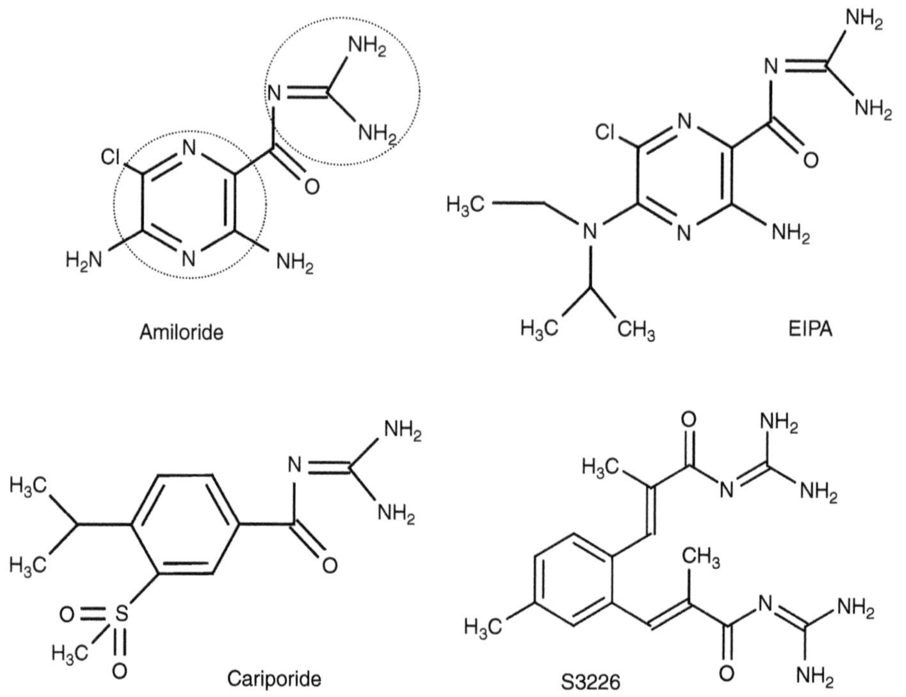

Figure 2 Structures of important pharmacological inhibitors of NHE. The pyrazine ring and guanidine moiety of amiloride are circled. The ionizable guanidine group is common to these inhibitors and may act as a competitor of extracellular sodium binding. EIPA shares the same core structure features of amiloride. Its 5′ alkyl substitutions confer increased potency over amiloride and increased specificity for NHE inhibition. The development of benzoylguanidine derivatives such as cariporide provided potent inhibitors of NHE that lack any inhibitory activity on Na/Ca^{2+} exchangers and Na^+ channels, and are more selective inhibitors of NHE-1 that are inactive against NHE-3 and NHE-5. Further development has lead to inhibitors that demonstrate high specificity for NHE-3, such as S3226.

inhibition by amiloride and related agents. The amiloride resistant NHE-3 isoform has a phenylalanine at the residue that corresponds with the leucine that is mutated to phenylalanine to produce amiloride resistance in NHE-1. There is also some evidence that the TM9 domain may contribute to amiloride sensitivity. Based on observations that the histidine modifier, diethyl pyrocarbonate, inhibits NHE-1, Wang and colleagues used a histidine mutation approach to identify several histidines in this region that are able to modify amiloride sensitivity (44). Thus, both TM4 and TM9 seem to participate in amiloride-mediated inhibition.

ISOFORM FUNCTION AND REGULATION

Sodium–Proton Exchangers of Endocellular Membranes

Sodium–proton exchangers NHE-6, -7, -8, and -9 represent a distinct evolutionary clade (17). Within this clade, NHE-6 and -7 show a high degree of homology (approximately 70% amino acid identity) with greatest conservation occurring in their TM domains. NHE-9 is ~55% identical to NHE-6 and -7. NHE-8 is the most evolutionarily remote isoform, being only 25% identical with the other endomembrane sodium–proton exchangers. The ubiquitous expression of members of this group is indicative of a housekeeping role. Indeed, when NHE-6 was first identified it was reported to have characteristics consistent with the long-sought mitochondrial NHE with the potential to fulfill mitochondrial proton exchanges required by Mitchell's chemiosomotic coupling model. This identification was based, in part, on homology with a yeast NHE for which evidence of a mitochondrial localization was developed (45). Subsequent cloning and sequencing of the human homolog, thereafter called NHE-6, allowed co-localization studies to be performed that suggested distribution of green fluorescent protein (GFP)-tagged NHE-6 to intra-cellular vesicles which overlapped the distribution of a mitochondrial marker dye (46). Further evidence in support of this assignment included the abundant distribution of NHE-6 to highly metabolically active tissues and the presence of a positively charged N-terminus that might serve as a mitochondrial targeting signal. However, studies in COS-7 cells showed that the acidic, putative mitochondrial targeting amino terminus of NHE-6, resulted in targeting of a GFP-fusion protein containing this portion of the NHE-6 to the endoplasmic reticulum. The amino terminal hydrophobic segment of NHE-6 was found to direct sorting to the secretory pathway and was subsequently cleaved (47). This evidence of NHE-6 localization to the secretory pathway, rather than mitochondrial membranes, was further substantiated by Brett and colleagues whose work with C-terminal GFP-tagged NHE-6 also supported co-distribution with markers of the endosomal compartment (48). Nakamura and colleagues have added more evidence against a mitochondrial role, but place the NHE-6 protein in the early endosomal, rather than secretory compartment where it was found to colocalize with the early endosome marker protein EEA1 (49). Consequently, the molecular identity of an authentic mitochondrial sodium–proton exchanger remains elusive.

NHE-7 is principally localized to the trans-Golgi network (TGN) and related endosomes, based on co-localization with TGN marker proteins (45,49). NHE-7 mediates the exchange of either Na^+ or K^+ for H^+. Since K^+ is the main intracellular cation, NHE-7 may serve as an H^+ efflux pathway from TGN and also contribute to the volume and growth of the TGN through K^+ influx from the cytoplasm to the TGN lumen. The pH of the vesicular compartments of the secretory and endocytosic pathways is different from that of the cytoplasm and appears to be tightly regulated and to influence function in these pathways. The vacuolar H-ATPase provides active transport of protons into the subcellular organelles. However, pH within these compartments seems to be principally determined by a leak mechanism in which K^+ is exchanged for H^+ by the NHE proteins of this compartment. In the secretory pathway pH declines along the pathway from about pH 7.1 in ER, ~pH 6.5 in the Golgi, ~pH 6.0 in the TGN, and ~pH 5.0 in secretory granules. Similarly, early and late endosomes become more acidic as their cargo moves towards the lysosomes (pH 6.5–4.5) (50–52). Sorting and post-translational modification of newly synthesized proteins and trafficking and proteolytic degradation of proteins in endocytosed compartments may be dependent on modification of the pH within these sub-cellular compartments (53). While the catalytic properties of NHE-6 have not yet been reported, the sequence similarity with NHE-7 suggest that they may overlap with the latter's catalytic and functional properties.

NHE-8 has also been recently shown to transport both Na^+ and K^+ in exchange for H^+ and over-expression was found to result in luminal alkalinization of the mid to trans-Golgi compartment in which it was found to reside (49). Similarly, the most recently identified member of the mammalian NHE family, NHE-9, has also been show to be associated with endomembranes where it co-localizes with the late endosomes (49). Thus, it appears that the endomembrane NHE's share unique, though partially overlapping distributions to membrane sub-compartments and, by virtue of their capacity to act as proton leak pathways, oppose the acidifying action of vacuolar H^+-ATPase to provide regulation of acidity and fluid volume of endosomal membranes, thereby supporting their specialized functions. Current knowledge of the regulation of activity of these isoforms is very limited.

Sodium–Proton Exchangers of the Plasma Membrane (Recycling)

Two members of the NHE family, NHE-3 and NHE-5, have been not only shown to be predominantly localized to the plasma membrane, but to also undergo internalization by clathrin-coated pit mechanisms (54,55). These two isoforms have distinct distribution profiles with NHE-3 being a major participant in the epithelial sodium reabsorptive process of the gut and kidney localizing to the apical membrane, while NHE-5 is a brain-specific isoform enriched in brain regions of high neuronal density. In addition to its apical membrane role in bulk sodium flux, NHE-3 may also provide pH regulation of early endosomes originating from apical membrane by clathrin-coated pit mechanisms. This pH regulation may contribute to receptor-mediated endocytosis, an important mechanism by which filtered urinary protein is recovered from the tubular lumen. NHE-3 inhibition reduces uptake of albumin by endocytosis, diminishes degradation of internalized protein and reduces the rate of endocytic vesicle fusion, suggesting integration between the ion transport and recycling functions of the exchanger (56,57).

Epithelial distribution of NHE-3 in the renal tubule is non-uniform with the proximal tubule of the kidney (the site of bulk sodium reabsorption) and the medullary thick ascending limb having the highest density. Use of specific NHE-3 inhibitor, S3226, demonstrates the important contribution of the isoform to proximal tubular reabsorption (58). Apical entry of luminal sodium is facilitated by the NHE-3 isoform, which uses protons provided by the intracellular action of carbonic anhydrase that generates bicarbonate and protons from water and carbon dioxide. Distribution to the gastrointestinal tract suggests an important role of this isoform in both gut absorptive as well as renal reabsorptive dimensions of body sodium balance. Development of the NHE-3 knockout mouse provides further support for this view. These animals have volume-contraction (reflected in increased renin and aldosterone levels), mild diarrhea with alkalinization of the gut contents, reduced proximal tubule fluid reabsorption, reduced blood pressure and mild acidosis (59,60).

The functional role of NHE-5 is much less well understood. When epitope-tagged NHE-5 was transiently expressed in neuroendocrine cells localization studies indicated the presence of NHE-5 in perinuclear vesicles and along cell processes (55). These vesicles co-distribute with transferrin, a marker of the recycling endosome compartment. Positional mapping approaches have suggested that NHE-5 may be a susceptibility gene for a neurological disease, paroxysmal kinesigenic dyskinesia, however, this positional candidate gene was not found to contain causative mutations in affected individuals (61).

NHE-3 regulation has been very well studied. Transporters involved in unidirectional epithelial reabsorption function in this role only when they are inserted in the plasma membrane. Thus, regulation of NHE-3 in bulk sodium reabsorption heavily exploits the effect of endosomal internalization to remove transport protein from the plasma membrane as a means of modulating V_{max} activity of the transporter. The apparatus to effect such regulation is rather complex. NHE-3 contains two serine residues in the C-terminus that are targets of regulatory phosphorylation, Ser^{552} and Ser^{605} (62). Agents such as dopamine and parathyroid hormone activate cAMP production leading to activation of protein kinase A (PKA), phosphorylation of the NHE-3 C-terminus and inhibition of NHE-3 activity (63–66). Inhibition of activity correlates with removal of a sub-population of NHE-3 from the apical membrane by clathrin-mediated internalization. The actin cytoskeleton appears to confer stable apical membrane localization on a subpopulation of renal epithelial NHE-3 that may escape clathrin-mediated internalization (67,68). This cytoskeletal interaction requires the sustained action of Rho GTPases. Disruption of apical microvilli using the Rho GTPase disruptor, TxB, occurs through altered cytoskeletal structure and leads to a rapid redistribution of NHE-3 from the apical membrane (69). The bridging of NHE-3 to the cytoskeleton results from interactions between ezrin, a protypical member of the ezrin/radixin/moesin (ERM) protein family that is abundant in apical microvilli, and actin filaments (70). In turn, ezrin interacts through its N-terminal domain with both of the NHE regulatory proteins, NHERF-1 and -2 (71). Ezrin may also act as a PKA anchor protein, allowing spatial coordination that facilitates phosphorylation of proteins in this complex (72). The two NHERF proteins mediate the PKA inhibitory action on NHE-3 in a manner that requires binding to the cytoplasmic tail of NHE-3 (73). This interaction then allows the proximity of PKA anchored by ezrin to phosphorylate the C-terminus of NHE-3 leading to inhibition.

Other avenues of ezrin-dependent regulation of NHE-3 may exist, and are suggested by experiments in which NHERF-1 knockout and expression of mutant NHERF-1 did not lead to altered apical content of NHE-3 (74,75). Ezrin is also a target of phosphorylation. This appears to result from a mean arterial pressure (MAP) kinase pathway leading to activation of Akt. Purified Akt is able to directly phosphorylate ezrin at THE567 and to activate NHE-3 by increasing translocation (76). Thus the membrane–cytoskeleton interactions between NHE-3, NHERF's, PKA, ezrin, and actin provide a focal point for convergence of regulatory mechanisms that act to control sodium entry and proton exit by altering the subcellular distribution of NHE-3 to or from the apical membrane, thereby endowing the membrane with a greater or lower V_{max} of NHE-3 activity.

Although much less well studied, regulation of NHE-5 may share some features with regulation of NHE-3. For example, NHE-5 appears to undergo clathrin-mediated endocytosis that requires a dynamin-dependent cytoskeletal involvement and is partially mediated by the action of phosphatidylinositol 3′-kinase (55). Mechanisms of internalization of NHE-5 overlap with that of internalizing seven-membrane-spanning G-protein coupled receptors in utilizing beta-arrestin as an adaptor protein to recruit other proteins of the internalization machinery (77). Arrestins recognize phospho-serine and phospho-threonine residues in the internal sequences of internalizing G-protein-coupled receptors and promote interactions with adaptor proteins and clathrin. Serine and threonine residues exist in the C-terminus of NHE-5 that are potential sites of phosphorylation leading to arrestin binding and this phosphorylation might be provided by PKA and/or PKC which have been shown to affect the activity of NHE-5 (78). However, at present, direct evidence linking these protein kinases to phosphorylation of NHE-5 and linking such phosphorylation to beta-arrestin recruitment is lacking. The precise function of NHE-5 is open to speculation. It may play a role in general neuronal pH and volume regulation and it may also function in neuron-specific actions, which might include acidification of early endosomes. Thus such endosomes containing both NHE-5 and liganded G-protein coupled receptors might permit NHE-5 to contribute to rapid de-phosphorylation and re-sensitization of the G protein-coupled receptors.

Sodium–Proton Exchangers Resident in the Plasma Membrane

NHE-1 is the most widely distributed and best-studied member of the sodium–proton antiporter family. It is present almost exclusively at the plasma membrane, but may concentrate within specific regions of the plasma membrane, for example near the intercalated disks and adjacent transverse tubules of cardiac muscle cells (79), and around lamellipodia in fibroblasts (80). This prototypical family member also serves the two classic functions of the NHE family: regulation of intracellular pH and of cell volume. Allosteric regulation by intracellular pH provides a key mechanism to counterbalance metabolic acidification. While restoration of cell volume during osmotic shrinkage exploits NHE-1-mediated sodium entry coupled with Cl^- and water uptake, providing an osmotic counter-response leading to increased water entry.

Activation of NHE-1 is extremely sensitive to pH. The exchanger is essentially inactive at physiological intracellular pH, but is rapidly activated by small declines in pH (81). While this predominant allosteric regulation by intracellular proton concentration is central, superimposed on it is regulation of NHE-1 by a range of signaling pathways, which appear to converge on the intracellular C-terminus of the protein. Some of these pathways act on NHE-1 by phosphorylation and constitutive phosphorylation of NHE-1 in quiescent cells is increased in response to growth factor stimulation. Three protein kinases, p160/ROCK, p90 ribosomal S6 kinase ($p90^{RSK}$) and Nck-interacting kinase (NIK) have been implicated directly in NHE-1 phosphorylation. The Rho-associated kinase p160/ROCK acts downstream of RhoA and may integrate signaling from integrin receptors and focal adhesion complexes that adjust exchanger activity in relation to surface attachments of the cell (82). Activation of cell growth by serum stimulates NHE-1 activity and this may be driven by the capacity of the MAP kinase target, $p90^{RSK}$ kinase, to phosphorylate the Ser^{703} residue on the C-terminus of NHE-1. Mutation of $p90^{RSK}$ to prevent its kinase activity inhibits the serum-induced phosphorylation of NHE-1 at Ser^{703} (83). The platelet-derived growth factor receptor–related kinase, NIK, contains two distinct regions that are able to bind to and phosphorylate NHE-1 and full activation of NHE-1 by NIK requires both binding and phosphorylation (84).

Other regulatory mechanisms targeting the C-terminus of NHE-1 may not require its phosphorylation. Activation of NHE-1 by osmotic stress (85,86) and by ATP depletion (87) occur without a change in exchanger phosphorylation. Similarly, NHE-1 interacts with calmodulin to permit calcium-modulation of exchanger activity. Two calmodulin binding sites exist in the C-terminal region of NHE-1 (88). The site at residues 636–656 has high affinity ($K_D \sim 20$ nM). One model of the interaction at this site draws on evidence that, in the absence of calmodulin binding, NHE-1 is constitutively active and proposes that calcium binding to calmodulin releases the exchanger from an auto-inhibited state and increases proton export (89). Like NHE-3, NHE-1 may also be regulated by interactions with cytoskeletal proteins that are bridged by the ERM protein ezrin. In contrast to NHE-3 where the ezrin interaction is mediated by NHERF proteins, NHE-1 binds directly to ezrin and ezrin and NHE-1 are both enriched in fibroblast membranes at the lamellipodia (90). While this interaction may influence NHE-1 activity, it may also serve to modify the cytoskeletal organization in this region.

NHE-2 is an important mediator of sodium–proton exchange in the apical epithelium of the gastrointestinal tract (91). Its renal distribution is limited to the cortical thick ascending limb, macula densa, distal convoluted tubules and connecting tubules (92,93). In the distal nephron, and perhaps also the loop of Henlé, NHE-2 may be the primary sodium–proton exchanger and consequently contributes to distal bicarbonate reabsorption (94). NHE-2 is not detected in the recycling endosomes and therefore, like

NHE-1, is likely to be a plasma membrane-resident transporter. The secondary role of NHE-2 in gut and renal sodium–proton exchange is suggested by the phenotype of young NHE-2 knockout mice that show relatively normal intestinal and renal transport function (59). In contrast, as these NHE-2 knockout animals mature from juvenile to adult animals they reveal progressive degeneration of gastric parietal and zymogenic cells (95) and reduced parotid gland secretion (96). The impressive gastric phenotype in mature NHE-2 knockout animals is associated principally with necrotic loss of parietal cells. The absence of disruption of acid secretion in young NHE-2 knockout animals points to an important role of this isoform in the persistence of viability of gastric parietal cells, rather than directly in acid secretion. Based on understanding of the biochemical properties of NHE-2, in particular its maximal activation by extracellular pH greater than nine (97), it has been proposed that the gastric role of this isoform may include a basolateral function to respond to the alkaline change in basolateral pH that accompanies acid secretion from the parietal cell (95). By working in unison with other transporters at this location, including the Na^+–K^+-ATPase, the Cl^-/HCO_3^- exchanger and perhaps the Na^+–K^+–$2Cl^-$ transporter, NHE-2 may participate in the maintenance of cell volume and ionic homeostasis necessary to support acid secretion (95).

NHE-4 is another non-recycling isoform that exhibits very high expression in stomach and much lower levels in kidney, pancreas, salivary glands, and some brain regions (9,98,99). In the kidney, NHE-4 exists in basolateral membranes of a wide range of nephron segments with greatest abundance in the thick ascending limb and distal convoluted tubule with lower abundance in collecting ducts and proximal tubule. In the stomach, NHE-4 protein is located in basolateral plasma membranes of cells lining the gastric glands (100). NHE-4 mRNA is abundant in parietal and chief cells and less abundant in mucous cells (101). The recent development of an NHE-4 knockout model has informed discussion of the gastrointestinal role of this isoform (102). Absence of NHE-4 results in greatly reduced gastric acid secretion, a phenotype not dissimilar to that obtained by deletion of the Cl^-/HCO_3^- transporter (AE2) that also localizes to the parietal cell basolateral membrane (103). It is proposed, therefore, that these two exchangers couple to provide support for the secretion of HCl at the brush border. In this paradigm, NHE-4 drives sodium entry and proton export at the basolateral surface while AE2 permits chloride entry with bicarbonate loss. The resulting sodium and chloride influx supports acid secretion in part by supporting the maintenance of cell volume while acid secretion at the brush border depletes cell volume. The entering Cl^- also supports acid secretion by becoming available for apical secretion. The entry of sodium via NHE-4 contributes substrate (sodium ions) used to drive the basolateral entry of potassium mediated by Na^+–K^+-ATPase. These potassium ions can then be secreted at the brush border to provide substrate for the apical K^+–H^+-ATPase that drives proton delivery from the parietal cell to the gastric lumen in exchange for luminal potassium. The complex combined functions of these transporters achieve both acid secretion and the maintenance of parietal cell volume during secretion. Loss of NHE-4 function interrupts these relationships and consequently places severe limits on the acid secretion capacity of the parietal cell.

REFERENCES

1. Post RL. Seeds of sodium, potassium ATPase. Annu Rev Physiol 1989; 51:1–15.
2. Skou JC. Nobel lecture. The identification of the sodium pump. Biosci Rep 1998; 18:155–69.

3. Mitchell P. Coupling of phosphorylation to electron and hydrogen transfer by a chemiosmotic type of mechanism. Nature 1961; 191:144–8.
4. Mitchell P, Moyle J. Proton translocation coupled to ATP hydrolysis in rat liver mitochondria. Eur J Biochem 1968; 4:530–9.
5. Harold FM, Papineau D. Cation transport and electrogenesis by *Streptococcus faecalis*. II. Proton and sodium extrusion. J Membr Biol 1972; 8:45–62.
6. Murer H, Hopfer U, Kinne R. Sodium/proton antiport in brush-border-membrane vesicles isolated from rat small intestine and kidney. Biochem J 1976; 154:597–604.
7. Pouyssegur J, Sardet C, Franchi A, et al. A specific mutation abolishing Na^+/H^+ antiport activity in hamster fibroblasts precludes growth at neutral and acidic pH. Proc Natl Acad Sci USA 1984; 81:4833–7.
8. Sardet C, Franchi A, Pouyssegur J. Molecular cloning, primary structure, and expression of the human growth factor-activatable Na^+/H^+ antiporter. Cell 1989; 56:271–80.
9. Orlowski J, Kandasamy RA, Shull GE. Molecular cloning of putative members of the Na/H exchanger gene family. cDNA cloning, deduced amino acid sequence, and mRNA tissue expression of the rat Na/H exchanger NHE-1 and two structurally related proteins. J Biol Chem 1992; 267:9331–9.
10. Tse CM, Brant SR, Walker MS, et al. Cloning and sequencing of a rabbit cDNA encoding an intestinal and kidney-specific Na^+/H^+ exchanger isoform (NHE-3). J Biol Chem 1992; 267:9340–6.
11. Tse CM, Levine SA, Yun CH, et al. Cloning and expression of a rabbit cDNA encoding a serum-activated ethylisopropylamiloride-resistant epithelial Na^+/H^+ exchanger isoform (NHE-2). J Biol Chem 1993; 268:11917–24.
12. Wang Z, Orlowski J, Shull GE. Primary structure and functional expression of a novel gastrointestinal isoform of the rat Na/H exchanger. J Biol Chem 1993; 268:11925–8.
13. Wang D, King SM, Quill TA, et al. A new sperm-specific Na^+/H^+ exchanger required for sperm motility and fertility. Nat Cell Biol 2003; 5:1117–22.
14. http://www.membranetransport.org
15. Busch W, Saier MH, Jr. The transporter classification (TC) system, 2002. Crit Rev Biochem Mol Biol 2002; 37:287–337.
16. Chang AB, Lin R, Keith Studley W, et al. Phylogeny as a guide to structure and function of membrane transport proteins. Mol Membr Biol 2004; 21:171–81.
17. Brett CL, Donowitz M, Rao R. Evolutionary origins of eukaryotic sodium/proton exchangers. Am J Physiol Cell Physiol 2005; 288:C223–39.
18. Claiborne JB, Blackston CR, Choe KP, et al. A mechanism for branchial acid excretion in marine fish: identification of multiple Na^+/H^+ antiporter (NHE) isoforms in gills of two seawater teleosts. J Exp Biol 1999; 202:315–24.
19. Giannakou ME, Dow JA. Characterization of the Drosophila melanogaster alkali-metal/proton exchanger (NHE) gene family. J Exp Biol 2001; 204:3703–16.
20. Nehrke K, Melvin JE. The NHX family of Na^+–H^+ exchangers in *Caenorhabditis elegans*. J Biol Chem 2002; 277:29036–44.
21. Nass R, Cunningham KW, Rao R. Intracellular sequestration of sodium by a novel Na^+/H^+ exchanger in yeast is enhanced by mutations in the plasma membrane H+-ATPase. Insights into mechanisms of sodium tolerance. J Biol Chem 1997; 272:26145–52.
22. Bowers K, Levi BP, Patel FI, et al. The sodium/proton exchanger Nhx1p is required for endosomal protein trafficking in the yeast *Saccharomyces cerevisiae*. Mol Biol Cell 2000; 11:4277–94.
23. Nass R, Rao R. Novel localization of a Na^+/H^+ exchanger in a late endosomal compartment of yeast. Implications for vacuole biogenesis. J Biol Chem 1998; 273:21054–60.
24. Nass R, Rao R. The yeast endosomal Na^+/H^+ exchanger, Nhx1, confers osmotolerance following acute hypertonic shock. Microbiology 1999; 145(Pt 11):3221–8.
25. Ohta M, Hayashi Y, Nakashima A, et al. Introduction of a Na^+/H^+ antiporter gene from Atriplex gmelini confers salt tolerance to rice. FEBS Lett 2002; 532:279–82.

26. Serrano R, Rodriguez-Navarro A. Ion homeostasis during salt stress in plants. Curr Opin Cell Biol 2001; 13:399–404.
27. Venema K, Quintero FJ, Pardo JM, et al. The arabidopsis Na^+/H^+ exchanger AtNHX1 catalyzes low affinity Na^+ and K^+ transport in reconstituted liposomes. J Biol Chem 2002; 277:2413–8.
28. Patel H, Barber DL. A developmentally regulated Na–H exchanger in Dictyostelium discoideum is necessary for cell polarity during chemotaxis. J Cell Biol 2005; 169:321–9.
29. Williams KA. Three-dimensional structure of the ion-coupled transport protein NhaA. Nature 2000; 403:112–5.
30. Winkel GK, Sardet C, Pouyssegur J, et al. Role of cytoplasmic domain of the Na^+/H^+ exchanger in hormonal activation. J Biol Chem 1993; 268:3396–400.
31. Counillon L, Pouyssegur J, Reithmeier RA. The Na^+/H^+ exchanger NHE-1 possesses N- and O-linked glycosylation restricted to the first N-terminal extracellular domain. Biochemistry 1994; 33:10463–9.
32. Scholz W, Albus U, Counillon L, et al. Protective effects of HOE642, a selective sodium–hydrogen exchange subtype 1 inhibitor, on cardiac ischaemia and reperfusion. Cardiovasc Res 1995; 29:260–8.
33. Wakabayashi S, Pang T, Su X, et al. A novel topology model of the human Na(+)/H(+) exchanger isoform 1. J Biol Chem 2000; 275:7942–9.
34. Fafournoux P, Noel J, Pouyssegur J. Evidence that Na^+/H^+ exchanger isoforms NHE1 and NHE3 exist as stable dimers in membranes with a high degree of specificity for homodimers. J Biol Chem 1994; 269:2589–96.
35. Tse CM, Levine SA, Yun CH, et al. Na^+/H^+ exchanger-2 is an O-linked but not an N-linked sialoglycoprotein. Biochemistry 1994; 33:12954–61.
36. Otsu K, Kinsella JL, Koh E, et al. Proton dependence of the partial reactions of the sodium–proton exchanger in renal brush border membranes. J Biol Chem 1992; 267:8089–96.
37. Wakabayashi S, Hisamitsu T, Pang T, et al. Mutations of Arg440 and Gly455/Gly456 oppositely change pH sensing of Na^+/H^+ exchanger 1. J Biol Chem 2003; 278:11828–35.
38. Touret N, Poujeol P, Counillon L. Second-site revertants of a low-sodium-affinity mutant of the Na^+/H^+ exchanger reveal the participation of TM4 into a highly constrained sodium-binding site. Biochemistry 2001; 40:5095–101.
39. Frelin C, Vigne P, Barbry P, et al. Interaction of guanidinium and guanidinium derivatives with the Na^+/H^+ exchange system. Eur J Biochem 1986; 154:241–5.
40. Masereel B, Pochet L, Laeckmann D. An overview of inhibitors of Na(+)/H(+) exchanger. Eur J Med Chem 2003; 38:547–54.
41. Schwark JR, Jansen HW, Lang HJ, et al. S3226, a novel inhibitor of Na^+/H^+ exchanger subtype 3 in various cell types. Pflugers Arch 1998; 436:797–800.
42. Grinstein S, Smith JD. Asymmetry of the Na^+/H^+ antiport of dog red cell ghosts. Sidedness of inhibition by amiloride. J Biol Chem 1987; 262:9088–92.
43. Counillon L, Franchi A, Pouyssegur J. A point mutation of the Na^+/H^+ exchanger gene (NHE1) and amplification of the mutated allele confer amiloride resistance upon chronic acidosis. Proc Natl Acad Sci USA 1993; 90:4508–12.
44. Wang D, Balkovetz DF, Warnock DG. Mutational analysis of transmembrane histidines in the amiloride-sensitive Na^+/H^+ exchanger. Am J Physiol 1995; 269:C392–402.
45. Numata M, Orlowski J. Molecular cloning and characterization of a novel $(Na^+, K^+)/H^+$ exchanger localized to the trans-Golgi network. J Biol Chem 2001; 276:17387–94.
46. Numata M, Petrecca K, Lake N, et al. Identification of a mitochondrial Na^+/H^+ exchanger. J Biol Chem 1998; 273:6951–9.
47. Miyazaki E, Sakaguchi M, Wakabayashi S, et al. NHE6 protein possesses a signal peptide destined for endoplasmic reticulum membrane and localizes in secretory organelles of the cell. J Biol Chem 2001; 276:49221–7.
48. Brett CL, Wei Y, Donowitz M, et al. Human Na(+)/H(+) exchanger isoform 6 is found in recycling endosomes of cells, not in mitochondria. Am J Physiol Cell Physiol 2002; 282:C1031–41.

49. Nakamura N, Tanaka S, Teko Y, et al. Four Na^+/H^+ exchanger isoforms are distributed to Golgi and post-Golgi compartments and are involved in organelle pH regulation. J Biol Chem 2005; 280:1561–72.
50. Futai M, Oka T, Sun-Wada G, et al. Luminal acidification of diverse organelles by V-ATPase in animal cells. J Exp Biol 2000; 203:107–16.
51. Mellman I. The importance of being acid: the role of acidification in intracellular membrane traffic. J Exp Biol 1992; 172:39–45.
52. Mellman I, Fuchs R, Helenius A. Acidification of the endocytic and exocytic pathways. Annu Rev Biochem 1986; 55:663–700.
53. Weisz OA. Acidification and protein traffic. Int Rev Cytol 2003; 226:259–319.
54. Chow CW, Khurana S, Woodside M, et al. The epithelial Na(+)/H(+) exchanger, NHE3, is internalized through a clathrin-mediated pathway. J Biol Chem 1999; 274:37551–8.
55. Szaszi K, Paulsen A, Szabo EZ, et al. Clathrin-mediated endocytosis and recycling of the neuron-specific Na^+/H^+ exchanger NHE5 isoform. Regulation by phosphatidylinositol 3′-kinase and the actin cytoskeleton. J Biol Chem 2002; 277:42623–32.
56. D'souza S, Garcia-Cabado A, Yu F, et al. The epithelial sodium–hydrogen antiporter Na^+/H^+ exchanger 3 accumulates and is functional in recycling endosomes. J Biol Chem 1998; 273:2035–43.
57. Gekle M, Freudinger R, Mildenberger S. Inhibition of $Na^+–H^+$ exchanger-3 interferes with apical receptor-mediated endocytosis via vesicle fusion. J Physiol 2001; 531:619–29.
58. Vallon V, Schwark JR, Richter K, et al. Role of Na(+)/H(+) exchanger NHE3 in nephron function: micropuncture studies with S3226, an inhibitor of NHE3. Am J Physiol Renal Physiol 2000; 278:F375–9.
59. Ledoussal C, Lorenz JN, Nieman ML, et al. Renal salt wasting in mice lacking NHE3 Na^+/H^+ exchanger but not in mice lacking NHE2. Am J Physiol Renal Physiol 2001; 281:F718–27.
60. Schultheis PJ, Clarke LL, Meneton P, et al. Renal and intestinal absorptive defects in mice lacking the NHE3 Na^+/H^+ exchanger. Nat Genet 1998; 19:282–5.
61. Spacey SD, Szczygielski BI, Mcrory JE, et al. Mutation analysis of the sodium/hydrogen exchanger gene (NHE5) in familial paroxysmal kinesigenic dyskinesia. J Neural Transm 2002; 109:1189–94.
62. Zhao H, Wiederkehr MR, Fan L, et al. Acute inhibition of Na/H exchanger NHE-3 by cAMP. Role of protein kinase A and NHE-3 phosphoserines 552 and 605. J Biol Chem 1999; 274:3978–87.
63. Bacic D, Kaissling B, Mcleroy P, et al. Dopamine acutely decreases apical membrane Na/H exchanger NHE3 protein in mouse renal proximal tubule. Kidney Int 2003; 64:2133–41.
64. Collazo R, Fan L, Hu MC, et al. Acute regulation of Na^+/H^+ exchanger NHE3 by parathyroid hormone via NHE3 phosphorylation and dynamin-dependent endocytosis. J Biol Chem 2000; 275:31601–8.
65. Hu MC, Fan L, Crowder LA, et al. Dopamine acutely stimulates Na^+/H^+ exchanger (NHE3) endocytosis via clathrin-coated vesicles: dependence on protein kinase A-mediated NHE3 phosphorylation. J Biol Chem 2001; 276:26906–15.
66. Wiederkehr MR, Di Sole F, Collazo R, et al. Characterization of acute inhibition of Na/H exchanger NHE-3 by dopamine in opossum kidney cells. Kidney Int 2001; 59:197–209.
67. Kurashima K, Szabo EZ, Lukacs G, et al. Endosomal recycling of the Na^+/H^+ exchanger NHE3 isoform is regulated by the phosphatidylinositol 3-kinase pathway. J Biol Chem 1998; 273:20828–36.
68. Szaszi K, Kurashima K, Kaibuchi K, et al. Role of the cytoskeleton in mediating cAMP-dependent protein kinase inhibition of the epithelial Na^+/H^+ exchanger NHE3. J Biol Chem 2001; 276:40761–8.
69. Alexander RT, Furuya W, Szaszi K, et al. Rho GTPases dictate the mobility of the Na/H exchanger NHE3 in epithelia: role in apical retention and targeting. Proc Natl Acad Sci USA 2005; 102:12253–8.

70. Yonemura S, Tsukita S, Tsukita S. Direct involvement of ezrin/radixin/moesin (ERM)-binding membrane proteins in the organization of microvilli in collaboration with activated ERM proteins. J Cell Biol 1999; 145:1497–509.
71. Yun CH, Lamprecht G, Forster DV, et al. NHE3 kinase A regulatory protein E3KARP binds the epithelial brush border Na^+/H^+ exchanger NHE3 and the cytoskeletal protein ezrin. J Biol Chem 1998; 273:25856–63.
72. Dransfield DT, Bradford AJ, Smith J, et al. Ezrin is a cyclic AMP-dependent protein kinase anchoring protein. EMBO J 1997; 16:35–43.
73. Weinman EJ, Steplock D, Shenolikar S. Acute regulation of NHE3 by protein kinase A requires a multiprotein signal complex. Kidney Int 2001; 60:450–4.
74. Weinman EJ, Steplock D, Shenolikar S. NHERF-1 uniquely transduces the cAMP signals that inhibit sodium–hydrogen exchange in mouse renal apical membranes. FEBS Lett 2003; 536:141–4.
75. Weinman EJ, Steplock D, Wade JB, et al. Ezrin binding domain-deficient NHERF attenuates cAMP-mediated inhibition of Na(+)/H(+) exchange in OK cells. Am J Physiol Renal Physiol 2001; 281:F374–80.
76. Shiue H, Musch MW, Wang Y, et al. Akt2 phosphorylates ezrin to trigger NHE3 translocation and activation. J Biol Chem 2005; 280:1688–95.
77. Szabo EZ, Numata M, Lukashova V, et al. beta-Arrestins bind and decrease cell-surface abundance of the Na^+/H^+ exchanger NHE5 isoform. Proc Natl Acad Sci USA 2005; 102:2790–5.
78. Attaphitaya S, Nehrke K, Melvin JE. Acute inhibition of brain-specific Na(+)/H(+) exchanger isoform 5 by protein kinases A and C and cell shrinkage. Am J Physiol Cell Physiol 2001; 281:C1146–57.
79. Petrecca K, Atanasiu R, Grinstein S, et al. Subcellular localization of the Na^+/H^+ exchanger NHE1 in rat myocardium. Am J Physiol 1999; 276:H709–17.
80. Grinstein S, Woodside M, Waddell TK, et al. Focal localization of the NHE-1 isoform of the Na^+/H^+ antiport: assessment of effects on intracellular pH. EMBO J 1993; 12:5209–18.
81. Paris S, Pouyssegur J. Biochemical characterization of the amiloride-sensitive Na^+/H^+ antiport in Chinese hamster lung fibroblasts. J Biol Chem 1983; 258:3503–8.
82. Tominaga T, Ishizaki T, Narumiya S, et al. p160ROCK mediates RhoA activation of Na–H exchange. EMBO J 1998; 17:4712–22.
83. Takahashi E, Abe J, Gallis B, et al. p90(RSK) is a serum-stimulated Na^+/H^+ exchanger isoform-1 kinase. Regulatory phosphorylation of serine 703 of Na^+/H^+ exchanger isoform-1. J Biol Chem 1999; 274:20206–14.
84. Yan W, Nehrke K, Choi J, et al. The Nck-interacting kinase (NIK) phosphorylates the Na^+–H^+ exchanger NHE1 and regulates NHE1 activation by platelet-derived growth factor. J Biol Chem 2001; 276:31349–56.
85. Grinstein S, Woodside M, Sardet C, et al. Activation of the Na^+/H^+ antiporter during cell volume regulation. Evidence for a phosphorylation-independent mechanism. J Biol Chem 1992; 267:23823–8.
86. Mcswine RL, Li J, Villereal ML. Examination of the role for Ca2+ in regulation and phosphorylation of the Na^+/H^+ antiporter NHE1 via mitogen and hypertonic stimulation. J Cell Physiol 1996; 168:8–17.
87. Goss GG, Woodside M, Wakabayashi S, et al. ATP dependence of NHE-1, the ubiquitous isoform of the Na^+/H^+ antiporter. Analysis of phosphorylation and subcellular localization. J Biol Chem 1994; 269:8741–8.
88. Bertrand B, Wakabayashi S, Ikeda T, et al. The Na^+/H^+ exchanger isoform 1 (NHE1) is a novel member of the calmodulin-binding proteins. Identification and characterization of calmodulin-binding sites. J Biol Chem 1994; 269:13703–9.
89. Wakabayashi S, Bertrand B, Ikeda T, et al. Mutation of calmodulin-binding site renders the Na^+/H^+ exchanger (NHE1) highly H(+)-sensitive and Ca2+ regulation-defective. J Biol Chem 1994; 269:13710–5.

90. Denker SP, Huang DC, Orlowski J, et al. Direct binding of the Na–H exchanger NHE1 to ERM proteins regulates the cortical cytoskeleton and cell shape independently of H(+) translocation. Mol Cell 2000; 6:1425–36.
91. Hoogerwerf WA, Tsao SC, Devuyst O, et al. NHE2 and NHE3 are human and rabbit intestinal brush-border proteins. Am J Physiol 1996; 270:G29–41.
92. Chambrey R, Warnock DG, Podevin RA, et al. Immunolocalization of the Na^+/H^+ exchanger isoform NHE2 in rat kidney. Am J Physiol 1998; 275:F379–86.
93. Peti-Peterdi J, Chambrey R, Bebok Z, et al. Macula densa Na(+)/H(+) exchange activities mediated by apical NHE2 and basolateral NHE4 isoforms. Am J Physiol Renal Physiol 2000; 278:F452–63.
94. Wang T, Hropot M, Aronson PS, et al. Role of NHE isoforms in mediating bicarbonate reabsorption along the nephron. Am J Physiol Renal Physiol 2001; 281:F1117–22.
95. Schultheis PJ, Clarke LL, Meneton P, et al. Targeted disruption of the murine Na^+/H^+ exchanger isoform 2 gene causes reduced viability of gastric parietal cells and loss of net acid secretion. J Clin Invest 1998; 101:1243–53.
96. Park K, Evans RL, Watson GE, et al. Defective fluid secretion and NaCl absorption in the parotid glands of Na^+/H^+ exchanger-deficient mice. J Biol Chem 2001; 276:27042–50.
97. Yu FH, Shull GE, Orlowski J. Functional properties of the rat Na/H exchanger NHE-2 isoform expressed in Na/H exchanger-deficient Chinese hamster ovary cells. J Biol Chem 1993; 268:25536–41.
98. Bookstein C, Musch MW, Depaoli A, et al. Characterization of the rat Na^+/H^+ exchanger isoform NHE4 and localization in rat hippocampus. Am J Physiol 1996; 271:C1629–38.
99. Park K, Olschowka JA, Richardson LA, et al. Expression of multiple Na^+/H^+ exchanger isoforms in rat parotid acinar and ductal cells. Am J Physiol 1999; 276:G470–8.
100. Pizzonia JH, Biemesderfer D, Abu-Alfa AK, et al. Immunochemical characterization of Na^+/H^+ exchanger isoform NHE4. Am J Physiol 1998; 275:F510–7.
101. Rossmann H, Sonnentag T, Heinzmann A, et al. Differential expression and regulation of Na(+)/H(+) exchanger isoforms in rabbit parietal and mucous cells. Am J Physiol Gastrointest Liver Physiol 2001; 281:G447–58.
102. Gawenis LR, Greeb JM, Prasad V, et al. Impaired gastric acid secretion in mice with a targeted disruption of the NHE4 Na^+/H^+ exchanger. J Biol Chem 2005; 280:12781–9.
103. Gawenis LR, Ledoussal C, Judd LM, et al. Mice with a targeted disruption of the AE2 Cl^-/HCO_3^- exchanger are achlorhydric. J Biol Chem 2004; 279:30531–9.

4

Renal Structure Proteins and Sodium Transport

Paolo Manunta and Maria Teresa Sciarrone
Division of Nephrology, Dialysis, and Hypertension, San Raffaele University Hospital "Vita-Salute," Milan, Italy

OVERVIEW OF TUBULE TRANSPORT

The regulation of sodium transport in the kidney is important for maintenance of extracellular fluid volume and arterial blood pressure regulation. A wealth of studies on the molecular identification of ion transporters has increased our understanding of how the urinary excretion is fine-tuned to meet homeostatic requirements. In fact the filtered load of human kidneys is impressive. The filtration rate amounts to 180 L/day, which corresponds to 1.7 kg of NaCl. This is approximately 11 times our total extracellular space. The largest part of this filtered load must be absorbed by renal tubules; this is paid by O_2 and fuel consumption. The overall O_2 consumption of both kidneys is fairly small, with approximately 20 L/day, which corresponds to 6 mol of ATP/day (on the basis of 1 mol O_2/6 mol ATP) (1). The major sodium transporters and channels in individual renal tubule segments have now been identified via micropuncture, physiological techniques, and complementary DNAs for all of the key sodium transporters, and channels expressed along the renal tubule have been cloned (2,3). Complementary DNA probes and antibodies are now being used to investigate the molecular basis of renal tubule sodium transport regulation. Approximately 60% to 70% of the filtered load of Na^+ and H_2O are absorbed in the proximal nephron (Fig. 1). The essential regulatory mechanisms include: the glomerulotubular balance and neural and hormonal control [sympathetic innervation, angiotensin II (AII), endothelin, parathyroid hormone (PTH), and other mediators].

The remaining 30% to 40% is delivered to the thick ascending limb of the loop of Henle (TAL). There, as much as 20% to 30% of the delivered Na^+, but no H_2O is absorbed (5).

The rate of absorption depends on the load. In addition, the absorption is also controlled by [β]-adrenergic receptor agonists, PTH, calcitonin, prostaglandin E2 (6,7).

Usually, a tubule fluid containing 30 to 120 mmol/L Na^+ is delivered to the macula densa segment. These tubule cells, which on their basal side are near the glomerulus, with its vascular pole, sense the lumen concentration of Na^+ or that of Cl^- (8,9). This signal is used by two regulatory loops: the tubuloglomerular feedback (TGF) and the secretion of renin from the renin producing cells of the afferent arteriole.

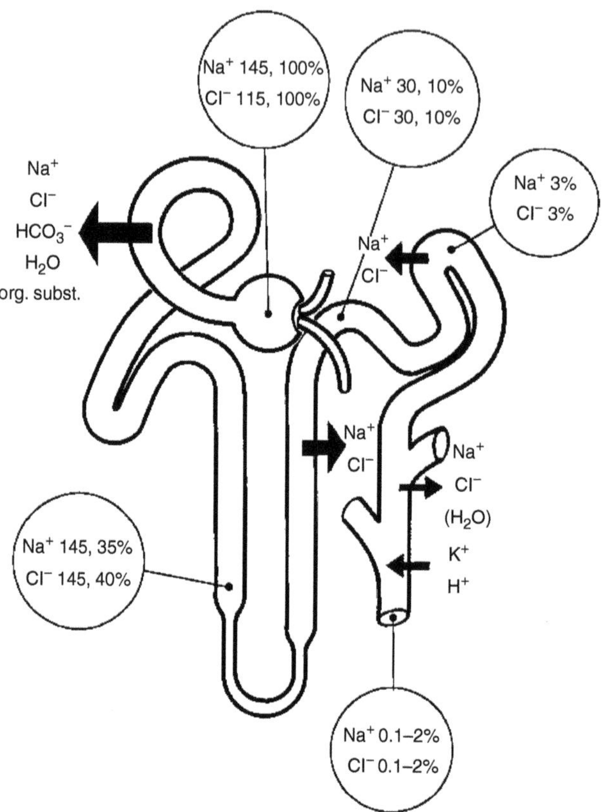

Figure 1 Na^+ and Cl^- absorption along the nephron. The numbers refer to millimoles per liter at the respective nephron site. For the distal tubule and collecting duct, no absolute concentrations are given because they can vary considerably. *Abbreviation*: Org. subst., organic substances. *Source*: From Ref. 4.

The Na^+ and water loads delivered to the distal tubule (DT) amount to approximately 10% and 25% of the filtered load, respectively. Here, another 5% to 10% is absorbed; this process is controlled by sympathetic innervation, bradykinin, and other hormones.

A small percentage of the filtered load of Na^+ and some 10% to 15% of the filtered load of H_2O are normally delivered to the collecting duct (CD). The absorption of Na^+ at this site is under control of aldosterone. Less than 1% of the filtered Na^+ is then lost in urine. Natriuretic hormone increases Na^+ excretion, but the precise mechanism is still not clarified (10).

PROXIMAL ABSORPTION

As in any other nephron segment, proximal absorption is mainly energized by the basolateral Na^+–K^+-ATPase. Most mammalian cell pump out Na^+ ions in exchange for extracellular K^+ ions by the action of Na^+–K^+-ATPase. This process is called active Na^+ transport because energy is expended in creating electrochemical gradients for Na^+ and K^+. This pump extrudes three Na^+ and takes up two K^+ for each ATP hydrolyzed (11).

The Na^+–K^+-ATPase is a highly-conserved integral membrane protein that is expressed in virtually all cells of higher organisms. As one measure of its importance, it has been estimated that roughly 25% of all cytoplasmic ATP is hydrolyzed by sodium pumps in resting humans. In nerve cells, approximately 70% of the ATP is consumed to fuel sodium pumps (12).

The ionic transport conducted by sodium pumps creates both an electrical and chemical gradient across the plasma membrane. This is critical not only for that cell but, in many cases, for directional fluid and electrolyte movement across epithelial sheets (13,14).

Export of sodium from the cell provides the driving force for several facilitated transporters, which import glucose, amino acids and other nutrients into the cell (13).

Translocation of sodium from one side of an epithelium to the other side creates an osmostic gradient that drives absorption of water. Important instances of this phenomenon can be found in the kidney.

Depending on cell type, there are between 800,000 and 30 million pumps on the surface of cells. They may be distributed fairly evenly, or clustered in certain membrane domains, as in the basolateral membranes of polarized epithelial cells in the kidney (15).

Abnormalities in the number or function of Na^+–K^+-ATPases are thought to be involved in several pathologic states, particular heart disease and hypertension. Well-studied examples of this linkage include:

- Several types of heart failure are associated with significant reductions in myocardial concentration of Na^+–K^+-ATPase.
- Excessive renal reabsorption of sodium due to over secretion of aldosterone has been associated with hypertension in humans.

The Na^+–K^+-ATPase is composed of two subunits. The α subunit ($\sim$113 kDa) is the action hero of the pair—it binds ATP and both sodium and potassium ions, and contains the phosphorylation site. The smaller β subunit ($\sim$35 kDa glycoprotein) is absolutely necessary for activity of the complex. It appears to be critical in facilitating the plasma membrane localization and activation of the α subunit. Several isoforms of both α and β subunits have been identified, but aside from kinetic characterizations and tissue distribution, little is known regarding their differential physiologic importance (15).

Several uncertainties remain in describing the structure of this molecule, but based on primary amino acid sequence, it is thought to possess 8 or 10 transmembrane domains. Considerable information is available to define the amino acids involved in ATP and cation binding.

Cation transport occurs in a cycle of conformational changes apparently triggered by phosphorylation of the pump. As currently understood, the sequence of events can be summarized as follows:

1. The pump, with bound ATP, binds three intracellular Na^+ ions.
2. Adenosine triphosphate (ATP) is hydrolyzed, leading to phosphorylation of a cytoplasmic loop of the pump and release of adenosine diphosphate (ADP).
3. A conformational change in the pump exposes the Na^+ ions to the outside, where they are released.
4. The pump binds two extracellular K^+ ions, leading somehow to dephosphorylation of the α subunit.
5. ATP binds and the pump reorients to release K^+ ions inside the cell.
6. The pump is ready to go again.

Expression of sodium pump activity is regulated at multiple levels and in both acute and chronic timeframes. A functional pump requires synthesis and assembly of both α and

β subunits. In many cells excessive β subunits are produced, making synthesis of α subunit the rate-limiting step in expression. It should come as no surprise that such controls are physiologically complex and involve the action of multiple hormones.

Rapid changes in pump activity appear to reflect modulations in kinetic properties, induced by a variety of intracellular signalling pathways. Phosphorylation of the α subunit enhances pump activity, presumably by increasing turnover rate or affinity for substrates. A number of hormones stimulate kinase or phosphatase activities within the cell that affect pump activity. Also, it appears that some cell types contain an intracellular pool of pumps that can be rapidly recruited to a functional state in the plasma membrane.

Acute hypertension rapidly inhibits proximal tubule (PT) Na^+–K^+-ATPase activity and sodium reabsorption 30% to 40%, increasing sodium and volume delivery to the TAL and macula densa, providing the error signal for TGF.

Major hormonal controls over pump activity can be summarized as follows (16):

1. Thyroid hormones appear to be a major player in maintaining steady-state concentrations of pumps in most tissues. This effect appears to result from stimulation of subunit gene transcription.
2. Aldosterone is a steroid hormone with major effects on sodium homeostasis. It stimulates both rapid and sustained increases in pump numbers within several tissues. The sustained effect is due to enhanced transcription of the genes for both subunits.
3. Catecholamines have varied effects, depending on the specific hormone and tissue. For example, dopamine inhibits Na^+–K^+-ATPase activity in kidney, while epinephrine stimulates pump activity in skeletal muscle. These effects seem to be mediated via phosphorylation or dephosphorylation of the pumps.
4. Insulin is a major regulator of potassium homeostasis and has multiple effects on sodium pump activity. Within minutes of elevated insulin secretion, pumps containing α-1 and 2 isoforms have increased affinity for sodium and increased turnover rate. Sustained elevation in insulin causes upregulation of α-2 synthesis. In skeletal muscle, insulin may also recruit pumps stored in the cytoplasm or activate latent pumps already present in the membrane.
5. Endogenous ouabain (EO): according to the growing experimental data we might postulate a double action of this endogenous cardiac glycosides on the Na^+–K^+-ATPase:
   a. *Natriuretic*, this effect occurs only at high concentrations (10^{-6} M) in rats or sheep (17) and is potentiated when combined with a condition of plasma volume expansion (18).
   b. Emerging evidence suggests that a more complex series of events, rather than a simple intrarenal inhibition of the Na pump, might be evoked in response to EO. Recently, has been shown that cardiotonic steroids activate intracellular signaling pathways through Na^+–K^+-ATPase–Src–Ras–reactive oxygen species and extracellular-regulated kinases within restricted membrane subdomains, referred to as caveolae. This signal has genomic effects leading to changes in gene expression involved in the hypertrophic growth response. In addition, long-term infusion of low doses of ouabain 10^{-9} produced hypertension and cardiac hypertrophy in rats (19). Moreover, a growing number of studies suggest that elevated levels of endogenous cardiac glycosides, as EO, may have a primary role in cardiac dysfunction and failure.

The inward gradient created for Na^+ by Na^+–K^+-ATPase activity is used to drive several secondary active transporters (carriers). Quantitatively speaking, the most important Na^+-coupled transporter in proximal nephron segment is the Na^+/H^+ exchanger (20). This exchanger exports H^+, which is buffered by HCO_3^- in the lumen. The carbonic acid formed is dehydrated to CO_2 by carbonic anhydrase located in the luminal membrane. Within the cell, CO_2 is rehydrated by cytosolic carbonic anhydrase and carbonic acid is formed. This dissociates and returns the H^+ for another cycle. Na^+ is pumped out by the Na^+–K^+-ATPase and HCO_3^- leaves the cell by a Na^+-coupled cotransporter $[Na^+(HCO_3^-)_3]$ (21). The driving force for this exit mechanism is provided by the basolateral membrane voltage (22). By this mechanism, Na^+ and HCO_3^- are absorbed transcellularly and the luminal HCO_3^- falls rapidly along the tubule axis.

The putative molecular structure of the Na^+/H^+ (NHE3) exchanger (23,24) contains an upper side that is extracellular and two protein kinase (PKA and PKC), which represent phosphorylation sites, respectively. This transporter is probably regulated by phosphorylation but also by controlled retrieval via a specific SH3 motif of this protein (25). Relevant regulatory factors are probably AII and sympathetic innervation, which upregulate Na^+ absorption. PTH and dopamine, on the other hand, reduce NHE3 activity and Na^+ absorption (26). One of the most important regulatory mechanisms is provided by cytosolic pH. Cytosolic acidosis activates the exchanger, and alkaline pH has the opposite effect. This provides the mechanism whereby HCO_3^- absorption is maximized in acidosis and reduced in alkalosis (27). The Na^+ gradient across the luminal membrane is also used by the sodium glucose cotransporter to absorb D-glucose (28). Very similar transport systems secure the absorption of amino acids, phosphate, sulfate, and lactate (26).

Near the end of the PT, tubule flow rate is reduced to one third that of filtered. The tubule fluid has a Na^+ concentration very similar to that of the filtrate. The Cl^- concentration is slightly increased and that of HCO_3^- has fallen to approximately 5 to 10 mmol/L.

ABSORPTION IN THE TAL

The TAL is the engine of the concentrating mechanism. Up to 20% to 30% of the filtered load of Na^+ and Cl^- are absorbed at this site (5,29). Also, the residual HCO_3^- can be absorbed in this segment. Since H_2O cannot follow the ions, because the luminal membrane is almost water tight, the lumen fluid becomes hypotonic along the axis of the TAL and the interstitium becomes hypertonic. This hypertonicity is used for H_2O absorption from the descending thin limb of the loop of Henle and CD.

The mechanism of Na^+ and Cl^- absorption in this nephron segment is driven by the basolateral Na^+–K^+-ATPase. In fact, these cells are a specifically rich source for this enzyme (30). Na^+ is taken up across the luminal membrane by the $Na^+2Cl^-K^+$ cotransporter. Na^+ is pumped out by the Na^+–K^+-ATPase. Cl^- leaves the cell via basolateral Cl^- channels and probably also by KCl symport (5). K^+ recycles across the luminal membrane via renal outer medullary potassium channel (ROMK)-type channels (31,32). This K^+ recycling together with the Cl^- exit across the basolateral membrane produces a lumen positive voltage. This voltage is used to drive Na^+ across the paracellular pathway in absorptive direction (5). Previous data suggests that up to 50% of the Na^+ absorption occurs via this pathway. Also note that Ca^{2+} and Mg^{2+} are absorbed in the TAL. It is not clear how many of these ions move between and how many across the cell. At any rate, abolition of Na^+Cl^- absorption in the TAL also abolishes the absorption of the divalent ions.

Many hormones act in the TAL. On the one hand, Vasopressin (AVP), PTH, calcitonin, glucagon and epinephrine have all been shown to increase absorption of Na^+ and Cl^-. Prostaglandin E2, on the other hand, reduces absorption (7,33,34). The absorption in the TAL depends largely on the delivered load (5). Reduced absorption in the PT thence leads to an increased absorption in the TAL. This is one of the reasons why diuretics acting in the PT lead to a very limited diuretic and saluretic response. Conversely, loop diuretics such as furosemide exert a strong diuretic effect especially if absorption in the PT is not enhanced (35).

The membrane topology of the $Na^+2Cl^-K^+$ cotransporter is closely related to the Na^+Cl^- cotransporter present in the DT (36). It should be noticed that the two proteins are clearly distinct with respect to their pharmacology (35). The $Na^+2Cl^-K^+$ cotransporter binds only loop diuretics, such as bumetanide, torasemide, piretanide, furosemide, and azosemide, with high affinity, but no thiazides. On the other hand, the Na^+Cl^- cotransporter binds only thiazides. The $Na^+2Cl^-K^+$ cotransporter has several phosphorylation sites that may be used for cAMP-dependent activation (37,38).

ABSORPTION IN THE DUCT TUBLE

The mechanisms of Na^+ and Cl^- absorption at this site are still not completely understood, because this nephron segment is composed of several cell types along its axis (39). The electroneutral Na^+ and Cl^- absorption at this site (40,41) is driven by the basolateral Na^+–K^+-ATPase. Na^+ is taken up across the luminal membrane by the Na^+Cl^- cotransporter (36). Na^+ is pumped out by the Na^+–K^+-ATPase. Cl^- leaves the cell, probably via basolateral K^+Cl^- symport. It is important to mention that Ca^{2+} absorption continues along this nephron segment and that the amount of Ca^{2+} absorption is enhanced when Na^+ and Cl^- absorption is blocked by thiazides (41). The rate of Na^+ and Cl^- absorption in this tubule segment is enhanced by epinephrine, norepinephrine and bradykinin (26). As in the TAL, the rate of absorption is also controlled by the load delivered.

It is clear that the $Na^+2Cl^-K^+$ cotransporter and the Na^+Cl^- cotransporter share a very high degree of homology. In fact, one might speculate that conspicuous areas of low homology may have to do with the K^+-binding site, which is present in the $Na^+2Cl^-K^+$ cotransporter but absent in the Na^+Cl^- cotransporter (42).

The regulation of the Na^+Cl^- cotransporter is not clear at this stage. Shortly after its discovery, mutations have been found in this protein which lead to Gitelman's syndrome (43,44). This important finding now makes easy the distinction between this and the related inherited disease, Bartter's syndrome. Clinically both syndromes differ with respect to their effects on renal Ca^{2+} excretion. Although Bartter's predictably causes calciuria, Gitelman's causes anticalciuria and hypercalcemia (43).

ABSORPTION IN THE CD

The CD is equipped with at least three types of cells (39). Intercalated A-type cells, on the one hand, are equipped with two types of proton pumps in the luminal membrane: the lysosomal type H^+-ATPase (45) and the gastric/colonic type of H^+/K^+-ATPase (46). Whereas the first type responds with strong upregulation in acidosis and enhances CD H^+ secretion, the latter type seems to be activated by hypokalemia and, therefore, apparently serves active K^+ absorption (46). The B-type intercalated cells, on the other hand, secrete HCO_3^- and are activated in metabolic alkalosis. The principal cells absorb Na^+ and secrete K^+. These cells are also the target of AVP and mediate aquaporin two-controlled water absorption (47).

Once again, the absorptive process is entirely dependent of the basolateral Na^+–K^+-ATPase. Na^+ enters the cell via Na^+ channels. The Na^+ influx through these channels has two consequences: (*i*) the lumen voltage turns lumen negative and (*ii*) the luminal membrane is strongly depolarized. This depolarization of the luminal membrane provides extra driving force for the secretion of K^+ through the ROMK-type K^+ channels present in the same membrane (48). The increase in lumen negative voltage is also proposed to be the key mechanism for the increased H^+ secretion via A-type cells. One important factor that determines the magnitude of Na^+ absorption is the load of Na^+ delivered to the CD (49). When this load is increased, the CD principal cells do their best to minimize renal losses of Na^+. In other words, Na^+ absorption is maximized, as are the secretion of K^+ and H^+. Another important factor that determines CD Na^+ absorption is the mineralocorticoid status. Aldosterone enhances CD Na^+ absorption. The mechanism whereby this occurs is not completely understood. With the molecular identification of epithelium sodium channel (ENaC) (50), it has now become possible to elucidate its regulation more closely. It turned out that the mRNA for ENaC itself, including all its described subunits ([α], [β], and [γ]), is not upregulated by aldosterone. Therefore, it is more likely that another protein controlling the residence or activity of ENaC in the luminal membrane is controlled by this hormone (51). In any case, the absorptive Na^+ current across the cell is enhanced by aldosterone, as is the secretion of K^+ and H^+. Hyperkalemia is another independent pathway to activate aldosterone secretion (26). The range of aldosterone control of urinary Na^+ is by the way fairly wide (26).

The role of atrial natriuretic peptide (ANP) on Na^+ absorption in the CD is still not entirely clear (26). ANP receptors are, however, present in the CD, and increased Na^+ permeability has been shown, especially for the inner medullary CD (26). The cyclic guanosine monophosphate-dependent kinase II, which is supposed to mediate the ANP effects, however, has been shown for the ascending thin limb of the loop of Henle (52).

SALT SENSITIVITY

The epidemiological evidence for the involvement of sodium in the pathogenesis of essential hypertension demonstrates an essential role for this element.

The evidence is and will continue to be indirect, because direct proof of the role of any ubiquitous environmental factor in the pathogenesis of a slowly developing disorder that follows polygenic inheritance is not easy.

Alterations in sodium balance and extracellular fluid volume have heterogeneous effects in normotensive and hypertensive humans (53). Studies in relatively large groups of subjects have yielded inconsistent evidence for a sure relationship between salt and blood pressure. When individual responses are examined, most studies demonstrate that blood pressure in some individuals is responsive (sensitive) to manipulation of sodium, whereas others are resistant (54,55).

Several different approaches to the identification of salt responsivity have been reported. These studies have revealed characteristics associated with salt sensitivity and resistance of blood pressure as well as some evidence regarding the mechanism that may be involved (56,57).

Recently genetic factors have been identified that may simplify the recognition of salt sensitivity.

Our group has been studying for many years adducin and its genetic polymorphisms and its involvement in salt sensitivity.

ADDUCIN, RENAL NA$^+$ REABSORPTION AND HYPERTENSION

Primary and even renal forms of hypertension are characterized by heterogeneity in terms of potential molecular mechanisms, pathophysiological and clinical patterns, and response to therapy. Furthermore, a network of feedback loops interacting with the renal, hormonal, hemodynamic, and nervous mechanisms that control blood pressure hampers the distinction between primary and secondary mechanisms. Therefore, appropriate animal models may facilitate elucidation of the hierarchical and temporal order of events linking a given molecular mechanism to hypertension (58). The usefulness of the animal model obviously depends on its similarity to the human condition. This implies a precise definition of the subset of patients whose pathophysiological and clinical profiles approximate to that of the model. We pursued this complex approach throughout a series of empirical observations that led us to propose adducin as a candidate gene for human hypertension. Adducin polymorphism is certainly one of the very few polymorphisms (59), if not the unique one (60), affecting blood pressure in two species (rat and human) that diverged 40 million years ago.

To discuss the adducin data within the framework of the multitude of interactive blood pressure-regulating mechanisms, this book chapter is subdivided as follows: (*i*) comparison of experimental results obtained in the Milan hypertensive rat strain (MHS) and its normotensive control (Milan normotensive rat strain, MNS) with observations in humans, focusing on renal intermediate phenotypes that are on the pathophysiological pathway linking a genetic mutation to the blood pressure phenotype; (*ii*) description of the molecular mechanisms affected by adducin; and (*iii*) characterization of those subsets of patients who develop high blood pressure following these mechanisms.

COMPARISON BETWEEN MHS MODEL AND HUMANS

The pathophysiological similarities across the two species when prehypertensive or early hypertensive individuals are compared with their respective normotensive controls are reported in Table 1. The glomerular filtration rate (GFR) of young prehypertensive MHS is definitely higher than that of MNS when measured at inulin concentrations of 0.1 mg/mL (61), whereas the opposite is true when 10 higher inulin concentrations are used (61). Definitely in adult MHS, GFR is similar to that of adult MNS. In humans, GFR is higher, similar or lower in young prehypertensive or early hypertensive patients compared with normotensive controls (61,62). Variability may be accounted for by the experimental conditions under which GFR is measured (63) and by genetic–molecular mechanisms, such as those operating in some rat strains showing a reduced GFR at the very early stage of hypertension (63). These findings highlight the importance of standardizing the experimental settings, the stage of hypertension, and the genetic and environmental backgrounds of the subjects to identify subsets of patients having a renal pathophysiological profile similar to that of the rat model (61,63,64).

The higher GFR and the lower plasma renin activity (PRA) at the prehypertensive phase, together with the renal sodium retention during development of hypertension, point to a primary increase in tubular sodium reabsorption in MHS as the cause of hypertension. This hypothesis is further strengthened by the following observations: (*i*) hypertension may be transplanted with the kidney in rats as well as in humans (65); (*ii*) in MHS, ion

Table 1 Comparison of Humans Either Prone to or at the Early Hypertensive Stage, with Rats of the Milan Strain

Intermediate phenotypes	Human essential	Milan hypertensive rat strain
Pressor effect of kidney transplantation	↑	↑
Renal blood flow	↑[a], =, ↓	= or ↑ in isolated kidney
Glomerular filtration rate	↑[a], =, ↓	↑
Na excretion after load	↑	↑
24-hr urinary output	↑	↑
Plasma renin	↓	↓
Urine kallikrein	↓	↓
Erythrocyte Na content	↓[a], =, ↑	↓
Net erythrocyte membrane Na transport	↑[a], =, ↓	↑

Higher (↑), lower (↓), or equal (=) in the hypertensive humans and rats wih the appropriate controls.
[a]In subsets of patients.

transport occurs at a faster rate across the membranes of renal tubular cells and erythrocytes than in MNS (66); and (*iii*) bone marrow transplantation experiments from MHS to irradiated MNS suggest that the erythrocyte membrane abnormalities of MHS are transplanted with the stem cells (66). In addition, in the MHS MNS F2 population, the blood pressure and erythrocyte phenotypes cosegregate (66). In a subset of hypertensive patients, erythrocyte Na^+–K^+–Cl^- cotransport and Na^+–Li countertransport occur at rates higher than the maximal values observed in normotensive controls (66). Furthermore, a subset of young offspring of hypertensive parents shows a lower intracellular sodium content than controls (Table 1) (66). When the renal tubular function of hypertensive patients with high erythrocyte Na^+–K^+–Cl^- cotransport is compared with that of normotensive subjects or patients with normal cotransport, the former shows lower fractional excretion of uric acid, lower PRA, and a larger natriuretic response to furosemide than the latter (66).

The widespread constitutive cellular abnormalities in sodium handling and volume observed in MHS and in a subgroup of hypertensive patients, both characterized by a common defect of renal tubular function, were suggestive of a protein alteration in the actin cytoskeleton. Indeed, the removal of the actin membrane skeleton from erythrocytes nullifies the differences in membrane ion transport between MHS and MNS erythrocytes (66). To detect subtle protein differences between the membrane cytoskeleton of the two strains, we cross-immunized MHS and MNS rats with the membrane skeleton. The antibodies raised in these experiments recognize a protein which we later identified as adducin, via screening of a cDNA expression library (66).

MOLECULAR MECHANISM OF ADDUCIN

Adducin is a heterodimeric cytoskeleton protein and consists of an α-subunit (Mr 103 kDa) and either a β-(Mr 97 kDa) or γ-subunit (Mr 90 kDa). Three genes (ADD1, ADD2, and ADD3, or Add1, Add2, and Add3, human and rat genes, respectively) that map to different chromosomes encode these subunits (67). Adducin promotes the organization of the spectrin-actin lattice by favoring the spectrin-actin binding and controlling the rate of actin polymerization as an end-capping actin protein

(67). Its function is calcium- and calmodulin-dependent (67). It is phosphorylated by protein kinases A and C, tyrosine, and (rho(-kinases (67). It is a member of the myristoylated alanine-rich C kinase substrate protein family, which is involved in signal transduction, cell-to-cell contact formation, and cell migration (67). Adducin is highly conserved through the different species, thus suggesting a role in basic cellular functions. The analysis of the full-length adducin cDNA sequence in the MHS and MNS strains revealed the presence of point mutations causing an amino acid substitution on the α-(F316Y) and the β-(Q529R) adducin subunits (68). We also detected a point mutation in the γ-adducin subunit of MHS (Q572K) (69). In the MHS MNS F2 hybrid population, mutation of the Add1 gene accounts for the 50% blood pressure difference between MHS and MNS. Add2 and Add3 gene mutations are not, per se, associated with hypertension but epistatically interact with that of Add1 in determining the blood pressure level of the F2 hybrids (70). Moreover, the transfer of a short chromosomal region including Add1 locus from MHS to MNS and vice versa raises the blood pressure in the MNS genetic background and reduces it in the reciprocal strain (71). In humans, two polymorphisms of the ADD1 gene lead to amino acid substitutions: G460W and S586C (72). Other polymorphisms occur in the human ADD2 and ADD3. The first linkage and case-control studies demonstrated an association of the ADD1 W allele with hypertension (72). Moreover, carriers of the ADD1 W allele, when compared with homozygotes for the ADD1 G allele, have a decreased erythrocyte sodium content and faster Na–K cotransport (73), in analogy with the findings in MHS. Cell culture and cell-free system experiments helped to elucidate the molecular mechanisms that, in humans and rats, make adducin mutation responsible for the abnormal cell sodium handling and ultimately for hypertension. In renal cells, transfection with the MHS Add1 Y increases the Na–K pump activity and causes a rearrangement of the actin cytoskeleton (74). In a cell-free system, rat-mutated adducin accelerates actin polymerization (74), and rat- and human (ADD1 W)-mutated adducins bind to and activate the Na^+–K^+ pump with higher affinity than the respective normal proteins (75). Studies on the dynamics of the endocytotic processes in transfected cells have provided an interpretation for the increased cellular expression and activity of the Na^+–K^+ pump caused by the expression of the α-adducin mutants (Fig. 2) (76). Cells transfected with either the human or rat hypertensive α-adducin compared with cells transfected with the wild-type variant show a higher Na^+–K^+ pump activity and an impaired Na^+–K^+ pump endocytosis in basal conditions (76) as well as in response to natriuretic signals such as dopamine (76). Clathrin-dependent endocytosis of membrane proteins is initiated by adaptor proteins (AP2), which simultaneously bind to cargo proteins, recruit clathrin, and promote formation of clathrin-coated vesicles, with the cooperation of many other proteins. This protein interaction is reduced by mutated α-adducin (76). Deficient endocytosis of the Na^+–K^+ pump might therefore be an important factor contributing to the increased renal tubular reabsorption observed in rats as well as in humans (77,78) carrying the mutated adducin variant. In fact, an efficient endocytosis of the sodium transporting proteins is crucial for blunting the rise in systemic arterial pressure (79).

RELATIONSHIP BETWEEN ADDUCIN AND HORMONES AFFECTING RENAL NA^+ HANDLING

The evaluation of this relationship is indispensable for assessing the role of a gene influencing the tubular Na^+ transport. Plasma and hypothalamic ouabain levels are higher

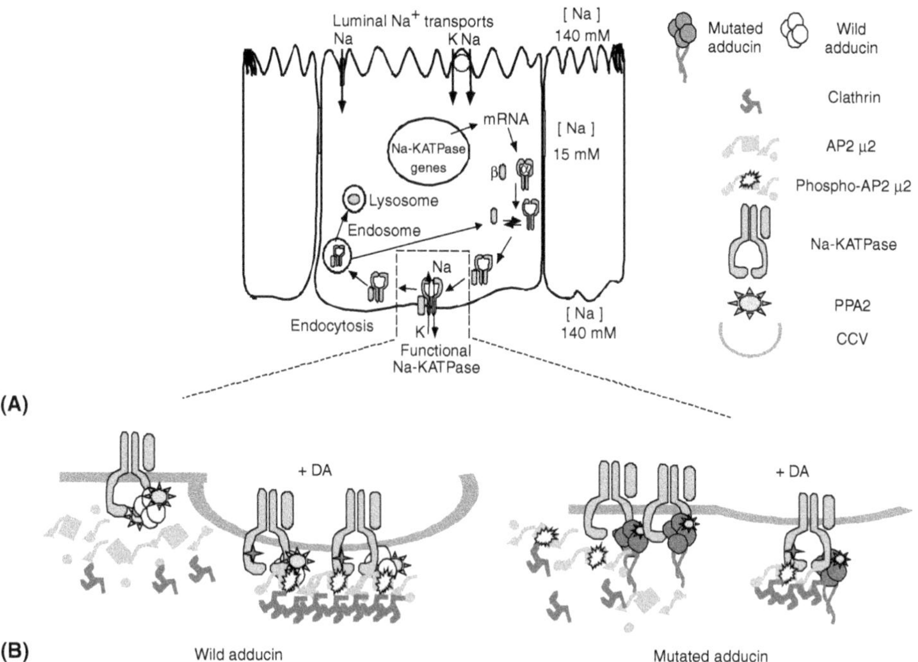

Figure 2 Influence of α-adducin polymorphism on Na–K pump endocytosis and renal Na reabsorption. (**A**) The process of insertion and removal (endocytosis) of the Na–K pump on basolateral renal cell membranes of a tubular cell. Reduced endocytosis increases the Na–K pump molecules on basolateral membrane thus leading to increased sodium reabsorption. (**B**) The interaction among some proteins involved in these processes. In basal condition, the PPA2 α-adducin association is reduced in cell transfected with mutated adducin (please note the smaller dimension of the phosphathase PPA2 protein symbol associated to mutated adducin). Since the phosphorylation state of a protein results from the balance between protein kinase and PPA2, the reduced PPA2-adducin association favors the AP2-μ2 phosphorylated state, thus impairing the phospho–dephospho cycle of AP2-μ2. This cycle promotes the association of AP2 to Na–K pump which is a key event for the recruitment of clathrin and the formation of clathrin coated vescicles. Therefore, the impairment of this cycle may represent the molecular mechanism underlying the reduced constitutive and dopamine-induced Na–K pump endocytosis observed in the presence of mutated adducin. This cartoon does not include another possible mechanism of deficient endocytosis represented by the less permissive, stiffer cortical actin cytoskeleton of cell transfected with the mutated adducin. *Abbreviations*: AP2, adaptor proteins; PPA2, protein phosphatase 2.

in MHS than in MNS (80). According to the Blaustein's hypothesis (81), we hypothesized that these changes may represent a counterregulatory mechanism triggered by a primary increase in Na^+ tubular reabsorption, which also contributes to increase blood pressure via an inhibition of the vascular Na^+–K^+ pump. However, subsequent findings disputed this hypothesis: (*i*) variation of plasma ouabain in rats, within concentrations found in MHS rat or hypertensive subjects induced by chronic infusion of ouabain, are able to increase blood pressure and Na^+–K^+ pump activity on the tubular cell basolateral membrane (19,82). Similar alterations of Na^+–K^+ activity were achieved by incubation of renal tubular cell culture with subnanomolar concentration of ouabain (82). A highly selective ouabain antagonist is able to block these effects on renal Na^+–K^+ pump both in cell culture and in the intact animal, where blood pressure is also normalized (83). These findings clearly demonstrate a primary effect of ouabain on Na^+ tubular reabsorption that may contribute to the hypertension in rats infused with ouabain, or in MHS, or in hypertensive humans. In congenic MNS rats harboring the MHS adducin locus (71), plasma ouabain is similar to that of MNS but blood pressure is higher. When challenged with a low salt diet, plasma ouabain increases in the congenic MNS rats but not in the parental MNS (83). This suggests that somehow the MHS Add1 is involved in the rise of ouabain after Na depletion. Plasma ouabain is increased on low salt diet also in humans (83,84).

In never treated early hypertensives, the plasma levels of renin, aldosterone and ouabain are lower in carriers of the mutated adducin compared to the other subjects (85). The down regulation of the hormones promoting hypertension and renal Na^+ retention at the early stages of hypertension suggests a counterregulatory mechanism that tends to limit the rise of blood pressure substained by other mechanisms including a primary increase in tubular Na^+ reabsorption. Studies in a predominantly normotensive general population showed an interesting interrelationship among plasma ouabain, blood pressure and 24 hours renal Na^+ excretion taken as an index of Na^+ intake (86). At lower Na^+ excretion, blood pressure is higher in subjects with plasma ouabain above the median value of the population than in subjects with plasma ouabain below this median value. Conversely at higher level of Na^+ excretion, blood pressure is lower in subjects with higher plasma ouabain (86). A dose-dependent effect of the mutated W ADD1 allele on plasma ouabain is found in the general population, being the plasma levels of homozygous homozygotes W allele carriers 20% higher than those of wild homozygotes carriers (86).

Taken together all these findings suggest a relationship between ADD1 polymorphism and plasma ouabain based on an interaction with the Na^+–K^+ pump. We may tentatively propose that ouabain and adducin polymorphism play a key role in the homeostatic regulation of blood pressure in response to variations in Na^+ intake and that an ouabain increase may limit either the rise of blood pressure at higher salt diet or the fall in blood pressure at low salt diet. The molecular mechanisms underlying the regulation of this set-point as well as the difference in the mutated adducin–plasma ouabain relationship between the general population and the never treated early hypertensives remain to be clarified.

CLINICALLY RELEVANT GENETIC INTERACTIONS

Since Adducin is present with different proportion of α-β or α-γ subunits in all tissues (i.e., α-β vassels, α-γ in the renal tubules) and these subunit are coded by genes located in different chromosomes, we have the biochemical and molecular basis to investigate the genetic interactions. Indeed, several studies carried out in rat and humans showed:

- an interactions between Add1 and Add2 (68) on blood pressure values
- as shown in Figure 3, an epistatic interaction between ADD1 and ADD3 on blood pressure (85) or pulse pressure (87) in humans,
- another interaction was found in never treated early hypertensive patients and in a predominantly normotensive population between adducin and angiotensin-converting enzyme (ACE). The effect of the W ADD1 allele on the fall in plasma renin (88) and on the increase in blood pressure after a sodium load (88), on the incidence of hypertension in a general population (89), on the intima-media thickness (90) and stiffness (91) of femoral artery, on the decrease of GFR (92) and on the increase in urine protein excretion (93), is augmented in the DD ACE genotype and is diminished in the ACE II genotype, when compared to the

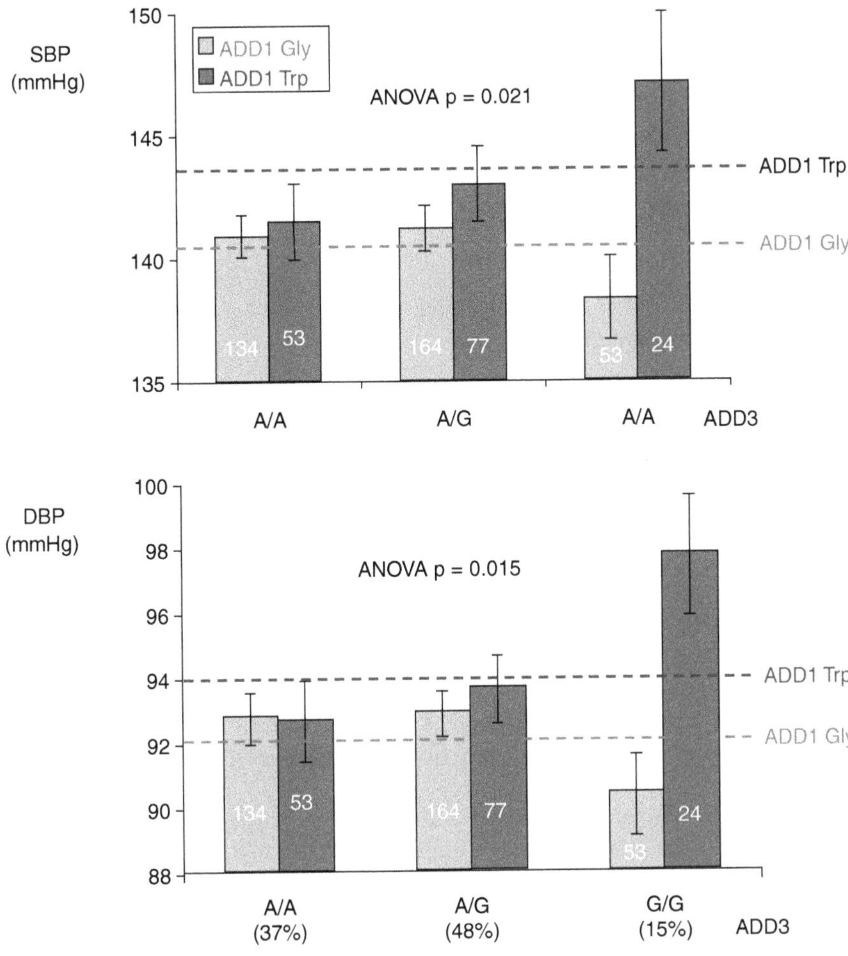

Figure 3 ADD1/ADD3 interaction. Systolic (SBP top panel) and DBP in carriers of Gly460Gly (black bars) and Gly460Trp + Trp460Trp (gray bars) ADD1 genotypes, subdivided according to the three ADD3 genotypes with their frequency in parentheses. To facilitate comparison, the dashed lines indicate the SBP and DBP of two ADD1 genotypes (lower blue line 460Gly and upper red line 460Trp) in the total hypertensive population. A significant interaction ANOVA $p = 0.020$ was found. Data are the means ± sem after correction for confounders basal metabolic index, age, sex. *Abbreviations*: DBP, diastolic blood pressure; SBP, systolic blood pressure.

average values of the general population. Cell surface ACE activity in fibroblasts isolated from patients with various ADD1 genotypes was higher in W ADD1 carriers than in wild ADD1 homozygous homozygotes (93). This may suggest that the W allele increases the number of ACE molecules on the plasma membrane similarly to the effect on Na^+–K^+ pump.

The bulk of data on isolated fibroblasts and on the various intermediate phenotypes measured in patients supports the hypothesis that the combination of these two genotypes may favor the development of a specific clinical entity characterized by consistent alterations at DNA, cellular, renal and cardiovascular phenotypes favoring the development of hypertension and organ damage. The proposal of this new clinical entity is also reinforced by the findings that combination of these genotypes also modulates the magnitude of blood pressure fall after diuretics (94). The strength of this proposal relies on the consistency among data collected from different contexts. The weakness is mainly due to lack of a proper follow-up on a large group of patients in whom all these characteristics are simultaneously measured in the same subjects.

RELATIONSHIP BETWEEN ADDUCIN AND CARDIOVASCULAR ORGAN DAMAGE

Two (95,96) out of three studies (97) demonstrate an association between W ADD1 allele and coronary disease in hypertensive patients. A fourth study (98) shows a lower frequency of this allele in myocardial infarction (MI) survivors aged <75 years compared to controls of the same age. It is therefore unclear whether these findings suggest a protective effect of the W ADD1 allele in controls or a high risk of premature death in W ADD1 allele carriers with MI. Ventricular hypertrophy has been shown to occur in WW ADD1 genotype (99). The intima-media thickness (87) and femoral artery stiffness (88) are increased in W ADD1 and D ACE carriers. A recent prospective study on 2235 Belgian residents followed for several years (100) shows that the W ADD1 allele may be a risk factor for total and cardiovascular morbidity and mortality when systolic blood pressure at baseline is included in the analysis as a continuous variable. The hazard ratio for cardiovascular complications associated with the W allele relative to wild homozygous homozygotes after adjustment for other risk factors is 2:94 $p=0.01$ in patients with stage two systolic hypertension (≥ 160 mmHg) and 0:83 $p=0.32$ in the other subjects. For each 10-year increment in age, the relative hazard ratio associated to the Trp allele increased by 39.7% (100).

W ADD1 allele frequency is around 8% in African populations (101), 12% in African Americans (102), 22% to 25% in Caucasians (72,89) and above 50% in Asian populations (103,104). How to reconcile this trend implying some positive effect on biological fitness with the "pathological" influence on cardiovascular and overall mortality? Two possibile mechanisms may be proposed. The W ADD1 allele may exert a protective effect at lower level of blood pressure (100) or at younger ages (105). Second, several studies on epistatic interaction show that the "pathological effect" of W ADD1 allele occurs in the presence of some other genotypes (for instance ACE DD) (88–92) while in the presence of other genotypes (for instance ACE II) the W allele may also reduce the value of pathological intermediate phenotypes below the level of the general population. Therefore, the increase in the frequency of the W allele in Caucasian or Asian populations may be due to the "positive" effect on biological fitness of this allele in specific subsets of population. According to the trade-off hypothesis (106), natural selection will increase the frequency of "mutations" that produce beneficial effect early in life even though these mutations may be deleterious later in life. This may also account for the high frequency of alleles such as the D ACE allele that certainly accelerates cardiovascular and renal damage at older ages (107).

CONCLUSIONS

The existence of gene modifiers (either enhancing or blunting the pathological effect of another gene variant) is a well-established fact in monogenic diseases and applies also to genes affecting renal sodium handling and blood pressure. Indeed, it is unlikely that a single gene polymorphism underlies a very heterogeneous syndrome such as primary hypertension, affecting up to 40% of the adult population of industrialized countries. Variation in the intrarenal formation of AII associated to ACE D/D allele may produce a synergistic effect with the ADD1 W allele on renal sodium excretion. Indeed, carriers of these allele combinations, compared with carriers of the W allele alone, have a more marked decrease of plasma renin for any level of sodium intake (88,94) associated with a larger increase of blood pressure during a saline load (88), a larger femoral intima-media thickness with a consequent variation in arterial stiffness (90,91), a lower renal function with a larger increase in urine protein excretion for the same phase of hypertension or age (92), and a greater fall in blood pressure with diuretics (94). The ACE/D allele seems to potentiate the clinical impact of ADD1 W allele. A practical way to "measure" the overall clinical impact of the ADD1 W allele, and then to estimate the size of the population that may be affected by this genetic mechanism, is to apply a very selective pharmacological tool able to interfere with the sequence of events triggered by this allele. Among the available drugs, diuretics are those that better approximate this tool. The selective beneficial effects of these drugs in reducing blood pressure and preventing MI and stroke in carriers of the ADD1 W allele (96) might be even greater if drugs interfering with adducin but devoid of the well-known side effects of diuretics are developed.

REFERENCES

1. Deetjen P, Kramer K. Die Abhängigkeit des O_2-Verbrauchs der Niere von der Na-Rückresorption. Pfluegers Arch Eur J Physiol 1961; 273:636–42.
2. Ullrich KJ, Greger R. Approaches to study tubule transport functions. In: Seldin DW, Giebisch G, eds. The Kidney: Physiology and Pathophysiology. New York: Raven Press, 1992:707–78.
3. Wright EM. The intestinal Na^+/glucose cotransporter. Annu Rev Physiol 1993; 55:575–89.
4. Greger R. Secondo me è giusto (ho controllato). Am J Med Sci 2005; 319(1):51.
5. Greger R. Ion transport mechanisms in thick ascending limb of Henle's loop of mammalian nephron. Physiol Rev 1985; 65:760–97.
6. Schlatter E, Greger R. cAMP increases the basolateral Cl^--conductance in the isolated perfused medullary thick ascending limb of Henle's loop of the mouse. Pfluegers Arch Eur J Physiol 1985; 405:367–76.
7. Wittner M, Di Stefano A. Effects of antidiuretic hormone, parathyroid hormone and glucagon on transepithelial voltage and resistance of the cortical and medullary thick ascending limb of Henle's loop of the mouse nephron. Pfluegers Arch Eur J Physiol 1990; 415:707–12.
8. Schnermann JB. Juxtaglomerular cell complex in the regulation of renal salt excretion. Am J Physiol 1998; 274:R263–79.
9. Schnermann JB, Briggs JP. Function of the juxtaglomerular apparatus: control of glomerular hemodynamics and renin secretion. In: Seldin DW, Giebisch G, eds. The Kidney: Physiology and Pathophysiology. New York: Raven Press, 1992:1249–90.
10. Ballermann BJ, Zeidel ML. Atrial natriuretic hormone. In: Seldin DW, Giebisch G, eds. The Kidney: Physiology and Pathophysiology. New York: Raven Press, 1992:1843–84.
11. Skou JC. The Na–K pump. News Physiol Sci 1992; 7:95–100.
12. Geering K. Na, K-ATPase. Curr Opin Nephrol Hypertens 1994; 6:434.
13. Greger R. Principles of renal transport, concentration and dilution of urine. In: Greger R, Windhorst U, eds. Comprehensive Human Physiology, from Cellular Mechanisms to Integration. New York: Springer, 1996:1489–516.
14. Lingrel JB, Kuntzweiler T. Na^+, K^+-ATPase. J Biol Chem 1994; 269:19659.
15. Jorgensen PL, Hakansson KO, Karlish SJD. Structure and mechanism of Na, K-ATPase: functional sites and their interactions. Annu Rev Physiol 2003; 65:817–49.
16. Ewart HS, Klip A. Hormonal regulation of the Na(+)–K(+)-ATPase: mechanisms underlying rapid and sustained changes in pump activity. Am J Physiol 1995; C269:C295.

17. Foulkes R, Ferrario RG, Salvati P, Bianchi G. Differences in ouabain-inducednatriuresis between isolated kidneys of Milan hypertensive and normotensiverats. Clin Sci 1992; 82:185–90.
18. Yates NA, McDougall JC. Effect of volume expansion on the natriuretic response to ouabain infusion. Renal Physiol Biochem 1995; 18:311–20.
19. Ferrandi M, Molinari I, Barassi P, Minotti E, Bianchi G, Ferrari P. Organ hypertrophic signaling within caveolae membrane subdomains triggered by ouabain and antagonized by PST 2238. J Biol Chem 2004; 279(32):33306–14.
20. Wakayabashi S, Shigekawa M, Pouysségur J. Molecular physiology of vertebrate Na^+/H^+ exchangers. Physiol Rev 1997; 77:51–74.
21. Romero MF, Hediger MA, Boulpaep EL, et al. Expression cloning and characterization of a renal electrogenic Na^+/HCO_3^- cotransporter. Nature 1997; 387:409–13.
22. Yoshitomi K, Burckhardt BC, Frömter E. Rheogenic sodium-bicarbonate cotransport in the peritubular cell membrane of rat renal proximal tubule. Pfluegers Arch Eur J Physiol 1985; 405:360–6.
23. Biemesderfer D, Pizzonia J, Abu-Alfa A, et al. NHE3: a Na^+/H^+ exchanger isoform of renal brush border. Am J Physiol 1993; 265:F736–42.
24. Tse CM, Brant SR, Walker MS, et al. Cloning and sequencing of a rabbit cDNA encoding an intestinal and kidney-specific Na^+/H^+ exchanger isoform (NHE-3). J Biol Chem 1992; 267:9340–6.
25. Yun CHC, Oh S, Zizak M, et al. cAMP-mediated inhibition of the epithelial brush border Na^+/H^+ exchanger, NHE3, requires an associated regulatory protein. Proc Natl Acad Sci USA 1997; 94:3010–5.
26. Greger R. Renal handling of individual solutes of the glomerular filtrate. In: Greger R, Windhorst U, eds. Comprehensive Human Physiology, from Cellular Mechanisms to Integration. New York: Springer, 1996:1517–44.
27. Aronson PS, Nee J, Suhm MA. Modifier role of internal H^+ in activating the Na^+–H^+ exchanger in renal microvillus membrane vesicles. Nature 1982; 299:161–3.
28. Hediger MA, Coady MJ, Ikeda TS, et al. Expression cloning and cDNA sequencing of the Na^+/glucose co-transporter. Nature 1987; 330:379–81.
29. Capasso G, Unwin R, Agulian S, et al. Bicarbonate transport along the loop of Henle I. Micropuncture studies of load and inhibitor sensitivity. J Clin Invest 1991; 88:430–7.
30. Jorgensen PL. Sodium potassium ion pump in kidney tubules. Physiol Rev 1980; 60:864–917.
31. Bleich M, Schlatter E, Greger R. The luminal K^+ channel of the thick ascending limb of Henle's loop. Pfluegers Arch Eur J Physiol 1990; 415:449–60.
32. Ho K, Nichols CG, Lederer WJ, et al. Cloning and expression of an inwardly rectifying ATP-regulated potassium channel. Nature 1993; 362:31–8.
33. Bailly C. Transducing pathways involved in the control of NaCl reabsorption in the thick ascending limb of Henle's loop. Kidney Int 1998; 65:S29–35.
34. Culpepper RM, Andreoli TE. Interactions among prostaglandin E2, antidiuretic hormone, and cyclic adenosine monophosphate in modulating Cl^- absorption in single mouse medullary thick ascending limbs of Henle. J Clin Invest 1983; 71:1588–601.
35. Greger R. Loop diuretics. In: Greger R, Knauf H, Mutschler E, eds. Handbook of Experimental Pharmacology; Diuretics. New York: Springer, 1995:221–74.
36. Gamba G, Slatzberg SN, Lombardi M, et al. Primary structure and functional expression of a cDNA encoding the thiazide-sensitive, electroneutral sodium–chloride cotransporter. Proc Natl Acad Sci USA 1993; 90:2749–53.
37. Gamba G, Miyanoshita A, Lombardi M, et al. Molecular cloning, primary structure, and characterization of two members of the mammalian electroneutral sodium–(potassium)–chloride cotransporter family expressed in kidney. J Biol Chem 1994; 269:17713–22.
38. Payne JA, Xu JC, Haas M, Lytle CY, Ward D, Forbush B. Primary structure, functional expression, and chromosomal localization of the bumetanide-sensitive Na–K–Cl cotransporter in human colon. J Biol Chem 1995; 270:17977–85.

39. Kriz W, Kaissling B. Structural organization of the mammalian kidney. In: Seldin DW, Giebisch G, eds. The Kidney: Physiology and Pathophysiology. New York: Raven Press, 1992:707–78.
40. Greger R. Chloride transport in thick ascending limb, distal convolution, and collecting duct. Annu Rev Physiol 1988; 50:111–22.
41. Velázquez H, Knauf H, Mutschler E. Thiazide diuretics. In: Greger R, Knauf H, Mutschler E, eds. Handbook Experimental Pharmacology: Diuretics. New York: Springer, 1995:275–334.
42. Greger R, Schlatter E. Presence of luminal K^+, a prerequisite for active NaCl transport in the thick ascending limb of Henle's loop of rabbit kidney. Pfluegers Arch Eur J Physiol 1981; 392:92–4.
43. Simon DB, Lifton RP. The molecular basis of inherited hypokalaemic alkalosis: Bartter's and Giltelman's syndromes. Am J Physiol 1998; 271:F961–6.
44. Takeuchi K, Kato T, Taniyama Y, et al. Three cases of Gitelman's syndrome possibly caused by different mutations in the thiazide-sensitive Na–Cl cotransporter. Intern Med 1997; 36:582–5.
45. Schuster VL. Function and regulation of collecting duct intercalated cells. Annu Rev Physiol 1993; 55:267–88.
46. Wingo CS, Cain BD. The renal H–K-ATPase: physiological significance and role in potassium homeostasis. Annu Rev Physiol 1993; 55:323–47.
47. Knepper MA. Molecular physiology of urinary concentrating mechanism: regulation of aquaporin water channels by vasopressin. Am J Physiol 1997; 272:F3–12.
48. Schlatter E, Bleich M, Hirsch J, et al. pH-sensitive K^+ channels in the distal nephron. Nephrol Dial Transplant 1993; 8:488–90.
49. Greger R. Why do loop diuretics cause hypokalaemia? Nephrol Dial Transplant 1997; 12:1799–801.
50. Canessa CM, Schild L, Buell G, et al. Amiloride-sensitive epithelial Na^+ channel is made of three homologous subunits. Nature 1994; 367:463–7.
51. Berger S, Bleich M, Schmid W, et al. Pathophysiology of mineralocorticoid receptor knock-out mice. Proc Natl Acad Sci USA 1998; 95:9424–9.
52. Gambaryan S, Hausler C, Markert T, et al. Expression of type II cGMP-dependent protein kinase in rat kidney is regulated by dehydration and correlated with renin gene expression. J Clin Invest 1996; 98:662–70.
53. Cutler JA, Follmann D, Allender PS. Randomized trias of sodium reduction: an overview. Am J Clin Nutr 1997; 65(Suppl.):643S–51.
54. Elliott P. Observational studies of salt and blood pressare. Hypertension 1991; 17(Suppl. 1):I-3–8.
55. Elliott P, Stamler J, Nichols R, et al. Intersalt revisited: further analyses of 24-hours sodium excretion and blood pressare within and accross populations. BMJ 1996; 312:1249–53.
56. Midgley JP, Matthew AG, Greenwood CM, Logan AG. Effect of reduced dietary sodium on blood pressare: a meta-analysis of randomized controlled trias. JAMA 1996; 275:1590–7.
57. Law MR, Frost CD, Wald NJ. By how much does dietary salt reduction lower blood pressure? I: analysis of observational data among populations BMJ 1991; 302:811–5.
58. Cowley AW. Genomics and homeostasis. Am J Physiol Regul Integr Comp Physiol 2003; 284:R611–27.
59. Hopkins PN, Hunt SC. Genetics of hypertension. Genet Med 2003; 5:413–29.
60. Luft FC. Molecular genetics of salt-sensitivity and hypertension. Drug Metab Dispos 2001; 29:500–4.
61. Ferrari P, Bianchi G. In: Laragh JH, Brenner BM, eds. Lessons from Experimental Genetic Hypertension. 2nd ed Hypertension: Pathophysiololgy, Diagnosis, and Management. 2nd ed., Vol. 74. New York: Raven Press, 1995:1261–79.
62. de Leeuw PW, Birkenhager WH. The renal circulation in essential hypertension. J Hypertens 1983; 1:321–31.
63. Cusi D, Bianchi G. Renal mechanisms of genetic hypertension: from the molecular level to the intact organism. Kidney Int 1996; 49:1754–9.

64. Bianchi G, Manunta P. Adducin, renal intermediate phenotypes, and hypertension. Hypertension 2004; 44:394–5.
65. Guidi E, Menghetti D, Milani S, Montagnino G, Palazzi P, Bianchi G. Hypertension may be transplanted with the kidney in humans: a long-term historical prospective follow-up of recipients grafted with kidneys coming from donors with or without hypertension in the family. J Am Soc Nephrol 1996; 7:1131–8.
66. Ferrari P, Bianchi G. In: Birkenhäger WH, Reid JL, eds. Pathophysiology of Hypertension. Membrane Ion Transports in Hypertension. Handbook of Hypertension. Vol. 17. Amsterdam, The Netherlands: Elsevier, 1997:935–74.
67. Matsuoka Y, Li X, Bennett V. Adducin: structure, function and regulation. Cell Mol Life Sci 2000; 57:884–95.
68. Bianchi G, Tripodi MG, Casari G, et al. Two point mutations within the adducin genes are involved in blood pressure variation. Proc Natl Acad Sci USA 1994; 91:3999–4003.
69. Tripodi MG, Szpirer C, Reina C, Szpirer J, Bianchi G. Polymorphism of [gamma]-adducin gene in genetic hypertension and mapping of the gene to rat chromosome 1q55. Biochem Biophys Res Comm 1997; 237:685–9.
70. Zagato L, Modica R, Florio M, et al. Genetic mapping of blood pressure quantitative trait loci in Milan hypertensive rats. Hypertension 2000; 36:734–9.
71. Tripodi MG, Florio M, Ferrandi M, et al. Effect of Add1 gene transfer on blood pressure in reciprocal congenic strains of Milan rats. Biochem Biophys Res Comm 2004; 324:562–8.
72. Cusi D, Barlassina C, Azzani T, et al. Polymorphisms of [alpha]-adducin and salt sensitivity in patients with essential hypertension. Lancet 1997; 349:1353–7.
73. Glorioso N, Filigheddu F, Cusi D, et al. alpha-Adducin 460Trp allele is associated with erythrocyte Na transport rate in North Sardinian primary hypertensives. Hypertension 2002; 39:357–62.
74. Tripodi MG, Valtorta F, Torielli L, et al. Hypertension-associated point mutations in the adducin [alpha] and [beta] subunits affect actin cytoskeleton and ion transport. J Clin Invest 1996; 97:2815–22.
75. Ferrandi M, Salardi S, Tripodi MG, et al. Evidence for an interaction between adducin and Na,K'ATPase: relation to genetic hypertension. Am J Physiol 1999; 277:1338–49.
76. Efendiev R, Krmar RT, Leibiger IB, et al. Hypertension-linked mutation in the adducin [alpha]-subunit affects AP2-μ2 phosphorylation and impairs Na^+,K^+-ATPase endocytosis. Circ Res 2004; 95:1100–8.
77. Manunta P, Cusi D, Barlassina C, Righetti M, Lanzani C, D'Amico M, Buzzi L, Citterio L, Stella P, Rivera R, Bianchi G. Alpha-Adducin polymorphisms and renal sodium handling in essential hypertensive patients. Kidney Int 1998 Jun; 53(6):1471–8.
78. Manunta P, Burnier M, D'Amico M, et al. Adducin polymorphism affects renal proximal tubule reabsorption in hypertension. Hypertension 1999; 33:694–7.
79. Magyar CE, Zhang Y, Holstein-Rathlou NH, McDonough AA. Proximal tubule Na transporter responses are the same during acute and chronic hypertension. Am J Physiol Renal Physiol 2000; 279:F358–69.
80. Ferrandi M, Minotti E, Salardi S, Florio M, Bianchi G, Ferrari P. Ouabainlike factor in the Milan hypertensive rats (MHS). Am J Physiol 1992; 263:739–48.
81. Blaustein MP. Sodium ions, calcium ions, and blood pressure regulation: a reassessment and hypothesis. Am J Physiol 1977; 232:C165–73.
82. Ferrari P, Torielli L, Ferrandi M, et al. PST 2238: a new antihypertensive compound that antagonizes the long-term pressor effect of ouabain. J Pharm Exp Ther 1998; 285(1):83–94.
83. Manunta P, Ballabeni C, Ferrandi M, et al. Modulation of endogenous ouabain response to salt challenge by α-adducin polymorphism in rats and humans. Hypertension 2002; 40:395.
84. Manunta P, Messaggio E, Ballabeni C, et al. Plasma ouabain-like factor during acute and chronic changes in sodium balance in essential hypertension. Hypertension 2001; 38:198–203.
85. Lanzani C, Citterio L, Jankaricova M, et al. Role of the adducin family genes in human essential hypertension. J Hypertens 2005; 23(3):543–9.

86. Wang JG, Staessen JA, Messaggio E, et al. Salt, endogenous ouabain and blood pressure interactions in the general population. J Hypertens 2003; 21(8):1475–81.
87. Cwynar M, Staessen JA, Ticha M. Epistatic interaction between alpha and gamma-adducin influences peripheral and central pulse pressures in white Europeans. J Hypertens 2004; 22(Suppl. 2):S72 (Abstract P1.186 2004).
88. Barlassina C, Schork NJ, Manunta P, et al. Synergistic effect of alpha-adducin and ACE genes causes blood pressure changes with body sodium and volume expansion. Kidney Int 2000; 57(3):1083–90.
89. Staessen JA, Wang JG, Brand E, et al. Effects of three candidate genes on prevalence and incidence of hypertension in a Caucasian population. J Hypertens 2001; 19(8):1349–58.
90. Balkestein EJ, Wang JG, Struijker-Boudier HA, et al. Carotid and femoral intima-media thickness in relation to three candidate genes in a Caucasian population. J Hypertens 2002; 20(8):1551–61.
91. Balkestein EJ, Staessen JA, Wang JG, et al. Carotid and femoral artery stiffness in relation to three candidate genes in a white population. Hypertension 2001; 38(5):1190–7.
92. Wang JG, Staessen JA, Tizzoni L, et al. Renal function in relation to three candidate genes. Am J Kidney Dis 2001; 38(6):1158–68.
93. Zagato L, Paroni R, Fermo I, et al. Influence of ACE and alpha-adducin (ADD1) polymorphisms on ACE activity incultured human skin fibroblasts. Hypertension 2002; 40(4):569–91.
94. Sciarrone MT, Stella P, Barlassina C, et al. ACE and alpha-adducin polymorphism as markers of individual response to diuretic therapy. Hypertension 2003; 41(3):398–403.
95. Morrison AC, Bray MS, Folsom AR, Boerwinkle E. ADD1 460W allele associated with cardiovascular disease in hypertensive individuals. Hypertension 2002; 39(6):1053–7.
96. Psaty BM, Doggen C, Vos HL, Vandenbroucke JP, Rosendaal FR. Association of the alpha-adducin polymorphism with blood pressure and risk of myocardial infarction. J Hum Hypertens 2000; 14(2):95–7.
97. Psaty BM, Smith NL, Heckbert SR, et al. Diuretic therapy, the alpha-adducin gene variant, and the risk of myocardial infarction or stroke in persons with treated hypertension. JAMA 2002; 287(13):1680–9.
98. Tobin MD, Braund PS, Burton PR, et al. Genotypes and haplotypes predisposing to myocardial infarction: a multilocus case-control study. Eur Heart J 2004; 25(6):459–67.
99. Winnicki M, Somers VK, Accurso V, et al. On behalf of the HARVEST Study Group. alpha-Adducin Gly460Trp polymorphism, left ventricular mass and plasma renin activity. J Hypertens 2002; 20(9):1771–7.
100. Li Y, Thijs L, Kuznetsova T, Zagato L, Struijiker-Boudier H, Bianchi G, Staessen JA. Cardiovascular risk and α-adducin Gly460Trp polimorphism and systolic pressure—a prospective population study. Hypertension 2005 Sep; 46(3):527–32 (Epub 2005 Jul 25).
101. Barlassina C, Norton GR, Samani NJ, et al. alpha-Adducin polymorphism in hypertensives of South African ancestry. Am J Hypertens 2000; 13(6 Pt 1):719–23.
102. Schork NJ, Chakravarti A, Thiel B, et al. Lack of association between a biallelic polymorphism in the adducin gene and blood pressure in whites and African Americans. Am J Hypertens 2000; 13(6 Pt 1):693–8.
103. Ju Z, Zhang H, Sun K, et al. alpha-Adducin gene polymorphism is associated with essential hypertension in Chinese: a case-control and family-based study. J Hypertens 2003; 21(10):1861–8.
104. Wang JG, Liu L, Zagato L, et al. Blood pressure in relation to three candidate genes in a Chinese population. J Hypertens 2004; 22(5):937–44.
105. Castellano M, Barlassina C, Muiesan ML, et al. alpha-Adducin gene polymorphism and cardiovascular phenotypes in a general population. J Hypertens 1997; 15(12 Pt 2):1707–10.
106. Partridge L, Gems D. Mechanisms of ageing: public or private? Nat Genet 2002; 3:165–75.
107. Staessen JA, Wang J-G, Ginocchio G, et al. The deletion/insertion polymorphism of the angiotensin converting enzyme and cardiovascular-renal risk. J Hypertens 1997; 15:1579–92.

5

Hormonal Control of Sodium Balance

Michel Burnier, Lionel Coltamai, and Bruno Vogt
Division of Nephrology and Hypertension Consultation, University Hospital, University of Lausanne, Lausanne, Switzerland

INTRODUCTION

The regulation of sodium balance results from a complex interplay between extrarenal and intrarenal factors affecting either salt intake or sodium excretion. These mechanisms are crucial to maintain body fluid homeostasis because the sodium ion is the main determinant of extracellular fluid volume. Most of these extra- and intrarenal factors are under the influence of endocrine, paracrine, and autocrine systems, which contribute to the regulation of sodium balance either through their effects on blood pressure and renal perfusion or because they exert direct effects on renal tubular transport systems. Some of these neurohormonal factors, such as the sympathetic nervous system, sex hormones, aldosterone, and steroids, are discussed elsewhere in this book. In this chapter we present the other main hormonal systems involved in the maintenance of sodium balance. These systems are divided into two categories, i.e., the vasoconstrictor and antinatriuretic systems such as the renin-angiotensin and the endothelin (ET) systems and the vasodilator and natriuretic systems illustrated by natriuretic peptides and nitric oxide (NO). Because most of these systems interact with each other to form a complex network enabling the fine tuning of sodium balance, an integrative view of the renal regulation of sodium balance will be developed by Montani et al. in Chapter 9.

THE RENIN-ANGIOTENSIN SYSTEM

The renin-angiotensin cascade that leads to the generation of angiotensin II (Ang II) is certainly one of the most important endocrine systems regulating sodium balance. This enzymatic cascade starts with the cleavage of angiotensinogen by renin to form angiotensin I (Ang I) (1). Because angiotensinogen concentrations in plasma are generally high, the main rate-limiting factor for the production of Ang I is the availability of active renin which is synthesized and released from the juxtaglomerular cells of the kidney. Ang I is then converted into Ang II by the angiotensin-converting enzyme (ACE) located on endothelial cells in several vascular beds, but particularly in the lung. Of note, several alternative pathways for the production of Ang I and II have been identified in some specific tissues. Thus, Ang II can be produced from Ang I in the heart under the effect of

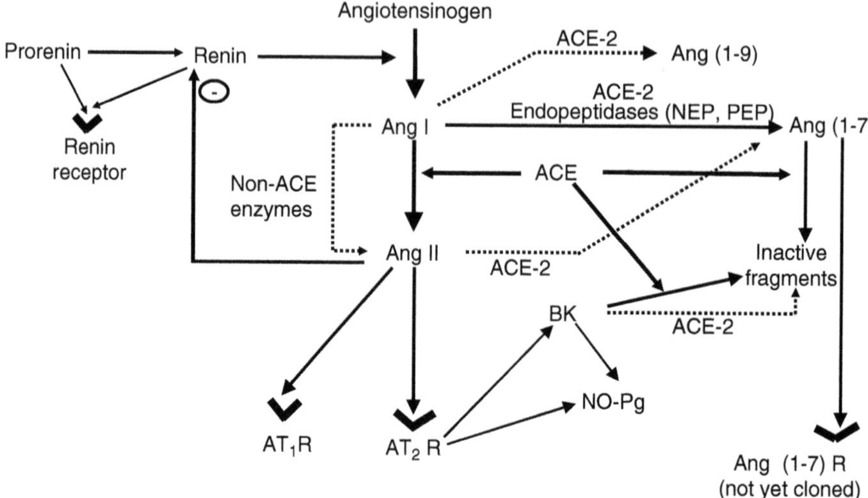

Figure 1 The renin-angiotensin system. *Abbreviations*: ACE, angiotensin-converting enzyme; ACE-2, angiotensin-converting enzyme 2; Ang, angiotensin; AT_1R, angiotensin II type 1 receptor; AT_2R, angiotensin II type 2 receptor; BK, bradykinin; NO, nitric oxide; PG, prostaglandins.

a chymostatin-sensitive chimase and angiotensin peptides can be produced by non-renin enzymes such as tonin, cathepsin, pepsin, trypsin, and kallikrein (2). Moreover, both Ang I and Ang II can be metabolized by an ACE-2 enzyme to form angiotensin 1–9 or angiotensin 1–7, a peptide with specific effects (Fig. 1) (3).

Ang II exerts its effects through the activation of specific receptors including the AT_1 and the AT_2 receptors and probably some other as yet undefined receptors (AT_n) (1,4). The AT_1 receptor mediates most of the Ang II effects such as vascular smooth muscle cells contraction, increase in cardiac contractility, stimulation of aldosterone release, stimulation of the sympathetic nervous system, regulation of thirst and salt appetite and the modulation of renal hemodynamics and sodium excretion. Ang II exerts an important negative feedback on renin secretion mediated by the AT_1 receptor. More recently, Ang II has also been shown to stimulate inflammation and atherosclerosis and to promote cell growth through the activation of the AT_1 receptor (5). The role of the AT_2 receptor is less well characterized but some properties linked to this receptor have been described as a vasodilatory and natriuretic effect, an inhibition of cell proliferation and growth and the stimulation of NO synthase. The numerous effects of Ang II are summarized in Table 1. Very recently, a renin/prorenin receptor has been identified, the function of which remains yet to be defined (6).

Central Effects of Ang II and Sodium Balance

Blood-borne Ang II exerts several actions on the brain that affect sodium balance. Among them, two central properties of Ang II have a major impact on sodium homeostasis, i.e., the ability of Ang II to stimulate thirst and salt hunger (7). In addition to these effects, systemically administered Ang II has been shown to enhance vasopressin and adreno-corticotropic hormone secretion and intracerebroventricular (ICV) injections of Ang II have been shown to increase or decrease sympathetic nerve activity, depending on the dose and the site of brain activation, and to raise blood pressure (8).

Table 1 Angiotensin II Receptors and Their Functions and Localization

Receptor	Actions	Localization
AT_1	Vasoconstriction Increases sodium retention Suppresses renin secretion Stimulates aldosterone release Increases thirst and sodium intake Increases endothelin secretion Increases vasopressin and ACTH release Activates the sympathetic nervous system Promotes myocyte hypertrophy Stimulates vascular and cardiac fibrosis Increases cardiac inotropic/contractile activity Chronotropic/arrythmogenic Stimulates plasminogen activator inhibitor 1 Stimulates growth factors (TGF-β, PDGF..) Stimulates matrix formation Stimulates superanoxide formation Stimulates inflammation Promotes atherosclerosis	Vessels, brain, heart, kidney, adrenal, nerves
AT_2	Antiproliferation/inhibition of cell growth Cell differentiation Tissue repair Apoptosis Vasodilatation (NO mediated ?) Kidney and urinary tract development Control of pressure/natriuresis Stimulate renal prostaglandins Stimulate renal bradykinin and nitric oxide	Adrenal, heart, brain, myometrum fetus injured tissues
AT_3	?	Neuroblastoma cells amphibians
AT_4	Renal vasodilator Stimulate plasminogen activator Inhibitor 1	Brain, heart, vessels lungs, prostate adrenal, kidney

Abbreviations: ACTH, adrenocorticotropic hormone; AT, angiotensin II; NO, nitric oxide; PDGF, platelet-derived growth factor; TGF-β, transforming growth factor-beta.

The effect of Ang II on sodium appetite has been demonstrated in several species (9). Interestingly, sodium intake increases only several hours after the central injection of Ang II. The exact mechanism of this effect on salt intake is not precisely elucidated: it may the consequence of the natriuretic effect of centrally administered Ang II. This effect on sodium intake can be blunted by the central administration of AT_1 and AT_2 receptor antagonists (10). When injected in the cerebral ventricules, Ang II has also been shown to induce a natriuresis that may be related to the increase in blood pressure or to changes in sympathetic nerve activity as well as to changes in vasopressin and renin activity. The natriuretic response to ICV Ang II is blocked by the central injection of an AT_1 receptor antagonist (11). Of note, the natriuretic response to ICV infusion of hypertonic saline is blocked by an AT_1 receptor antagonist suggesting the possibility of a centrally active angiotensinergic AT_1 system involved (12).

As mentioned earlier, Ang II also has a major impact on thirst. Indeed, in many species, the intracerebral injection of Ang II produces an almost immediate increase in thirst and copious water drinking (9). One site of action of Ang II has been postulated to explain this effect, i.e., the stimulation of the median preoptic nucleus in the anterior wall of the third ventricle.

Renal Effects of Ang II and Sodium Balance

The major influence of the renin-angiotensin system on sodium and water homeostasis results from the effects of Ang II on the kidney. All the components of the system are abundantly present in the kidney, which is the major source of renin. Intrarenal Ang II receptors are widely distributed within the kidney on the luminal and basolateral membranes of several segments of the nephron as well as on the renal microvasculature in both the cortex and medulla. On the vascular side, Ang II receptors (mainly AT_1) have been localized to afferent and efferent arterioles, to the glomeruli in mesangial cells, podocytes and even epithelial cells, to vasa recta bundles and arcuate arteries. With these particular locations, Ang II play an important role in the regulation of renal hemodynamics, glomerular filtration rate (GFR) and regulatory mechanisms such as the tubuloglomerular feedback (TGF) mechanism. On epithelial cells, Ang II receptors or AT_1 transcripts have been found in proximal tubule brush border and basolateral membranes, distal tubule, collecting ducts, medullary thick ascending limb (MTAL), medullary collecting ducts and macula densa cells. The AT_2 receptor has also been identified in the kidney (13). It is highly expressed during the fetal life and decreases in adulthood. It has been found in glomeruli, proximal tubules, collecting ducts and some parts of the renal vasculature.

Interestingly, much higher concentrations of Ang II have been measured within the kidney than in the plasma (14). Particularly, high concentrations of Ang II have been found in the proximal tubular fluid and in the renal interstitial fluid. In the proximal tubule, Ang II concentrations have been found to exceed the concentration in plasma (i.e., of the glomerular filtrate) suggesting that Ang II is secreted or formed in the lumen of the proximal tubule (14). It is also possible that Ang I is secreted and metabolized by the tubular ACE to generate Ang II in the lumen. The high concentration of Ang II in the interstitial fluid is more difficult to explain. Some data suggest that both Ang I and Ang II are formed intrarenally and derived from locally formed substrates (14). There may be also a translocation of intracellular Ang II into the renal instertitial space. It has been postulated that the ability of the kidney to produce high concentrations of Ang II in these compartments enables the kidney to adapt more accurately and rapidly to changes in renal hemodynamics and sodium balance and hence to maintain the body fluid and sodium homeostasis (14).

The renin-angiotensin system contributes to the regulation of sodium balance in several ways (Fig. 2). The first is the regulation of renal hemodynamics and in particular the control of GFR through its powerful vasoconstrictor effects on afferent and efferent arterioles with a more pronounced effect on efferent arteries. Ang II also influences glomerular function through a reduction in glomerular filtration coefficient (Kf), an effect that may be linked to the impact of Ang II on mesangial cells and perhaps on glomerular epithelial cells. Studies have also demonstrated that Ang II affects the medullary hemodynamics (15). This vascular medullary response to Ang II is modulated by NO, prostaglandins, and kinins. The microcirculation of the renal medulla has several important roles including tissue oxygenation and maintenance of salt and water balance through the countercurrent exchange system (15).

Ang II is a major regulator of proximal sodium reabsorption via activation of AT_1 receptors present on both basolateral and luminal membranes (13). In isolated perfused tubules, the effect of peritubular Ang II on proximal tubular sodium handling actually depends on the concentration of the peptide. At low concentrations (10^{-12}–10^{-10} M),

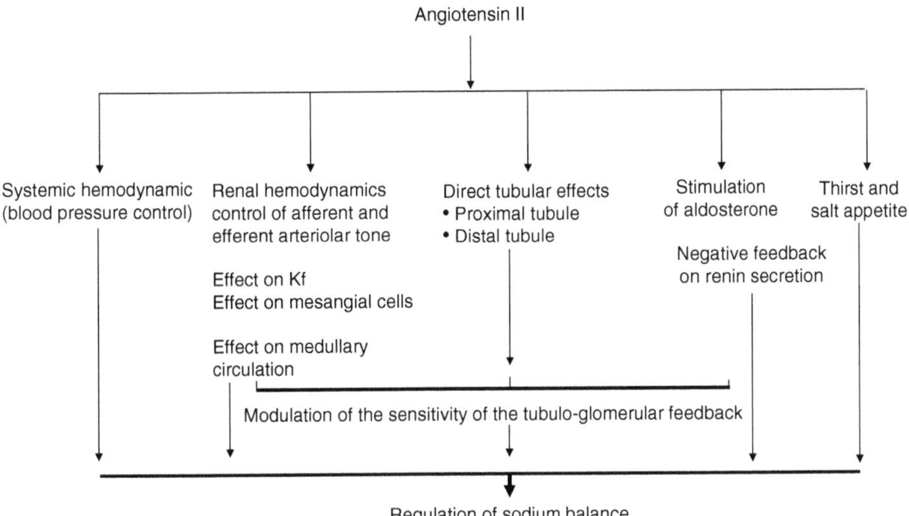

Figure 2 Systemic, renal, and central effects whereby angiotensin II contributes to the maintenance of sodium balance.

Ang II increases proximal tubular reabsorption of sodium whereas at high concentrations (10^{-7} M) it inhibits the reabsorption rate (16). Ang II exerts proximal tubule transport effects via activation of luminal membrane AT_1 receptors. Intraluminal Ang II enhances proximal tubule and bicarbonate reabsorption through stimulatory actions on the sodium/hydrogen exchanger (Na^+/H^+) (17). There are also indications that Ang II regulates the reabsorption rate in the distal tubule where AT_1 receptors have been located. In this nephron segment, addition of Ang II to the distal tubular fluid has been found to increase net bicarbonate and fluid reabsorption (18). Ang II is also one of the main circulating factors stimulating aldosterone release which directly regulates sodium excretion in the late segments of the nephron. There is also some evidence that Ang II may stimulate the amiloride-sensitive sodium channel activity in the cortical collecting duct (19) and in the colon (20).

The renal vascular and tubular effects of Ang II are not entirely dissociated. They are rather synergistic and provide a powerful regulation of sodium excretion. The TGF mechanism is the perfect example of an adaptation of the balance between the tubular reabsorption capacities and the filtered load through the regulation of GFR. Through this mechanism, flow-dependent changes in tubular fluid solute concentration at the level of the macula densa in the terminal part of the loop of Henle are sensed and signals are transmitted to the afferent arterioles in order to constrict or dilate the arterioles to maintain stability of the filtered load. Several factors contribute to this regulatory mechanism including adenosine, NO, and prostaglandins (21). Among them, Ang II has been shown to modulate the sensitivity of the TGF mechanism (22). This effect of Ang II is mediated both by the vascular effect of the peptide on vascular smooth muscle cells of afferent arterioles and by the effect of Ang II on the Na/H exchange system in cells of the macula densa (23).

Another approach to demonstrate the impact of the renin-angiotensin system on sodium balance is the investigation of the renal impact of drugs interfering directly with the system such as ACE inhibitors, Ang II AT_1 receptor antagonists and more recently renin inhibitors. Both ACE inhibitors and AT_1 receptor antagonists have been shown to increase renal blood flow and GFR and to enhance sodium excretion in animals (24).

In humans, similar results have been observed with significant increases in renal blood flow and urinary sodium excretion but the effect on sodium balance was obtained even in the absence of any change in GFR, an observation which would confirm the direct effect of Ang II on tubular sodium reabsorption (25).

ENDOTHELIN

ET is a very potent endogenous vasoconstrictor produced by the endothelium and identified by Yanagisawa et al. in 1988 (26). There are three isoforms of ET (i.e., ET-1,-2 and -3) but ET-1 is the only relevant peptide in humans. ET is derived from pro-ET which is cleaved into a big-ET and then converted to the active ET-1 by an ET-converting enzyme. Several stimuli induce ET release by endothelial cells, including shear stress, thrombin, Ang II, vasopressin, catecholamines, and hypoxia (Fig. 3) (27). The effects of ET are mediated by two receptors, i.e., the endothelin A (ET-A) and endothelin B (ET-B) receptors. The ET-A receptor is widely distributed and it is the principal receptor located on vascular smooth muscle cells and cardiomyocytes. In these cells, activation of ET-A receptors leads to an activation of phospholipase C, an increase in intracellular calcium and hence, to cell contraction. The ET-B receptor is located on both vascular smooth muscle and endothelial cells. In endothelial cells, activation of ET-B receptors releases vasodilating substances such as NO, prostacyclin, and adrenomedullin. In the vasculature, activation of the ET-B receptor induces a vasoconstriction. ET-1 production is modulated by several factors. Thus, in mesangial cells, for example, an increase in ET-1 is induced by

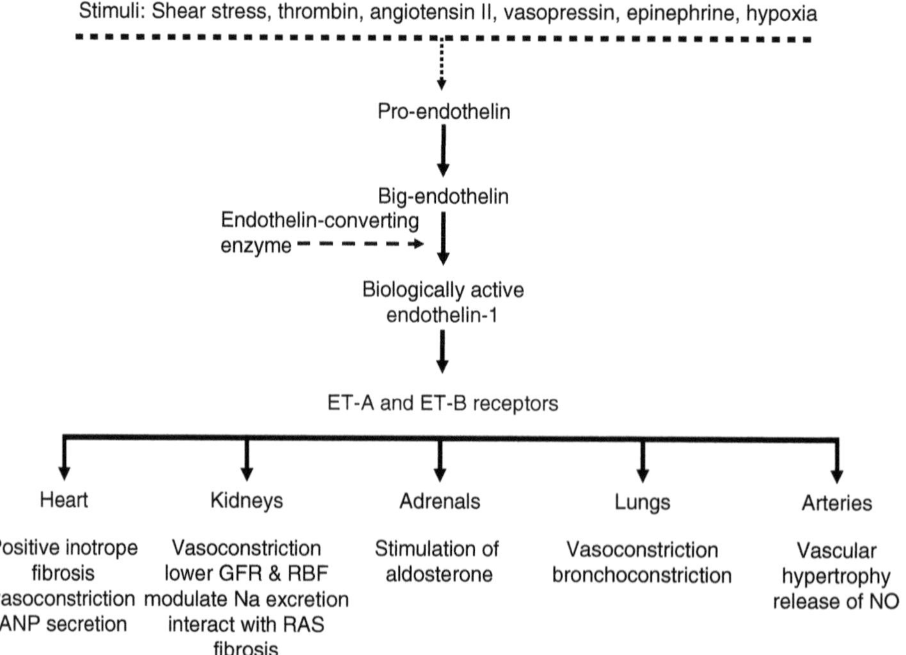

Figure 3 Stimuli contributing to endothelin release by endothelial cells. *Abbreviations*: ANP, atrial natriuretic peptide; ET-A, ET-B, endothelin A and B receptors; GFR, glomerular filtration rate; NO, nitric oxide; RAS, renin-angiotensin system; RBF, renal blood flow.

Ang II, vasopressin, thrombin, insulin, thromboxane A2, and tumor necrosis factor whereas a decrease in ET-1 production is induced by atrial natriuretic peptide (ANP), brain natriuretic peptide (BNP), cyclic guanosine monophosphate (cGMP), and cyclic adenosine monophosphate or heparin.

If vasoconstriction is the hallmark of ET's action, several other biological properties of ET have been described. Thus, renal function appears to be particularly responsive to the effects of ET (28). Administration of "pressor" concentrations of ET-1 (in nM) in animals and humans has been shown to decrease GFR and renal blood flow through the stimulation of vascular smooth muscle cells and contraction of mesangial cells and to reduce urinary sodium excretion secondary to the changes in renal hemodynamics (28). However, some studies have suggested that ET infusion decreases urinary sodium excretion independently of the changes in renal hemodynamics (29,30). Thus ET could mediate an antinatriuresis via direct effects on renal tubular sodium transport. In accordance with these data, subpressor doses of ET have been found to cause a natriuresis in rats through a direct inhibition of renal tubular sodium transport (29,30). These data would indicate that there is a dose-dependent effect of ET in renal sodium transport, a high dose producing sodium retention and a low dose inducing natriuresis. Thus, it has been postulated that systemically administered ET acts as an endocrine system and is antinatriuretic whereas lower local concentrations of ET act as a paracrine/autocrine system and are natriuretic.

The renal medulla is a major site of ET-1 synthesis and receptor expression in the kidney (Table 2) (29). In this area, the production of ET-1 is higher than anywhere else in the body. In the medulla, ET-1 contracts vasa recta and inhibits collecting duct and MTAL sodium chloride and water transport. Several lines of evidence indicate that the major effect of ET on sodium balance occurs in this region of the kidney (29). Application of ET-1 on the basolateral side of the cortical collecting tubule (CCT) increases luminal membrane voltage and resistance in microperfused rabbit CCT suggesting an inhibition of apical sodium transport by ET-1. In rabbit inner medulla collecting duct, ET has been reported to inhibit the activity of the Na/K-ATPase, an effect partially mediated by cyclooxygenase metabolites (31). ET-1 has also been shown to regulate amiloride-sensitive sodium channels with a different impact on channel activity depending on the concentration of ET (32). Interestingly, collecting duct ET-1 knockout mice were produced in which the ET-1 gene was selectively disrupted in principal cells (33). This selective knockout of the ET-1 gene in the collecting duct had no effect on sodium excretion in mice on a normal sodium diet but these mice had an impaired ability to excrete sodium when placed on a high sodium diet suggesting that ET-1 produced primarily from medullary collecting duct mediates, via autocrine and paracrine pathways, is part of the renal response to acute

Table 2 Expression of the Endothelin System in the Kidney

Cell type	ET1 synthesis	ET receptor expression	ET receptor subtype
Collecting duct	++++	++++	B$\gg$A
Thick ascending limb	++	++	B
Endothelial cells	++	++	B
Vascular smooth muscle	—	++	B
Descending thin limb	—	+	?
Ascending thin limb	—	—	—
Medullary interstitial cell	—	++	A and B

Abbreviation: ET, endothelin.
Source: From Ref. 31.

sodium loading. Of note, these transgenic rats deficient in ET-1, specifically in the collecting duct develop salt-sensitive hypertension (33).

Most studies investigating the effect of ET on sodium excretion indicate that natriuresis and diuresis are linked to the activation of ET-B receptors. However, ET-A receptors have also been localized in the inner medulla cortical duct. These ET-A receptors have also been knocked out in mice but this receptor knockout had no effect on sodium excretion on a normal or high sodium diet (34).

ET-1 is also an important regulator of sodium transport in the MTAL, an effect which appears to be mediated by NO (34). ET can also facilitate natriuresis through an increase in medullary blood flow (35). Indeed, intravenous infusion of ET-1 has been shown to decrease renal cortical blood flow but increase medullary blood flow through an activation of ET-B receptors. This effect is mediated in part by prostaglandins and NO. The effect of ET-1 on the renal medulla is mostly evident on a high sodium intake (36).

As mentioned previously, ET-1 interacts very closely with NO via activation of ET-B receptors. In the endothelium, ET-1 promotes the release of NO and thereby maintains a balance between the vasodilatory effect of NO and the vasoconstrictor effect of ET-1 itself (37). Thus, in all tissues, the vasoconstrictor effects of exogenous ET-1 are significantly enhanced when NO production is inhibited. There is also a close interaction between ET and the renin-angiotensin-aldosterone system (38). Ang II enhances the vascular responsiveness to exogenous ET-1, increases the release of ET-1 and the expression of preproendothelin in endothelial cells. Some of the effects of Ang II on cardiac tissue may actually be mediated by ET-1. In the heart, ET-1 has been found to stimulate aldosterone synthesis (39,40) and there is some evidence that ET-1 interferes with renin secretion (41).

Taken together, these data demonstrate that ET is a powerful peptide, which regulates not only systemic and renal hemodynamics but also body sodium homeostasis. Not surprisingly, ET is implicated in the pathogenesis of several diseases in which alterations of sodium balance has been shown to play a critical pathophysiological role such as hypertension, renal glomerular diseases, diabetic nephropathy, and cyclosporine nephrotoxicity.

VASOPRESSIN

Arginine–vasopressin has been recognized as one of the most potent vasoconstrictor peptide through the activation of V_1 vascular receptors. Moreover, vasopressin is a crucial determinant of fluid balance mediated by its activity on renal V_2 receptors. The molecular mechanisms whereby vasopressin regulates water excretion are now well established (42,43). Indeed, vasopressin has been shown to control water permeability in the collecting duct through the regulation of the water channels, aquaporin 2 and 3. More recent data have shown that vasopressin also possess antinatriuretic actions in the kidney, actions that are linked mainly to the activity of the renal V_2 receptor (44,45). Thus, vasopressin has been reported to increase sodium reabsorption in the thick ascending limb and in the collecting duct (44,46,47). The activity of the Na–K–2Cl cotransporter as well as the epithelial sodium channel (ENaC) have been found to be increased by vasopressin (45,47–49). In Brattelboro rats which lack vasopressin, water restriction or the injection of the V_2 receptor agonist desamino-8-D-arginine vasopressin (dDAVP) resulted in a significant increase abundance for the Na–K–2Cl cotransporter and for two subunits of ENaC, i.e., the β and γ subunits (49). Some sodium transporter such as the α subunit of ENaC and the thiazide-sensitive cotransporter were increased by dDAVP but not by water restriction (49). Nicco et al. have shown that the vasopressin-induced increase in ENaC subunits occurred in the renal cortex and in the lung but not in the rectum which does not have V_2 receptors (50). Interestingly, vasopressin had no effect on sodium transport systems in the proximal tubule (51). A V_2-mediated sodium reabsorption has also been observed in healthy subjects and in patients with central or nephrogenic diabetes insipidus (45). In humans, the antinatriuretic response to dDAVP also results from a direct tubular effect as it was found to be independent of any changes in hemodynamics.

DOPAMINE

Dopamine is mainly synthesized not only in noradrenergic and dopaminergic nerves but also in non-neural tissues such as the gut and the kidney (52). In the kidney, dopamine is produced essentially by the proximal tubules by decarboxylation of L-3,4 dihydroxyphenylalanine (L-DOPA) transported into proximal tubular cells from the blood (53). Within the tubule, dopamine is not transformed into norepinephrine because the cell lacks dopamine β-hydroxylase. Dopamine exerts autocrine and paracrine effects mediated by D_1- and D_3-receptors (52). On a high sodium intake, dopamine acts on the proximal tubule and on jejunal cells to decrease sodium transport via the D_1 receptor reinforced by the D_3 receptor (54,55). The autocrine and paracrine regulation of sodium excretion by dopamine is due to direct tubular effects and not renal hemodynamic changes induced by dopamine (56–59). In this respect, the impact of locally produced dopamine differs from that obtained with a systemic infusion of dopamine. One important observation is that dopamine interacts with Ang II by producing opposite effects both on renal hemodynamics and on renal sodium handling (60). Thus, the natriuretic effect of D_1 receptors is increased when Ang II levels are low or when the renin-angiotensin system is blocked with an Ang II receptor antagonist. Interestingly, D_1 receptor activation downregulates the expression of angiotensin AT_1 receptors and conversely Ang II increases the expression of D_1 receptors through its effect on AT_1 receptors (61,62).

Of note, the failure of the autocrine and paracrine effects of dopamine may result in the development of hypertension due to the lack of inhibition of sodium transport mechanism such as the Na^+/H^+ exchanger 3, the Na bicarbonate cotransporter and the Na^+/K^+-ATPase in the proximal tubule and thick ascending limb of Henle (52).

NITRIC OXIDE

Besides ET, endothelial cells are also producing NO, a potent vasorelaxant factor which contributes to the local regulation of vascular tone. NO is formed by the enzyme nitric oxide synthase (NOS) from the amino-acid L-arginine (63). Once formed, NO diffuses to the underlying vascular smooth muscle cells, activates soluble guanylate cyclase and produces a vasorelaxation. Three forms of NOS have been described: a neuronal NOS present in neural cells, an inducible NOS and an endothelial NOS (eNOS) (64,65). In the vessels, NO is released from endothelial cells in response to physical stimuli (shear stress and hypoxia) and by the stimulation of endothelial receptors such as bradykinin and muscarinic receptors (Fig. 4). NOS activity can be inhibited using endogenous analogues of L-arginine such as asymmetric dimethylarginine or *N*-monomethyl-L-arginine. Some of these analogues are increased in disease states, for example, in patients with chronic renal failure (66).

During the last 10 years, evidence has accumulated suggesting that NO participates in the regulation of vascular and renal functions and thereby contributes to the control of extra-cellular fluid volume by the kidney. There are two pathways whereby NO could

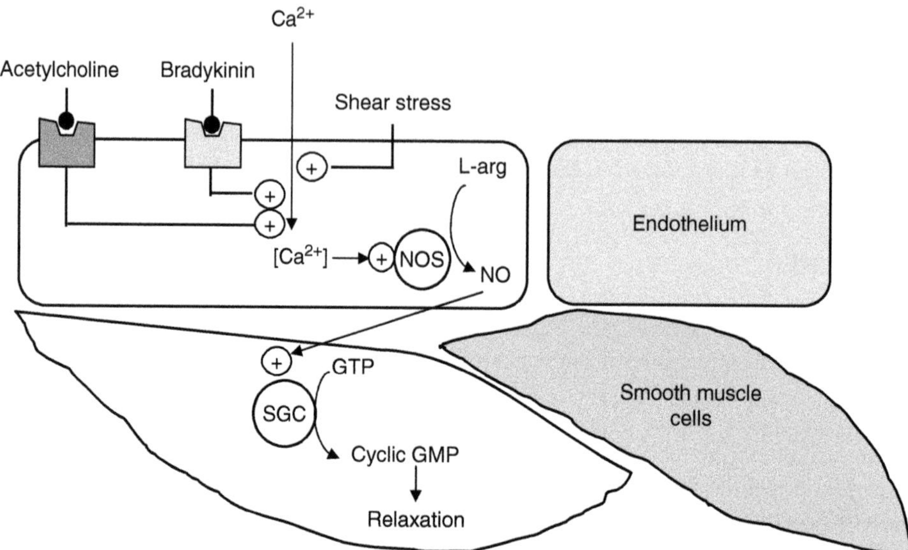

Figure 4 Mechanisms of nitric oxide release by the endothelial cells. *Abbreviations*: GMP, guanosine monophosphate; GTP, guanosine triphosphate; L-arg, L-arginine; NO, nitric oxide; NOS, nitric oxide synthase; SGC, soluble guanylate cyclase.

contribute to the regulation of sodium balance, that is, (*i*) the activation of the eNOS which reacts to short-term changes in renal perfusion pressure or shear stress and follows the acute changes in Ang II actions and (*ii*) the neuronal NOS (nNOS) of the macula densa which reacts to the long-term changes in distal delivery of sodium and regulates renin synthesis and release.

eNOS and the Regulation of Renal Perfusion Pressure

The eNOS enzyme has been localized throughout the renal vasculature and in the glomerulus (64,67) and like in the rest of the vasculature, eNOS is activated mainly by shear stress and pressure stretch. Ang II and transforming growth factor-beta (TGF-β) have also been found to stimulate eNOS mRNA in the kidney. In the renal vasculature, NO is released to oppose the intrinsic property of the vessel to react to an increase in perfusion pressure with a vasoconstriction. Thus, NO counterbalances the intrinsic myogenic mechanism of the vasculature. NO also interferes with the TGF mechanism which autoregulates renal blood flow and GFR (68). Thus, administration of NOS inhibitors has been shown to result in a strong enhancement of the TGF responsiveness suggesting a tonic depression of the TGF response under physiological conditions. The pressure–natriuresis phenomenon is reduced significantly with the applicaton of a NOS inhibitor (69). Similar observations were made after acute volume expansion with isotonic saline (70). In this experimental conditions, the natriuretic response to volume expansion was blunted when NOS was blocked by L-NAME (71). In one of this study, the change in fractional excretion of lithium was lower during L-NAME than during the control period suggesting an effect of NO synthesis inhibition on proximal tubular sodium reabsorption (72). Altogether, these data suggest that NO modulate the afferent arteriole autoregulatory process and thereby regulates sodium excretion in some physiological conditions such as acute volume expansion.

NO also interacts with the renin-angiotensin system and particularly with the renal hemodynamic effects of Ang II. Thus, in the rabbit, NOS blockade has been found to increase the sensitivity of afferent arterioles to Ang II (73). This would indicate that even under physiological conditions, the tonic influence of Ang II is counterbalanced by the vasodilating properties of NO. Thus, the renal vasoconstrictive effects of Ang II are always more pronounced during NOS inhibition.

nNOS and the Macula Densa

Another pathway whereby NO can affect sodium balance is the interaction with renin synthesis and release (74). The nNOS is expressed in the juxtaglomerular apparatus as well as in the renal medulla and in nerve terminals. nNOS has also been localized in cells of the efferent arterioles but not in the afferent arteriole. Macula densa nNOS expression is regulated in parallel with renin expression in a variety of conditions such as the administration of furosemide or the application of a low sodium diet (75). These data indicate that macula densa NOS expression varies simultaneously with renin gene expression during variations in the distal delivery of sodium. The interaction between NO and renin secretion is relatively complex and multiple contradictory results have been published which appear to be due to difference in the duration of NOS inhibition and the dosage of NOS inhibitors. Yet, the studies performed on the overall effect of NO on renin secretion in vivo, in isolated kidneys and in vitro, suggest that the tonic effects of NO on renin secretion is primarily stimulatory. NO appears to be an enhancer of renin secretion and synthesis rather than a specific activator. There is a close relation between Ang II, macula densa NO and sodium delivery in the distal tubule so that an increase in distal delivery of sodium leads to a decreased nNOS activity and reduced renin secretion enabling to maintain sodium balance as illustrated in (Fig. 5).

In summary, the NO system participates in the maintenance of sodium in several different ways: through the activity of eNOS, the NO system regulates the renal hemodynamic response to increases in perfusion pressure and hence sodium excretion whereas through the neuronal NOS located in the macula densa, the NO system influences renin secretion and thereby responds to changes in the distal delivery of sodium. With these two mechanisms the NO system contributes to the regulation of sodium and fluid balance.

NATRIURETIC PEPTIDES

In the 1980s, DeBold and collaborators discovered that rat atrial extracts had potent natriuretic and vasodilatory properties (76). This original finding led to the identification of the ANP and subsequently to the recognition of a family of four distinct natriuretic peptides: ANP (17 amino-acids), BNP (32 amino-acids), c-type natriuretic peptide (CNP) (22 amino acids), and urodilatin (32 amino acids). ANP is synthesized and secreted predominantly by the atria. BNP was initially isolated from pig's and dog's brains but it is produced essentially by cardiomyocytes (77). CNP has been localized in the brain and in the heart but also in several other peripheral tissues including the kidney, the adrenal glands and the endothelium. Urodilatin has been isolated from human urine and has been found only in the kidney (78).

ANP and BNP are released from the heart mainly in response to changes in atrial or ventricular stretch (Fig. 6). However, plasma levels of natriuretic peptides are also influenced by the body position and the salt intake and can be modulated by paracrine factors such as ET which is one of the most potent stimuli for ANP secretion or NO which

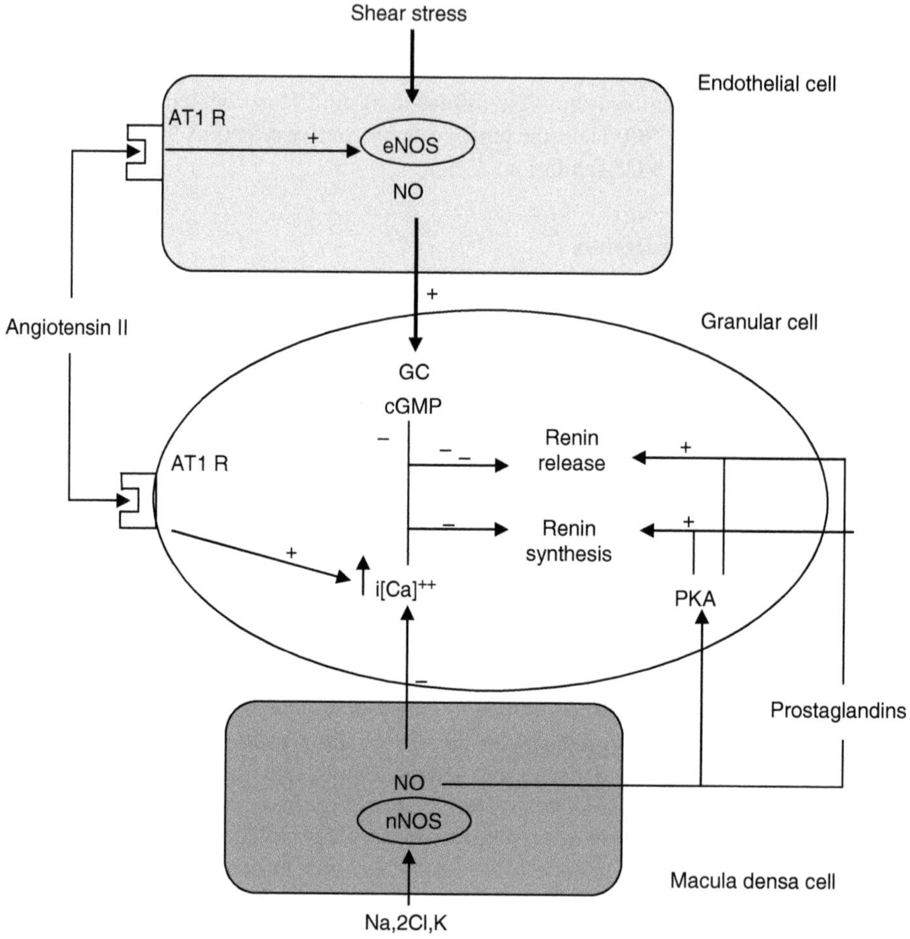

Figure 5 Schematic representation of the control of renin secretion by NO. *Abbreviations*: AT_1R, angiotensin II type 1 receptor; cGMP, cyclic guanosine monophosphate; eNOS, endothelial nitric oxide synthase; GC, guanylate cyclase; NO, nitric oxide; nNOS, neuronal nitric oxide; PKA, protein kinase A.

has been shown to inhibit ANP secretion. Other factors such as Ang II, vasopressin, and adrenergic agonists, opioids or calcitonin gene-related peptide could contribute to stimulate or inhibit ANP secretion in some clinical conditions (79). Natriuretic peptides act by stimulating specific receptors (natriuretic peptide receptor A, B, and C). These receptors are widely distributed throughout the body including endothelium, smooth muscle cells, heart, adrenal gland, lung, brain, adipose tissue, and in the kidney (79). Natriuretic peptides are degraded by the neutral endopeptidase 24.11 and by a receptor-mediated clearance via the C receptor. Along with the vasculature, the kidney is one of the prime target of the physiological effects of ANPs. ANP also causes intravascular volume contraction as documented by increases in hematocrit and serum albumin when administered to binephrectomized rats (80). ANP has an inhibitory action on aldosterone and renin secretion (81). ANP and BNP antagonize the vasoconstriction induced by

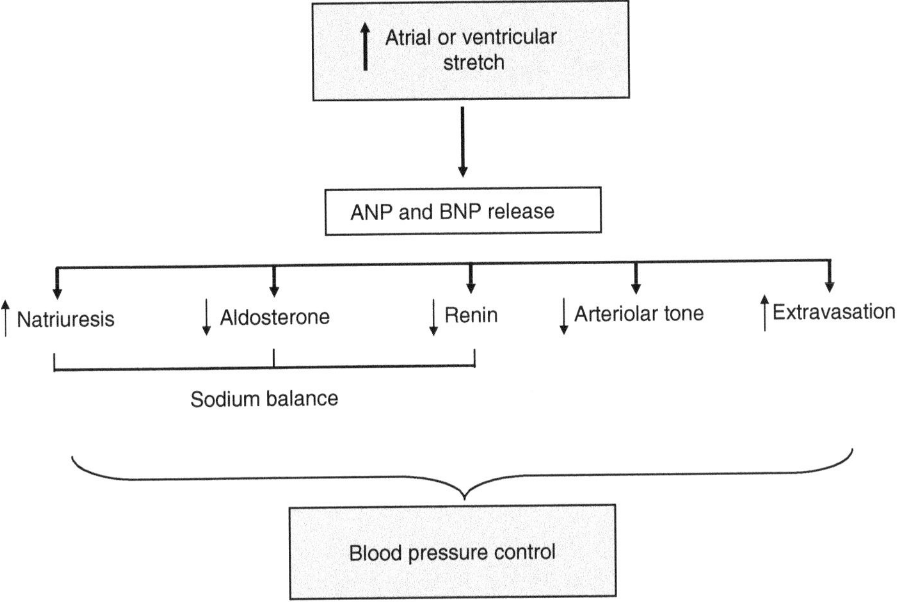

Figure 6 Mechanisms whereby ANP and BNP may affect sodium balance and blood pressure regulation. *Abbreviations*: ANP, atrial natriuretic peptide; BNP, brain natriuretic peptide.

the infusion of norepinephrine or Ang II (82). There is also some evidence that the central effects of ANP contribute to fluid and electrolyte balance and to the regulation of systemic hemodynamics (83). These central effects of ANP are mediated by an interaction between ANP and sympathetic tone in the brain stem.

Most studies assessing the role of natriuretic peptides on renal function have been conducted using ANP. The early studies performed in animals have shown that ANP increases urinary sodium and effect which has been attributed essentially to an increase in intraglomerular pressure, ANP producing a vasodilation of the afferent arteriole and a relative vasoconstriction of efferent arterioles; hence filtration fraction is increased by ANP (84,85). In addition, ANP has been found to relax mesangial cells and increase the filtration surface of glomeruli. However, in the original studies, ANP did not cause any change in GFR and yet, an increase in sodium excretion was found suggesting a direct tubular effect of ANP (86). When infused in healthy subjects, exogenous ANP has also been shown to increase sodium excretion in the absence of any change in GFR (87).

The impact of ANP on proximal sodium reabsorption has been relatively controversial. Some studies reported no effect on proximal sodium handling whereas others suggested that ANP reduced proximal sodium reabsorption (87–89). Some other studies suggested that ANP has no effect on basal sodium transport in the proximal tubule but decreases the effect of Ang II and norepinephrine which increase sodium transport in this nephron segment. In the proximal tubule, ANP has been shown to decrease the activity of the Na^+/H^+ exchanger and to inhibit the Na/K-ATPase (90). ANP may also inhibit an apical K channel. Of note, although ANP receptors have been identified on the proximal tubule, the impact of ANP on sodium handling by this tubule may be indirect. Indeed, the natriuretic effect of ANP is blunted by the administration of dopamine D1 receptor antagonists (91). This would suggest that dopamine is perhaps a mediator of the proximal tubular effects of ANP.

The proximal tubule does not appear to be the major tubular site of action of ANP. ANP has been reported to stimulate cGMP accumulation in the MTAL but not in the cortical thick ascending limb (90). The inner medullary collecting duct is probably the main site of action of ANP. This nephron segment contains the higher density of ANP receptors and in this segment, ANP has been found to cause a marked decrease in sodium reabsorption (92).

BNP has similar natriuretic properties than ANP. At low doses, BNP induces a natriuretic response without any change in renal hemodynamics. However, at higher doses, BNP increases GFR and decreases renal blood flow, an effect which is probably linked to the vasodilatory effect of BNP and to the decrease in blood pressure. At high doses, BNP rather produce sodium retention in response to the fall in blood pressure. Of note, the intrarenal distribution of BNP receptors differs from that of ANP receptors suggesting different functions within the kidney. C-natriuretic peptide has much less natriuretic effect than ANP or BNP. In contrast, urodilatin which is synthesized in the distal tubule, produces a greater natriuretic response than ANP probably because its tissue half-life is longer than that of ANP. Urodilatin reproduces the effects of ANP on the inner medullary collecting duct.

Taken together, these data demonstrate that natriuretic peptides have a key role in the regulation of sodium excretion. Hence, these peptides contribute to the regulation of fluid volume and blood pressure. In accordance with these important properties, mice lacking the ANP gene and ANP-receptor knockout mice develop hypertension, the former being salt-sensitive. After acute volume expansion, these mice show little increase in sodium excretion suggesting a maladaptive regulation of sodium balance.

THE KALLIKREIN–KININ SYSTEM

The kallikrein–kinin system consists of proteases (kallikreins) that release kinins from the low molecular weight and high molecular weight (HMW) kininogen, the precursor protein (93). Kininogen is synthesized primarily by the liver but mRNA for the HMW kininogen has been identified in endothelial cells. Kallikreins are present in plasma where they generate bradykinin from the HMW kininogen and in tissues, particularly in the kidney. Tissue kallikrein cleaves a low molecular weight kininogen to release lys-bradykinin (kallidin). Kallidin is then metabolized through an aminopeptidase into bradykinin. Kinins act by stimulating specific receptors (kinin B1, B2, and B3 receptors). The B1 receptor is involved in the chronic inflammatory and pain-producing response to kinins. The B2 receptor mediates most of the other actions of kinins. In the circulation and tissues, kinins are destroyed by aminopeptidases and carboxypeptidases. The dipeptidase kininase II (ACE) is the most important metabolizing enzyme within the cardiovascular and renal systems.

The kallikrein–kinin system is abundantly present in the kidney. In humans, approximately 50% of the urinary kallikrein is in the inactive form. Renal kallikrein releases kinins in vitro from both low molecular weight and HMW kininogen. Over 90% of the kallikrein in the kidney is found in the cortex. Scicli et al. (94) have shown that kallikrein is incorporated in the urine in the distal tubule and Ostarvik et al. (95) have found in the rat that kidney kallikrein is localized in the convoluted distal tubules from the macula densa to the collecting ducts but no kallikrein was localized in the collecting duct. In fact, all the components of the system, i.e., tissue kallikrein, low molecular weight kininogen, bradykinin B_2 receptors, renal kininases and an inhibitor of tissue kallikrein (kallistatin) are secreted and distributed in the distal tubule from the connecting tubule to the collecting duct. Considerable amounts of kinins are found in the urine which are formed within the kidney and in the urine. Indeed, the proximal tubule is so rich in kininases that circulating and filtered kinins are rapidly degraded and do not reach the distal tubule (96). The nephron is also rich in aminopeptidases which transform kallidin into bradykinin. Taken together, these observations suggest that the kallikrein–kinin system in the kidney is mainly localized in the distal nephron.

The synthesis, activity and release of renal kallikrein mRNA and protein levels are influenced by several hormonal systems including mineralocorticoids, glucocorticoids, testosterone, thyroxine, insulin, vasopressin, cathecholamines, and Ang II. Sodium restriction and a high potassium diet have also been associated with increased excretion of urinary kallikrein suggesting an activation of the renal system by these electrolytes.

When infused into the renal artery or intravenously in dogs or men, bradykinin or kallidin causes an increase in renal blood flow (97,98). This change in renal flow is mainly due to an increase in papillary blood flow rather than cortical blood flow (99) and it has been related to the release of prostaglandins and NO. Kinins infusion also induces diuresis and natriuresis without any change in GFR. The natriuretic response may result from several mechanisms. Kinins stimulate the synthesis of prostaglandins in the collecting duct and renal medulla (PGE_2) and in the arterioles (PGI_2), an effect which has been linked to the activation of phospholipase A_2 (100). As for the renal vasodilation, part of the natriuretic properties of kinins may thus be mediated through the release of prostaglandins. In accordance with this proposal, studies have shown that the natriuretic response to kinins can be blocked by non-steroidal anti-inflammatory drugs such as indomethacin. This mechanism remains however controversial. Kinins do not affect proximal sodium and water reabsorption in outer cortical nephrons available for micropuncture (97). Interestingly, the enteral administration of ebelactone B, a selective inhibitor of carboxypeptidase Y-like exopeptidase (a major kininase in urine) has been shown to promote sodium and water excretion, again suggesting that inhibition of kinins degradation in the tubular lumen induces diuresis and natriuresis (101). Hence, the natriuretic effect of kinins appear to be mediated essentially through an effect on the distal part of the nephron or eventually to changes in deep nephron reabsorption. Of note, urinary kallikrein has been shown in vitro to convert inactive renin to active renin and renal kallikrein has been reported to activate renin in vivo (102). Hence the catalytic effect of kallikrein on renin may also affect sodium balance indirectly.

Recently, Katori and Majima have hypothesized that a deficit in the renal kallikrein–kinin system is a cause of salt-sensitive hypertension (103). In support of their hypothesis, a lower urinary excretion of active kallikrein in the urine of salt-sensitive hypertensives was found in comparison to salt-resistant patients (104). Moreover, rats congenitally deficient in kininogen (105) as well as mice in which the bradykinin B2 receptor has been disrupted (106) were found to be more salt-sensitive than their controls. However, this latter observation remains controversial as it was not confirmed when blood pressure was measured using telemetry (107). Bradykinin B2 receptor knockout mice display a significantly higher blood pressure, reduced renal blood flow and an increased renal vascular resistance when receiving a high sodium diet (108).

INSULIN

Early in vivo and ex vivo experiments performed in animals have well demonstrated the antinatriuretic and antidiuretic properties of insulin (Fig. 7). In the isolated perfused dog kidney, insulin was found to decrease sodium excretion independent of changes in

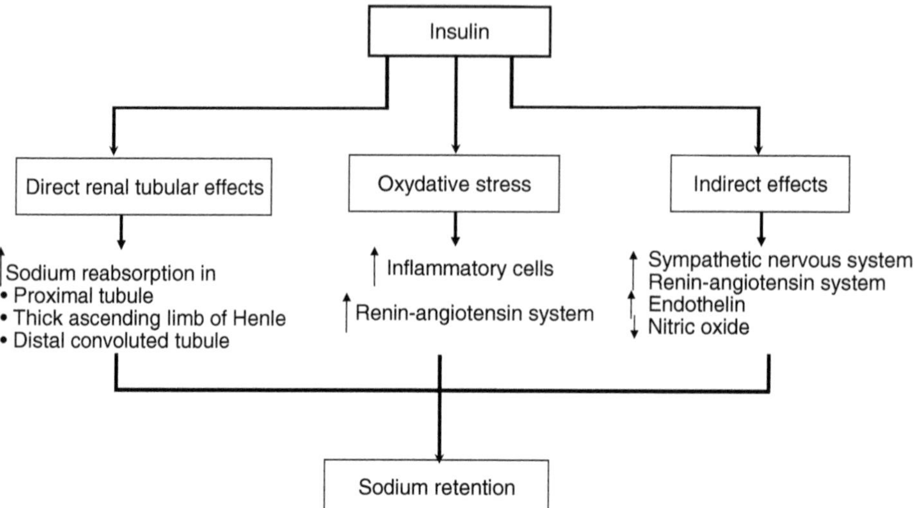

Figure 7 Mechanisms whereby insulin affects sodium balance in health and disease.

GFR, renal hemodynamics and sympathetic nerve activity suggesting a direct effect of insulin on tubular sodium transport (109). More recently, the long-term effect (seven days) of an intrarenal infusion of insulin was investigated in instrumented dogs. These experiments demonstrated once again that insulin promotes sodium retention without any effect on potassium excretion (110). In humans, the renal effect of insulin was characterized 30 years ago by De Fronzo et al. (111) (for a recent review see Ref. 112). An infusion of exogenous insulin reduced urinary sodium excretion by almost 50% with no effect on plasma glucose or the filtered load of glucose. In addition, the decrease in sodium excretion was not accompanied by any changes in GFR, renal hemodynamics and plasma aldosterone levels suggesting again a direct impact of the hormone on tubular sodium handling. In one study, no change in lithium clearance, a marker of proximal sodium handling, was found upon infusion of insulin (113). Yet, in a second study, the fall in urinary sodium excretion induced by hyperinsulinemia paralleled a decrease in urinary uric acid excretion, an observation which would suggest an impact of insulin on sodium handling by the proximal segments of the nephron (114).

In fact, binding of insulin is greatest in the thick ascending limb of Henle and in the distal convoluted tubule (115). In the rat, there is rather evidence that insulin acts on the proximal tubule and in vitro studies have found that insulin stimulates the Na^+/H^+ exchange and the activity of the Na/K-ATPase in the proximal tubule (116). These data were however not confirmed by human studies which suggested a distal effect of insulin (113,114). The effect of insulin on the distal tubule has recently been supported by the demonstration that insulin stimulates serum and glucocorticoid-mediated kinase isoform-1 activity in the epithelial cells resulting in a ENaC-mediated sodium reabsorption (117). Insulin can also promote sodium retention by indirect mechanisms. These include the stimulation of the renin-angiotensin system and the activation of the sympathetic nervous system (118,119). At last, a high plasma glucose and the presence of glucose in the urine can also increase sodium reabsorption. In this case, sodium is reabsorbed in the proximal tubule due to an activation of the Na–glucose cotransport (116,120).

OTHER FACTORS

Besides the above-mentioned factors involved in the regulation of sodium balance, several other systems can contribute to maintenance of sodium either directly or indirectly. For example, thyroid hormones have a major impact on renal function including on sodium and water excretion. Thyroid hormones have been shown to be essential for the function of the Na/K-ATPase in the kidney (121,122). They interact closely with the renin-angiotensin system as well as with NO and ET. Growth hormone may also have an impact on sodium homeostasis. Indeed, an excess of growth hormone has been shown to cause vascular hypertrophy, to activate the sympathetic nervous system, and to promote renal sodium retention (123). Oxidative stress defined as an imbalance between reactive oxygen species and antioxidant substances of the organism in favor of the former is also linked to alterations in renal sodium handling (124). Thus, oxidative stress promotes sodium retention in the kidney. This effect is mediated by the accumulation of inflammatory cells (T cells and macrophages) in the renal interstitium and hence the production of Ang II. This latter increases sodium retention via the hemodynamic and tubular mechanisms discussed earlier in this chapter. Oxidative stress also affects renal and medullary microcirculation and thereby influences sodium excretion (125). Thus, administration of an inhibitor of superoxide dismutase (SOD) has been shown to cause sodium retention whereas a SOD mimetic has been reported to cause the opposite effect (125). Moreover, prevention of oxidative stress has been shown to protect salt-sensitive rats against a rise in blood pressure and the development of renal interstitial fibrosis (126).

CONCLUSIONS

The endocrine and autocrine systems presented in this chapter confirm the multiplicity and the complexity of the mechanisms existing to control sodium balance. This probably reflects the importance of regulating extracellular fluid volume and plasma osmolality within a narrow range. There is no clearly defined hierarchy among these systems but some endocrine systems probably have a greater impact on sodium and water homeostasis and hence, on the maintenance of blood pressure. This can be demonstrated using a selective blockade of several hormonal systems consecutively. For example, in dehydrated rats, vasopressin inhibition and blockade of the sympathetic nervous system induce almost no fall in blood pressure as long as the renin-angiotensin system is present and active (127). In contrast, dehydrated rats with a blocked renin-angiotensin system are unable to maintain their blood pressure even though the vasopressin and sympathetic nervous system are activated. This would suggest that in some clinical conditions, certain endocrine factors predominate and are perhaps more important for the sodium and water homeostasis. However, few studies have actually investigated the relative role of the various regulatory systems involved in the maintenance of sodium and fluid balance.

REFERENCES

1. Carey RM, Siragy HM. Newly recognized components of the renin-angiotensin system: potential roles in cardiovascular and renal regulation. Endocr Rev 2003; 24:261–71.
2. Nussberger J. Circulating versus tissue angiotensin II. In: Epstein M, Brunner H-R, eds. Angiotensin II Receptor Antanonists. Philadelphia, PA: Hanley and Belfus, Inc., 2001:69.
3. Der Sarkissian S, Huentelman MJ, Stewart J, Katovich MJ, Raizada MK. ACE2: a novel therapeutic target for cardiovascular diseases. Prog Biophys Mol Biol 2006; 91:163–98.

4. Timmermans PB, Wong PC, Chiu AT, et al. Angiotensin II receptors and angiotensin II receptor antagonists. Pharmacol Rev 1993; 45:205–51.
5. Cheng ZJ, Vapaatalo H, Mervaala E. Angiotensin II and vascular inflammation. Med Sci Monit 2005; 11:RA194–205.
6. Nguyen G, Burckle C, Sraer JD. The renin receptor: the facts, the promise and the hope. Curr Opin Nephrol Hypertens 2003; 12:51–5.
7. Buggy J, Fisher AE. Evidence for a dual central role for angiotensin in water and sodium intake. Nature 1974; 250:733–5.
8. Reid IA. Actions of angiotensin II on the brain: mechanisms and physiologic role. Am J Physiol 1984; 246:F533–43.
9. Fitzsimons JT. Angiotensin, thirst, and sodium appetite. Physiol Rev 1998; 78:583–686.
10. Rowland NE, Rozelle A, Riley PJ, Fregly MJ. Effect of nonpeptide angiotensin receptor antagonists on water intake and salt appetite in rats. Brain Res Bull 1992; 29:389–93.
11. McKinley MJ, Evered M, Mathai M, Coghlan JP. Effects of central losartan on plasma renin and centrally mediated natriuresis. Kidney Int 1994; 46:1479–82.
12. Rohmeiss P, Beyer C, Hocher B, et al. Osmotically induced natriuresis and blood pressure response involves angiotensin AT1 receptors in the subfornical organ. J Hypertens 1995; 13:1399–404.
13. Miyata N, Park F, Li XF, Cowley AW, Jr. Distribution of angiotensin AT1 and AT2 receptor subtypes in the rat kidney. Am J Physiol 1999; 277:F437–46.
14. Navar LG, Nishiyama A. Why are angiotensin concentrations so high in the kidney? Curr Opin Nephrol Hypertens 2004; 13:107–15.
15. Pallone TL, Zhang Z, Rhinehart K. Physiology of the renal medullary microcirculation. Am J Physiol Renal Physiol 2003; 284:F253–66.
16. Harris PJ, Navar LG. Tubular transport responses to angiotensin. Am J Physiol 1985; 248:F621–30.
17. Saccomani G, Mitchell KD, Navar LG. Angiotensin II stimulation of Na(+)–H+ exchange in proximal tubule cells. Am J Physiol 1990; 258:F1188–95.
18. Wang T, Giebisch G. Effects of angiotensin II on electrolyte transport in the early and late distal tubule in rat kidney. Am J Physiol 1996; 271:F143–9.
19. Peti-Peterdi J, Warnock DG, Bell PD. Angiotensin II directly stimulates ENaC activity in the cortical collecting duct via AT(1) receptors. J Am Soc Nephrol 2002; 13:1131–5.
20. Wang Q, Horisberger JD, Maillard M, Brunner HR, Rossier BC, Burnier M. Salt- and angiotensin II-dependent variations in amiloride-sensitive rectal potential difference in mice. Clin Exp Pharmacol Physiol 2000; 27:60–6.
21. Navar LG. Integrating multiple paracrine regulators of renal microvascular dynamics. Am J Physiol 1998; 274:F433–44.
22. Schnermann J, Briggs J. Role of the renin-angiotensin system in tubuloglomerular feedback. Fed Proc 1986; 45:1426–30.
23. Peti-Peterdi J, Bell PD. Regulation of macula densa Na:H exchange by angiotensin II. Kidney Int 1998; 54:2021–8.
24. Burnier M, Waeber B, Brunner HR. The advantages of angiotensin II antagonism. J Hypertens Suppl 1994; 12:S7–15.
25. Burnier M, Roch-Ramel F, Brunner HR. Renal effects of angiotensin II receptor blockade in normotensive subjects. Kidney Int 1996; 49:1787–90.
26. Yanagisawa M, Kurihara H, Kimura S, et al. A novel potent vasoconstrictor peptide produced by vascular endothelial cells. Nature 1988; 332:411–5.
27. Luscher TF, Seo BG, Buhler FR. Potential role of endothelin in hypertension. Controversy on endothelin in hypertension. Hypertension 1993; 21:752–7.
28. Rabelink TJ, Kaasjager KA, Boer P, Stroes EG, Braam B, Koomans HA. Effects of endothelin-1 on renal function in humans: implications for physiology and pathophysiology. Kidney Int 1994; 46:376–81.
29. Kohan DE. The renal medullary endothelin system in control of sodium and water excretion and systemic blood pressure. Curr Opin Nephrol Hypertens 2006; 15:34–40.

30. Kohan DE. Endothelins in the normal and diseased kidney. Am J Kidney Dis 1997; 29:2–26.
31. Zeidel ML, Brady HR, Kone BC, Gullans SR, Brenner BM. Endothelin, a peptide inhibitor of Na(+)–K(+)-ATPase in intact renal tubular epithelial cells. Am J Physiol 1989; 257:C1101–7.
32. Gilmore ES, Stutts MJ, Milgram SL. SRC family kinases mediate epithelial Na+ channel inhibition by endothelin. J Biol Chem 2001; 276:42610–7.
33. Ahn D, Ge Y, Stricklett PK, et al. Collecting duct-specific knockout of endothelin-1 causes hypertension and sodium retention. J Clin Invest 2004; 114:504–11.
34. Ge Y, Stricklett PK, Hughes AK, Yanagisawa M, Kohan DE. Collecting duct-specific knockout of the endothelin A receptor alters renal vasopressin responsiveness, but not sodium excretion or blood pressure. Am J Physiol Renal Physiol 2005; 289:F692–8.
35. Schiffrin EL. The angiotensin–endothelin relationship: does it play a role in cardiovascular and renal pathophysiology? J Hypertens 2003; 21:2245–7.
36. Gariepy CE, Ohuchi T, Williams SC, Richardson JA, Yanagisawa M. Salt-sensitive hypertension in endothelin-B receptor-deficient rats. J Clin Invest 2000; 105:925–33.
37. Intengan HD, Schiffrin EL. Structure and mechanical properties of resistance arteries in hypertension: role of adhesion molecules and extracellular matrix determinants. Hypertension 2000; 36:312–8.
38. Nakov R, Pfarr E, Eberle S. Darusentan: an effective endothelin A receptor antagonist for treatment of hypertension. Am J Hypertens 2002; 15:583–9.
39. Rossi GP, Andreis PG, Neri G, Tortorella C, Pelizzo MR, Nussdorfer GG. Endothelin-1 stimulates aldosterone synthesis in Conn's adenomas via both A and B receptors coupled with the protein kinase C- and cyclooxygenase-dependent signaling pathways. J Investig Med 2000; 48(5):343–50.
40. Rossi GP, Sacchetto A, Cesari M, Pessina AC. Interactions between endothelin-1 and the renin-angiotensin-aldosterone system. Cardiovasc Res 1999; 43(2):300–7.
41. Ryan MJ, Black TA, Millard SL, Gross KW, Hajduczok G. Endothelin-1 increases calcium and attenuates renin gene expression in As4.1 cells. Am J Physiol Heart Circ Physiol 2002; 283(6):H2458–65.
42. Share L. Role of vasopressin in cardiovascular regulation. Physiol Rev 1988; 68:1248–84.
43. Bankir L. Antidiuretic action of vasopressin: quantitative aspects and interaction between V1a and V2 receptor-mediated effects. Cardiovasc Res 2001; 51:372–90.
44. Zuber AM, Singer D, Penninger JM, Rossier BC, Firsov D. Increased renal responsiveness to vasopressin and enhanced V2 receptor signaling in RGS2-/- mice. J Am Soc Nephrol 2007; 18:1672–8.
45. Bankir L, Fernandes S, Bardoux P, Bouby N, Bichet DG. Vasopressin-V2 receptor stimulation reduces sodium excretion in healthy humans. J Am Soc Nephrol 2005; 16:1920–8.
46. Peterson LN, De Rouffignac C, Sonnenberg H, Levine DZ. Thick ascending limb response to dDAVP and atrial natriuretic factor in vivo. Am J Physiol 1987; 252:F374–81.
47. Kim GH, Ecelbarger CA, Mitchell C, Packer RK, Wade JB, Knepper MA. Vasopressin increases Na–K–2Cl cotransporter expression in thick ascending limb of Henle's loop. Am J Physiol 1999; 276:F96–103.
48. Djelidi S, Fay M, Cluzeaud F, et al. Transcriptional regulation of sodium transport by vasopressin in renal cells. J Biol Chem 1997; 272:32919–24.
49. Sauter D, Fernandes S, Goncalves-Mendes N, et al. Long-term effects of vasopressin on the subcellular localization of ENaC in the renal collecting system. Kidney Int 2006; 69:1024–32.
50. Nicco C, Wittner M, DiStefano A, Jounier S, Bankir L, Bouby N. Chronic exposure to vasopressin upregulates ENaC and sodium transport in the rat renal collecting duct and lung. Hypertension 2001; 38:1143–9.
51. de Rouffignac C, Imbert-Teboul M. Effects of antidiuretic hormone on renal reabsorption of electrolytes. Adv Nephrol Necker Hosp 1984; 13:297–317.
52. Zeng C, Zhang M, Asico LD, Eisner GM, Jose PA. The dopaminergic system in hypertension. Clin Sci (Lond) 2007; 112:583–97.

53. Ibarra FR, Aguirre J, Nowicki S, Barontini M, Arrizurieta EE, Armando I. Demethylation of 3-*O*-methyldopa in the kidney: a possible source for dopamine in urine. Am J Physiol 1996; 270:F862–8.
54. Agnoli GC, Cacciari M, Garutti C, Ikonomu E, Lenzi P, Marchetti G. Effects of extracellular fluid volume changes on renal response to low-dose dopamine infusion in normal women. Clin Physiol 1987; 7:465–79.
55. Ragsdale NV, Lynd M, Chevalier RL, Felder RA, Peach MJ, Carey RM. Selective peripheral dopamine-1 receptor stimulation. Differential responses to sodium loading and depletion in humans. Hypertension 1990; 15:914–21.
56. Albrecht FE, Drago J, Felder RA, et al. Role of the D1A dopamine receptor in the pathogenesis of genetic hypertension. J Clin Invest 1996; 97:2283–8.
57. Amenta F, Barili P, Bronzetti E, Ricci A. Dopamine D1-like receptor subtypes in the rat kidney: a microanatomical study. Clin Exp Hypertens 1999; 21:17–23.
58. Hughes JM, Beck TR, Rose CE, Jr., Carey RM. The effect of selective dopamine-1 receptor stimulation on renal and adrenal function in man. J Clin Endocrinol Metab 1988; 66:518–25.
59. Jose PA, Felder RA, Holloway RR, Eisner GM. Dopamine receptors modulate sodium excretion in denervated kidney. Am J Physiol 1986; 250:F1033–8.
60. Cheng HF, Becker BN, Harris RC. Dopamine decreases expression of type-1 angiotensin II receptors in renal proximal tubule. J Clin Invest 1996; 97:2745–52.
61. Salomone LJ, Howell NL, McGrath HE, et al. Intrarenal dopamine D1-like receptor stimulation induces natriuresis via an angiotensin type-2 receptor mechanism. Hypertension 2007; 49:155–61.
62. Carey RM, Wang ZQ, Siragy HM. Role of the angiotensin type 2 receptor in the regulation of blood pressure and renal function. Hypertension 2000; 35:155–63.
63. Palmer RM, Ferrige AG, Moncada S. Nitric oxide release accounts for the biological activity of endothelium-derived relaxing factor. Nature 1987; 327:524–6.
64. Forstermann U, Closs EI, Pollock JS, et al. Nitric oxide synthase isozymes. Characterization, purification, molecular cloning, and functions. Hypertension 1994; 23:1121–31.
65. Griffith OW, Stuehr DJ. Nitric oxide synthases: properties and catalytic mechanism. Annu Rev Physiol 1995; 57:707–36.
66. Gross SS, Wolin MS. Nitric oxide: pathophysiological mechanisms. Annu Rev Physiol 1995; 57:737–69.
67. Ujiie K, Yuen J, Hogarth L, Danziger R, Star RA. Localization and regulation of endothelial NO synthase mRNA expression in rat kidney. Am J Physiol 1994; 267:F296–302.
68. Wilcox CS, Welch WJ, Murad F, et al. Nitric oxide synthase in macula densa regulates glomerular capillary pressure. Proc Natl Acad Sci USA 1992; 89:11993–7.
69. Wangensteen R, Rodriguez-Gomez I, Moreno JM, Chamorro V, Osuna A, Vargas F. Role of neuronal nitric oxide synthase in response to hypertonic saline loading in rats. Acta Physiol Scand 2004; 182:389–95.
70. Ng CW, De Matteo R, Badoer E. Effect of muscimol and L-NAME in the PVN on the RSNA response to volume expansion in conscious rabbits. Am J Physiol Renal Physiol 2004; 287:F739–46.
71. Brown R, Ollerstam A, Persson AE. Neuronal nitric oxide synthase inhibition sensitizes the tubuloglomerular feedback mechanism after volume expansion. Kidney Int 2004; 65: 1349–56.
72. Llinas MT, Gonzalez JD, Salazar FJ. Interactions between angiotensin and nitric oxide in the renal response to volume expansion. Am J Physiol 1995; 269:R504–10.
73. Wang D, Chen Y, Chabrashvili T, et al. Role of oxidative stress in endothelial dysfunction and enhanced responses to angiotensin II of afferent arterioles from rabbits infused with angiotensin II. J Am Soc Nephrol 2003; 14:2783–9.
74. Reid IA. Role of nitric oxide in the regulation of renin and vasopressin secretion. Front Neuroendocrinol 1994; 15:351–83.
75. Castrop H, Schweda F, Mizel D, et al. Permissive role of nitric oxide in macula densa control of renin secretion. Am J Physiol Renal Physiol 2004; 286:F848–57.

76. de Bold AJ, Borenstein HB, Veress AT, Sonnenberg H. A rapid and potent natriuretic response to intravenous injection of atrial myocardial extract in rats. Life Sci 1981; 28:89–94.
77. Iida T, Hirata Y, Takemura N, Togashi K, Nakagawa S, Marumo F. Brain natriuretic peptide is cosecreted with atrial natriuretic peptide from porcine cardiocytes. FEBS Lett 1990; 260:98–100.
78. Schulz-Knappe P, Forssmann K, Herbst F, Hock D, Pipkorn R, Forssmann WG. Isolation and structural analysis of "urodilatin," a new peptide of the cardiodilatin-(ANP)-family, extracted from human urine. Klin Wochenschr 1988; 66:752–9.
79. Nakao K, Ogawa Y, Suga S, Imura H. Molecular biology and biochemistry of the natriuretic peptide system. II: natriuretic peptide receptors. J Hypertens 1992; 10:1111–4.
80. Fluckiger JP, Waeber B, Matsueda G, Delaloye B, Nussberger J, Brunner HR. Effect of atriopeptin III on hematocrit and volemia of nephrectomized rats. Am J Physiol 1986; 251:H880–3.
81. Volpe M, Odell G, Kleinert HD, et al. Effect of atrial natriuretic factor on blood pressure, renin, and aldosterone in Goldblatt hypertension. Hypertension 1985; 7:I43–8.
82. Kleinert HD, Maack T, Atlas SA, Januszewicz A, Sealey JE, Laragh JH. Atrial natriuretic factor inhibits angiotensin-, norepinephrine-, and potassium-induced vascular contractility. Hypertension 1984; 6:I143–7.
83. de Wardener HE. The hypothalamus and hypertension. Physiol Rev 2001; 81:1599–658.
84. Maack T. Role of atrial natriuretic factor in volume control. Kidney Int 1996; 49:1732–7.
85. Loutzenhiser R, Hayashi K, Epstein M. Atrial natriuretic peptide reverses afferent arteriolar vasoconstriction and potentiates efferent arteriolar vasoconstriction in the isolated perfused rat kidney. J Pharmacol Exp Ther 1988; 246:522–8.
86. Maack T, Marion DN, Camargo MJ, et al. Effects of auriculin (atrial natriuretic factor) on blood pressure, renal function, and the renin–aldosterone system in dogs. Am J Med 1984; 77:1069–75.
87. Biollaz J, Bidiville J, Diezi J, et al. Site of the action of a synthetic atrial natriuretic peptide evaluated in humans. Kidney Int 1987; 32:537–46.
88. Eiskjaer H, Nielsen CB, Pedersen EB. Pressure-dependent distal tubular action of atrial natriuretic peptide in healthy humans. J Hypertens 1996; 14:99–106.
89. Eiskjaer H, Nielsen CB, Sorensen SS, Pedersen EB. Renal and hormonal actions of atrial natriuretic peptide during angiotensin II or noradrenaline infusion in man. Eur J Clin Invest 1996; 26:584–95.
90. Beltowski J, Wojcicka G. Regulation of renal tubular sodium transport by cardiac natriuretic peptides: two decades of research. Med Sci Monit 2002; 8:RA39–52.
91. Holtback U, Kruse MS, Brismar H, Aperia A. Intrarenal dopamine coordinates the effect of antinatriuretic and natriuretic factors. Acta Physiol Scand 2000; 168:215–8.
92. Zeidel ML, Kikeri D, Silva P, Burrowes M, Brenner BM. Atrial natriuretic peptides inhibit conductive sodium uptake by rabbit inner medullary collecting duct cells. J Clin Invest 1988; 82:1067–74.
93. Regoli D, Calo G, Rizzi A, et al. Bradykinin receptors and receptor ligands (with special emphasis on vascular receptors). Regul Pept 1996; 65:83–9.
94. Scicli AG, Carretero OA, Hampton A, Cortes P, Oza NB. Site of kininogenase secretion in the dog nephron. Am J Physiol 1976; 230:533–6.
95. Orstavik TB, Brandtzaeg P, Nustad K, Halvorsen KM. Cellular localization of kallikreins in rat submandibular and sublingual salivary glands: immunofluorescence tracing related to histological characteristics. Acta Histochem 1975; 54:183–92.
96. Hall ER, Kato J, Erdos EG, Robinson CJ, Oshima G. Angiotensin i-converting enzyme in the nephron. Life Sci 1976; 18:1299–303.
97. Stein JH, Congbalay RC, Karsh DL, Osgood RW, Ferris TF. The effect of bradykinin on proximal tubular sodium reabsorption in the dog: evidence for functional nephron heterogeneity. J Clin Invest 1972; 51:1709–21.
98. Adetuyibi A, Mills IH. Relation between urinary kallikrein and renal function, hypertension, and excretion of sodium and water in man. Lancet 1972; 2:203–7.

99. Mattson DL, Cowley AW, Jr. Kinin actions on renal papillary blood flow and sodium excretion. Hypertension 1993; 21:961–5.
100. Nasjletti A, Malik KU. Relationships between the kallikrein–kinin and prostaglandin systems. Life Sci 1979; 25:99–109.
101. Majima M, Kuribayashi Y, Ikeda Y, et al. Diuretic and natriuretic effect of ebelactone B in anesthetized rats by inhibition of a urinary carboxypeptidase Y-like kininase. Jpn J Pharmacol 1994; 65:79–82.
102. Sealey JE, Atlas SA, Laragh JH. Linking the kallikrein and renin systems via activation of inactive renin: new data and a hypothesis. Am J Med 1978; 65:994–1000.
103. Katori M, Majima M. A missing link between a high salt intake and blood pressure increase. J Pharmacol Sci 2006; 100:370–90.
104. Ferri C, Bellini C, Carlomagno A, Perrone A, Santucci A. Urinary kallikrein and salt sensitivity in essential hypertensive males. Kidney Int 1994; 46:780–8.
105. Majima M, Yoshida O, Mihara H, et al. High sensitivity to salt in kininogen-deficient brown Norway Katholiek rats. Hypertension 1993; 22:705–14.
106. Alfie ME, Yang XP, Hess F, Carretero OA. Salt-sensitive hypertension in bradykinin B2 receptor knockout mice. Biochem Biophys Res Commun 1996; 224:625–30.
107. Milia AF, Gross V, Plehm R, et al. Normal blood pressure and renal function in mice lacking the bradykinin B(2) receptor. Hypertension 2001; 37:1473–9.
108. Alfie ME, Sigmon DH, Pomposiello SI, Carretero OA. Effect of high salt intake in mutant mice lacking bradykinin-B2 receptors. Hypertension 1997; 29:483–7.
109. Nizet A, Lefebvre P, Crabbe J. Control by insulin of sodium potassium and water excretion by the isolated dog kidney. Pflugers Arch 1971; 323:11–20.
110. Hall JE, Brands MW, Mizelle HL, Gaillard CA, Hildebrandt DA. Chronic intrarenal hyperinsulinemia does not cause hypertension. Am J Physiol 1991; 260:F663–9.
111. DeFronzo RA. The effect of insulin on renal sodium metabolism. A review with clinical implications. Diabetologia 1981; 21:165–71.
112. Sarafidis PA, Bakris GL. The antinatriuretic effect of insulin: an unappreciated mechanism for hypertension associated with insulin resistance? Am J Nephrol 2007; 27:44–54.
113. Skott P, Hother-Nielsen O, Bruun NE, et al. Effects of insulin on kidney function and sodium excretion in healthy subjects. Diabetologia 1989; 32:694–9.
114. Stenvinkel P, Bolinder J, Alvestrand A. Effects of insulin on renal haemodynamics and the proximal and distal tubular sodium handling in healthy subjects. Diabetologia 1992; 35:1042–8.
115. Butlen D, Vadrot S, Roseau S, Morel F. Insulin receptors along the rat nephron: [125I] insulin binding in microdissected glomeruli and tubules. Pflugers Arch 1988; 412:604–12.
116. Baum M. Insulin stimulates volume absorption in the rabbit proximal convoluted tubule. J Clin Invest 1987; 79:1104–9.
117. Pearce D. The role of SGK1 in hormone-regulated sodium transport. Trends Endocrinol Metab 2001; 12:341–7.
118. Tuck ML, Bounoua F, Eslami P, Nyby MD, Eggena P, Corry DB. Insulin stimulates endogenous angiotensin II production via a mitogen-activated protein kinase pathway in vascular smooth muscle cells. J Hypertens 2004; 22:1779–85.
119. Landsberg L. Insulin-mediated sympathetic stimulation: role in the pathogenesis of obesity-related hypertension (or, how insulin affects blood pressure, and why). J Hypertens 2001; 19:523–8.
120. Bank N, Aynedjian HS. Progressive increases in luminal glucose stimulate proximal sodium absorption in normal and diabetic rats. J Clin Invest 1990; 86:309–16.
121. Vargas F, Moreno JM, Rodriguez-Gomez I, et al. Vascular and renal function in experimental thyroid disorders. Eur J Endocrinol 2006; 154:197–212.
122. Barlet C, Doucet A. Triiodothyronine enhances renal response to aldosterone in the rabbit collecting tubule. J Clin Invest 1987; 79:629–31.
123. Bondanelli M, Ambrosio MR, degli Uberti EC. Pathogenesis and prevalence of hypertension in acromegaly. Pituitary 2001; 4:239–49.

124. Wilcox CS. Oxidative stress and nitric oxide deficiency in the kidney: a critical link to hypertension? Am J Physiol Regul Integr Comp Physiol 2005; 289:R913–35.
125. Zou AP, Li N, Cowley AW, Jr. Production and actions of superoxide in the renal medulla. Hypertension 2001; 37:547–53.
126. Park JB, Touyz RM, Chen X, Schiffrin EL. Chronic treatment with a superoxide dismutase mimetic prevents vascular remodeling and progression of hypertension in salt-loaded stroke-prone spontaneously hypertensive rats. Am J Hypertens 2002; 15:78–84.
127. Burnier M, Biollaz J, Brunner DB, Brunner HR. Blood pressure maintenance in awake dehydrated rats: renin, vasopressin, and sympathetic activity. Am J Physiol 1983; 245:H203–9.

6
Neural Control of Sodium Balance

Edward J. Johns
Department of Physiology, University College Cork, Cork, Republic of Ireland

INTRODUCTION

Cardiovascular homeostasis is maintained by a balance between the volume of blood in the vascular system, the effectiveness of the heart as a pump and the ability of the kidney to ensure that the level of fluid reabsorption and excretion are appropriate. If any one arm of this cardiovascular–renal axis is deficient, then there will be a development of a chronically elevated blood pressure; that is, hypertension. Hypertension is present in up to 20% of the adult population of many developed countries placing these individuals at risk of stroke and heart attacks creating a major demand on the healthcare system (1).

The kidney is the key element in the regulation of extracellular fluid volume and a variety of important mechanisms exist to ensure that there is a dynamic and rapid response when sodium and water intake occurs during everyday activity (2). At the kidney, some 20% of the total renal blood flow is filtered at the glomerulae of the cortex and as the filtrate passes along the nephron it is subjected to processing such as the reabsorption of water and sodium together with the secretion of metabolites and waste products. It is the reabsorption of sodium, the major extracellular electrolyte, and water that determines extracellular fluid balance and hence cardiovascular homeostasis. The major part of fluid reabsorption takes place along the highly permeable proximal tubule, with differing proportions of sodium, chloride, bicarbonate, and water being transported at the pars convoluta and pars recta segments. A further component of fluid reabsorption takes place along the thick limb of the ascending loop of Henle where sodium, chloride, and potassium are transported. It is along the low permeability distal tubule that the fine adjustments and separate regulation of water as against sodium reabsorption is determined by humoral regulation; that is, antidiuretic hormone for water and aldosterone for sodium transport.

FACTORS INFLUENCING FLUID REABSORPTION

The bulk reabsorption of fluid along the proximal tubule is a primary determinant of extracellular fluid volume and is subjected to a degree of control by three distinct elements: hydrostatic pressure within the renal interstitium; humoral, autocrine and paracrine factors; and the renal sympathetic nerves.

Pressure Natriuresis

There is now good evidence showing that there is a linear relationship between blood pressure at the kidney and the level of sodium and water excretion (3), thus, as pressure rises, the level of sodium excretion increases. It is now considered that as hydrostatic pressure within the conducting arteries (interlobar, arcuate and to a degree interlobular arteries) increases, it is transmitted into the renal interstitium and to the peritubular capillaries of the cortex where it contributes to the Starling's forces thereby decreasing the rate of fluid flux across the tubules. It is important to point out that in response to changes in blood pressure over a normal range renal hemodynamics change very little. This phenomenon is termed autoregulation and is exhibited in relation to both renal blood flow and glomerular filtration rate and occurs when the balance between the afferent and efferent arteriolar resistances is kept constant to ensure that glomerular filtration pressure, and hence filtration rate, remains unchanged. Clearly, in the longer term a raised blood (hydrostatic) pressure will result in an increased fluid loss with the result that eventually blood pressure will be normalized and equilibrium will again be reestablished. This view was proposed and developed by Guyton and evaluated both by modeling and experimental approaches (4). The relationships are illustrated in Figure 1 where a normal curve has an almost infinite slope but in different states, for example raised renal nerve activity or increased angiotensin II the basal levels of blood pressure is elevated, the slope becomes finite and a salt sensitive hypertension appears.

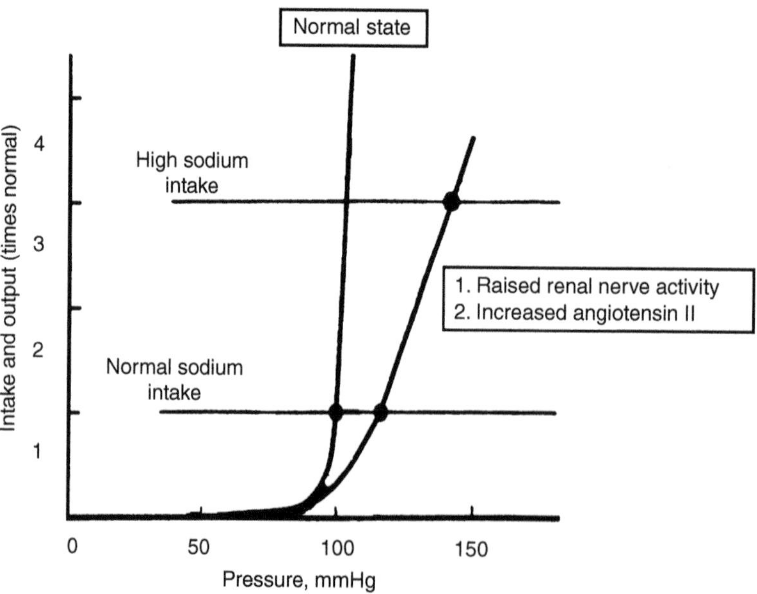

Figure 1 This illustrates the relationship between sodium intake and blood pressure in normal states and when the kidney is subjected to an elevated level of renal sympathetic nerve activity or raised angiotensin II levels. *Source*: From Ref. 4.

Humoral Factors

The absolute level of tubular epithelial cell fluid reabsorption is also influenced by humoral factors circulating in the plasma, but there are a number of autocrine and paracrine factors generated within the kidney itself which have an intrarenal homeostatic regulatory function. Examples of such factors are nitric oxide, reactive oxygen species and prostacyclins. One important factor is the peptide angiotensin II which is present at high concentrations within the renal interstitium and is able to stimulate sodium transport across the tubular epithelial cells (5). It is important to recognize that, in terms of the pressure natriuresis relationships, the peptide will shift the relationship to the right, that is, at each pressure level fluid reabsorption will be elevated. The question remains open as to whether it is the circulating or interstitial angiotensin II which regulates proximal tubular fluid transport, but it is likely to be both as factors determining the level of renin release and angiotensin II generation have the same directional action on both sources of the peptide.

Renal Sympathetic Nerves

The kidney receives a dense innervation of sympathetic nerve fibers, which is high compared to other organs, and the post-ganglionic fibers originate from the aorticorenal, splanchnic, coeliac and superior mesenteric ganglia (6). A cartoon depicting the origins and relationships of the renal sympathetic nerves are shown in Figure 2.

The nerve fibers are typical of those of the autonomic nervous system in that they possess varicosities which contain the neurotransmitter noradrenaline. As the fibers enter the kidney at the hilus, they distribute initially along the blood vessels but as the cortex is reached they infiltrate amongst both the vascular and tubular elements.

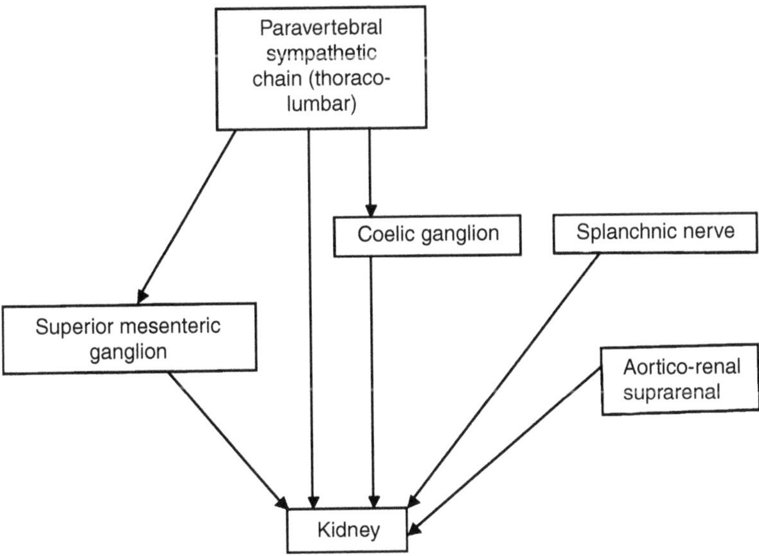

Figure 2 This depicts the origins and routes of passage of the nerves from the sympathetic chain (paravertebral ganglia) via prevertebral ganglia to the kidney.

FUNCTIONS OF THE RENAL SYMPATHETIC NERVES

Actions of the Renal Nerves

As the action potential passes along the nerve fiber, the depolarization causes the release of noradrenaline from the varicosities into the neuroeffector junction which then diffuses onto the post-synaptic membrane and interacts with its receptors. Figure 3 provides a diagrammatic scheme of the interaction of the nerves with the various end point of function. At the vascular smooth muscle cells, noradrenaline causes a vasoconstriction of the resistance arterioles via activation of α_1-adrenoceptors (7,8). This nerve induced increase in afferent arteriolar resistance will result in a decrease in total renal blood flow. By contrast, the increase in efferent arteriolar resistance will have variable effects in which a modest rise in efferent resistance will ensure that glomerular filtration pressure, and hence filtration, will be maintained in the face of a decrease in renal blood flow. However, at high levels of renal sympathetic nerve activity, the increased resistance at both arteriolar beds will decrease both renal blood flow and glomerular filtration rate.

At the granular renin containing cells of the juxtaglomerular apparatus, the noradrenaline acts on β_1-adrenoceptors to stimulate renin secretion and there is a direct proportionality between the level of nerve activity and the magnitude of renin secretion. It is those tubular elements of the nephron which reside in the cortex and outer medulla that are primarily influenced by noradrenaline released from the renal sympathetic nerves. The neurotransmitter released in close proximity to the proximal tubules act most probably at the basolateral membrane to stimulate α_1-adrenoceptors (9,10). The ligand binding

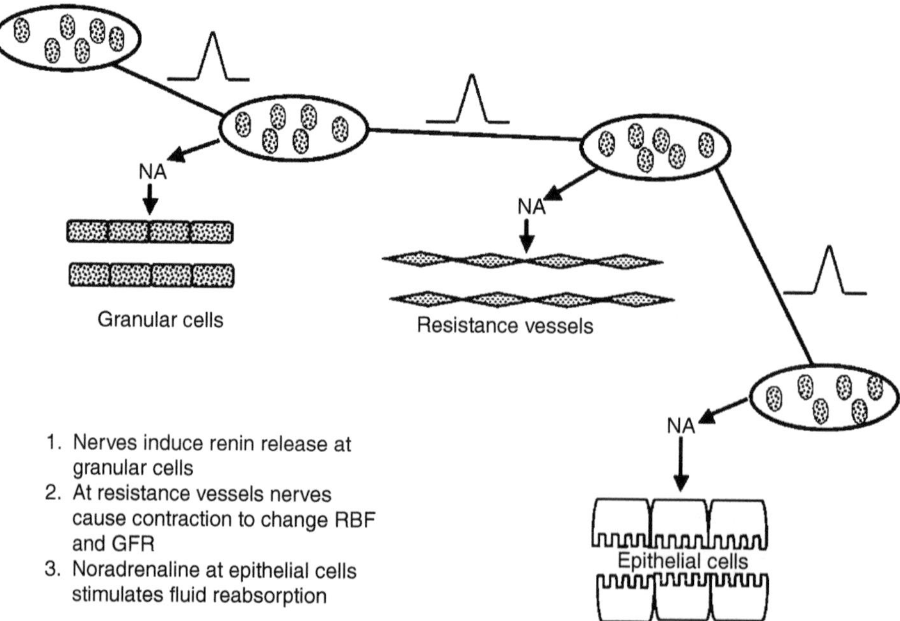
NA
NA
Granular cells
Resistance vessels
NA
1. Nerves induce renin release at granular cells
2. At resistance vessels nerves cause contraction to change RBF and GFR
3. Noradrenaline at epithelial cells stimulates fluid reabsorption
Epithelial cells

Figure 3 This illustrates how NA release from the varicosities of the sympathetic nerve fibers act on the renin-containing granular cells to stimulate renin secretion, at the vascular smooth muscle cells of the afferent and efferent arterioles to determine GFR and RBF, and at the epithelial cells of the proximal tubule and the thick ascending limb of the loop of Henle to stimulate sodium and water reabsorption. *Abbreviations*: GFR, glomerular filtration rate; NA, noradrenaline; RBF, renal blood flow.

initiates intracellular signaling pathways leading to an increase in activity of the sodium/potassium ATPase on the basolateral membrane, and the sodium/hydrogen exchanger on the apical membrane which results in a raised sodium and water transport across the epithelial cells (11,12). At the thick limb of the ascending loop of Henle, renal sympathetic nerve stimulation at low rates has been found to increase fluid transport (13), comprising water, sodium, chloride and potassium. The situation at the distal tubule has received much less attention and the impact of the nerves at this site has not been investigated in detail.

It is important to appreciate that the impact of the renal sympathetic nerves on these different end-points of renal function does not occur to the same degree. These relationships are illustrated in Figure 4 which shows the responses in renal hemodynamics, renin release and sodium excretion subsequent to electrical stimulation of the renal nerves. Experimental evidence has accrued demonstrating that at very low levels of electrical stimulation of the renal sympathetic nerves there are modest increases in renin secretion with small decreases in sodium excretion but no meaningful changes in either renal blood flow or glomerular filtration rate. Nonetheless, such small changes if they exist over a prolonged period of time, could have a major impact on the level of extracellular fluid volume and hence blood pressure. It is not until the renal sympathetic nerves are stimulated at quite high rates that there are marked reductions in both renal blood flow and glomerular filtration rate (14). It is likely that activation of the nerves to this degree only occurs under situations of extreme stress or severe exercise levels, but this will occur over

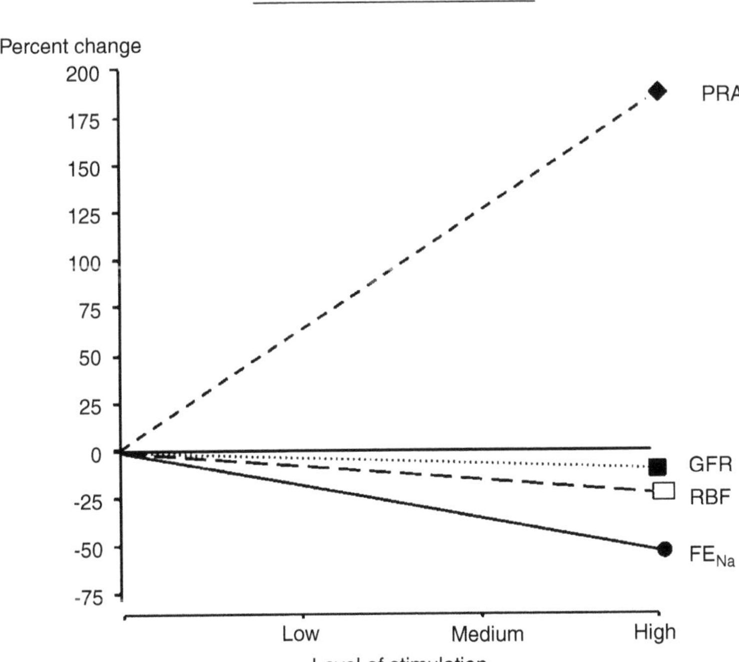

Figure 4 This demonstrates how increasing levels of electrical stimulation of the renal sympathetic nerves, from low to medium and high frequencies, cause a progressive increase in PRA and at the same time a decrease in FE$_{Na}$, an indicator of sodium reabsorption, RBF, and GFR. *Abbreviations*: FE$_{Na}$, fractional sodium excretion; GFR, glomerular filtration rate; PRA, plasma renin activity; RBF, renal blood flow.

a relatively short period of time and unlikely to have a long-term effect on cardiovascular homeostasis.

Reflex Activation of the Renal Sympathetic Nerves

Activity within the renal sympathetic nerves and the subsequent modulation of kidney function is regulated reflexly due to sensory information arising from a number of sources, the cardiovascular baroreceptors, from somatic and visceral sensory receptors, as well as input from the higher cortical centers sensing environmental stressors. The various inputs are shown in Figure 5. One of the primary means whereby renal sympathetic nerve activity is regulated reflexly is via the cardiovascular baroreceptors. Thus, a reduction in arterial pressure at the carotid sinuses and aortic arch decreases afferent baroreceptor nerve activity which will reflexly increase electrical activity within the renal sympathetic nerves with the result that tubular sodium reabsorption and renin release will be raised (15,16). By contrast, stretch or expansion of circulating volume activates the low pressure baroreceptors of the heart and lungs, which leads to a reflex decrease in renal sympathetic nerve activity and a subsequent renal nerve-dependent decrease in tubular sodium reabsorption and renin release (17–19).

There is accumulating evidence that the somatic sensory system also contributes in an important way as stimulation of mechano- and chemoreceptors in the muscle and thermoreceptors and nociceptors of the skin increases sympathetic outflow to most organs, including the kidney (20). There is now a body of evidence originating from experimental studies demonstrating that electrical activation of somatic afferent nerves or subcutaneous chemical stimulation using capsaicin causes renal nerve-dependent increases in renin release and decreases in sodium excretion in the face of minimal changes in renal hemodynamics (21,22). Chemo- and mechanoreceptors have also been identified in visceral organs, including the liver, most probably forming the basis of the hepatorenal

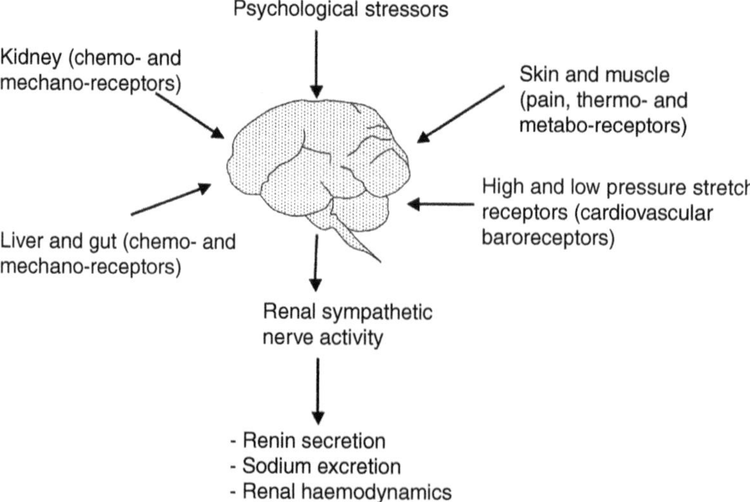

Figure 5 This shows the various sensory systems that supply afferent information to the autonomic centers of the brain. Within the central nervous system, this information is integrated in order to generate an appropriate level of sympathetic nerve activity to the kidney to ensure that renal function is regulated and homeostasis is maintained.

reflex (23,24), gut (25) and the kidney itself (26), with the latter probably forming the basis of the renorenal reflexes. Activation of these visceral receptors leads to a reflex increase in renal sympathetic nerve traffic although the functional responses have not been examined in detail as yet. It should be pointed out that a number of studies have demonstrated that following carotid sinus denervation or bilateral cervical vagotomy, the magnitude of the renal sympathetic nerve activity responses and renal nerve-dependent functional responses to somatic and visceral stimulation are potentiated (21,25). Together, these reports indicate that both the high and low pressure baroreceptors of the cardiovascular system under normal conditions exert another level of control, which is a tonic inhibitory regulation over the ability of the somatic and visceral sensory systems to influence the neural regulation of kidney function. Thus, the actual level of sympathetic outflow to the kidney is the end result of integration arising from a range of sensory inputs from different systems in the body. Moreover, it is evident that normal everyday behavior, that is, physical activity, feeding and drinking, will result in sensory signals passing to the central nervous system which will ensure that an appropriate alteration in renal sympathetic nerve activity takes place in order that any load of sodium or water is appropriately mobilized and excreted.

ANGIOTENSIN II AND THE BRAIN

The Brain Renin-Angiotensin System

It is becoming evident that the baroreceptor and somatosensory control of the sympathetic nerve activity by the central nervous system can be influenced by angiotensin II. There are two possible means whereby this might arise, either via circulating angiotensin II, or by angiotensin II generated locally within the brain at specific nuclei. It is now accepted that in the areas of the circumventricular organs the blood-brain barrier is leaky (27) enabling circulating angiotensin II to act on nuclei within this region which have been shown to contain a high density of angiotensin II receptors (28). At these sites the peptide is able to influence fluid balance, it stimulates drinking, induces anti-diuretic hormone release and causes an increased sodium reabsorption and renin release (27).

The second means whereby angiotensin II may influence autonomic control is that generated within the brain itself, as all components of the renin–angiotensin system are present, that is, renin, angiotensinogen, converting enzyme and angiotensin II receptors (29). The content of angiotensinogen in brain tissue is high and it has been reported to be some 30% of that which is found in the liver. Interestingly, mRNA for angiotensinogen has been found to exist almost exclusively in the astrocytes and the question arises as to whether the protein is metabolized by peptidases intracellularly generating angiotensin II, which is then released into the interstitium, or whether the angiotensinogen protein is released into the extracellular space where angiotensin II may be produced. Immunocytochemistry evaluations, in situ hybridization studies and mRNA measurements of angiotensin II receptors have shown them to be present or their genes expressed on those nuclei involved with autonomic control, that is, the nucleus tractus solitarius (NTS), rostral and caudal venterolateral medulla (RVLM and CVLM) and paraventricular nucleus (PVN) as well as nuclei of the subfornical organs and the area postrema which, as indicated above, are most likely subject to the action of circulating angiotensin (30,31). Indeed, local administration of angiotensin II onto the NTS and RVLM is excitatory and produces a sympathetically mediated pressor response, but when applied to the CVLM it causes a sympathoinhibition, thus, angiotensin II may have different actions and consequences dependent on its site of production and action (32,33).

The role played by angiotensin II within the brain in modulating autonomic control is only now being elucidated and the exact interactions within these areas remain a subject for debate (34,35). Attention initially was directed to the cardiovascular baroreceptors and a number of reports provided evidence showing that the baroreflex control of heart rate was marginally influenced by the levels of brain angiotensin II. However, the baroreflex control of renal sympathetic nerve activity was subjected to a tonic inhibitory control by angiotensin II as the slope and sensitivity of the baroreflex gain curves were enhanced (14,36). A somewhat different scenario was revealed when the sympathoexcitatory responses to somatosensory stimulation was examined. In this instance, blockade of angiotensin II receptors within the brain by giving the AT_1-receptor antagonist losartan intracerebroventricular (ICV) prevented the renal nerve-mediated antinatriuresis and antidiuresis resulting from somatosensory activation with capsaicin while replacing angiotensin II ICV restored the renal nerve-dependent functional responses suggesting that this particular reflex was actually facilitated by angiotensin II levels in the brain (37). It is important to recognize that angiotensin II may influence the central pathways in several ways, not only by increasing or decreasing basal levels of electrical activity within different neurones, but they may also attenuate or enhance the sensitivity of the neurones to sensory information arising from the periphery. The crucial issue is to appreciate that factors determining the level of angiotensin II within the central nervous system could then impact on the degree of autonomic control exerted at the kidney.

Dietary Sodium and the Brain Renin-Angiotensin System

An important link between the autonomic control of the cardiovascular system and brain levels of angiotensin II appears to be the level of dietary sodium intake. Many early studies demonstrated that in relation to the renal renin–angiotensin system, an increase in dietary sodium intake suppresses both renal renin content as well as circulating levels of angiotensin II whereas a decrease in dietary sodium intake stimulated renin secretion and angiotensin II levels in the plasma. Importantly, an increase in sodium intake has been found to decrease angiotensin II receptor density in peripheral blood vessels but concomitantly there was a rise in angiotensin II receptor density in the brain (38,39). To a degree, it remains unclear as to whether in the brain the upregulation of angiotensin II receptor density reflects a local increase or decrease in angiotensin II concentration.

An early report by Leenen et al. (40) demonstrated that increasing dietary sodium intake in rats over the developing phase, from four to eight weeks of age, led to an enhanced baroreflex gain associated with a resetting to a higher pressure for renal nerve activity, but not for heart rate. This importance of dietary sodium intake during development has been reinforced by recent reports (41,42) which showed that in rats fed a high, but not a normal or low salt diet, from four to eight weeks of age, a low dose infusion of angiotensin II ICV over five days caused a sustained increase in blood pressure associated with an antinatriuresis. The rises in blood pressure and fluid retention were prevented if the animals were subjected to a bilateral renal denervation which was consistent with the view that a rise in angiotensin II levels caused a sympathoexcitation which at the kidney caused an increased sodium retention which would contribute to the elevated blood pressure. Strikingly, this angiotensin II induced hypertension did not occur in mature rats, between 8 and 12 weeks old when exposed to the four weeks of high-salt diet. These studies highlight the fact that the impact of the elevated sodium intake was greater in young compared with older mature animals suggesting that the dietary intake influenced the brain before plasticity had been lost, with the consequence of a more potent autonomic control of the cardiovascular system and the kidney.

The exact sites within the brain where the manipulation of dietary sodium intake may change the impact of brain angiotensin II on neural pathways have yet to be fully explored. DiBona and coworkers (43) subjected mature rats to two weeks of either low, normal or high dietary sodium intakes and microinjected an AT_1-receptor antagonist onto RVLM neurons and demonstrated that in the animals on a low salt diet, blood pressure fell and the baroreflex and the renal sympathetic baroreflex gain curve operated over a lower pressure range. However, this effect of blocking angiotensin II receptors was not apparent in those animals on either a normal or high-salt diet. This approach was extended by this group (44) who went on to examine the role of the PVN by injecting bicucculine onto the nucleus to cause a rise in blood pressure and a renal sympathoexcitation. These findings demonstrated that the responses were dependent upon local angiotensin II as the responses were blocked following local microinjection of an AT_1 receptor antagonist onto the PVN. Of great significance was the observation that the bicucculine induced blood pressure and renal sympathetic nerve responses were larger in the rats on a low dietary sodium intake but were blunted in animals provided with an elevated dietary sodium intake. There now remains uncertainty as to the exact mechanisms which underlie this impact of sodium diet on the relationships between the neural control of the kidney and brain levels of angiotensin II and its receptors but this remains an important area for future investigation.

NEURAL CONTROL OF SODIUM BALANCE

Renal Nerves and Sodium Balance

A great deal of evidence has accrued demonstrating that the renal sympathetic nerves can exert a direct regulation of the sodium reabsorption at a tubular level. It has to be acknowledged that the majority of these studies have been carried out in acutely anesthetized animals where there may be an artificial elevation in basal levels of sympathetic activity which may bias the role of the renal sympathetic nerves. Moreover, in many of these short term studies the contribution of the renal sympathetic nerves in physiological reflexes have been examined but exactly how these findings may be extrapolated into the chronic situation remains to be clarified. Thus, it is less clear as to the role of the renal sympathetic nerves in the maintenance of sodium balance in everyday conditions when there is fluctuation in intake of sodium in the food and the need for a dynamic response in order to ensure that sodium balance is maintained within narrow limits.

Neural Impact on Long-Term Sodium Balance

There are a number of key studies in conscious animal studies which have attempted to provide support for the view that the renal sympathetic nerves can be implicated in the normal control of sodium balance. The general approach has been to use conscious chronically instrumented animals, which in itself is technically demanding; moreover, the challenge of either an increased or decreased sodium intake has to be evaluated under acute dynamic situations where it is likely that the renal nerves acting at the proximal tubule may come into play, rather than the longer term where other humoral mechanisms will be evoked, for example, activation of the renin–angiotensin system, stimulation of aldosterone secretion and compensatory reabsorption of sodium at the distal tubule. One of the first approaches was to examine the excretory responses to a sodium challenge in intact kidneys compared to kidneys subjected to prior denervation. There are now reports in rats (45), dogs (46–48) and humans (49,50) which have demonstrated a deficit in sodium retaining ability in response to a reduction in dietary sodium intake if the kidneys were denervated. Moreover, in these studies it was evident that the degree of reduction in sodium intake had to be quite severe in order to generate a clear distinction between innervated versus the denervated kidneys. Nonetheless, a role for the renal nerves was convincingly demonstrated in these reports. Perhaps one of the most influential observations was that of Greenberg et al. (51), using the conscious chronically instrumented rat, in which a controlled increase in sodium load, via an intravenous infusion, resulted in a longer lag time to achieve sodium balance in the denervated rats compared to the intact rats. The situation in man is difficult to ascertain, primarily because of the limited situations in which the adrenergic control of the kidney can be manipulated and the sodium intake can be varied. This has meant that information has been gathered from reports where an extreme situation pertains or a pathophysiological state exists. Thus, Gill and Bartter (49) demonstrated that following ganglion blockade with guanethidine, there was a relatively higher sodium excretion when the patients were exposed to a low dietary sodium intake, indicative of a loss in renal nerve-dependent sodium retention. Wilcox et al. (50) in a study of patients with autonomic failure, observed that these patients underwent an inappropriate loss of sodium when exposed to a low dietary sodium intake. Together, these observations indicate that the renal sympathetic nerves contribute importantly to the immediate dynamic response to control sodium balance in response to a fluctuating sodium intake while other humoral systems are likely to be implicated in the longer term adjustments necessary for the maintenance of total body sodium.

There are a number of conscious animal studies which support this view. Kaplan and Rapoport (52) undertook a unilateral denervation in dogs and demonstrated that there was an increased sodium excretion from the denervated kidney compared to the innervated kidney when the dogs were given a sodium load, and that this difference was exacerbated if the animals were concomitantly relatively dehydrated. In a somewhat different scenario, Hall and coworkers (53,54) using a fat-fed dog model of obesity found that the hypertension and sodium retention, which occurred as obesity developed, was prevented if the animals were subjected to a renal denervation. Furthermore, in a somewhat different setting, Lohmeirer and coworkers found in dogs subjected to a slow sub-pressor intravenous infusion of angiotensin II that sodium excretion was enhanced in the innervated compared to the denervated kidney, that is, a suppression of activity in the renal sympathetic nerves was effective in mobilizing sodium in an attempt to restore blood pressure (55,56). Thus, albeit under more pathophysiological conditions where renal sympathetic nerve activity may be elevated, the nerves significantly contribute to the reabsorption of sodium which impacts on sodium balance and the level of blood pressure within the animals.

CONCLUSIONS

The conclusions to be drawn from these studies is that control of sodium handling by the kidney is exerted not only through the renal sympathetic nerves but also via humoral mechanisms to a greater or lesser degree, and whether the neural or humoral mechanism will be dependent upon the prevailing conditions, whether over the short term or longer term. Nonetheless, it is apparent that the reflex regulation of renal sympathetic nerve activity and the neural regulation of sodium reabsorption remain key elements in the homeostatic response to maintaining sodium balance and total body sodium.

REFERENCES

1. Swales JD. Hypertension in the political arena. Hypertension 2000; 35(6):1179–82.
2. Boron WF, Boulpaep EL. Medical Physiology. London/New York/Sydney: Saunders, 2003.
3. Granger JP, Alexander BT, Llinas M. Mechanisms of pressure natriuresis. Curr Hypertens Rep 2002; 4(2):152–9.
4. Guyton AC. Kidneys and fluids in pressure regulation. Small volume but large pressure changes. Hypertension 1992; 19(Suppl. 1):I2–8.
5. Ichihara A, Kobori H, Nishiyama A, Navar LG. Renal renin–angiotensin system. Contrib Nephrol 2004; 143:117–30.
6. DiBona GF, Kopp UC. Neural control of renal function. Physiol Rev 1997; 77(1):75–197.
7. Johns EJ. The physiology and pharmacology of the renal nerves. Pol Arch Med Wewn 1991; 85(3):141–9.
8. Sattar MA, Johns EJ. Evidence for an alpha 1-adrenoceptor subtype mediating adrenergic vasoconstriction in Wistar normotensive and stroke-prone spontaneously hypertensive rat kidney. J Cardiovasc Pharmacol 1994; 23(2):232–9.
9. Hesse IF, Johns EJ. The subtype of alpha-adrenoceptor involved in the neural control of renal tubular sodium reabsorption in the rabbit. J Physiol 1984; 352:527–38.
10. Johns EJ, Manitius J. An investigation into the neural regulation of calcium excretion by the rat kidney. J Physiol 1987; 383:745–55.
11. Bello-Reuss E, Colindres RE, Pastoriza-Munoz E, Mueller RA, Gottschalk CW. Effects of acute unilateral renal denervation in the rat. J Clin Invest 1975; 56(1):208–17.
12. Wu XC, Johns EJ. Interactions between nitric oxide and superoxide on the neural regulation of proximal fluid reabsorption in hypertensive rats. Exp Physiol 2004; 89(3):255–61.
13. DiBona GF, Sawin LL. Effect of renal nerve stimulation on NaCl and H_2O transport in Henle's loop of the rat. Am J Physiol 1982; 243(6):F576–80.
14. Johns EJ. The autonomic nervous system and pressure–natriuresis in cardiovascular–renal interactions in response to salt. Clin Auton Res 2002; 12(4):256–63.
15. DiBona GF, Johns EJ. A study of the role of renal nerves in the renal responses to 60 degree head-up tilt in the anaesthetized dog. J Physiol 1980; 299:117–26.
16. Zambraski EJ, Dibona GF, Kaloyanides GJ. Effect of sympathetic blocking agents on the antinatriuresis of reflex renal nerve stimulation. J Pharmacol Exp Ther 1976; 198(2):464–72.
17. DiBona GF, Sawin LL. Exaggerated natriuresis in experimental hypertension. Proc Soc Exp Biol Med 1986; 182(1):43–51.
18. Gilmore JP, Echtenkamp S, Wesley CR, Zucker IH. Atrial receptor modulation of renal nerve activity in the nonhuman primate. Am J Physiol 1982; 242(6):F592–8.
19. Miki K, Hayashida Y, Shiraki K. Role of cardiac–renal neural reflex in regulating sodium excretion during water immersion in conscious dogs. J Physiol 2002; 545(Pt 1):305–12.
20. Zhang T, Johns EJ. Somatosensory influences on renal sympathetic nerve activity in anesthetized Wistar and hypertensive rats. Am J Physiol 1997; 272(3 Pt 2):R982–90.
21. Davis G, Johns EJ. Effect of somatic nerve stimulation on the kidney in intact, vagotomized and carotid sinus-denervated rats. J Physiol 1991; 432:573–84.
22. Zhang T, Huang C, Johns EJ. Neural regulation of kidney function by the somatosensory system in normotensive and hypertensive rats. Am J Physiol 1997; 273(5 Pt 2):R1749–57.
23. Kostreva DR, Castaner A, Kampine JP. Reflex effects of hepatic baroreceptors on renal and cardiac sympathetic nerve activity. Am J Physiol 1980; 238(5):R390–4.
24. Morita H, Nishida Y, Hosomi H. Neural control of urinary sodium excretion during hypertonic NaCl load in conscious rabbits: role of renal and hepatic nerves and baroreceptors. J Auton Nerv Syst 1991; 34(2–3):157–69.
25. Weaver LC, Genovesi S, Stella A, Zanchetti A. Neural, hemodynamic, and renal responses to stimulation of intestinal receptors. Am J Physiol 1987; 253(5 Pt 2):H1167–76.
26. Kopp UC, Cicha MZ, Nakamura K, Nusing RM, Smith LA, Hokfelt T. Activation of EP4 receptors contributes to prostaglandin E2-mediated stimulation of renal sensory nerves. Am J Physiol Renal Physiol 2004; 287(6):F1269–82.

27. McKinley MJ, Pennington GL, Oldfield BJ. Anteroventral wall of the third ventricle and dorsal lamina terminalis: headquarters for control of body fluid homeostasis? Clin Exp Pharmacol Physiol 1996; 23(4):271–81.
28. Mendelsohn FA, Quirion R, Saavedra JM, Aguilera G, Catt KJ. Autoradiographic localization of angiotensin II receptors in rat brain. Proc Natl Acad Sci USA 1984; 81(5):1575–9.
29. Wright JW, Harding JW. Important role for angiotensin III and IV in the brain renin–angiotensin system. Brain Res Brain Res Rev 1997; 25(1):96–124.
30. Allen AM, Moeller I, Jenkins TA, et al. Angiotensin receptors in the nervous system. Brain Res Bull 1998; 47(1):17–28.
31. Phillips MI, Speakman EA, Kimura B. Levels of angiotensin and molecular biology of the tissue renin angiotensin systems. Regul Pept 1993; 43(1–2):1–20.
32. Head GA. Role of AT1 receptors in the central control of sympathetic vasomotor function. Clin Exp Pharmacol Physiol Suppl 1996; 3:S93–8.
33. Head GA, Mayorov DN. Central angiotensin and baroreceptor control of circulation. Ann NY Acad Sci 2001; 940:361–79.
34. Dampney RA, Fontes MA, Hirooka Y, Horiuchi J, Potts PD, Tagawa T. Role of angiotensin II receptors in the regulation of vasomotor neurons in the ventrolateral medulla. Clin Exp Pharmacol Physiol 2002; 29(5–6):467–72.
35. Horiuchi J, Dampney RA. Evidence for tonic disinhibition of RVLM sympathoexcitatory neurons from the caudal pressor area. Auton Neurosci 2002; 99(2):102–10.
36. Johns EJ. Angiotensin II in the brain and the autonomic control of the kidney. Exp Physiol 2005; 90(2):163–8.
37. Huang C, Johns EJ. Role of ANG II in mediating somatosensory-induced renal nerve-dependent antinatriuresis in the rat. Am J Physiol 1998; 275(1 Pt 2):R194–202.
38. Strehlow K, Nickenig G, Roeling J, et al. AT(1) receptor regulation in salt-sensitive hypertension. Am J Physiol 1999; 277(5 Pt 2):H1701–7.
39. Wang JM, Veerasingham SJ, Tan J, Leenen FH. Effects of high salt intake on brain AT1 receptor densities in Dahl rats. Am J Physiol Heart Circ Physiol 2003; 285(5):H1949–55.
40. Huang BS, Leenen FH. Sympathoexcitatory and pressor responses to increased brain sodium and ouabain are mediated via brain ANG II. Am J Physiol 1996; 270(1 Pt 2):H275–80.
41. Camara AK, Osborn JL. AT1 receptors mediate chronic central nervous system AII hypertension in rats fed high sodium chloride diet from weaning. J Auton Nerv Syst 1998; 72(1):16–23.
42. Osborn JL, Camara AK. Renal neurogenic mediation of intracerebroventricular angiotensin II hypertension in rats raised on high sodium chloride diet. Hypertension 1997; 30(3 Pt 1):331–6.
43. DiBona GF, Jones SY. Sodium intake influences hemodynamic and neural responses to angiotensin receptor blockade in rostral ventrolateral medulla. Hypertension 2001; 37(4):1114–23.
44. DiBona GF, Jones SY. Effect of dietary sodium intake on the responses to bicuculline in the paraventricular nucleus of rats. Hypertension 2001; 38(2):192–7.
45. DiBona GF, Sawin LL. Renal nerves in renal adaptation to dietary sodium restriction. Am J Physiol 1983; 245(3):F322–8.
46. Brubacher ES, Vander AJ. Sodium deprivation and renin secretion in unanesthetized dogs. Am J Physiol 1968; 214(1):15–21.
47. Gotshall RW, Davis JO, Shade RE, Spielman W, Johnson JA, Braverman B. Effects of renal denervation on renin release in sodium-depleted dogs. Am J Physiol 1973; 225(2):344–9.
48. Kaczmarczyk G, Mohnhaupt R, Reinhardt HW. Renal sodium handling in intact and renal denervated dogs. Pflugers Arch 1986; 407(4):382–7.
49. Gill JR, Bartter FC. Adrenergic nervous system in sodium metabolism. II. Effects of guanethidine on the renal response to sodium deprivation in normal man. N Engl J Med 1966; 275(26):1466–71.
50. Wilcox CS, Aminoff MJ, Slater JD. Sodium homeostasis in patients with autonomic failure. Clin Sci Mol Med 1977; 53(4):321–8.

51. Greenberg SG, Tershner S, Osborn JL. Neurogenic regulation of rate of achieving sodium balance after increasing sodium intake. Am J Physiol 1991; 261(2 Pt 2):F300–7.
52. Kaplan SA, Rapoport S. Urinary excretion of sodium and chloride after splanchnicotomy; effect on the proximal tubule. Am J Physiol 1951; 164(1):175–81.
53. Hall JE, Hildebrandt DA, Kuo J. Obesity hypertension: role of leptin and sympathetic nervous system. Am J Hypertens 2001; 14(6 Pt 2):103S–15.
54. Kassab S, Kato T, Wilkins FC, Chen R, Hall JE, Granger JP. Renal denervation attenuates the sodium retention and hypertension associated with obesity. Hypertension 1995; 25(4 Pt 2): 893–7.
55. Lohmeier TE, Hildebrandt DA. Renal nerves promote sodium excretion in angiotensin-induced hypertension. Hypertension 1998; 31(1 Pt 2):429–34.
56. Lohmeier TE, Hildebrandt DA, Warren S, May PJ, Cunningham JT. Recent insights into the interactions between the baroreflex and the kidneys in hypertension. Am J Physiol Regul Integr Comp Physiol 2005; 288(4):R828–36.

7
Aldosterone and Mineralocorticoid Receptors

Nicolette Farman
Faculté de Médecine, Xavier Bichat, Paris, France

INTRODUCTION

The steroid hormone aldosterone plays a major role in the control of blood pressure and extracellular volume homeostasia (1–4). Aldosterone is synthesized in the glomerular zone of the adrenal cortex in response to hyperkalemia or sodium depletion, as the end point of activation of the renin-angiotensin system. Its biosynthesis from cholesterol depends on several enzymes, many of which belong to the cytochrome P 450 family; the biosynthetic pathways, their regulation and pathophysiological aspects will not be exposed here (see Ref. 5 for a recent overview). Considerable work has been achieved to improve the understanding of the molecular and cellular events involved in aldosterone actions, in normal as well as in pathological situations (1–4,6–9). It is well established that aldosterone stimulates renal sodium reabsorption and potassium excretion. These effects are observed one to two hours after hormone administration, a delay necessary for hormonally mediated activation of sodium transporters and regulation of transcription of target genes. As illustrated schematically in Figure 1, aldosterone binds to the mineralocorticoid receptor (MR), which is a ligand-dependent transcription factor (6,10,11); once translocated into the nucleus, the hormone–receptor complexes bind to glucocorticoid response elements (GRE) within the promotor region of early aldosterone-induced genes to modulate their transcription (there is no mineralocorticoid-specific response element; mineralocorticoid, glucocorticoid, androgen as well as progesterone receptors bind to the same GREs). This will trigger an increase in the activity and number of sodium transporters or channels. In a typical target cell for aldosterone, such as the renal collecting duct (CD) principal cell, the sodium of the tubular fluid enters the cell through amiloride-sensitive apical sodium channels (ENaC, epithelium sodium channel), and is then extruded from the cell to the peritubular space by the Na–K-ATPase located in the basolateral membrane (8,9,12). Detailed information on ENaC, the rate-limiting step for transepithelial sodium transport, is provided in Reference 12 and in Chapter 2 of this book. ENaC and Na–K-ATPase are coordinately activated in the presence of aldosterone, leading to an initial increase in transepithelial sodium reabsorption via the transcellular route, followed by augmented biosynthesis of some of their subunits (αENaC and α1Na–K-ATPase in the kidney).

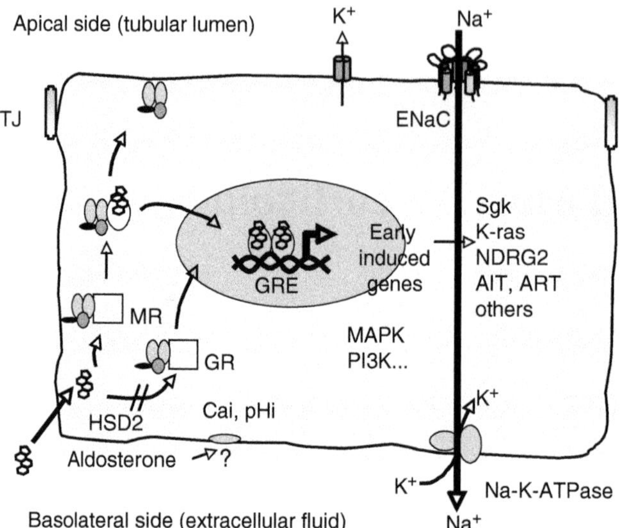

Figure 1 Schematic view of the mechanism of action of aldosterone in principal cells of the collecting duct. *Abbreviations*: AIT, aldosterone induced transcripts; ART, aldosterone repressed transcripts; ENaC, epithelium sodium channel; GR, glucocorticoid receptor; GRE, glucocorticoid response elements; HSD2, 11β hydroxysteroid dehydrogenase type 2; MR, mineralocorticoid receptor; NDRG2, N-Myc downstream regulated gene 2; sgk, serum and glucocorticoid-regulated kinase; TJ, tight junctions.

In addition to ENaC, aldosterone stimulates sodium reabsorption in the distal tubule through enhanced expression of the thiazide-sensitive NaCl cotransporter (NCC) (13). Regulation of this transporter will be detailed elsewhere in this book. Mineralocorticoids are known to increase the apical potassium conductance of the CD (14–16). It is not fully established yet how aldosterone stimulates K secretory channel activity. The best channel candidate is rat, renal outer medullary potassium channel, (ROMK) or Kir 1.1. The apical ROMK channels mediate the downhill movement of K from the intracellular compartment to the lumen of the distal tubule and CD. Intracellular K is determined mainly by the Na–K-ATPase pump, and the aldosterone-induced increase in apical Na entry via ENaC provides a driving force for K secretion. There is no evidence that aldosterone directly modulates ROMK biosynthesis. Interestingly, it has been shown that the serum and glucocorticoid kinase1 (sgk1) can phosphorylate ROMK and can stimulate K secretion through an increase in ROMK surface expression (17).

Aldosterone acts in the distal parts of the nephron [the MR is expressed in the distal tubule, the connecting tubule and the CD (18)], after the bulk of sodium reabsorption that occurs in the proximal tubule and loop of Henle (Fig. 2). This effect is however critical: variations in aldosteronemia lead to precise and physiologically relevant adjustments of sodium reabsorption. Alterations in these adjustments, as observed in Addison's disease, in syndromes of resistance to aldosterone (such as pseudohypoaldosteronism) or hyperaldosteronism, illustrate the critical role of aldosterone in the regulation of sodium handling. Aldosterone-mediated regulations are essentially studied in the CD, the prototype of mineralocorticoid-sensitive cell. Experimental access to distal tubule or connecting tubule is technically very difficult in vivo and there are no satisfactory cell models representative of these epithelia. The relative contributions of different

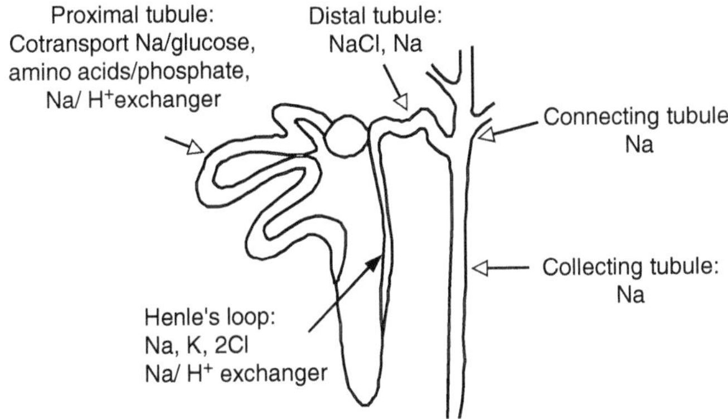

Figure 2 Routes of sodium reabsorption along the nephron.

parts of the aldosterone-sensitive distal nephron (Fig. 2) to sodium reabsorption merit some comments. The distal convoluted tubule accounts for a much larger fraction of sodium reabsorption (6–7% of the filtered load of sodium) than the following connecting tubule and CD (1–2%). As an illustration to this notion, the CD-specific knockout of ENaC (19) did not impair sodium and potassium balance of mice, even after low sodium diet (that enhances plasma aldosterone levels). This result indicates that sodium transport through the preceding distal tubule and connecting tubule can fully compensate for the lack of ENaC in the CD. It is likely that NCC-mediated sodium reabsorption represents a major component of the anti-natriuretic action of aldosterone.

The classical schematic view of aldosterone action has to be revisited, in view of the complexity of the biological responses that have been elucidated more recently.

The MR has been cloned in 1987 (20), and it was subsequently evidenced that the MR displays similar high affinity (in the nanomolar range) for aldosterone and glucocorticoid hormones, which are much more abundant in the plasma (100–1000 fold) than aldosterone (Fig. 3). This should lead to permanent occupancy of the MR by glucocorticoid hormones, inducing permanent maximal sodium retention, independent of plasma aldosterone levels. Several mechanisms ensuring in vivo mineralocorticoid selectivity have been highlighted. The main mechanism (21–23) involves the enzyme 11β hydroxysteroid dehydrogenase type 2 (11-HSD2), which metabolizes circulating glucocorticoid hormones (cortisol in man, corticosterone in rodents) into inactive 11-dehydro-derivatives (cortisone, 11-dehydrocorticosterone) with very low affinity for the MR (Fig. 3). 11-HSD2 is coexpressed with the MR in cells of the distal nephron, allowing efficient MR protection (7,8). Any reduction in its activity leads to excessive renal sodium reabsorption and hypertension, as seen in the syndrome of apparent mineralocorticoid excess (due to inactivating mutations of the gene) or in liquorice intoxication (through inhibition of 11-HSD2 catalytic activity). This will be reviewed in Chapter 8 of this book. Many drugs or factors (including components of food or xenobiotics) downregulate 11-HSD2 activity, thus possibly contributing to hypertension (23). Polymorphisms of the human 11-HSD2 gene have been reported, but their links to essential hypertension are still controversial. On the other hand, reduced catalytic activity of the enzyme has been evidenced in patients suffering from essential hypertension (24). Unfortunately almost no 11-HSD2 "enhancing" factors have been identified; they would however represent important and novel tools in hypertension therapy to restore 11-HSD2

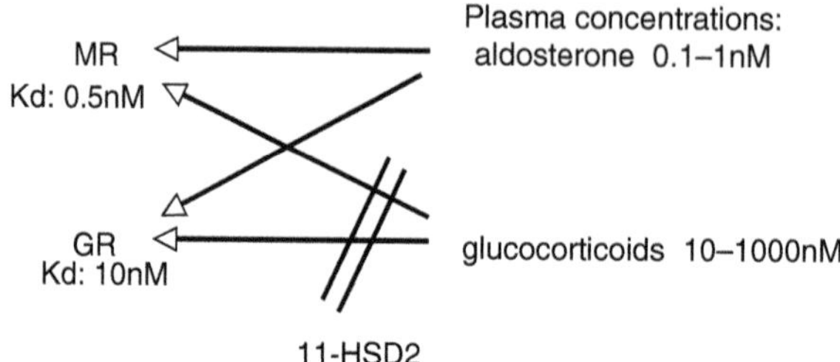

-Relative amounts of MR, GR, and 11-HSD2 vary in a cell-specific manner

-MR and GR form dimers with distinct transcriptional activities:
MR/MR, GR/GR, MR/GR, and each receptor can be occupied by each hormone

Figure 3 Complexity of corticosteroid action: two ligands for two receptors. The mineralocorticoid receptor has similar high affinity (0.5 nM) for aldosterone and for glucocorticoid hormones. The glucocorticoid receptor exhibits lower affinity (10 nM) for each of these steroids. The enzyme 11-hydroxysteroid dehydrogenase 2 metabolizes glucocorticoid hormones into derivatives with very low affinity for the MR and for the GR. Several hormone–receptor complexes can form, depending on the cell context and environment.

activity levels in situations of partial deficiency. Aldosterone target cells also express the glucocorticoid receptor (GR), in addition to MR and 11-HSD2. Glucocorticoid metabolites produced by 11-HSD2 are inactive on MR and also on GR; thus effective protection of MR by the enzyme should preclude any glucocorticoid effect via their own receptor in aldosterone-sensitive cells. This is hardly conceivable in view of the important functions of the GR. It can be proposed that functional compartmentalization of 11-HSD2 within the cell could restrict 11-HSD2 to the vicinity of MR, not GR, allowing glucocorticoid effects in addition to MR protection. Although 11-HSD2 plays a key role in mineralocorticoid selectivity, other factors also intervene (7,8) such as the intrinsic properties of the MR, its capacity to form homo-or heterodimer (with the GR) or its interaction with other transcription factors.

THE MINERALOCORTICOID RECEPTOR: STRUCTURE–FUNCTION RELATIONSHIPS

The human MR (hMR) gene is located in chromosome 4q31.1 and spans over more than 400 kb; it is composed of 10 exons, with two alternative (1 α and 1 β) untranslated exon 1, leading to two distinct mRNA isoforms that differ in their 5′ untranslated region (Fig. 4). Both isoforms are expressed in human tissues at somewhat distinct levels (25), but we ignore most of their functional relevance; they are translated into the same 984 amino acids protein (Fig. 4). Some MR variants have been reported; among them, the delta five to six MR that lacks the ligand-binding domain (LBD), might be a modulator of MR function in pathological states (26). The MR belongs to the superfamily of nuclear receptors, (including MR and GR, androgen, estrogen, progesterone, vitamin D, thyroid and retinoic acid receptors as well as several orphan receptors), all having a common organization (27). Nuclear receptors are ligand-dependent transcription factors. Some of their domains are highly conserved between members of this superfamily, such as the DNA-binding domain (DBD) and the LBD. In particular, the MR and the GR share high

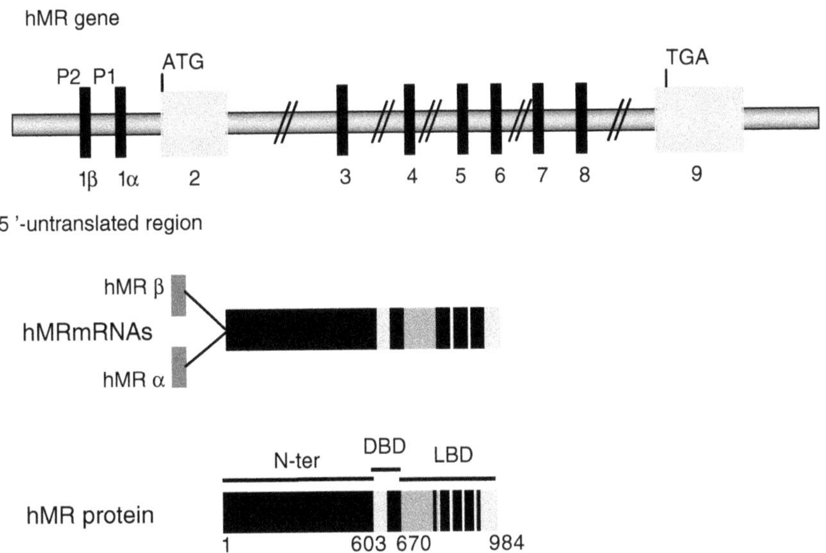

Figure 4 Human mineralocorticoid receptor gene, mRNAs and protein. P1 and P2 refer to the alternate promoters, leading to expression of isoforms α or β. The protein includes an N-terminal region, a DNA-binding domain, and a ligand-binding domain.

homology within the DBD (94% identity) and the LBD (57% identity), while their N-terminal regions are divergent (less than 15% identity). Such divergence may be an important determinant of the differences in transcriptional activities between MR and GR. Because of the structural homology of their LBD, it is easier to understand the numerous observations on cross occupancies of MR and GR by aldosterone and glucocorticoid hormones. The structure of the LBD of the hMR has been elucidated (28). Three-dimensional modeling and mutagenesis have shown that it is organized in 12α helices and one β sheet, with identification of the amino acids that are critical for ligand binding. In the absence of ligand, the LBD binds several chaperone proteins (as hsp90, hsp70, immunophilins***). Aldosterone binding triggers MR conformational changes, dissociation of chaperone proteins and nuclear translocation of the hormone–receptor complex. Upon aldosterone binding, the LBD is compacted, by establishing many polar and hydrophobic contacts that stabilize the C-terminal H12 helix in its active conformation, allowing binding of cofactors (coactivators or corepressors) of transcription. The MR antagonists (spironolactone, progesterone) do not accommodate properly into the hydrophobic pocket of the LBD (loss of critical contacts), precluding rotation of H12 and coactivator recruitment. Very recently, crystal structures of the MR LBD have been obtained (29,30) that allow to progress in the understanding of the structure-function relationships of normal and mutant MRs and the mechanism of activation and antagonism. These novel findings will be helpful to explain the previously reported characteristics of MR when bound to various ligands. Indeed, aldosterone, antialdosterone molecules (such as spironolactone) or glucocorticoids binding to MR confer distinct properties to the complex, despite the fact that the receptor displays the same affinity for all these ligands (8,10,11,31,32). It has been shown that aldosterone–MR complexes are much more stable than cortisol–MR (or spironolactone–MR) complexes. The efficiency of nuclear translocation of MR–ligand complexes is higher in the presence of aldosterone than of glucocorticoids. MR sensitivity to chymotrypsin proteolysis is also ligand-dependent.

The MR can transactivate a reporter gene (for example the promoter of the mouse mammary tumor virus coupled to luciferase) more efficiently when bound to aldosterone than to other ligands (concentrations of aldosterone ten-fold lower than of glucocorticoid hormones are sufficient to transactivate reporter genes). Altogether these observations suggested that the "active" conformation of MR (i.e., efficient to interact with the transcriptional machinery) was ligand-dependent, with aldosterone being more efficient than glucocorticoid hormones. Thus, it appears that the receptor itself plays a role in mineralocorticoid selectivity.

MR AND TRANSCRIPTIONAL COFACTORS

The MR interacts with the transcriptional machinery, as other steroid receptors (6,10). We will underline some elements that are more specific for MR, as novel factors possibly contributing to its specific signaling. Coactivators/corepressors interact with steroid receptors and modify their transcriptional activities. Several of these coactivators are common to most nuclear receptors. Some GR-coregulators have been also shown to modulate aldosterone-dependent MR transcriptional activity (10), as GR-interacting protein 1, transcriptional intermediary factor 1α, steroid receptor coactivator 1. Of interest, other coregulators appear to exert selective regulation of MR activity. Among them, protein inhibitor of activated signal transduction 1 (PIAS1), a sumo-ligase, is a ligand-dependent specific repressor of hMR transactivation activity, while GR transactivation is unaffected (33). PIAS1 interacts with the N-terminal region of the hMR and it can sumoylate it. Very recently a coactivator specific for hMR has been identified: eleven-nineteen lysine-rich leukemia (ELL), a RNA polymerase II elongation factor (34). Interestingly, ELL is a potent coactivator of MR, but it strongly represses GR transactivation and has no effect on other steroid receptors (as the androgen and the progesterone receptor). Src1 may also discriminate between MR and GR signaling (35). Such cofactors may be important to modify selectively MR activity in a tissue-specific and ligand-dependent manner; further studies are needed to evaluate their in vivo relevance to aldosterone-MR signaling.

DIMERIZATION

The MR binds to DNA regulatory elements (promotors) as dimers, which may be homodimers (MR–MR) or heterodimers, together with other receptors, particularly the GR (36). In transfection experiments (where the relative amounts of MR and GR was varied) it has been shown that transcriptional activity varies according to the dimer formed: homodimers MR–MR or GR–GR, or MR–GR heterodimers (36–39). This phenomenon likely occurs in vivo, and may be at the origin (at least partly) of the complex and tissue-specific effects of corticosteroid hormones (36–39). For example, several authors have proposed that full mineralocorticoid effects on sodium transport require occupancy of both MR and GR (simultaneously or successively). Conversely MR may inhibit GR through heterodimer formation (38). Since each of these receptors may bind aldosterone and glucocorticoid hormones, it offers a great regulatory flexibility due to the different possible combinations of receptor–ligand complexes (Fig. 3):

- MR–MR, occupied by aldosterone alone, or partly by glucocorticoid hormones,
- GR–GR, occupied by glucocorticoids alone, or partly by aldosterone,
- MR–GR, with variable proportions of each ligand.

These variable associations should depend on the cellular context and on the respective intracellular concentration of each ligand (indeed, some glucocorticoid hormones are likely to be present in the cell, despite the very high metabolizing efficiency of 11-HSD2). In addition, the relative amounts of MR and GR vary among cell types (7,8,40). Other non-receptor transcription factors also intervene to modulate MR activity, as those of the AP1 family (6).

POST-TRANSLATIONAL MODIFICATIONS OF MR

MR activity may also depend on post-translational modifications that are not fully characterized. The MR exhibits several putative phosphorylation sites, but little is known about their contribution to MR activity (41). It has been shown recently (42) that protein kinase Cα (PKCα) dependent phosphorylation of MR on serine residues occurs shortly after exposure to low doses of aldosterone, while the glucocorticoid dexamethazone is uneffective to do so. However it is ignored if serine-phosphorylation modifies per se the properties of the MR. It has also been reported that protein kinase A activation leads to enhanced MR activity (presumably through phosphorylation of an associated protein rather than of the MR itself). Other post-translational modifications have been reported (10), as sumoylation and acetylation that remain to be explored further.

GENETIC DEFECTS OF MR GENE

Mutations of the hMR have been identified in human pathology. Several inactivating mutations of MR were evidenced in the autosomal-dominant form (or in some sporadic forms) of type I pseudohypoaldosteronism (type I PHA), a rare syndrome of mineralocorticoid resistance characterized by renal salt wasting, dehydration and failure to thrive in newborns (43–45). Mutations have been found in all functional domains of the receptor, and the loss of function of one MR allele is sufficient to induce a salt-loosing syndrome. Interestingly, affected children can be clinically cured by sodium supplementation, although the renal defect persists all life-long and induces persistent up-regulation of the renin-angiotensin–aldosterone system. A mouse model of type I PHA was created by invalidation of the MR (46): the MR knockout mice die a few days after birth from severe dehydration and renal salt wasting, but some animals may be rescued by sodium chloride loading, thus mimicking the type I PHA evolution.

A gain-of-function mutation of hMR (S810L) leading to severe hypertension has been found in young subjects of a single pedigree (47). Analysis of transfection assays of the mutated MR showed that the S810L MR mutant can be paradoxically activated by classical antagonists of the normal (wild type) receptor, as spironolactone or as progesterone (explaining exacerbation of the hypertension during pregnancy), and also by cortisone (the normally inactive metabolite of cortisol produced by renal 11-HSD2). These rare genetic diseases highlight the crucial role of MR in regulating renal salt reabsorption and blood pressure in humans. It should be noted that the search for mutations in the hMR gene in essential hypertension has been negative so far. However recent genome-wide scan from the Hypertension Genetic Epidemiology Network indicated that the maximum logarithm of odds for early-onset hypertension in African Americans was, in part, on chromosome 4 at 153cM and overlies the MR (48).

TISSUE-SPECIFIC EXPRESSION OF MR; PATHOPHYSIOLOGICAL INSIGHTS

At variance with the almost ubiquitous expression of GR, MR expression is restricted to some tissues. They can be classified schematically as classical target tissues (i.e., epitheliums where aldosterone controls sodium reabsorption) and as new targets (where MR has been evidenced, but its function remains elusive).

Classical target tissues include the terminal parts of the nephron (distal tubule, connecting tubule and CD), the colonic epithelium and the excretory ducts of sweat and salivary glands (6–8). In these tissues, there seems to be no or very little regulation of MR expression [the level of MR transcripts does not vary in the presence or absence of circulating corticosteroid hormones (40)]. However, aldosterone triggers differential gene regulations in these classical target tissues. For example, as a result of variations in plasma aldosterone (adrenalectomized rats compared to aldosterone-injected rats) aldosterone increases the level of mRNA expression of the sole α subunit of the amiloride-sensitive sodium channel ENaC in the kidney, while in the colon the regulated subunits are the β and the γ subunits (49). These distinct effects are probably due to differential interactions of MR with yet unidentified tissue-specific transcription factors.

The presence of MR has been clearly assessed in other tissues, in particular in non-epithelial cells, devoid of vectorialized sodium transport processes. This is the case for neurons (in particular in the hippocampus), for cardiomyocytes, blood vessels or adipocytes, as well as skin keratinocytes (10,50–52). The nature of aldosterone action in these tissues is actively investigated, in normal as well as in pathological situations. Although beyond the scope of this chapter, some of them will be briefly evoked. Neuronal effects of aldosterone (50) may be important for cognitive processes and memory, for response to stress (including central blood pressure control). Direct cardiovascular effects of aldosterone (beside the cardiovascular consequences of an altered functioning of the renin-angiotensin system) have been suggested (53,54). Indeed, cardiomyocytes do express MR (51); cardiac synthesis of aldosterone has been reported (55), raising the question of a local production and action independent of adrenal production of corticosteroid hormones. There are data in favor of an involvement of aldosterone in the constitution of cardiac remodeling and fibrosis (54). Exposure of uninephrectomized rats to aldosterone and high-salt diet leads to cardiac fibrosis that can be prevented by spironolactone. In apparent contradiction is the observation that reduced expression of the cardiac MR by an inducible antisense strategy in transgenic mice (56) also produces cardiac fibrosis [while MR overexpression does not (57)]. These observations indicate that modifications of the levels of the ligand are far from being equivalent to changes in receptor expression levels. Future work will be important to dissect the pathological mechanisms triggered in these distinct effects and their clinical relevance. As an illustration of the difficulty to understand the primum movens of aldosterone/MR-induced pathology, it is should be noted that the sole elevation of plasma aldosterone is not sufficient to trigger cardiac remodeling, even in the presence of an additional salt load. Indeed patients with type I PHA or transgenic mice with rescued knockout of the α subunit of ENaC (58) exhibit chronic hyperaldosteronism, but do not present cardiac remodeling. Importantly, the RALES and the EPHESUS studies have demonstrated the beneficial effect of MR-antagonists (spironolactone, eplerenone) in large cohorts of patients with severe heart failure; a striking reduction in mortality was observed, that may be attributed, at least in part, to reduction of cardiac electrical disturbances (59,60). Consistent with this feature, mouse models of MR overexpression also exhibit arrhythmias (57,61,62). It must be recognized that the mechanisms of spironolactone-mediated improvements are far from being understood; they may depend on yet unknown targets in addition to MR antagonism.

Recent studies have investigated the links between aldosterone and the progression of renal injury; it is proposed that the underlying mechanisms include oxidative stress and endothelial dysfunction as well as inflammation (63). Profibrotic effects of aldosterone may be related to aldosterone modulation of plasminogen activator inhibitor 1 or TGF β (63). Interestingly, it has been recently reported that aldosterone stimulates the proliferation of mesangial cells by a mechanism involving MR occupancy and activation of mitogen-activated protein kinase (MAPK) 1/2 and cyclin A and D1 (64,65).

EARLY EVENTS IN ALDOSTERONE ACTION: ACTIVATION OF SEVERAL KINASES

The increase in sodium transport elicited by aldosterone is preceded by a series of events that are still under debate (Fig. 5). Within the first hour following hormone addition to cultured renal cells, several signaling cascades are activated and the question is raised to know whether they involve the MR or non-genomic effects. In Madin–Darby canine kidney or Chinese Hamster Ovary cells that do not (or marginally) express the MR, aldosterone

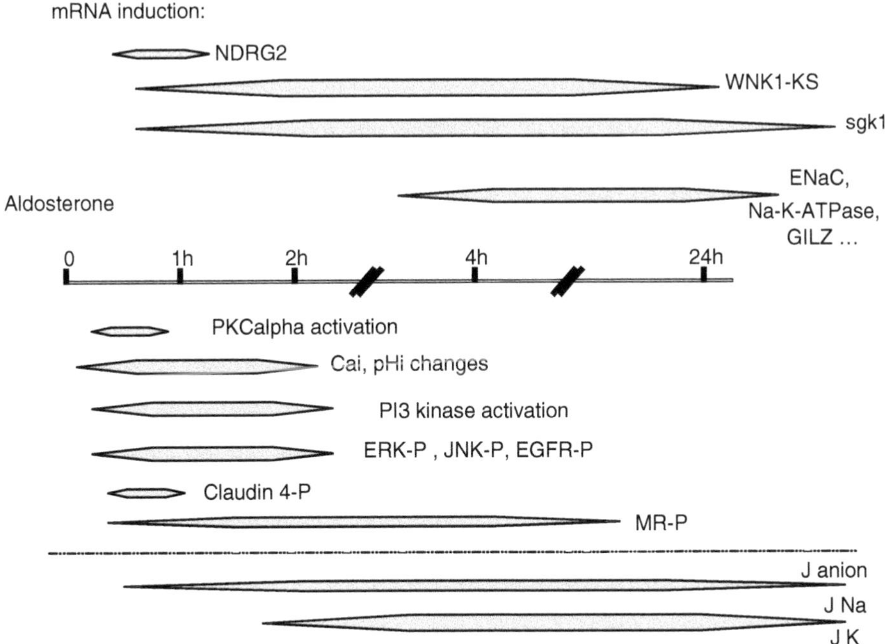

Figure 5 Schematic representation of sequential aldosterone-induced signaling and ion transport in mammalian target cells. *Abbreviations*: EGFR, epidermal growth factor receptor; ENaC, epithelium sodium channel; ERK, extracellular signal-regulated kinase; GILZ, glucocorticoid-induced leucine zipper; J anion, transepithelial anion flux; J K, transepithelial potassium flux; J Na, transepithelial sodium flux; JNK, c-Jun N-terminal kinase; NDRG2, N-Myc downstream-regulated gene 2; P, phosphorylated form of the protein; PI3 kinase, phosphatidylinositol 3 kinase; PKC, proteine kinase C; sgk1, serum and glucocorticoid-regulated kinase 1; WNK1-KS, with no lysine kinase 1-kidney-specific.

stimulates epidermal growth factor receptorphosphorylation and extracellular-regulated kinases 1/2 activation (66–68). This is accompanied by stimulation of Na/H exchange and by an increase in cytosolic calcium. It is considered that such rapid aldosterone signaling is via non-genomic pathway, since it was not prevented by inhibitors of transcription or translation or by spironolactone. In A6 amphibian cells, aldosterone activates the MAPK 1/2 and the PI3 kinase (phosphatidylinositol 3 kinase) cascades that are both necessary for sodium transport in this model; the latter cascade is a major pathway mediating aldosterone action on Na transport, as it provides a link between the transcriptionallyinduced K-Ras and sgk phosphorylation and activation (6,69,70). Other kinases are rapidly activated (or induced, see below) upon aldosterone exposure, as sgk (6), the Src kinase (71), kidney-specific With No Lysine Kinase (72) and PKCα (42). On the whole, a series of proteins undergo phosphorylation during the early phase of aldosterone action; although the nature of the kinase involved is not determined in each case, these events appear to participate to establish a novel functional status of the target cell that allows stimulation of sodium transport later on.

EARLY EVENTS IN ALDOSTERONE ACTION: ALDOSTERONE-REGULATED GENES

The development of screening methods for differentially expressed genes has led to the discovery of several mRNAs whose expression is influenced shortly after aldosterone exposure, as shown in amphibian (A6 cells) or mammalian cell lines issued from the renal CD, or in vivo situations (animal models). None of them have been validated in humans, partly because they correspond to acute major changes (hormone-deprived vs. hormone-treated tissues or cells), and not to the subtle physiological variations of plasma aldosterone levels as it occurs in vivo. Nevertheless, these gene products are interesting, not only from a fundamental point of view, but also because they are potential candidate genes or therapeutical targets in human pathologies with disturbed salt handling. It should be noted that there is only a limited overlap of identified genes between studies, due to the different models used, to variable experimental treatments (concentrations of aldosterone, duration of treatment), and to the intrinsic complexity of the biological response. Indeed it is likely that several interacting gene networks are regulated by aldosterone, in a precisely tuned time- and tissue-dependent manner. In many cases, search for induced genes has been done in the presence of relatively high doses of aldosterone (occupying the GR in addition to MR), thus precluding any firm conclusion on the mineralo versus glucocorticoid specificity of the observed transcript modification. This statement has its own limitations, if one considers that both corticosteroids may be needed to get a full response, and/or if these hormones control a partially overlapping network of genes. Only some of the genes involved in the early aldosterone response will be mentioned here (more extensive comments may be found in Refs. 2 and 6 and in other chapters of this book).

The sgk1 is considered as the prototype of aldosterone-(and glucocorticoid) induced gene in CD cells, where it is strongly upregulated within 15 to -30 minutes. (73,74). It plays a critical role in the regulation of ENaC expression at the apical surface of the epithelium, as it phosphorylates the ubiquitin-ligase Nedd-4-2 (which is responsible for ENaC retrieval from the apical membrane and its subsequent entry in the ubiquitination pathway); this results in a reduced affinity of Nedd-4-2 for ENaC leading to stabilization of sodium channels at the cell surface. Mice with sgk1 knockout exhibit renal sodium loss when placed on a low sodium diet, indicating the pivotal role of sgk1 in the control of Na reabsorption (75).

The oncogene K-ras is induced within 1hr in the presence of aldosterone in A6 cells and coinjection of its cRNA together with those of the ENaC subunits in *Xenopus* oocytes leads to an increase in sodium current (76). K-ras stimulates ENaC activity via the PI3 kinase pathway cascade. K-ras induction has not been shown in mammalian cells.

N-Myc downstream regulated gene 2 (NDRG2) is rapidly (15 minutes) and specifically upregulated by aldosterone in rat kidney CD in vivo and in rat cortical collecting duct (RCCD2) cells (77). As other members of the novel NDRG gene family, its function is unknown, and may be related to proliferation/differentiation processes. Because of its homology with MESK, a Drosophila gene modulating the Ras pathway, it can be proposed that NDRG2 could be the mammalian counterpart of K-ras.

Corticosteroid hormone-induced factor (CHIF) was originally cloned as a glucocorticoid-induced gene in rat colon. It belongs to a novel family of regulatory proteins (FXYD); CHIF exerts a fine tuning of the Na–K-ATPase activity in the distal nephron, by modulating sodium pump affinities for sodium and potassium (78). CHIF may participate to the late phase of aldosterone/glucocorticoid actions.

GILZ (Glucocorticoid-induced leucine zipper) is one of the aldosterone-regulated transcripts identified by serial analysis of gene expression of the mpkCCD mouse CD cell line, among 34 induced and 29 repressed transcripts (79). GILZ is induced by aldosterone in rat kidney CD (80). GILZ is a transcription factor that interferes with the function of AP-1 and NF-κB (nuclear factor κB) in T lymphocytes and exerts anti-inflammatory and immunosuppressive effects in macrophages (81,82). It may be a protein that links aldosterone and inflammatory processes.

Several other genes issued from differential screenings have been identified, and future work should allow to discriminate those that are pertinent for the regulation of sodium transport. It will be also important to investigate the links between early phosphorylation events, activation of signaling cascades, rapid transcriptional responses and the late phase of aldosterone action (Fig. 5).

GENOMIC VERSUS NONGENOMIC ACTIONS OF ALDOSTERONE

From a general point of view, it is clear that rapid effects of aldosterone do occur, that precede the classical delayed increase in sodium transport. However their in vivo relevance in animals or humans still needs confirmation. There are divergent views concerning their mechanism. Some of them seem to involve very early transcriptional events mediated by the MR, or unconventional (and yet not understood) other effects via the MR, or activation of a membrane receptor. Despite deep efforts to clone a membrane mineralocorticoid-binding protein, there is no evidence so far for such a receptor (83–86). However, there is increasing evidence suggesting that important steroid-induced signaling events are triggered independent of transcription (87). Further work should allow us to know whether this is the case for aldosterone, as it may also provide a link between early aldosterone-stimulated signaling cascades and the classical genomic responses.

ALDOSTERONE AND TIGHT JUNCTIONS

Aldosterone regulates sodium transport that occurs through the trans-cellular route in epithelia with high electrical resistance. In addition, it has been proposed that the hormone could also affect paracellular permeability. It is conceivable that this pathway could participate to the efficiency of sodium reabsorption, by limiting sodium backflux and allowing chloride reabsorption. Paracellular permeability of tight epithelia (as the CD) depends on the properties of tight junctions (TJ) that behave as a barrier with selective pores (88). The TJ proteins claudins play a major role in determining the charge selectivity and conductance properties of the paracellular pathway. The claudin family includes more than 20 members that are expressed in a precise tissue-specific manner, conferring variable properties to the TJ among epithelia. It was recently shown that the paracellular charge-selectivity properties of TJ of RCCD2 cells could be modified within 15 to 20 minutes. by aldosterone, as anion (but not sodium) permeability was increased within this delay (89). This was accompanied by a mineralocorticoid-specific phosphorylation of the TJ protein claudin 4. Thus the TJ appears as a novel target for aldosterone that should merit further investigations.

GENERAL CONSIDERATIONS AND PERSPECTIVES

The MR and the GR share some regulatory activities, while others are distinct. These two receptors have diverged relatively late during evolution, originating from serial duplications of ancestral steroid receptors (90). GR sequences appeared first and an MR-related sequence was found in ray-finned fish. Both MR and GR have been identified in teleost fish (as rainbow trout), with cortisol as ligand. It is generally admitted that aldosterone, the main mineralocorticoid in land animals, is not synthesized in fish. An ortholog of 11-HSD2 was also identified in medaka, trout, and zebra fish (91). Thus it appears that mineralocorticoid-related control of osmoregulation was initially achieved through variable metabolization of cortisol regulating GR and MR occupancy rather than through differential ligands. In mammals, GR and MR are not redundant, despite their structural homologies: the salt-loosing phenotype of MR knockout mice develop despite the presence of the GR (46), and conversely GR knockout mice are not rescued by the endogenous MR (92).

Several aspects of MR activation remain to be investigated. They include possible dimerization with other steroid receptors, interaction with several transcription factors, identification of splice variants and novel hMR mutants, elucidation of the mechanisms controlling MR trafficking in and out of the nucleus, drug design of specific and selective antagonists, impact of post-translational modifications on MR properties, novel functions in non epithelial target tissues or unclassical target cells. Molecular and functional characterization of early aldosterone-regulated genes and signaling cascades should bring insights in the understanding of sodium transport and possibly in the pathophysiology of hypertension. Additional information should arise from transcriptomic and proteomic investigations of the consequences of long-term perturbations of corticosteroid hormones and of MR and GR expression levels.

REFERENCES

1. Bonvalet JP. Regulation of sodium transport by steroid hormones. Kidney Int 1998; 53:S49–56.
2. Connell JM, Davies E. The new biology of aldosterone. J Endocrinol 2005; 186:1–20.
3. Eaton DC, Malik B, Saxena NC, Al-Khalili OK, Yue G. Mechanisms of aldosterone's action on epithelial Na+ transport. J Membr Biol 2001; 184:313–9.
4. Freel EM, Connell JM. Mechanisms of hypertension: the expanding role of aldosterone. J Am Soc Nephrol 2004; 15:1993–2001.
5. Bassett MH, White PC, Rainey W. The regulation of aldosterone synthase expression. Mol Cell Endocrinol 2004; 217:67–74.

6. Bhargava A, Pearce D. Mechanisms of mineralocorticoid action: determinants of receptor specificity and actions of regulated gene products. Trends Endocrinol Metab 2004; 15:147–53.
7. Farman N, Bocchi B. Mineralocorticoid selectivity: molecular and cellular aspects. Kidney Int 2000; 57:1364–9.
8. Farman N, Rafestin-Oblin ME. Multiple aspects of mineralocorticoid selectivity. Am J Physiol 2001; 280:F181–92.
9. Stockand JD. New ideas about aldosterone signaling in epithelia. Am J Physiol 2002; 282:F559–76.
10. Pascual-Le Tallec L, Lombes M. The mineralocorticoid receptor: a journey exploring its diversity and specificity of action. Mol Endocrinol 2005; 19:2211–21.
11. Rogerson FM, Brennan FE, Fuller PJ. Mineralocorticoid receptor binding, structure and function. Mol Cell Endocrinol 2004; 217:203–12.
12. Rossier BC, Pradervand S, Schild L, Hummler E. Epithelial sodium channel and the control of sodium balance: interaction between genetic and environmental factors. Annu Rev Physiol 2002; 64:877–97.
13. Kim GH, Masilamani S, Turner R, Mitchell C, Wade JB, Knepper MA. The thiazide-sensitive Na-Cl cotransporter is an aldosterone-induced protein. Proc Natl Acad Sci USA 1998; 95:14552–7.
14. Palmer LG, Frindt G. Aldosterone and potassium secretion by the cortical collecting duct. Kidney Int 2000; 57:1324–8.
15. Wang W. Renal potassium channels: recent developments. Curr Opin Nephrol Hypertens 2004; 13:549–55.
16. Wang W, Sackin H, Giebisch G. Renal potassium channels and their regulation. Annu Rev Physiol 1992; 54:81–96.
17. Yoo D, Kim BY, Campo C, et al. Cell surface expression of the ROMK (Kir 1.1) channel is regulated by the aldosterone-induced kinase, SGK-1, and protein kinase A. J Biol Chem 2003; 278:23066–75.
18. Farman N, Oblin ME, Lombes M, et al. Immunolocalization of gluco- and mineralocorticoid receptors in rabbit kidney. Am J Physiol 1991; 260(2 Pt 1):C226–33.
19. Rubera I, Loffing J, Palmer LG, et al. Collecting duct-specific gene inactivation of alpha ENaC in the mouse kidney does not impair sodium and potassium balance. J Clin Invest 2003; 112:554–65.
20. Arriza JL, Weinberger C, Cerelli G, et al. Cloning of human mineralocorticoid receptor complementary DNA: structural and functional kinship with the glucocorticoid receptor. Science 1987; 237:268–75.
21. Edwards CRW, Stewart PM, Burt D, et al. Localisation of 11β-hydroxysteroid dehydrogenase-tissue specific protector of the mineralocorticoid receptor. Lancet 1988; 2:986–9.
22. Funder JW, Pearce PT, Smith R, Smith AI. Mineralocorticoid action: target tissue specificity is enzyme, not receptor, mediated. Science 1988; 242:583–5.
23. Stewart PM, Krozowski ZS. 11 beta-Hydroxysteroid dehydrogenase. Vitam Horm 1999; 57:249–324.
24. Bocchi B, Kenouch S, Lamarre-Cliche M, et al. Impaired 11-beta hydroxysteroid dehydrogenase type 2 activity in sweat gland ducts in human essential hypertension. Hypertension 2004; 43(4):803–8.
25. Zennaro MC, Farman N, Bonvalet JP, Lombes M. Tissue-specific expression of alpha and beta messenger ribonucleic acid isoforms of the human mineralocorticoid receptor in normal and pathological states. J Clin Endocrinol Metab 1997; 82:1345–52.
26. Zennaro MC, Souque A, Viengchareun S, Poisson E, Lombes M. A new human MR splice variant is a ligand-independent transactivator modulating corticosteroid action. Mol Endocrinol 2001; 15:1586–98.
27. Mangelsdorf DJ, Thummel C, Beato M, et al. Overview: the nuclear receptor superfamily: the second decade. Cell 1995; 83:835–9.
28. Fagart J, Wurtz JM, Souque A, Hellal-Levy C, Moras D, Rafestin-Oblin ME. Antagonism in the human mineralocorticoid receptor. EMBO J 1998; 17:3317–25.

29. Fagart J, Huyet J, Pinon GM, Rochel M, Mayer C, Rafestin-Oblin ME. Crystal structure of a mutant mineralocorticoid receptor responsible for hypertension. Nat Struct Mol Biol 2005; 12:554–5.
30. Bledsoe RK, Madauss KP, Holt JA, et al. A ligand-mediated hydrogen bond network required for the activation of the mineralocorticoid receptor. J Biol Chem 2005; 280:31283–93.
31. Arriza JL, Simerly RB, Swanson LW, Evans RM. The neuronal mineralocorticoid receptor as a mediator of glucocorticoid response. Neuron 1988; 1:887–900.
32. Couette B, Fagart J, Jalaguier S, Lombes L, Souque A, Rafestin-Oblin ME. The ligand induced conformational change of the mineralocorticoid receptor occurs within its heterooligomeric structure. Biochem J 1996; 315:421–7.
33. Le Tallec LP, Kirsh O, Lecomte MC, et al. Protein inhibitor of activated signal transducer and activator of transcription 1 interacts with the N-terminal domain of mineralocorticoid receptor and represses its transcriptional activity: implication of small ubiquitin-related modifier 1 modification. Mol Endocrinol 2003; 17:2529–42.
34. Pascual-Le Tallec L, Simone F, Viengchareun S, Meduri G, Thirman MJ, Lombes M. The elongation factor ELL (eleven-nineteen lysine-rich leukemia) is a selective coregulator for steroid receptor functions. Mol Endocrinol 2005; 19:1158–69.
35. Meijer OC, Kalkhoven E, van der Laan S, et al. Steroid receptor coactivator-1 splice variants differentially affect corticosteroid receptor signaling. Endocrinology 2005; 146:1438–48.
36. Trapp T, Holsboer F. Heterodimerization between mineralocorticoid and glucocorticoid receptors increases the functional diversity of corticosteroid action. Trends Pharmacol Sci 1996; 17:145–9.
37. Lim-Tio SS, Keightley MC, Fuller PJ. Determinants of specificity of transactivation by mineralocorticoid or glucocorticoid receptor. Endocrinology 1997; 138:2537–43.
38. Liu WH, Wang J, Sauter NK, et al. Steroid receptor heterodimerization demonstrated in vitro and in vivo. Proc Natl Acad Sci USA 1995; 92:12480–4.
39. Rupprecht R, Arriza JL, Spengler D, et al. Transactivation and synergistic properties of the mineralocorticoid receptor—relationship to the glucocorticoid receptor. Mol Endocrinol 1993; 7:597–603.
40. Escoubet B, Coureau C, Blot-Chabaud M, et al. Corticosteroid receptor mRNA expression is unaffected by corticosteroids in rat kidney, heart, and colon. Am J Physiol 1996; 39:C1343–53.
41. Galigniana MD. Native rat kidney mineralocorticoid receptor is a phosphoprotein whose transformation to a DNA-binding form is induced by phosphatases. Biochem J 1998; 333:555–63.
42. Le Moellic C, Ouvrard-Pascaud A, Capurro C, et al. Early nongenomic events in aldosterone action in renal collecting duct cells: PKCalpha activation, mineralocorticoid receptor phosphorylation, and cross-talk with the genomic response. J Am Soc Nephrol 2004; 15:1145–60.
43. Geller DS. Mineralocorticoid resistance. Clin Endocrinol (Oxf) 2005; 62:513–20.
44. Zennaro MC, Lombes M. Mineralocorticoid resistance. Trends Endocrinol Metab 2004; 15:264–70.
45. Sartorato P, Khaldi Y, Lapeyraque AL, et al. Inactivating mutations of the mineralocorticoid receptor in Type I pseudohypoaldosteronism. Mol Cell Endocrinol 2004; 217:119–25.
46. Berger S, Bleich M, Schmid W, et al. Mineralocorticoid receptor knockout mice: pathophysiology of Na+ metabolism. Proc Natl Acad Sci USA 1998; 95:9424–9.
47. Geller DS, Farhi A, Pinkerton N, et al. Activating mineralocorticoid receptor mutation in hypertension exacerbated by pregnancy. Science 2000; 289:119–23.
48. Wilk JB, Djousse L, Arnett DK, et al. Genome-wide linkage analyses for age at diagnosis of hypertension and early-onset hypertension in the HyperGEN study. Am J Hypertens 2004; 17:839–44.
49. Escoubet B, Coureau C, Bonvalet JP, Farman N. Noncoordinate regulation of epithelial Na channel and Na pump subunit mRNAs in kidney and colon by aldosterone. Am J Physiol 1997; 272:C1482–91.

50. Joels M, de Kloet ER. Corticosteroid hormones: endocrine messengers in the brain. News Physiol Sci 1995; 10:71–6.
51. Lombes M, Alfaidy N, Eugene E, Lessana A, Farman N, Bonvalet JP. Prerequisite for cardiac aldosterone action. Mineralocorticoid receptor and 11β-hydroxysteroid dehydrogenase in the human heart. Circulation 1995; 92:175–82.
52. Kenouch S, Lombes M, Delahaye F, Eugene E, Bonvalet JP, Farman N. Human skin as target for aldosterone: coexpression of mineralocorticoid receptors and 11 beta-hydroxysteroid dehydrogenase. J Clin Endocrinol Metab 1994; 79:1334–41.
53. Brilla CG, Weber KT. Mineralocorticoid excess, dietary sodium, and myocardial fibrosis. J Lab Clin Med 1992; 120:893–901.
54. Funder JW. Aldosterone, mineralocorticoid receptors and vascular inflammation. Mol Cell Endocrinol 2004; 217:263–9.
55. Mizuno Y, Yoshimura M, Yasue H, et al. Aldosterone production is activated in failing ventricle in humans. Circulation 2001; 103:72–7.
56. Beggah AT, Escoubet B, Puttini S, et al. Reversible cardiac fibrosis and heart failure induced by conditional expression of an antisense mRNA of the mineralocorticoid receptor in cardiomyocytes. Proc Natl Acad Sci USA 2002; 99:7160–5.
57. Le Menuet D, Isnard R, Bichara M, et al. Alteration of cardiac and renal functions in transgenic mice overexpressing human mineralocorticoid receptor. J Biol Chem 2001; 276:38911–20.
58. Wang Q, Clement S, Gabbiani G, et al. Chronic hyperaldosteronism in a transgenic mouse model fails to induce cardiac remodeling and fibrosis under a normal-salt diet. Am J Physiol 2004; 286:F1178–84.
59. Pitt B, Zannad F, Remme WJ, et al. The effect of spironolactone on morbidity and mortality in patients with severe heart failure. N Engl J Med 1999; 341:709–16.
60. Pitt B, Remme W, Zannad F, et al. Eplerenone, a selective aldosterone blocker, in patients with left ventricular dysfunction after myocardial infarction. N Engl J Med 2003; 348:1309–21.
61. Ouvrard-Pascaud A, Sainte-Marie Y, Benitah JP, Perrier R, Soukaseum C, Cat AN, Royer A, Le Quang K, Charpentier F, Demolombe S, et al. Conditional mineralocorticoid receptor expression in the heart leads to life-threatening arrhythmias. Circulation 2005; 111:3025–33.
62. Le Menuet D, Viengchareun S, Muffat-Joly M, Zennaro MC, Lombes M. Expression and function of the human mineralocorticoid receptor: lessons from transgenic mouse models. Mol Cell Endocrinol 2004; 217:127–36.
63. Hostetter TH, Ibrahim HN. Aldosterone in chronic kidney and cardiac disease. J Am Soc Nephrol 2003; 14:2395–401.
64. Terada Y, Kobayashi T, Kuwana H, et al. Aldosterone stimulates proliferation of mesangial cells by activating mitogen-activated protein kinase 1/2, cyclin D1, and cyclin A. J Am Soc Nephrol 2005; 16:2296–305.
65. Miyata K, Rahman M, Shokoji T, et al. Aldosterone stimulates reactive oxygen species production through activation of NADPH oxidase in rat mesangial cells. J Am Soc Nephrol 2005; 16(10):2906–12.
66. Gekle M, Freudinger R, Mildenberger S, Schenk K, Marschitz I, Schramek H. Rapid activation of Na+/H+-exchange in MDCK cells by aldosterone involves MAP-kinase ERK1/2. Pflugers Arch 2001; 441:781–6.
67. Grossmann C, Freudinger R, Mildenberger S, Krug AW, Gekle M. Evidence for epidermal growth factor receptor as negative-feedback control in aldosterone-induced Na+ reabsorption. Am J Physiol 2004; 286:F1226–31.
68. Krug AW, Grossmann C, Schuster C, et al. Aldosterone stimulates epidermal growth factor receptor expression. J Biol Chem 2003; 278:43060–6.
69. Mastroberardino L, Spindler B, Forster I, et al. Ras pathway activates epithelial Na+ channel and decreases its surface expression in *Xenopus* oocytes. Mol Cell Biochem 1998; 9:3417–27.
70. Staruschenko A, Patel P, Tong Q, Medina JL, Stockand JD. Ras activates the epithelial Na(+) channel through phosphoinositide 3-OH kinase signaling. J Biol Chem 2004; 279:37771–8.
71. Braun S, Losel R, Wehling M, Boldyreff B. Aldosterone rapidly activates Src kinase in M-1 cells involving the mineralocorticoid receptor and HSP84. FEBS Lett 2004; 570:69–72.

72. Naray-Fejes-Toth A, Snyder PM, Fejes-Toth G. The kidney-specific WNK1 isoform is induced by aldosterone and stimulates epithelial sodium channel-mediated Na+ transport. Proc Natl Acad Sci USA 2004; 101:17434–9.
73. Pearce D. SGK1 regulation of epithelial sodium transport. Cell Physiol Biochem 2003; 13:13–20.
74. McCormick JA, Bhalla V, Pao AC, Pearce D. SGK1: a rapid aldosterone-induced regulator of renal sodium reabsorption. Physiology (Bethesda) 2005; 20:134–9.
75. Wulff P, Vallon V, Huang DY, et al. Impaired renal Na(+) retention in the sgk1-knockout mouse. J Clin Invest 2002; 110:1263–8.
76. Spindler B, Mastroberardino L, Custer M, Verrey F. Characterization of early aldosterone-induced RNAs identified in A6 kidney epithelia. Pflugers Arch 1997; 434:323–31.
77. Boulkroun S, Fay M, Zennaro MC, et al. Characterization of rat NDRG2 (N-Myc downstream regulated gene 2), a novel early mineralocorticoid-specific induced gene. J Biol Chem 2002; 277:31506–15.
78. Garty H, Lindzen M, Fuzesi M, et al. A specific functional interaction between CHIF and Na, K-ATPase: role of FXYD proteins in the cellular regulation of the pump. Ann NY Acad Sci 2003; 986:395–400.
79. Robert-Nicoud M, Flahaut M, Elalouf JM, et al. Transcriptome of a mouse kidney cortical collecting duct cell line: effects of aldosterone and vasopressin. Proc Natl Acad Sci USA 2001; 98:2712–6.
80. Muller OG, Parnova RG, Centeno G, Rossier BC, Firsov D, Horisberger JD. Mineralocorticoid effects in the kidney: correlation between alphaENaC, GILZ, and Sgk-1 mRNA expression and urinary excretion of Na+ and K+. J Am Soc Nephrol 2003; 14:1107–15.
81. Ayroldi E, Migliorati G, Bruscoli S, et al. Modulation of T-cell activation by the glucocorticoid-induced leucine zipper factor via inhibition of nuclear factor kappaB. Blood 2001; 98:743–53.
82. Berrebi D, Bruscoli S, Cohen N, et al. Synthesis of glucocorticoid-induced leucine zipper (GILZ) by macrophages: an anti-inflammatory and immunosuppressive mechanism shared by glucocorticoids and IL-10. Blood 2003; 101:729–38.
83. Chun TY, Pratt JH. Non-genomic effects of aldosterone: new actions and questions. Trends Endocrinol Metab 2004; 15:353–4.
84. Falkenstein E, Tillmann HC, Christ M, Feuring M, Wehling M. Multiple actions of steroid hormones—a focus on rapid, nongenomic effects. Pharmacol Rev 2000; 52:513–56.
85. Funder JW. The nongenomic actions of aldosterone. Endocr Rev 2005; 26(3):313–21.
86. Harvey BJ, Condliffe S, Doolan CM. Sex and salt hormones: rapid effects in epithelia. News Physiol Sci 2001; 16:174–7.
87. Hammes SR. The further redefining of steroid-mediated signaling. Proc Natl Acad Sci USA 2003; 100:2168–70.
88. Van Itallie CM, Anderson JM. The molecular physiology of tight junction pores. Physiology (Bethesda) 2004; 19:331–8.
89. Le Moellic C, Boulkroun S, Gonzalez-Nunez D, et al. Aldosterone and tight junctions: modulation of claudin-4 phosphorylation in renal collecting duct cells. Am J Physiol Cell Physiol 2005; 289(6):C1513–21.
90. Baker ME. Co-evolution of steroidogenic and steroid-inactivating enzymes and adrenal and sex steroid receptors. Mol Cell Endocrinol 2004; 215:55–62.
91. Baker ME. Evolutionary analysis of 11beta-hydroxysteroid dehydrogenase-type 1, -type 2, -type 3 and 17beta-hydroxysteroid dehydrogenase-type 2 in fish. FEBS Lett 2004; 10(574): 167–70.
92. Tronche F, Kellendonk C, Reichardt HM, Schutz G. Genetic dissection of glucocorticoid receptor function in mice. Curr Opin Genet Dev 1998; 8:532–8.

8
11β-Hydroxysteroid Dehydrogenase

Paolo Ferrari
Department of Nephrology, Fremantle Hospital and School of Medicine and Pharmacology, University of Western Australia, Perth, Australia

John W. Funder
Prince Henry's Institute of Medical Research, Clayton, Victoria, Australia

INTRODUCTION

Over 30 years ago Werder et al. described a case of a 3-year-old girl with short stature, polydipsia and polyuria without obvious external abnormalities (including genitalia), and who had features of mineralocorticoid hypertension with hypokalemia and metabolic alkalosis (1). She had suppressed plasma renin and aldosterone; gas-chromatographic analysis of her urinary steroid profile excluded hypertensive forms of congenital adrenal hyperplasia, but showed an unexpected steroid profile (1). The author did not appreciate the underlying defect affecting that girl, a syndrome later recognized and biochemically characterized by Ulick and New (2,3). At that time radiological investigation of the adrenal was limited, and to contrast the adrenal with surrounding tissue translumbar retroperitoneal carbon dioxide insufflation was used (4); this procedure revealed no enlargement of the patient's adrenal. Subsequently the patient withdrew from further medical evaluation and management, her whereabouts unknown, until 25 years later she presented with intracranial haemorrhage and end-stage renal disease (ESRD). We have analyzed her relevant DNA sequences and found (unpublished) that she was a compound heterozygote, with two mutations in the gene encoding the enzyme 11β-hydroxysteroid dehydrogenase type 2 (11βHSD2), an enzyme that plays a crucial role in mineralocorticoid regulated renal sodium transport. In this overview we briefly discuss the subsequent cloning, physiology, pathophysiology, and clinical relevance of the 11β-hydroxysteroid dehydrogenase (11βHSD) enzymes.

UNMASKING A NEW BIOLOGICAL PRINCIPLE

The severe juvenile low-renin hypertension first described in 1974 (1) and later characterized biochemically and termed apparent mineralocorticoid excess (AME) by New et al. (2,3) unveiled a new biological principle. The classical view of hormone action in target organs was that of hormone signaling by the binding of ligand to a specific, cognate receptor. When aldosterone enters the cell, it binds to the mineralocorticoid receptor (MR), and thereafter the ligand-receptor complex is translocated into the nucleus. Binding to hormone response elements increases the transcription of genes encoding specific aldosterone-inducible proteins, such as rate-limiting subunits of the apical epithelial sodium channel (Fig. 1A). In response sodium influx causes intracellular sodium (Na^+) to rise; this increase in substrate increases turnover of Na^+/K^+-ATPase, which in turn increases Na^+ reabsorption and potassium (K^+) excretion. The increased Na^+ reabsorption leads to volume expansion and contributes to hypertension.

Although cortisol and aldosterone have the same affinity for MR, in mineralocorticoid target organs only aldosterone acts as the physiologic agonist (Fig. 1B). The latter is protected from activation by glucocorticoids through the agency of a gatekeeper enzyme, the microsomal 11βHSD2 enzyme, evidence that mineralocorticoid target tissue specificity is enzyme, not receptor, mediated (Figs. 1 and 2) (5). MR and glucocorticoid receptors (GR) have a high degree of sequence identity (6), 94% in the central DNA-binding domain and 57% in the C-terminal ligand-binding domain. With the cloning and expression of the MR (6) it was confirmed that aldosterone and cortisol have similar binding affinities for MR in vitro (7,8). Circulating levels of cortisol in humans and corticosterone in rodents are three orders of magnitude higher than aldosterone levels, despite which in vivo only aldosterone acts as a physiologic agonist of the MR. This paradox was apparently solved by the discovery of the enzyme 11βHSD (5,8), which converts biologically active 11-hydroxysteroids to their inactive 11-keto-steroid forms, thus conferring ligand specificity on MR; in addition, it stoichometrically generates nicotinamide adenine dinucleotide (NADH), which appears to be crucial in maintaining glucocorticoid-occupied MR in an inactive state, by mechanisms which remain to be established (9). Cyclization of the 11-hydroxyl group with the 18-aldehyde group of aldosterone renders the physiological mineralocorticoid not a substrate for 11βHSD. Of the two cloned 11βHSD isoforms, only the 11βHSD2 acts in this way to protect MR; when 11βHSD2 activity is decreased, reflecting inhibition or mutation, cortisol is able to stimulate MR and induces the state of AME (Fig. 1C).

CLONING AND BIOCHEMISTRY

The 11βHSD enzymes catalyze the interconversion of cortisol and cortisone in humans (Fig. 2), and of corticosterone and dehydrocorticosterone in rodents (5). Cortisone and dehydrocorticosterone show minimal biological activity per se, reflecting their negligible affinity for GR and MR. Two kinetically distinct forms of 11βHSD (11βHSD1 and 11βHSD2) have been cloned and are differentiated by directionality in vivo, cofactor specificity and tissue expression (Table 1) (10–14). 11β-hydroxysteroid dehydrogenase type 1 (11βHSD1) activity and expression are found in most tissues; its K_m for cortisol is more than an order of magnitude higher than that of 11βHSD2; it is reduced nicotinamide adenine dinucleotide phosphate preferring, and has been shown to have overwhelmingly reductase activity in vivo (Table 1). The roles of 11βHSD1 have been investigated in mice lacking 11βHSD1, which are unable to convert 11-dehydrocorticosterone to corticosterone in vivo, confirming 11βHSD1 as the sole 11-reductase in the mouse; such animals show reduced activation of a variety

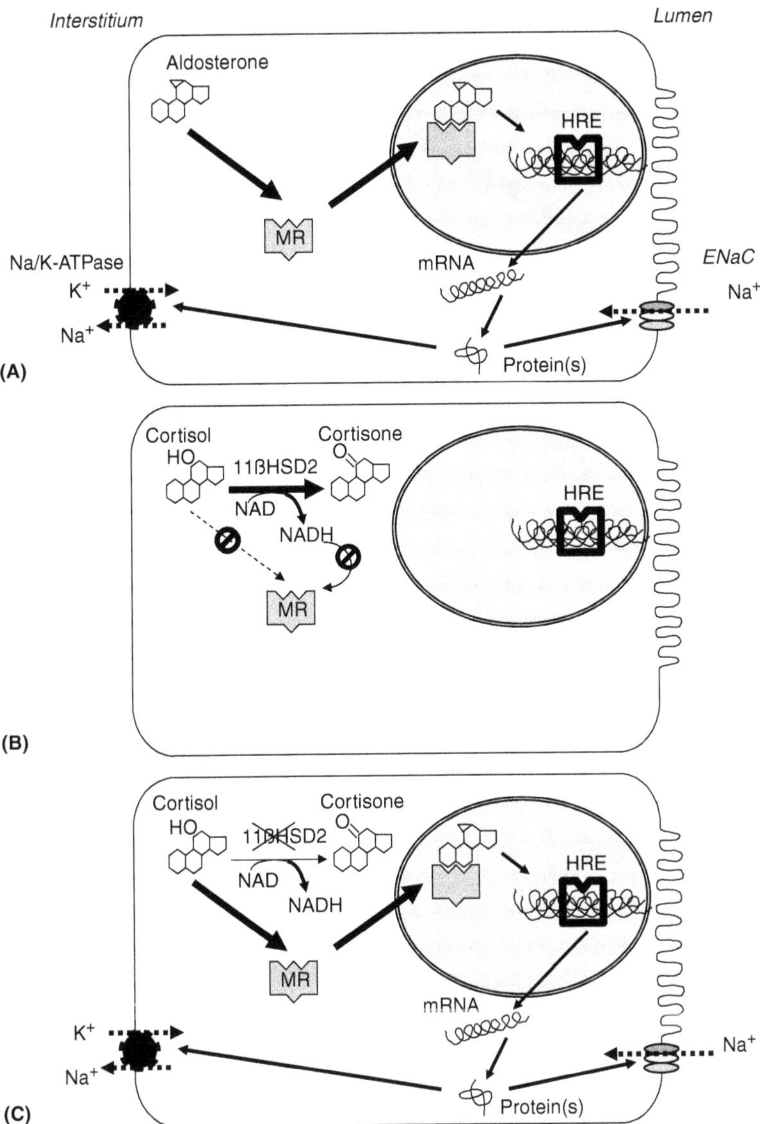

Figure 1 Mineralocorticoid action in renal cells of the CCD: (**A**) When aldosterone enters the CCD cell, it binds to the MR, and thereafter the ligand-receptor complex is translocated into the nucleus. Binding to its hormone response element increases the transcription of genes encoding specific aldosterone-inducible proteins, such as the rate-limiting subunits of the apical epithelial sodium channel, sgk-1 and basolateral Na/K-ATPase. In turn, this stimulates sodium (Na^+) reabsorption and potassium (K^+) excretion. (**B**) When cortisol enters the CCD cell the enzyme 11βHSD2 largely (~90%) converts it to inactive cortisone and generates high levels of NADH, thereby protecting the MR by from activation by cortisol. (**C**) When 11βHSD2 activity is decreased as a consequence of inherited or acquired reduction in enzymatic activity, the intracellular cortisol level increases further, but the level of NADH plummets, leading to activation of the MR by cortisol. The resulting glucocorticoid activation of MR produces Na^+ retention, volume expansion and hypertension. *Abbreviations*: CCD, cortical collecting duct; MR, mineralocorticoid receptor; NADH, nicotinamide adenine dinucleotide; 11βHSD2, 11β-hydroxysteroid dehydrogenase type 2.

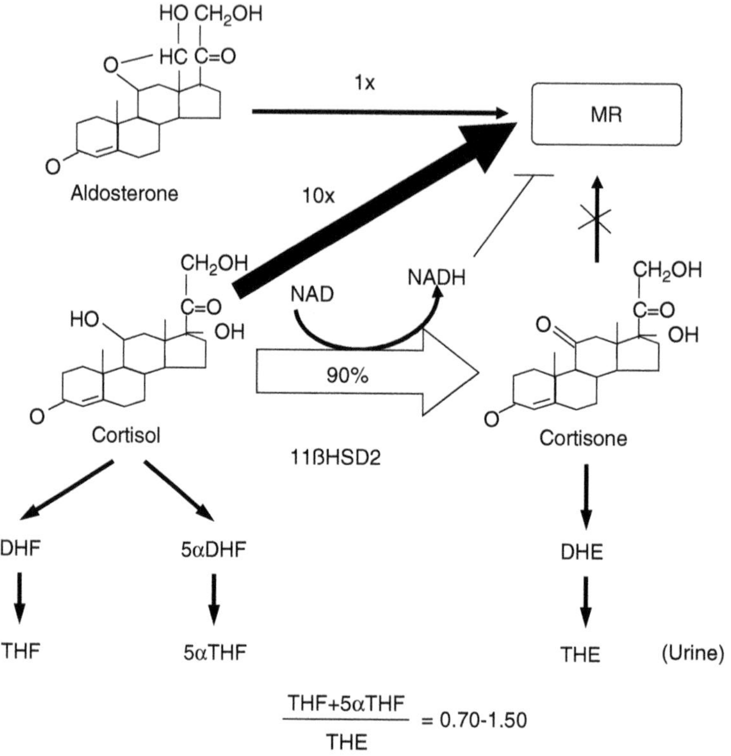

Figure 2 Peripheral cortisol metabolism and mineralocorticoid receptor selectivity: Cortisol and aldosterone bind with equal affinity to the MR. Plasma concentrations of cortisol are 1000× higher than those of aldosterone, but in MR-target cells the NAD-dependent 11βHSD2 debulks intracellular cortisol and generates high levels of NADH. Generated NADH maintains cortisol·MR complexes in an inactive state and permits aldosterone to selectively activate the receptor, despite 10× higher intracellular cortisol levels. The hemiacetal conformation of the 11-hydroxyl group with the 18-aldehyde group of aldosterone renders this steroid a poor substrate for the enzyme. Cortisol and cortisone are substrates for a series of enzymatic activities in the liver. These include reduction of Δ^4 double bond yielding 5α- and 5β-dihydrocortisol and dihydrocortisone, and reduction of 3-keto group, producing THF and THE. The activity of the 11βHSD2 enzyme can be assessed in vivo by measuring the urinary (THF+5αTHF)/THE ratio by gas chromatography and mass spectrometry. In normal subjects this ratio ranges between 0.7 and 1.5. *Abbreviations*: MR, mineralocorticoid receptor; 11βHSD2, 11β-hydroxysteroid dehydrogenase type 2; THE, tetrahydrocortisone; THF, 5α- and 5β-tetrahydrocortisol.

glucocorticoid-induced responses (15,16). 11βHSD1-deficient mice have elevated circulating levels of plasma corticosterone and adrenal hyperplasia, but also show attenuated glucocorticoid-induced activation of gluconeogenic enzymes in response to fasting, and lower glucose levels in response to obesity or stress. They also have improved lipid profiles, hepatic insulin sensitization, and a potentially atheroprotective phenotype (17).

In contrast, 11βHSD2 has been identified to date in a limited range of tissues (12–14). It has a low K_m for cortisol (40–50 nM), and even lower for corticosterone (~4 nM), is nicotinamide adenine dinucleotide (NAD) requiring and shows only dehydrogenase activity for endogenous glucocorticoids (Fig. 2, Table 1) (12–14), although reduction of dehydrodexamethasone has been demonstrated in vitro (18,19). Importantly,

Table 1 11βHSD Isoenzymes

	11βHSD type 1	11βHSD type 2
Molecular biology		
Chromosome	1	16
Gene structure	30 kb, 6 exons	6.2 kb, 5 exons
mRNA	1902 bases	1944 bases
Amino acids	292, 34 kDa	405, 45 kDa
Enzyme kinetics		
Activity	Bi-directional, reductase in vivo	Dehydrogenase only
Substrate affinity	Low (K_m μM range)	High (K_m nM range)
Cofactor specificity	NADP/NADPH	NAD
Expression		
Tissue localization	Ubiquitous, mainly liver, lung, adipose tissue, brain, gonads	Kidney, colon, sweat glands, placenta
Cellular localization	Microsomal	Microsomal, MR positive cells
Function	Elevation of cellular cortisol concentration	Protection of the MR

Abbreviations: MR, mineralocorticoid receptor; 11βHSD, 11β-hydroxysteroid dehydrogenase.

immunohistochemical studies have consistently localized 11βHSD2 to a restricted range of tissues-distal renal tubules, distal colon, sweat and salivary glands, placenta and vascular wall (12–14,20,21).

PHYSIOLOGY AND PATHOPHYSIOLOGY OF 11βHSD2

Localization and Expression

Odermatt et al. co-expressed epitope-tagged MR and 11βHSD2 in HEK-293 cells lacking 11βHSD2 activity and analyzed their subcellular localization by fluorescence microscopy (22). When co-expressed with 11βHSD2 the MR displayed a reticular distribution pattern, absent ligand, suggesting association of MR with 11βHSD2 at the endoplasmic reticulum membrane. Aldosterone induced rapid nuclear translocation of MR, with the enzyme remaining tethered in the cytoplasmic compartment. In parallel studies (23), green fluorescent protein tagged MR were expressed in similar cells, and absent steroid MR were similarly shown to be predominantly cytoplasmic. Addition of aldosterone, corticosterone, and, to some extent, spironolactone all served to move MR intranuclear, rapidly with aldosterone, less rapidly with corticosterone, and slowly and partially with spironolactone (23).

Experimental Blockade

In addition to the syndrome of AME, in which patients show reduced or absent 11βHSD2 activity, the enzyme can be blocked by licorice (which contains glycyrrhizin), and by the erstwhile anti-peptic ulcer drug carbenoxolone, the hemisuccinate of glycyrrhetinic acid. These agents are non-selective, in that they block both 11βHSD1 and 11βHSD2, and in addition other steroid- and prostaglandin-metabolizing enzymes. More or less selective blockers of 11βHSD1 have been developed, on the basis of lowering the intracellular conversion of cortisone to cortisol in tissues where the enzyme is expressed in abundance (e.g., liver) as a therapeutic approach to diabetes, known to be induced/exacerbated by glucocorticoid-induced glucoconeogenesis. As noted above, such inhibitors have been shown to have beneficial effects on diabetes in mice (24–26), and to ameliorate the metabolic syndrome and the progression of diabetes in diet-induced obese mice (27). Topical 11βHSD1 selective inhibitors may also play a useful therapeutic role in glaucoma (28).

Aldosterone, Blood Pressure and Salt

Normal regulation of fluid and electrolyte homeostasis in mammals is regulated in a negative-feedback loop by the renin–angiotensin–aldosterone system (29), and by the direct effects of plasma [K^+] on aldosterone secretion (30). Renin is released by the juxtaglomerular cells of the afferent arterioles and macula densa cells of the kidney, and aldosterone is produced by the adrenal glands. Plasma concentrations of renin and angiotensin II rise in response to contraction of intravascular volume and reduction in renal perfusion, and are lowered by intravascular volume expansion. To maintain blood pressure and organ perfusion healthy subjects respond to salt deficiency by an increase in renin and aldosterone secretion to minimize urinary Na^+ and water loss, and respond to K^+ loading by a direct effect on the adrenal to raise aldosterone secretion rate and thus K^+ excretion. Complex organisms on the planet evolved in the Na^+-rich aqueous environment of the sea (31), and terrestrial life thus necessitated the development of mechanisms to retain Na^+ (32). Fractional regulation of salt and water balance involves the kidney (33,34), and in particular the renal medulla, which develops very differently between species, and is more prominent in species with a high urinary concentrating capacity (35). Nephron elements such as the loop of Henle and the collecting duct, which function to concentrate the urine by increasing Na^+ and water reabsorption, are found in humans and other terrestrial mammals, but are absent or rudimentarily developed in fish and amphibians. This evolutionary adaptation of the nephron underlines the central role of the kidney in the homeostatic regulation of Na^+ and water balance and thus maintenance the blood pressure (32).

Most species, including humans, evolved in a Na^+ poor, K^+ rich context (33,34), and thus needed to retain as much dietary salt as possible, and conversely to shed potassium. It has been estimated that in the first 10 million years of existence, as hunters and gatherers, humans enjoyed a dietary salt intake of approximately 1 g daily ($\sim$17 meq). Given the variable availability of salt, particularly inland, humans developed regulatory mechanisms to prevent loss of Na^+ through the kidney and other epithelia, in which aldosterone, MR and 11βHSD2 are crucial elements. It is important to note that MR preceded terrestrial evolution and are clearly present in fish, which lack the capacity to make aldosterone. Cortisol is thus the evolutionary driver for MR (36); a possibly useful question might thus be why epithelial Na^+/K^+ balance regulation pressed into service an existing receptor, which recognized a "novel" ligand (aldosterone) with affinity equivalent to that of cortisol, protected in epithelia by the coexpression of 11βHSD2 at very high levels, rather than evolving an aldosterone-specific MR. In contrast with the evolutionary state of relative Na^+ paucity, species that were able to transport or mine salt, or balance Na^+ and K^+ intake by meat eating, appear unable to suppress aldosterone to a degree sufficient to obviate a pattern of deleterious effects seen experimentally magnified in animals administered exogenous aldosterone and maintained on 0.9% NaCl solution to drink (37). This possible inability to lower aldosterone appropriately in the face of a normal (Western) Na^+ intake (150–500 meq/day), coupled with an undampened Na^+ appetite, may thus be a major contributing factor to human cardiovascular disease (38).

MR Blockade

Recently, it has become clear that blockade of aldosterone action is not coterminous with MR blockade. This reflects the equivalent affinity of MR for aldosterone and cortisol, the predominant occupancy (39) but not activation of MR by glucocorticoids even in "protected" tissues expressing 11βHSD2, and the activation of MR by glucocorticoids in the context of tissue damage and reactive oxygen species generation (40) or a similar change in intracellular redox state following 11βHSD2 blockade (41). In various clinical trials RALES, EPHESUS, 4E (42–44) starting aldosterone levels were low normal, and Na^+ status unremarkable: in all instances, however, MR blockade in addition to standard of care was attended by substantial clinical improvement. It has long been thought that blockade of angiotensin generation by angiotensin converting enzyme inhibitors, or of its action by type 1 angiotensin II receptor blockers, was sufficient to keep aldosterone levels within the normal range despite diuretic use. The phenomenon of aldosterone breakthrough (often ignorantly termed "escape") was instanced as evidence for the need for additional MR blockade, even though such breakthrough is not inevitable. In fact, the evidence is now difficult to ignore that whereas inappropriate MR activation in tissues such as blood vessels and cardiomyocytes is presumably caused by aldosterone in primary aldosteronism, in the context of tissue damage it appears caused by normal levels of endogenous glucocorticoids, with aldosterone levels appropriate for salt status.

CLINICAL RELEVANCE OF 11βHSD

Mutations in the 11βHSD2

Inherited deficiency in 11βHSD2 causes impaired peripheral metabolism of cortisol, presenting with juvenile hypertension, hypokalaemia and suppressed circulating renin and aldosterone (1–3), the syndrome of so-called AME. Typical clinical signs and symptoms of AME include low birth weight and failure to thrive, severe hypertension, hypokalaemia, suppressed plasma renin activity with hypoaldosteronaemia, polyuria, polydipsia and nephrocalcinosis. The disease is inherited as an autosomal recessive trait, and various mutations in the HSD11B2 gene have subsequently been shown to cause 11βHSD2 deficiency. Signs and symptoms of the syndrome can be partially or fully reversed by treatment with the MR-antagonist spironolactone (2,45–47), evidence for the crucial role of 11βHSD2 in MR protection (48,49).

Normally plasma cortisol levels are in the sub-micromolar range, while aldosterone levels are sub-nanomolar; even in 11βHSD protected cells intracellular levels of glucocorticoid are $\sim 10\times$ those of aldosterone (39). In AME, deficient 11βHSD2 enzyme activity further elevates intracellular glucocorticoid levels, but crucially does not generate the levels of NADH needed to keep the cortisol MR complexes inactive. The resultant MR activation produces Na^+ retention, volume expansion, hypokalaemia and suppression of plasma renin and aldosterone secretion. Thus, the hallmark of the disease is a state of excess mineralocorticoid activity in the absence of aldosterone, and the abnormal urinary steroid profile of an increased ratio of cortisol to cortisone metabolites, or urinary free cortisol to cortisone.

11βHSD2 in the kidney is primarily expressed in the cells of the cortical collecting duct (21,48,49); in contrast, the liver is the principal site for cortisone to cortisol conversion by 11βHSD1. Both cortisol and cortisone are substrates for a series of enzymatic activities in the liver, including the reduction of Δ^4 double bond to reduction of 3-keto group and reduction of 20-keto group, most of which metabolites are excreted in the urine as glucuronides, with only a small part excreted unconjugated, mainly as 3-*oxo*-4-ene steroids (50). The activity of the 11βHSD2 enzyme can be reliably assessed in vivo by measuring the ratio of biologically active cortisol (F) to inactive cortisone (E), or their tetrahydrometabolites (THF and THE), in the urine by gas chromatography with mass spectrometry (51,52). An increase in urinary free F/E or urinary (THF + 5αTHF)/THE ratio thus indicates decreased 11βHSD2 activity (53).

In the last decade the molecular basis of the syndrome of AME has been elucidated (54–71). We and others have identified mutations in the gene encoding 11βHSD2, revealing to date more than 35 different non-silent mutations in the HSD11B2 gene (Fig. 3). Most of the known mutations have been found in exons 3, 4 or 5 of the HSD11B2 gene, with the exception of the R74G and P75,Δ1nt in exon 1 (70) and L114,Δ6nt mutant in exon 2 (67). A few mutations were found to leave the amino acid sequence unchanged, but potentially to cause aberrant splicing; sequence analysis of a de novo base transversion, 771C>G in exon 4 (V254V, TGC to TGG) creates a canonical donor splice site (70).

Most of the patients described had characteristic signs of severe 11βHSD2 deficiency (Fig. 4). Birth weights were significantly lower than that of their unaffected sibs, and the patients were short, underweight and hypertensive for their age. The in vivo activity of 11βHSD2, as assessed by urinary excretion ratio of the cortisol (THF + 5αTHF) to cortisone (THE) metabolites, is characteristically abnormal, with ratios of 6-60, whereas the normal ratio is ~1.0. In vitro expression studies showed that most of the mutations described result in an 11βHSD2 protein with absent enzymatic activity (Fig. 4)

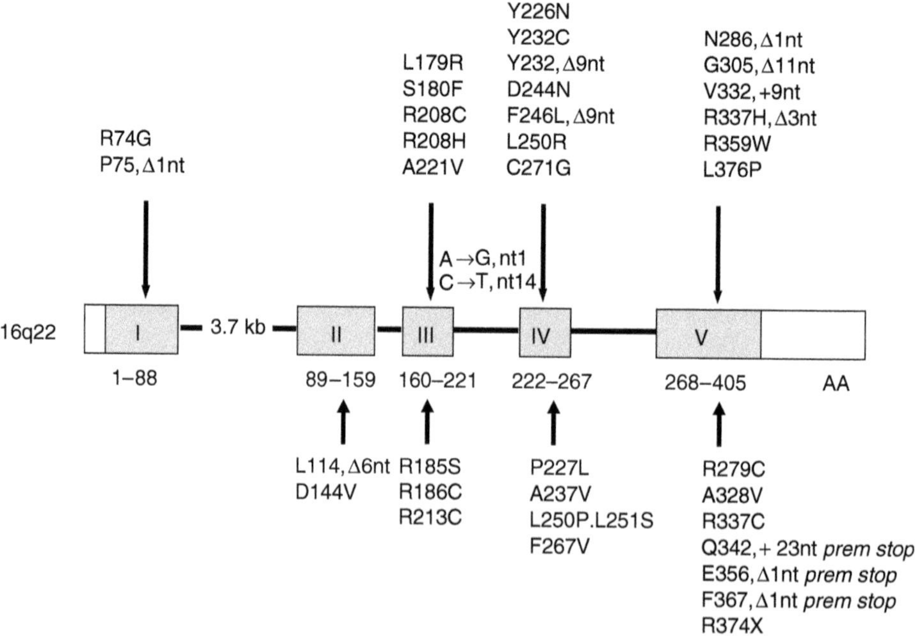

Figure 3 Location of HSD11B2 gene mutations: The HSD11B2 gene is located on chromosome 16 and consists of 5 exons, labeled I through V (gray boxes). Introns are represented by the lines and the untranslated regions by the open boxes. Numbers below the exons indicate the AA number. Mutations are listed relative to their position in the gene. Those shown below the gene are mutations investigated by the authors, with mutations reported above the gene reported by others. *Abbreviations*: AA, amino acid; HSD11B2, 11β-hydroxysteroid dehydrogenase type 2.

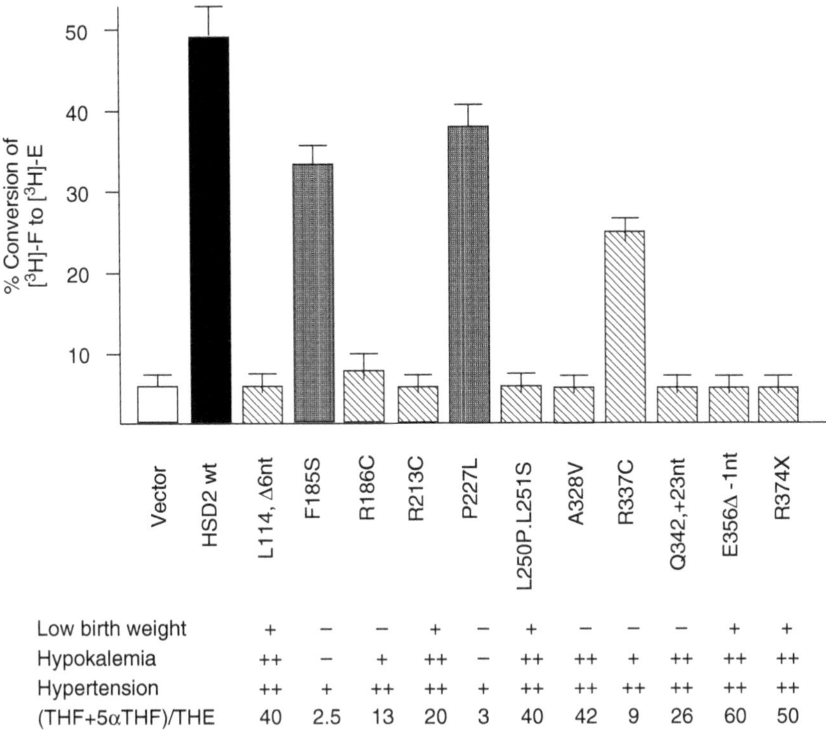

	L114, Δ6nt	F185S	R186C	R213C	P227L	L250P.L251S	A328V	R337C	Q342,+23nt	E356Δ -1nt	R374X
Low birth weight	+	−	−	+	−	+	−	−	−	+	+
Hypokalemia	++	−	+	++	−	++	++	+	++	++	++
Hypertension	++	+	++	++	+	++	++	++	++	++	++
(THF+5αTHF)/THE	40	2.5	13	20	3	40	42	9	26	60	50

Figure 4 Genotype-phenotype correlations in apparent mineralocorticoid excess: The bars show the results of in vitro enzymatic activity assays using CHOP cells transfected with mutant plasmids of the HSD11B2 gene. Transfected cells were incubated for two hours with [^{3}H]-cortisol, with [^{3}H]-cortisol and [^{3}H]-cortisone from the supernatant at the end of incubation separated by chromatography and quantified. Birth weight, blood pressure, serum potassium and in vivo 11βHSD2 activity (assessed by the urinary (THF+5αTHF)/THE ratio) are correlated with the genotype and in vitro 11βHSD2 activity. When in vitro enzymatic activity is completely abolished as a consequence of mutations in the HSD11B2 gene carriers of the mutation almost invariably show classical AME with severe hypokalemia, hypertension and a markedly increased (THF+5αTHF)/THE ratio. In milder cases with isolated hypertension the identified mutation produces only a moderate reduction in 11βHSD2 activity. *Abbreviations*: CHOP, chinese hamster ovary cells expressing polymona antigen; 11βHSD2, 11β-hydroxysteroid dehydrogenase type 2; THE, tetrahydrocortisone; THF, tetrahydrocortisol.

(54–58,60,62,65,70). Nevertheless, patients with homozygous mutations from different families show varying degrees of severity in terms of clinical and biochemical features (Fig. 4; personal observation and Refs. 55, 57, 58, 61, 63, 64, 67). We have, in addition, reported a form of low-renin hypertension with a mutation producing mild deficiency in 11βHSD2 activity without the phenotypic features of AME (64). From clinical observations and in vitro cotransfection studies, 11βHSD2 activity appears mildly impaired in heterozygotes (57), predisposing to isolated hypertension of later onset. Recently, the heterozygous father of a child with AME in a Brazilian kindred was found to have hypertension with no other characteristic signs of AME (62). Thus, depending on the degree of loss of enzyme activity, 11βHSD2 mutations can cause a spectrum of hypertension ranging from a severe, life-threatening disease in early childhood to a milder form diagnosed only in adults.

This view is supported by the clarification of the molecular basis of the so-called AME type II (66,72). In AME type II the urinary ratio of (THF + 5αTHF)/THE is almost normal, with the main abnormality in cortisol metabolism defective in A-ring reduction (72), on which basis a defect other than in 11βHSD2 was thought to be the underlying cause. However, patients with AME type II have prolonged plasma half-life of [11α-^{3}H]-cortisol, as in classic AME; molecular analysis of a large pedigree with AME type II from Sardinia showed a C945T mutation, resulting in the substitution of a cysteine for an arginine at codon 279 (R279C mutation) in 11βHSD2. In vitro expression of the mutant enzyme showed an identical K_m for cortisol as the wild-type enzyme, while the maximum velocity was reduced by approximately 35% (73). Inhibition of 11βHSD2 activity by glycyrrhetinic acid results in an acquired form of AME associated with an increase in the urinary (THF + 5αTHF)/THE ratio similar to that observed in AME type II (53,74).

11βHSD2 in "Essential" Hypertension: Activity, Microsatellites, and Polymorphisms

Although patients with essential hypertension lack overt signs of mineralocorticoid excess, the demonstration of more subtle changes such as low renin levels in some patients, a positive correlation between blood pressure and serum Na^+ levels, plus a negative correlation with potassium levels in other patients, suggests that a mineralocorticoid effect may be contributing to hypertension in a subset of these individuals (75). Variations in 11βHSD2 activity can be assessed by the ratio of urinary cortisol to cortisone metabolites, and by plasma cortisol half-life. Recent studies have reported that the half-life of cortisol is significantly prolonged, the excretion of urinary cortisol metabolites increased and the vasoconstrictor response to glucocorticoids enhanced in some patients with essential hypertension (76,77). In the "4 corner study" impaired conversion of cortisol to inactive metabolites has also been reported in young men with higher blood pressure whose parents also had high blood pressure (78), and another study found a positive association between urinary free cortisol and salt-resistant hypertension (73); other authors, however, could not confirm these observations (79,80). There are several possible explanations for this discrepancy, notably the differences in the ethnic groups, age, selection criteria and the methods used to assess 11βHSD2 function. Nevertheless, taken together, these studies suggest that 11βHSD2 may play some role in a subset of patients with essential hypertension.

Since steroid hormones modulate renal Na^+ retention, it is possible that variations in 11βHSD2 activity may be responsible for the sensitivity of blood pressure to changes in dietary salt intake. A salt-sensitive response of blood pressure has been observed in not only patients with hypertension, but also in some young normotensive individuals (81). These subjects also display a number of traits, including suppression of the renin–angiotensin system, which can also be found in some patients with essential hypertension (82); it has therefore been suggested that salt-sensitive individuals may be genetically predisposed to the development of hypertension (83). Preliminary data suggest that impaired 11βHSD2 activity is associated with an increased susceptibility of blood pressure to salt load (84), an observation in line with the well-established concept that low-renin hypertension is generally considered as a salt-sensitive form of high blood pressure (83); low ratios of urinary steroid metabolites were also found to be associated with a low prevalence of salt-sensitivity in young Caucasian males (84). These findings are in apparent contrast with the observation of Litchfield et al. (73), that subjects with highest urinary free cortisol show the least sensitivity of blood pressure to dietary salt. In this study of urinary free cortisol [but not cortisone or (THF + 5αTHF)/THE ratios] were measured, thereby not allowing a direct evaluation of 11βHSD2 activity; reduced 11βHSD2 activity correlates with a decrease urinary excretion of free cortisone rather than an increased urinary free cortisol excretion (51). Thus, measuring cortisone and its metabolites or (THF+5αTHF)/THE in urine seems to be the most appropriate assay of renal 11βHSD2 activity.

Other observations on the metabolism of glucocorticoid hormones seem to link 11βHSD2 function with hypertension. Low birth weight and/or stillbirth (61) are often found in patients with AME. It seems likely that 11βHSD2 protects the foetus against the excessive levels of maternal glucocorticoids (85,86); deficient fetal (placental) 11βHSD2 would therefore allow increased levels of glucocorticoids to cross the placenta and thus inhibit foetal growth. In humans, low birth weight is a risk factor for the development of essential hypertension in adult life (87–89); some clinical and experimental observations suggest that decreased activity of placental 11βHSD2 reduces birth weight and produces hypertensive adult offspring (88–90). A mild form of 11βHSD2 deficiency could therefore present as a low birth weight infant with the onset of hypertension in later life.

The exact mechanisms mediating cortisol-induced hypertension are still not fully understood, in that the Na^+ retention and increase in blood pressure induced by exogenous cortisol has been reported not to be reversed by spironolactone (90,91). Since spironolactone acts by competitive inhibition of binding to MR (92), it is possible that the doses of cortisol given in these studies (90,91) were sufficiently high to give circulating levels that compete with spironolactone for MR. Nevertheless, other renal or extrarenal effects of cortisol upon GR have to be considered. Although MR in the central nervous system have been implicated in the pathogenesis of mineralocorticoid hypertension (93,94), there appears to be no pathophysiological role for 11βHSD; experimentally, the hypertension produced by intracerebroventricular administration of very low doses of aldosterone can be progressively blocked by one to twofold injected in the cerebral ventricules corticosterone (95). Correction of hypertension by kidney transplantation in a patient with AME (96) argues against a role for central nervous system MR in the pathogenesis of hypertension related to 11βHSD2 deficiency.

A few years ago we reported on a girl with AME, homozygous for a gene mutation resulting in a mild deficiency in 11βHSD2 (64). The only relevant findings were hypertension and suppressed plasma renin levels, without hypokalaemia and the other phenotypic features that could support the diagnosis of AME. This case illustrates that a mutation leading to decreased 11βHSD2 activity can masquerade as essential hypertension. It is thus possible that a subset of patients among essential hypertensive population may suffer from a subtle form of AME; there have been few attempts to analyze whether an association exists between HSD11B2 gene activity and essential hypertension.

One of the leading causes of ESRD in African-Americans is low-renin hypertension, a form of salt-dependent hypertension; is therefore conceivable that impaired 11βHSD2 activity might be more prevalent among this population. Watson et al. reported a genetic association of a HSD11B2 flanking microsatellite and hypertension in African-Americans with ESRD (97). An association between a polymorphic marker in exon 3 [Glu178/Glu (G534A)] of the HSD11B2 gene and ESRD was also recently described, although this marker was not associated with essential hypertension in humans (98). Since this mutation would not alter the amino acid sequence, and therefore is not expected to affect 11βHSD2 activity, the mechanisms underlying the association of ESRD with this polymorphic marker are unclear. Structural analysis of the HSD11B2 gene in patients with ESRD demonstrated that the frequency of homozygosity for mutated alleles of the gene is less than 1/250,000 in Caucasians (99).

Brand et al. analyzed a polymorphic CA-repeat microsatellite marker near the HSD11B2 gene in a large series of families with essential hypertension, but found no correlation between this marker and blood pressure in their cohort (100). We analyzed the same polymorphic marker in salt-sensitive subjects and found a positive association between the short allele A7 homozygosity and salt-sensitivity, and a negative correlation with allele pair A7/A8 of the microsatellite marker (84), findings later confirmed by Agarwal et al. (101). This suggests that the activity of the 11βHSD2 enzyme may be genetically determined by variants in the HSD11B2 promoter or by the presence of undetected mutations in the HSD11B2 gene itself, an issue deserving further investigation. The apparently divergent findings of some of these studies may be explained by the lack of selection for the blood pressure response to salt-load in the patients studied by Brand et al. (100).

Licorice

Licorice root has been used in Europe since prehistoric times, and is well documented in written form from the time of the ancient Greeks. Licorice root and extracts have been used in medical herb products, sweeteners and mouth fresheners (102). The active ingredient of licorice is glycyrrhizic acid, which is hydrolysed into its aglycone glycyrrhetinic acid in vivo. Licorice products are made from peeled and unpeeled dried root, which are powdered or finely cut; these formulations have different concentrations of glycyrrhizic acid, which can vary from trace amounts to 20% based on the extraction process. Carbenoxolone, the hemisuccinate of glcyrrhetinic acid, was previously successfully used to treat patients with peptic ulceration (103).

Licorice possesses additional endocrine effects including glucocorticoid activity, antiandrogen effects, and estrogenic activity (103–105). Patients consuming excessive quantities of licorice present with hypertension and hypokalaemia (105–107), which may be severe enough to cause myopathy and cardiac arrhythmias. Both plasma renin activity and aldosterone levels are suppressed (53) and exchangeable Na^+ levels are increased. The condition responds to spironolactone and is reversible upon stopping licorice ingestion (53,108). Glycyrrhizic and glycyrrhetinic acids have very low affinity for MR, but are very potent competitive inhibitors of 11βHSD2 (Ki of approx. 5–10 nM) (109). Licorice administration to normal volunteers results in a mineralocorticoid excess state, an increase in the urinary THF + 5αTHF/THE ratio, an increase in plasma cortisol half-life, and a decrease in circulating cortisone values, indicative of inhibition of 11βHSD2 in vivo (53,74). It is now clear that licorice induces an acquired and milder form of AME, causing its mineralocorticoid effects through inhibition of 11βHSD2 rather than directly occupying and activating MR.

RELEVANCE AND OUTLOOK

Whereas mutation or inhibition of 11βHSD2 has been clearly shown to produce a congenital or acquired syndrome of mineralocorticoid excess, the questions remaining are the extent to which subtle abnormalities in MR/11βHSD2 mechanisms may contribute to essential hypertension. Abnormalities in 11βHSD1 action have proven clinically more complex, in that a double mutation in 11βHSD1 and hexose 6 phosphate dehydrogenase (H6PDH) appears to be required for a phenotype (110,111). Patients with so-called cortisone reductase deficiency (CRD), who are unable to convert cortisone to cortisol, have an allele of 11βHSD1, which is present in 4% of the normal, unaffected population: subsequent sequencing of H6PDH showed mutations in exon 5 of the gene in all phenotypically affected patients. CRD thus appears to be a digenic disease; the genetic studies point to an intimate link between H6PDH and 11βHSD1 function, and the possibility that the 4% of the normal population may thus be at least in part protected from the metabolic syndrome.

11βHSD1 knockout mice appear protected against features of the metabolic syndrome, and 11βHSD1 selective antagonists similarly reduce signs of the metabolic syndrome and the progression of atherosclerosis in diet-induced obese mice. Very recently H6PDH knockout mice showed reduced weight gain when fed a high-fat diet and resting hypoglycemia (109), consistent with the demonstrated lack of 11βHSD1 activity: in addition, however, they showed consistent and concomitant type 2 fiber myopathy, a phenotype not seen in 11βHSD1 knockout mice and presumably reflecting roles for H6PDH over and above those involved in providing reducing equivalents for 11βHSD1 activity.

Finally, paradoxically, though 11βHSD2 received the lion's share of the scientific attention in the 1990s, it now appears clear that 11βHSD1 is a much more promising therapeutic target, given the epidemic in type 2 diabetes, alone and as a component of the metabolic syndrome. This is not to minimize the pathophysiological role of inappropriate MR activation in the cardiovascular system; the physiological remit of 11βHSD2 is to ensure that this does not happen in epithelia, and very importantly in the vessel wall. In terms of therapeutic intervention, however, it would appear that MR is the logical target in this context, whereas 11βHSD1 modulation of GR activation is the logical target in ameliorating the pathophysiologic responses involved in the disorders characterizing the metabolic syndrome.

REFERENCES

1. Werder EA, Zachmann M, Vollmin JA, Veyrat R, Prader A. Unusual steroid excretion in a child with low renin hypertension. Res Steroids 1974; 6:385–9.
2. New MI, Levine LS, Biglieri EG, Pareira J, Ulick S. Evidence for an unidentified steroid in a child with apparent mineralocorticoid hypertension. J Clin Endocrinol Metab 1977; 44:924–33.
3. Ulick S, Levine LS, Gunczler P, et al. A syndrome of apparent mineralocorticoid excess associated with defects in the peripheral metabolism of cortisol. J Clin Endocrinol Metab 1979; 49:757–64.
4. McLachlan MS, Beales JS. Retroperitoneal pneumography in the investigation of adrenal disease. Clin Radiol 1971; 22:188–97.
5. Funder JW, Pearce PT, Smith R, Smith AI. Mineralocorticoid action: target tissue specificity is enzyme, not receptor, mediated. Science 1988; 242:583–5.
6. Arriza JL, Weinberger C, Cerelli G, et al. Cloning of human mineralocorticoid receptor complementary DNA: structural and functional kinship with the glucocorticoid receptor. Science 1987; 237:268–75.
7. Krozowski ZS, Funder JW. Renal mineralocorticoid receptors and hippocampal corticosterone- binding species have identical intrinsic steroid specificity. Proc Natl Acad Sci USA 1983; 80:6056–60.
8. Edwards CR, Stewart PM, Burt D, et al. Localisation of 11β-hydroxysteroid dehydrogenase-tissue specific protector of the mineralocorticoid receptor. Lancet 1988; 2:986–9.
9. Funder JW. RALES, EPHESUS and redox. J Steroid Biochem Mol Biol 2005; 93:121–5.
10. Agarwal AK, Monder C, Eckstein B, White PC. Cloning and expression of rat cDNA encoding corticosteroid 11β-dehydrogenase. J Biol Chem 1989; 264:18939–43.

11. Tannin GM, Agarwal AK, Monder C, New MI, White PC. The human gene for 11β-hydroxysteroid dehydrogenase. Structure, tissue distribution, and chromosomal localization. J Biol Chem 1991; 266:16653–8.
12. Walker BR, Campbell JC, Williams BC, Edwards CR. Tissue-specific distribution of the NAD(+)-dependent isoform of 11β-hydroxysteroid dehydrogenase. Endocrinology 1992; 131:970–2.
13. Albiston AL, Obeyesekere VR, Smith RE, Krozowski ZS. Cloning and tissue distribution of the human 11β-hydroxysteroid dehydrogenase type 2 enzyme. Mol Cell Endocrinol 1994; 105:R11–7.
14. Agarwal AK, Mune T, Monder C, White PC. Cloning of cDNA encoding an NAD(+)-dependent isoform of 11β-hydroxysteroid dehydrogenase in sheep kidney. Endocr Res 1995; 21:389–97.
15. Kotelevtsev Y, Holmes MC, Burchell A, et al. 11β-hydroxysteroid dehydrogenase type 1 knockout mice show attenuated glucocorticoid-inducible responses and resist hyperglycemia on obesity or stress. Proc Natl Acad Sci USA 1997; 94:14924–9.
16. Holmes MC, Kotelevtsev Y, Mullins JJ, Seckl JR. Phenotypic analysis of mice bearing targeted deletions of 11β-hydroxysteroid dehydrogenases 1 and 2 genes. Mol Cell Endocrinol 2001; 171:15–20.
17. Morton NM, Holmes MC, Fievet C, et al. Improved lipid and lipoprotein profile, hepatic insulin sensitivity, and glucose tolerance in 11β-hydroxysteroid dehydrogenase type 1 null mice. J Biol Chem 2001; 276:41293–300.
18. Ferrari P, Smith RE, Funder JW, Krozowski ZS. Substrate and inhibitor specificity of the cloned human 11β-hydroxysteroid dehydrogenase type 2 isoform. Am J Physiol 1996; 270:E900–4.
19. Li KX, Obeyesekere VR, Krozowski ZS, Ferrari P. Oxoreductase and dehydrogenase activities of the human and rat 11β-hydroxysteroid dehydrogenase type 2 enzyme. Endocrinology 1997; 138:2948–52.
20. Naray-Fejes-Toth A, Watlington CO, Fejes-Toth G. 11β-hydroxysteroid dehydrogenase activity in the renal target cells of aldosterone. Endocrinology 1991; 129:17–21.
21. Krozowski Z, MaGuire JA, Stein-Oakley AN, Dowling J, Smith RE, Andrews RK. Immunohistochemical localization of the 11β-hydroxysteroid dehydrogenase type II enzyme in human kidney and placenta. J Clin Endocrinol Metab 1995; 80:2203–9.
22. Odermatt A, Arnold P, Frey FJ. The intracellular localization of the mineralocorticoid receptor is regulated by 11β-hydroxysteroid dehydrogenase type 2. J Biol Chem 2001; 276:28484–92.
23. Fejes-Toth G, Pearce D, Naray-Fejes-Toth A. Subcellular localization of mineralocorticoid receptors in living cells: effects of receptor agonists and antagonists. Proc Natl Acad Sci USA 1998; 95:2973–8.
24. Alberts P, Engblom L, Edling N, et al. Selective inhibition of 11beta-hydroxysteroid dehydrogenase type 1 decreases blood glucose concentrations in hyperglycaemic mice. Diabetologia 2002; 45:1528–32.
25. Barf T, Vallgarda J, Emond R, et al. Arylsulfonamidothiazoles as a new class of potential antidiabetic drugs. Discovery of potent and selective inhibitors of the 11beta-hydroxysteroid dehydrogenase type 1. J Med Chem 2002; 45:3813–5.
26. Alberts P, Nilsson C, Selen G, et al. Selective inhibition of 11 beta-hydroxysteroid dehydrogenase type 1 improves hepatic insulin sensitivity in hyperglycemic mice strains. Endocrinology 2003; 144:4755–62.
27. Hermanowski-Vosatka A, Balkovec JM, Cheng K, et al. 11beta-HSD1 inhibition ameliorates metabolic syndrome and prevents progression of atherosclerosis in mice. J Exp Med 2005; 202:517–27.
28. Rauz S, Cheung CM, Wood PJ, et al. Inhibition of 11β-hydroxysteroid dehydrogenase type 1 lowers intraocular pressure in patients with ocular hypertension. QJM 2003; 96:481–90.
29. Corvol P, Michel JB, Evin G, Gardes J, Bensala-Alaoui A, Menard J. The role of the renin–angiotensin system in blood pressure regulation in normotensive animals and man. J Hypertens Suppl 1984; 2:S25–30.

30. Funder JW, Blair-West JR, Coghlan JP, Denton DA, Scoggins BS, Wright RD. Effect of (K+) on the secretion of aldosterone. Endocrinology 1969; 85:381–4
31. Griffith RW. Freshwater or marine origin of the vertebrates? Comp Biochem Physiol A 1987; 87:523–31.
32. Cirillo M, Capasso G, Di Leo VA, De Santo NG. A history of salt. Am J Nephrol 1994; 14:426–31.
33. Smith HW. Renal physiology. In: Fishman AP, Richards WR, eds. Circulation of the Blood: Men and Ideas. New York: Oxford University Press, 1964:545–606.
34. Frassetto L, Morris RC, Jr., Sellmeyer DE, Todd K, Sebastian A. Diet, evolution and aging—the pathophysiologic effects of the post-agricultural inversion of the potassium-to-sodium and base-to-chloride ratios in the human diet. Eur J Nutr 2001; 40:200–13.
35. Kriz W. Structural organization of the renal medulla: comparative and functional aspects. Am J Physiol 1981; 241:R3–16.
36. Hu X, Funder JW. The evolution of mineralocorticoid receptors. Mol Endocrinol 2006; 20:1471–78 .
37. Rocha R, Funder JW. The pathophysiology of aldosterone in the cardiovascular system. Ann NY Acad Sci 2002; 970:89–100.
38. Ferrari P, Bonny O. Forms of mineralocorticoid hypertension. Vitam Horm 2003; 66:113–56.
39. Funder J, Myles K. Exclusion of corticosterone from epithelial mineralocorticoid receptors is insufficient for selectivity of aldosterone action: in vivo binding studies. Endocrinology 1996; 137:5264–8.
40. Ward MR, Kanellakis P, Ramsey D, Funder J, Bobik A. Eplerenone suppresses constrictive remodeling and collagen accumulation after angioplasty in porcine coronary arteries. Circulation 2001; 104:467–72.
41. Young MJ, Moussa L, Dilley R, Funder JW. Early inflammatory responses in experimental cardiac hypertrophy and fibrosis: effects of 11β-hydroxysteroid dehydrogenase inactivation. Endocrinology 2003; 144:1121–5.
42. Pitt B, Zannad F, Remme WJ, et al. The effect of spironolactone on morbidity and mortality in patients with severe heart failure. Randomized Aldactone Evaluation Study Investigators. N Engl J Med 1999; 341:709–17.
43. Pitt B, Reichek N, Willenbrock R, et al. Effects of eplerenone, enalapril, and eplerenone/enalapril in patients with essential hypertension and left ventricular hypertrophy: the 4E-left ventricular hypertrophy study. Circulation 2003; 108:1831–8.
44. Pitt B, Remme W, Zannad F, et al. Eplerenone, a selective aldosterone blocker, in patients with left ventricular dysfunction after myocardial infarction. N Engl J Med 2003; 348:1309–21.
45. Mantero F, Opocher G, Rocco S, Carpene G, Armanini D. Long-term treatment of mineralocorticoid excess syndromes. Steroids 1995; 60:81–6.
46. Ferrari P, Krozowski Z. Role of the 11β-hydroxysteroid dehydrogenase type 2 in blood pressure regulation. Kidney Int 2000; 57:1374–81.
47. Ferrari P, Bianchetti M, Frey FJ. Juvenile hypertension, the role of genetically altered steroid metabolism. Horm Res 2001; 55:213–23.
48. Whitworth JA, Stewart PM, Burt D, Atherden SM, Edwards CR. The kidney is the major site of cortisone production in man. Clin Endocrinol (Oxf) 1989; 31:355–61.
49. Mercer WR, Krozowski ZS. Localization of an 11β-hydroxysteroid dehydrogenase activity to the distal nephron. Evidence for the existence of two species of dehydrogenase in the rat kidney. Endocrinology 1992; 130:540–3.
50. Palermo M, Gomez-Sanchez C, Roitman E, Shackleton CH. Quantitation of cortisol and related 3-*oxo*-4-ene steroids in urine using gas chromatography/mass spectrometry with stable isotope-labeled internal standards. Steroids 1996; 61:583–9.
51. Palermo M, Shackleton CH, Mantero F, Stewart PM. Urinary free cortisone and the assessment of 11β-hydroxysteroid dehydrogenase activity in man. Clin Endocrinol 1996; 45:605–11.

52. Shackleton CH. Mass spectrometry in the diagnosis of steroid-related disorders and in hypertension research. J Steroid Biochem Mol Biol 1993; 45:127–40.
53. Ferrari P, Sansonnens A, Dick B, Frey FJ. In vivo 11βHSD-2 activity: variability, salt-sensitivity, and effect of licorice. Hypertension 2001; 38:1330–6.
54. Wilson RC, Krozowski ZS, Li K, et al. A mutation in the HSD11B2 gene in a family with apparent mineralocorticoid excess. J Clin Endocrinol Metab 1995; 80:2263–6.
55. Obeyesekere VR, Ferrari P, Andrews RK, et al. The R337C mutation generates a high K_m 11β-hydroxysteroid dehydrogenase type II enzyme in a family with apparent mineralocorticoid excess. J Clin Endocrinol Metab 1995; 80:3381–3.
56. Mune T, Rogerson FM, Nikkila H, Agarwal AK, White PC. Human hypertension caused by mutations in the kidney isozyme of 11β-hydroxysteroid dehydrogenase. Nat Genet 1995; 10:394–9.
57. Ferrari P, Obeyesekere VR, Li K, et al. Point mutations abolish 11β-hydroxysteroid dehydrogenase type II activity in three families with the congenital syndrome of apparent mineralocorticoid excess. Mol Cell Endocrinol 1996; 119:21–4.
58. Ferrari P, Obeyesekere VR, Li K, Andrews RK, Krozowski ZS. The 11β-hydroxysteroid dehydrogenase type II enzyme: biochemical consequences of the congenital R337C mutation. Steroids 1996; 61:197–200.
59. Stewart PM, Krozowski ZS, Gupta A, et al. Hypertension in the syndrome of apparent mineralocorticoid excess due to mutation of the 11β-hydroxysteroid dehydrogenase type 2 gene. Lancet 1996; 347:88–91.
60. Kitanaka S, Katsumata N, Tanae A, et al. A new compound heterozygous mutation in the 11β-hydroxysteroid dehydrogenase type 2 gene in a case of apparent mineralocorticoid excess. J Clin Endocrinol Metab 1997; 82:4054–8.
61. Krozowski ZS, Stewart PM, Obeyesekere VR, Li K, Ferrari P. Mutations in the 11β-hydroxysteroid dehydrogenase type II enzyme associated with hypertension and possibly stillbirth. Clin Exp Hypertens 1997; 19:519–29.
62. Li A, Li KX, Marui S, et al. Apparent mineralocorticoid excess in a Brazilian kindred: hypertension in the heterozygote state. J Hypertens 1997; 15:1397–402.
63. Rogoff D, Smolenicka Z, Bergada I, et al. The codon 213 of the 11β-hydroxysteroid dehydrogenase type 2 gene is a hot spot for mutations in apparent mineralocorticoid excess. J Clin Endocrinol Metab 1998; 83:4391–3.
64. Wilson RC, Dave-Sharma S, Wei JQ, et al. A genetic defect resulting in mild low-renin hypertension. Proc Natl Acad Sci USA 1998; 95:10200–5.
65. Dave-Sharma S, Wilson RC, Harbison MD, et al. Examination of genotype and phenotype relationships in 14 patients with apparent mineralocorticoid excess. J Clin Endocrinol Metab 1998; 83:2244–54.
66. Li A, Tedde R, Krozowski ZS, et al. Molecular basis for hypertension in the "type II variant" of apparent mineralocorticoid excess. Am J Hum Genet 1998; 63:370–9.
67. Odermatt A, Dick B, Arnold P, et al. A mutation in the cofactor-binding domain of 11β-hydroxysteroid dehydrogenase type 2 associated with mineralocorticoid hypertension. J Clin Endocrinol Metab 2001; 86:1247–52.
68. Carvajal CA, Gonzalez AA, Romero DG, et al. Two homozygous mutations in the 11β-hydroxysteroid dehydrogenase type 2 gene in a case of apparent mineralocorticoid excess. J Clin Endocrinol Metab 2003; 88:2501–7.
69. Lavery GG, Ronconi V, Draper N, et al. Late-onset apparent mineralocorticoid excess caused by novel compound heterozygous mutations in the HSD11B2 gene. Hypertension 2003; 42:123–9.
70. Quinkler M, Bappal B, Draper N, et al. Molecular basis for the apparent mineralocorticoid excess syndrome in the Oman population. Mol Cell Endocrinol 2004; 217:143–9.
71. Lin-Su K, Zhou P, Arora N, Betensky BP, New MI, Wilson RC. In vitro expression studies of a novel mutation delta299 in a patient affected with apparent mineralocorticoid excess. J Clin Endocrinol Metab 2004; 89:2024–7.

72. Mantero F, Tedde R, Opocher G, Dessi Fulgheri P, Arnaldi G, Ulick S. Apparent mineralocorticoid excess type II. Steroids 1994; 59:80–3.
73. Litchfield WR, Hunt SC, Jeunemaitre X, et al. Increased urinary free cortisol: a potential intermediate phenotype of essential hypertension. Hypertension 1998; 31:569–74.
74. Stewart PM, Wallace AM, Valentino R, Burt D, Shackleton CH, Edwards CR. Mineralocorticoid activity of liquorice: 11β-hydroxysteroid dehydrogenase deficiency comes of age. Lancet 1987; 2:821–4.
75. Beretta-Piccoli C, Davies DL, Boddy K, et al. Relation of arterial pressure with body sodium, body potassium and plasma potassium in essential hypertension. Clin Sci 1982; 63:257–70.
76. Walker BR, Stewart PM, Shackleton CH, Padfield PL, Edwards CR. Deficient inactivation of cortisol by 11β-hydroxysteroid dehydrogenase in essential hypertension. Clin Endocrinol 1993; 39:221–7.
77. Soro A, Ingram MC, Tonolo G, Glorioso N, Fraser R. Evidence of coexisting changes in 11β-hydroxysteroid dehydrogenase and 5 beta-reductase activity in subjects with untreated essential hypertension. Hypertension 1995; 25:67–70.
78. Walker BR, Phillips DI, Noon JP, et al. Increased glucocorticoid activity in men with cardiovascular risk factors. Hypertension 1998; 31:891–5.
79. Iki K, Miyamori I, Hatakeyama H, et al. The activities of 5β-reductase and 11β-hydroxysteroid dehydrogenase in essential hypertension. Steroids 1994; 59:656–60.
80. Santini DL, Lorenzo BJ, Koufis T, Reidenberg MM. Cortisol metabolism in hypertensive patients who do and do not develop hypokalemia from diuretics. Am J Hypertens 1995; 8:516–9.
81. Sullivan JM. Salt sensitivity. Definition, conception, methodology, and long-term issues. Hypertension 1991; 17:I61–8.
82. Weinberger MH. Salt sensitivity of blood pressure in humans. Hypertension 1996; 27:481–90.
83. Sharma AM. Salt sensitivity as a phenotype for genetic studies of human hypertension. Nephrol Dial Transplant 1996; 11:927–9.
84. Lovati E, Ferrari P, Dick B, et al. Molecular basis of human salt-sensitivity: the role of the 11β-hydroxysteroid dehydrogenase type 2. J Clin Endocrinol Metab 1999; 84:3745–9.
85. Burton PJ, Waddell BJ. 11β-hydroxysteroid dehydrogenase in the rat placenta: developmental changes and the effects of altered glucocorticoid exposure. J Endocrinol 1994; 143:505–13.
86. Barker DJ, Osmond C, Golding J, Kuh D, Wadsworth ME. Growth in utero, blood pressure in childhood and adult life, and mortality from cardiovascular disease. BMJ 1989; 298:564–7.
87. Lindsay RS, Lindsay RM, Waddell BJ, Seckl JR. Prenatal glucocorticoid exposure leads to offspring hyperglycaemia in the rat: studies with the 11β-hydroxysteroid dehydrogenase inhibitor carbenoxolone. Diabetologia 1996; 39:1299–305.
88. Edwards CR, Benediktsson R, Lindsay RS, Seckl JR. Dysfunction of placental glucocorticoid barrier: link between fetal environment and adult hypertension? Lancet 1993; 341:355–7.
89. Seckl JR, Benediktsson R, Lindsay RS, Brown RW. Placental 11β-hydroxysteroid dehydrogenase and the programming of hypertension. J Steroid Biochem Mol Biol 1995; 55:447–55.
90. Montrella-Waybill M, Clore JN, Schoolwerth AC, Watlington CO. Evidence that high dose cortisol-induced Na+ retention in man is not mediated by the mineralocorticoid receptor. J Clin Endocrinol Metab 1991; 72:1060–6.
91. Williamson PM, Kelly JJ, Whitworth JA. Dose–response relationships and mineralocorticoid activity in cortisol-induced hypertension in humans. J Hypertens Suppl 1996; 14:S37–41.
92. Fanestil DD. Mode of spirolactone action: competitive inhibition of aldosterone binding to kidney mineralocorticoid receptors. Biochem Pharmacol 1968; 17:2240–2.
93. Gomez-Sanchez EP, Gomez-Sanchez CE. Central hypertensinogenic effects of glycyrrhizic acid and carbenoxolone. Am J Physiol 1992; 263:E1125–30.
94. Funder JW. Mineralocorticoid receptors in the central nervous system. J Steroid Biochem Mol Biol 1996; 56:179–83.
95. Gomez-Sanchez EP, Venkataraman MT, Thwaites D, Fort C. ICV infusion of corticosterone antagonizes ICV-aldosterone hypertension. Am J Physiol 1990; 258:E649–53.

96. Palermo M, Cossu M, Shackleton CH. Cure of apparent mineralocorticoid excess by kidney transplantation. N Engl J Med 1998; 339:1787–8.
97. Watson B, Jr., Bergman SM, Myracle A, Callen DF, Acton RT, Warnock DG. Genetic association of 11β-hydroxysteroid dehydrogenase type 2 (HSD11B2) flanking microsatellites with essential hypertension in blacks. Hypertension 1996; 28:478–82.
98. Smolenicka Z, Bach E, Schaer A, et al. A new polymorphic restriction site in the human 11β-hydroxysteroid dehydrogenase type 2 gene. J Clin Endocrinol Metab 1998; 83:1814–7.
99. Zaehner T, Plueshke V, Frey BM, Frey FJ, Ferrari P. Structural analysis of the 11β-hydroxysteroid dehydrogenase type 2 gene in end-stage renal disease. Kidney Int 2000; 58:1413–9.
100. Brand E, Kato N, Chatelain N, et al. Structural analysis and evaluation of the 11β-hydroxysteroid dehydrogenase type 2 (11βHSD2) gene in human essential hypertension. J Hypertens 1998; 16:1627–33.
101. Agarwal AK, Giacchetti G, Lavery G, et al. CA-Repeat polymorphism in intron 1 of HSD11B2: effects on gene expression and salt sensitivity. Hypertension 2000; 36:187–94.
102. Fiore C, Eisenhut M, Ragazzi E, Zanchin G, Armanini D. A history of the therapeutic use of liquorice in Europe. J Ethnopharmacol 2005; 99:317–24.
103. Henman FD. Inhibition of peptic activity by carbenoxolone and glycyrrhetinic acid. Gut 1970; 11:344–51.
104. Stewart PM, Whorwood CB, Walker BR. Steroid hormones and hypertension: the cortisol-cortisone shuttle. Steroids 1993; 58:614–20.
105. MacKenzie MA, Hoefnagels WH, Jansen RW, Benraad TJ, Kloppenborg PW. The influence of glycyrrhetinic acid on plasma cortisol and cortisone in healthy young volunteers. J Clin Endocrinol Metab 1990; 70:1637–43.
106. Whorwood CB, Sheppard MC, Stewart PM. Licorice inhibits 11β-hydroxysteroid dehydrogenase messenger ribonucleic acid levels and potentiates glucocorticoid hormone action. Endocrinology 1993; 132:2287–92.
107. Morris DJ. Liquorice: new insights into mineralocorticoid and glucocorticoid hypertension. R I Med 1993; 76:251–4.
108. Bernardi M, D'Intino PE, Trevisani F, et al. Effects of prolonged ingestion of graded doses of licorice by healthy volunteers. Life Sci 1994; 55:863–72.
109. Stewart PM, Murry BA, Mason JI. Human kidney 11β-hydroxysteroid dehydrogenase is a high affinity nicotinamide adenine dinucleotide-dependent enzyme and differs from the cloned type I isoform. J Clin Endocrinol Metab 1994; 79:480–4.
110. Draper N, Walker EA, Bujalska IJ, et al. Mutations in the genes encoding 11β-hydroxysteroid dehydrogenase type 1 and hexose-6-phosphate dehydrogenase interact to cause cortisone reductase deficiency. Nat Genet 2003; 34:434–9.
111. Lavery GG, Walker EA, Draper N, et al. Hexose-6-phosphate dehydrogenase knockout mice lack 11β-hydroxysteroid dehydrogenase type 1-mediated glucocorticoid generation. J Biol Chem 2006; 281:6546–51.

9

Integrative Renal Regulation of Sodium Excretion

Jean-Pierre Montani
Division of Physiology, Department of Medicine, University of Fribourg, Fribourg, Switzerland

Bruce N. Van Vliet
Division of Basic Medical Sciences, Faculty of Medicine, Memorial University of Newfoundland, St. John's, Newfoundland, Canada

THE IMPORTANCE OF ACHIEVING SODIUM BALANCE

Precise adjustments in renal sodium excretion are required to achieve salt balance in the face of wide fluctuations in sodium chloride (salt) intake. To maintain stable conditions in our internal environment, the *milieu intérieur* of Claude Bernard, it is crucial in a nongrowing individual to have a perfect balance between inputs into the body and outputs out of the body. This concept is at the basis of the body's homeostasis and is certainly not restricted to the handling of minerals such as sodium, potassium, or calcium. It applies in a general way to all "unchanged" molecules or to molecules situated at the end of the body's metabolic catabolic pathways, such as water (water lost by the body must be compensated by an equal amount of water ingested or produced endogenously by the metabolism), CO_2 (endogenous production must be exhaled by the lungs), fixed acids (endogenously produced H^+ by the catabolism of energy substrates must be eliminated in equal amounts by the kidneys), creatinine (production of creatinine by the muscles must be matched by an equal excretion into the urine) or urea (urea resulting from the degradation of proteins by the liver must be found in equal amounts in the urine). Any imbalance between input and output, if maintained in the long term, will result in a potentially damaging accumulation or depletion of the incriminating variable. This concept of "output must equal input" is often not understood by medical students, leading to conceptual aberrations that daily urinary creatinine excretion must be reduced in renal insufficiency or that sodium excretion must remain permanently elevated with chronic diuretic treatment.

Normally, there is little loss of sodium by extrarenal sources, 2 to 3 mmol/day by sweat and epithelial desquamation, and 2 to 3 mmol/day with the feces. The kidney thus becomes the central organ to adjust sodium excretion in order to achieve sodium balance. Without mechanisms to achieve sodium balance, every time sodium intake is increased above normal, sodium intake would exceed sodium excretion and the body would accumulate sodium leading to extracellular fluid accumulation (due to concomitant renal water retention and increased water intake as a regulatory response to control plasma osmolality) and a resultant increase in blood pressure (BP). Conversely, when sodium intake is decreased below normal, the lack of renal adjustments would lead to hypovolemia and a drop in BP, endangering survival.

Salt Intake May Vary Widely in Healthy Individuals

From the viewpoint of human evolution, the addition of salt to our diet is a relatively recent event. For several millions of years our hunter-gatherer ancestors ate a diet estimated to contain less than 1 g of salt per day (1,2). Very strong mechanisms for salt conservation were thus needed to maintain salt balance at a level sufficient to regulate the amount of fluid in our bodies. Without those mechanisms, our ancestors would have never survived the additional stresses associated with starvation or hemorrhage, and would not have the required hemodynamic reserve for fight or flight reactions. A minimal intake of salt is required to compensate for obligatory salt losses by urine, sweat, feces and epithelial desquamation. When animals are put on a diet that is extremely poor in sodium, they exhibit hypovolemia possibly with impaired exercise performance, thus becoming easier prey for predators. Salt depletion also endangers survival of the species due to poor reproductive functions with decreased fertility, decreased number of pups in the litter and decreased pup size (3).

The deliberate use of salt for food preservation, beginning about 10,000 years ago, was a major milestone in human history as it facilitated the preservation of food, allowing humans to settle down for agriculture, farming, and life in sedentary communities. In ancient times, salt was a very precious commodity. Roman soldiers were often paid with salt (and hence the origin of the word "salary"). The sale of salt was heavily controlled and taxed by kings and governments throughout the ages. Today, supply of salt is plentiful with average dietary values of about 10 g/day in industrialized and urbanized countries, rising to about 30 g/day (with individual levels up to 60 g/day) in northern Japan (4). Analysis of salt intakes in a large international epidemiological comparative study in 52 centers worldwide, the INTERSALT study (5,6), revealed wide fluctuations in salt intake among healthy individuals. Within the same individual, there are also normal day-to-day fluctuations in salt intake (up to 10-fold) (7). In our own personal lives, we have all experienced days in which we ate very little due to stress, flu, or simply lack of time in a busy life, and other days in which we indulge in a nice meal with friends, enjoying dried meat, bread and Swiss cheese fondue.

Sodium Balance is Usually Achieved within a Few Days of a Change in Salt Intake

As most ingested salt is excreted in the urine, the kidney is the key organ to adjust sodium excretion in order to achieve sodium balance. In healthy individuals, matching output to input is usually achieved within a few days of a change in sodium intake. Figure 1 is a composite figure from various data in the literature illustrating the effects of a 10-fold increase in sodium intake from a low sodium intake (30 mmol/day) to a high sodium intake (300 mmol/day). Sodium excretion does not rise instantaneously, but there must be signals to the kidneys so that sodium excretion increases progressively to match the new intake. Those signals come from the temporary imbalance between output and input, resulting in a gain in body sodium (and water via control of plasma osmolality), thus raising extra-cellular fluid volume (ECFV) and hence body weight. Conversely, when sodium intake is brought back to the original level, sodium excretion remains temporarily elevated,

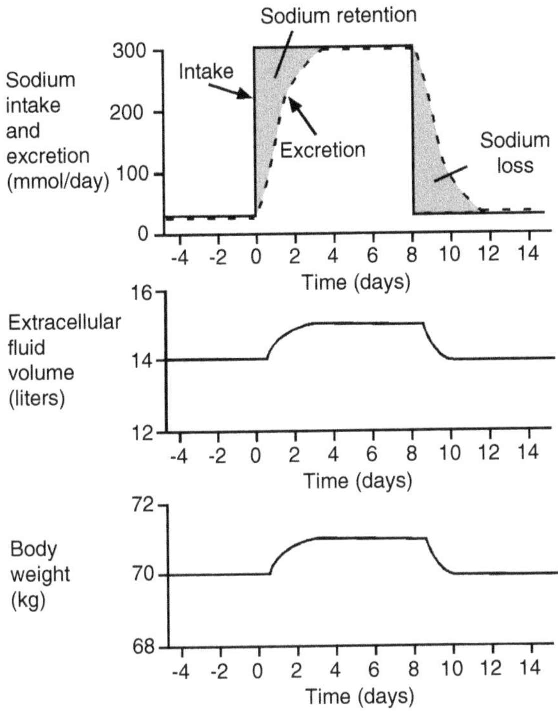

Figure 1 Effect of a marked change in sodium intake on sodium excretion, extracellular fluid volume, and body weight.

resulting in net sodium loss and a return of ECFV and body weight to normal. The amounts of sodium gained during the change to a high salt intake and subsequently lost during the return to a low salt intake are equal, bringing the body to the same original conditions.

Achieving sodium balance within a few days requires relatively intact renal, neurohormonal and cardiovascular functions. This is best illustrated by analyzing the changes in ECFV in response to an increased salt intake in patients with mild and severe chronic renal failure (CRF). When sodium intake is increased, normal subjects achieved salt balance within three to five days with only a mild increase in ECFV (Fig. 2) whereas patients with CRF required much more time, resulting in a profound increase in ECFV (8,9). A delay in reaching sodium balance may also be seen during impairment of the neural control to the kidney. For example, in rats instrumented for continuous collection of urine on an hourly basis, the time required for achieving sodium balance after a step increase in sodium intake (from 0.3 to 5.0 mmol/day) was greater in rats with denervated kidneys than in rats with intact renal nerves, resulting in a greater cumulative sodium balance (10). Sinoaortic baroreceptor denervated rats also show a greater degree of cumulative sodium balance when dietary sodium intake is increased compared with control rats (11). Dogs administered aldosterone show sodium retention for two or three days at most, rapidly escaping to the sodium-retaining properties of this mineralocorticoid (12,13). If the heart is weak and cannot generate higher cardiac output (CO) and BP, however, sodium retention is much prolonged (14) and sodium balance is eventually reached unless the amount of volume retention is so great that it leads to decompensated heart failure. Time to reach sodium balance during a step increase in salt intake is also prolonged in patients with mild or more severe congestive heart failure with a time course similar to Figure 2.

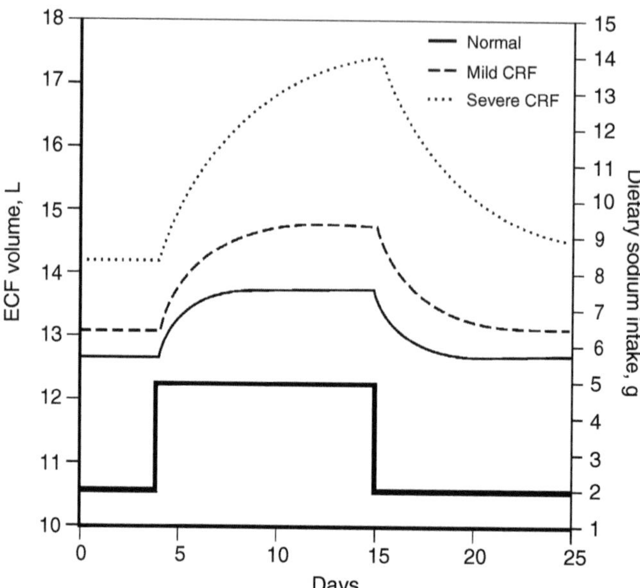

Figure 2 Effect of an increase in sodium intake on extracellular fluid (ECF) volume in normal subjects and in patients with mild or severe chronic renal failure (CRF). *Source*: From Ref. 8.

One cannot rely solely on the time to reach sodium balance to predict an impairment of the neurohormonal control of sodium balance. For example, a decrease in vascular capacity [such as found during norepinephrine (NE) or angiotensin infusion] requires less of an increase in blood volume to increase mean arterial pressure and thus may explain why sodium balance is rapidly reached when sodium intake is increased during a background of angiotensin hypertension (15).

Sodium balance is usually reached rapidly even if there is a strong stimulus in favor of sodium excretion. This is illustrated in Figure 3 by analyzing the ON and OFF transients

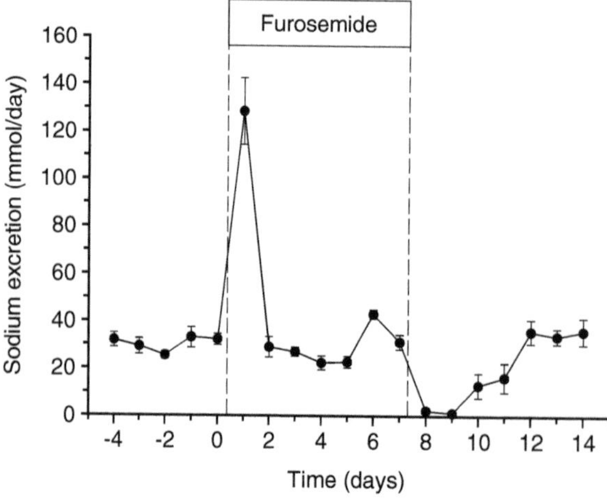

Figure 3 Effect of a seven-day continuous intravenous infusion of furosemide (2.5 μg/kg/min) on sodium excretion. Data are from four dogs.

of a chronic diuretic treatment. When furosemide, a potent loop diuretic, was administrated by a continuous intravenous infusion to dogs maintained on a fixed sodium intake of ~35 mmol/day, sodium excretion increased markedly on the first day of furosemide administration, resulting in a sodium loss of about 100 mmol (Montani, unpublished observations). But by the second day, sodium excretion was back to normal, at the expense of hemoconcentration (elevated hematocrit and plasma protein concentration) and stimulation of antinatriuretic systems (plasma renin activity and plasma aldosterone). When the infusion of furosemide was stopped one week later, there was a marked sodium retention that lasted for several days. The amounts of sodium lost at the beginning of diuretic treatment, and subsequently regained after cessation of diuretic administration were approximately equal, bringing the body to the same original conditions. This example illustrates that sodium balance is usually rapidly achieved, even if there is a strong stimulus for sodium loss. Similarly, sodium retention due to angiotensin II (Ang II) or aldosterone administration in intact animals is only seen during the first few days of hormonal administration, sodium balance being eventually reached despite continuing hormonal administration. All these examples stress the fact that analysis of sodium excretion in steady-state conditions will not bring any useful information other than reflect the level of sodium intake. Indeed, in steady-state conditions, the sole determinant of sodium excretion is sodium intake, independent of the level of any natriuretic or antinatriuretic factor affecting the kidney.

MECHANISMS FOR ACHIEVING SODIUM BALANCE

In the earlier chapters of this book, we have learned how various neurohormonal factors and transport proteins can affect renal sodium reabsorption and contribute to sodium balance. Indeed, it is clear that a great many factors can influence renal sodium excretion, including a number of autocrine and paracrine factors generated within the kidney itself. However, in understanding the regulation of sodium excretion, it is critical to recognize that there is one mechanism that resides within the kidney itself, which is not only capable of making powerful adjustments of sodium excretion, but also automatically linking sodium excretion to the regulation of ECFV and BP. This mechanism is referred to as the acute pressure–natriuresis relationship or mechanism. The pressure–natriuresis relationship is so central to the regulation of sodium excretion that the many other factors and mechanisms that influence sodium excretion are often considered to act chiefly by modifying this relationship (16).

The Central Role of Pressure–Natriuresis and Diuresis

Acute changes in renal perfusion pressure (RPP) lead to profound changes in sodium excretion, as illustrated by the solid curve in Figure 4A. Increases in BP cause increased sodium excretion (i.e., natriuresis) and reductions in BP cause reduced sodium excretion or even complete cessation of urine flow at low BP levels. This *acute* pressure–natriuresis relationship has been known for a long time (17) and has been reported in isolated kidneys (17,18), anesthetized animals (19) and conscious animals (20). The intrarenal mechanisms underlying this phenomenon have been reviewed elsewhere (21,22). Briefly, an increase in RPP leads to an increased medullary blood flow due to the poor autoregulatory properties of the renal inner medulla. As a consequence, vasa recta intravascular pressure increases, favoring movement of fluid into the medullary interstitium. Since the kidney is enclosed in a capsule with very low compliance, any increase of the interstitial fluid

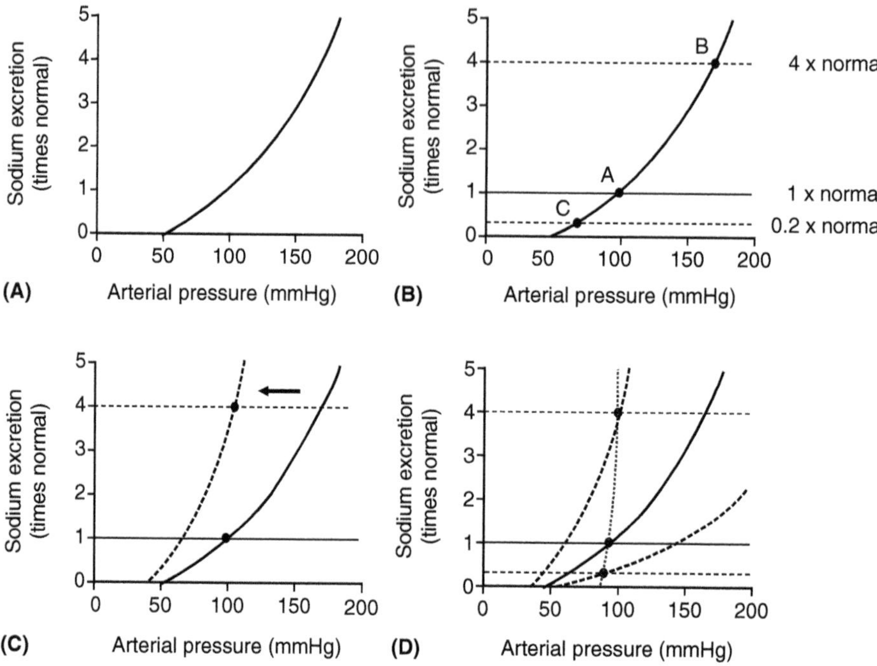

Figure 4 The concept of acute pressure–natriuresis and how adjustments of this relationship facilitate sodium balance during sustained changes in salt intake. (**A**) The basic pressure–natriuresis curve (PNC). (**B**) Three levels of salt intake are depicted (normal, 0.2×normal, and 4×normal). Equilibrium is reached at the intersection between the PNC and the corresponding level of salt excretion that matches salt intake. (**C**) Left shift of the PNC during a high salt intake. (**D**) Joining the intersection points reveals an almost vertical chronic pressure–natriuresis relationship (see the dotted line), i.e., the chronic renal function curve. The modulation of the PNC during alterations in salt intakes allows the body to achieve sodium balance with minimal changes in arterial pressure.

volume leads to an increase in renal hydrostatic fluid pressure that is transmitted to the entire kidney, diminishing thereby tubular sodium reabsorption via classical Starling forces.

To understand the role of the pressure–natriuresis in sodium balance and long-term BP control, the view of the cardiovascular system must not be restricted to a simple closed circuit consisting of a pump (the heart) and a series of tubes of various resistances (the vasculature), a simplistic model in which all that counts for BP control is the strength of the heart and the resistance of the peripheral vasculature. Rather, the cardiovascular system must be viewed as a system with an input from the outside (fluid and salt intakes) and an output to the outside (urinary excretion). Any change in the input would alter blood volume and thereby BP, which in turn leads to changes in the output via pressure–natriuresis.

Fluid Volume Equilibrium is Reached When Salt Excretion is Equal to Salt Intake

The pressure–natriuresis curve (PNC) of Figure 4A is at the center of blood volume and BP control. If the body gains too much fluid (e.g., acute volume load), BP increases.

This leads to increased excretion of salt and water via the pressure–natriuresis mechanism, bringing blood volume and BP back toward normal. Conversely, if one loses fluids (e.g., hemorrhage), BP decreases and the kidneys retain salt and water, which helps to bring blood volume and BP back to normal. In this analysis, the level at which BP stabilizes depends on the level of salt intake. As in steady-state conditions sodium balance can only be achieved when input equals output, BP will stabilize at a value that allows sodium excretion (determined by the pressure–natriuresis mechanism) to match perfectly sodium intake. For a normal level of salt intake (1×normal), only a BP value of about 100 mmHg (point A in Fig. 4B) is high enough, but not too high, to lead to a urinary excretion of sodium of 1×normal. Equilibrium is thus reached at the intersection point of the PNC with the corresponding level of salt intake, as shown in Figure 4B.

Based on this concept, one can understand the general *renal body fluid feedback mechanism* (16,23–25) as illustrated in the block diagram of Figure 5. Any imbalance between intake and output of salt will lead to a cascade of events that oppose the initial disturbance, a classical negative feedback loop. For example, if salt intake is greater than salt excretion (block A), there is a positive rate of change of the ECFV (ΔECFV), which integrated over time (block B) results in an increase in ECFV and, in turn, to an increase in blood volume (block C). The greater blood volume increases mean circulatory filling pressure (which represents the degree of filling of the whole circulation, i.e., the ratio of blood volume to vascular capacity), as shown by the relationship depicted in block D. This results in a right and upward shift of the equilibrium point (block E) in Guyton's classic graphical analysis of the cardiac function curve and the venous return curve (26), yielding

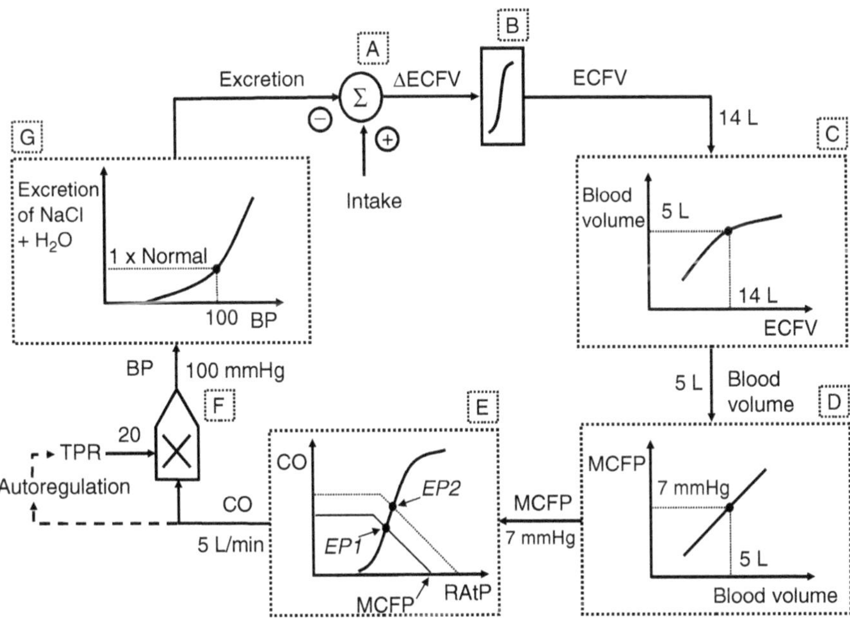

Figure 5 The renal body fluid feedback mechanism for control of blood volume and in the face of large changes in salt intake. See text for a detailed explanation of each block (A to G) of the block diagram. *Abbreviations*: BP, blood pressure; CO, cardiac output; ECFV, extracellular fluid volume; EP, equilibrium point; MCFP, mean circulatory filling pressure; RAtP, right atrial pressure; TPR, total peripheral resistance.

both an increase in right atrial pressure and an increase in venous return. The resulting increase in CO raises BP (block F). In turn, by the way of the pressure–natriuresis mechanism, the higher BP increases salt output (block G), which opposes the effects of the initial increase in salt intake. The system acts very slowly (hours or days), but it is extremely effective (in engineering terms, it has an infinite "gain") and corrects completely any error in salt balance.

At this stage, this simplified feedback loop may not explain the whole story. According to this analysis, a fourfold increase in salt intake would lead to volume retention until BP increases to well over 150 mmHg (point B in Fig. 4B). Sodium balance would be reached, but at the expense of profound volume retention and tremendous hypertension. Similarly, a diet poor in sodium (e.g., one-fifth of normal) would require a drop in BP by 30 or 40 mmHg (point C in Fig. 4B) to achieve a state of sodium balance. Yet, this sensitivity to salt does not fit with the small variations in BP, which are normally observed when animals (27) and humans (28) are subjected to large variations of salt intake. Clearly, additional mechanisms must normally come into play.

The Pressure–Natriuresis Relationship is Modulated by Changes in Salt Intake

The PNC depicted in Figure 4A is not immovable. In fact, it becomes steeper and is shifted to the left during high salt intake (Fig. 4C). This change in the pressure–natriuresis relationship represents the sum of many adjustments of renal function that allows the body to achieve sodium balance with minimal increases in BP. Conversely, during low salt intake, the PNC becomes flatter and is shifted to the right. Joining the equilibrium points at the various salt intakes now reveals a very steep "chronic" relationship with little change in BP (Fig. 4D). That is, the chronic relationship between salt intake and BP has become relatively salt-*in*sensitive.

Experimentally, the chronic pressure–natriuresis relationship is measured by imposing a level of salt intake on a subject for several days until salt balance is established and then measuring the resultant BP level. This process is repeated for a variety of salt intakes, each level of salt intake contributing one point to the chronic pressure–natriuresis relationship, also known as the "chronic renal function curve" (steep dotted line of Fig. 4D). In contrast to the acute pressure–natriuresis mechanism which represents a property of the renal tissues that can be demonstrated even in isolated perfused kidneys, the chronic pressure–natriuresis relationship represents the performance of the entire renal body fluid feedback system at equilibrium: that is, after the many control mechanisms affecting renal function and BP have exerted their influence, after salt balance has been established, and after BP has stabilized. Because the chronic renal function curve describes the pressure–natriuresis relationship when salt intake and renal salt excretion are equal, the *Y*-axis on a chronic renal function curve simultaneously represents both salt intake and salt excretion.

Various neurohormonal mechanisms contribute to the adjustment of the acute PNC with varying salt intakes, such as renal nerve sympathetic activity, natriuretic and antinatriuretic hormones. Above all, modulation of the renin–angiotensin system (RAS) plays a crucial role in the adaptation to changes in salt intake, with suppression of the RAS at high salt intake facilitating sodium excretion, and stimulation of the RAS at low salt intake contributing to sodium conservation (29). The importance of this modulation is illustrated by the dramatic salt-induced changes in BP, which occur when the RAS is blocked with an angiotensin-converting enzyme (ACE) inhibitor or when circulating Ang II levels are fixed with an intravenous infusion of angiotensin (27).

By which Mechanisms Do Ang II Levels Vary with Changes in Salt Intake?

The sequence of events is presented in the block diagram of Figure 6. The initial increase in salt intake (salt with little water) leads to an increased plasma osmolality, resulting in thirst and drinking, as well as renal water retention via stimulation of vasopressin release, resulting in an increase in ECFV. This leads to an increase in blood volume. From there on, a complex but logical sequence of events takes place. The greater blood volume increases mean circulatory filling pressure, resulting in both an increase in right atrial pressure and an increase in venous return, as described in the block diagram of Figure 5.

The greater right atrial pressure stretches the right atrium, loading low pressure receptors that cause reflex reductions in renal nerve sympathetic activity. Atrial stretch leads also to a direct increased release of atrial natriuretic peptide (ANP), a hormone that has a direct inhibitory action on renin release (and aldosterone secretion). By its vasodilatory action on preglomerular vessels, ANP also promotes an increase in glomerular filtration rate (GFR).

The greater venous return increases CO and thus arterial pressure, which in turn leads to three events: (*i*) loading of arterial carotid and aortic baroreceptors, resulting in a decreased renal sympathetic nerve activity; (*ii*) mechanical stretch of preglomerular vessels; (*iii*) increase in delivery of fluid and salt to the macula densa mediated by the small increase in GFR (favored by physical forces and accentuated by the vasodilatory ability of ANP on the afferent arteriole). Altogether, these three events promote a decrease in renin release and thus in Ang II levels.

In parallel, the slight increase in plasma NaCl concentration (Fig. 6) increases the filtered load of sodium chloride, but also reduces tubular sodium reabsorption

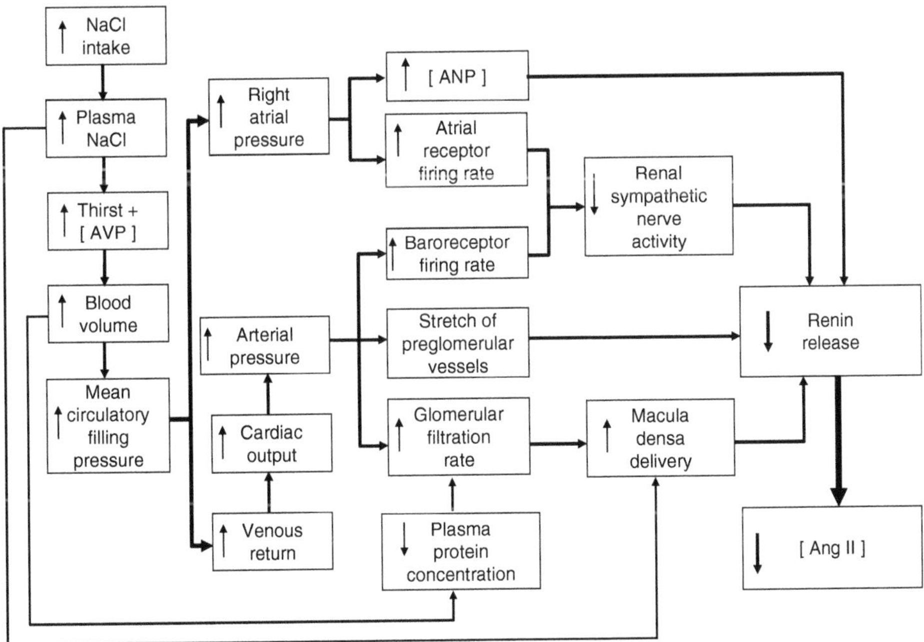

Figure 6 Block diagram illustrating the mechanisms whereby an increase in salt intake leads to a decrease in Ang II formation. *Abbreviations*: Ang II, angiotensin II; ANP, atrial natriuretic peptide; AVP, arginine vasopressin.

independently of a change in GFR (30). In turn, the expected increases in macula densa delivery would decrease renin release. A small increase in plasma sodium concentration with sustained higher salt intakes has indeed been documented in normotensive and hypertensive rats (31) and in longitudinal studies in dogs (27,32,33) and humans (34,35). An increase in plasma sodium is also seen after the ingestion of a single salty meal (36). Thus, the small increase in plasma sodium with salt could also contribute to sodium balance. Finally, the increase in blood volume decreases, at least acutely, plasma protein concentration, which alters Starling physical forces at the level of glomerular and peritubular capillaries, favoring an increased glomerular filtration and a decreased proximal tubular reabsorption (37).

A similar block diagram can be applied, but in the reverse direction, to explain the increased Ang II levels during low salt intake. Volume depletion leads to a decrease in filling pressures and arterial pressure. Unloading of atrial and arterial baroreceptors, decreased ANP concentration, decreased preglomerular stretch and decreased salt delivery to the macula densa all contribute to the stimulation of renin release.

EXPERIMENTAL SUPPORT FOR THE ROLE OF PRESSURE–NATRIURESIS

The control of sodium excretion is thus tightly linked to the control of blood volume and arterial pressure via the PNC that lies at the center of the renal body fluid feedback mechanism. The dominance of this mechanism in achieving sodium balance arises from the cumulative nature of its actions. Any long-lasting imbalance between salt intake and salt excretion leads to a progressive amplification of the changes in ECFV and blood volume, and thus to a parallel change in BP as long as BP remains away from the equilibrium level predicted by the PNC. Several lines of evidence are consistent with the renal body fluid feedback mechanism.

The Inability to Modulate the PNC Leads to Salt Sensitivity

As depicted in Figure 4D, if the PNC were to remain relatively fixed instead of becoming steeper with a higher salt intake or flatter with a lower salt intake, one would expect the development of a marked salt sensitivity. This is what precisely happens when normal variations of the activity of RAS with changing salt intakes are prevented from occurring, either by inhibiting the ACE with captopril or by fixing circulating Ang II levels with an exogenous intravenous infusion of Ang II. Dogs submitted to four different levels of salt intake lasting for one week each, from 5 mmol/day to as high as 500 mmol/day, achieved sodium balance with very little change in BP when the RAS was intact (27). However, with ACE inhibition, the lack of activation of the RAS during low salt intake led to a dramatic decrease in mean arterial pressure to less than 70 mmHg, as shown in Figure 7. At high salt intake, ACE inhibition was not effective in lowering BP since renin levels are already suppressed with high salt intakes. On the other hand, infusion of Ang II at 5 ng/kg/min, producing circulating Ang II levels only slightly higher than what is seen during sodium restriction, led to very little increase in BP at a low salt intake. At high salt intakes, however, Ang II infusion prevented the expected suppression of the RAS, leading to a relatively fixed PNC and severe hypertension, with a mean arterial pressure of about 150 mmHg with the highest salt intake of 500 mmol/day.

Thus one of the major roles of the RAS is to prevent a large drop in BP (and ECFV) during low salt intakes, and a large increase in BP (and ECFV) during high salt intakes. In other words, when the ability to suppress renin at high salt intakes is lost,

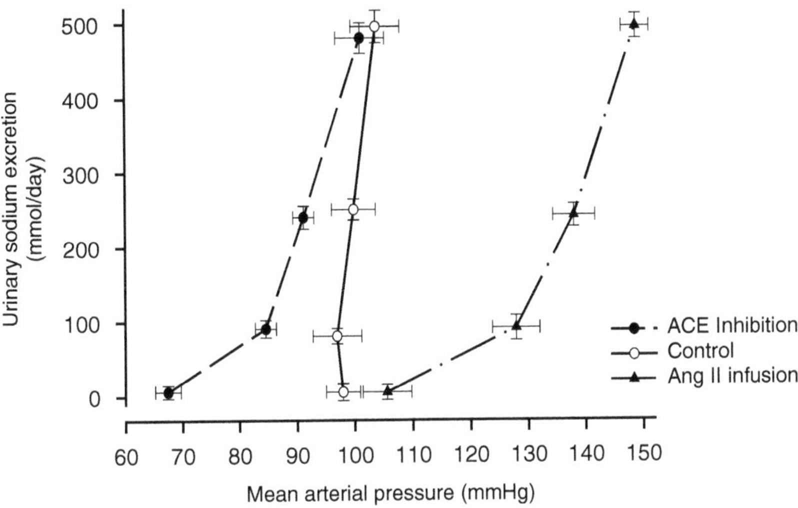

Figure 7 Steady-state relationships between mean arterial pressure and urinary sodium excretion in dogs subjected to varying salt intakes from 5 to 500 mmol/day, lasting one week at every level. The dogs were studied in three conditions: (*i*) with an intact RAS; (*ii*) during chronic blockade of the RAS with captopril; (*iii*) during fixed elevated circulating levels of Ang II via an intravenous infusion of Ang II at 5 ng/kg/min. *Abbreviations*: ACE, angiotensin-converting enzyme; Ang II, angiotensin II; RAS, renin–angiotensin system. *Source*: From Ref. 27.

volume-dependent salt sensitivity develops. This may particularly occur in the following two situations:

1. *Aging*. Circulating levels of renin decrease steadily with age (38), possibly related to the observed decrease in glomerular number and size that occur with aging (39). The response of renin in older individuals is also blunted when the RAS is either stimulated (volume contraction) or inhibited (volume expansion) (40). The lower basal levels of plasma renin activity and poor reactivity of the RAS may help explain the higher prevalence of salt sensitivity in older subjects.
2. *Low-renin essential hypertension*. About one-quarter of all essential hypertensive patients have low renin levels that are poorly stimulated by a low salt intake (41). Because renin levels are low to start with, the inability to further suppress renin at high salt intake may explain the salt sensitivity frequently observed in low-renin essential hypertension.

At the other end of the PNC, the concept of RAS modulation is particularly useful to understand the increased effectiveness of ACE inhibitors or angiotensin receptor blockers in lowering BP if the antihypertensive treatment is combined with a reduction in salt intake or with the use of diuretics.

BP "Follows" the Kidney in Renal Transplant Experiments

According to the renal body fluid feedback theory, hypertension should occur every time the PNC is shifted to the right (parallel shift or with a greater slope), as higher BP levels are required to achieve sodium balance. If the theory is correct, one would expect BP of normotensive rats to increase if rats are transplanted with kidneys of various strains of genetically hypertensive rats (spontaneously hypertensive rats, stroke-prone spontaneously hypertensive rats, Dahl, Milan, Prague) whereas hypertension of those strains would be corrected by kidney transplantation from a normotensive donor. Earlier transplantation studies (42,43) support this hypothesis (for review, see Ref. 44). More recent studies have refined the approach further, circumventing potential pitfalls such as rejection phenomena, the need for immunosuppressants and the use of indirect methods of BP assessment (45). In such experiments, the BP level of animals receiving a transplanted kidney was shown to be strongly influenced by the BP level of the donor animal: implantation of a hypertensive kidney elevated the BP level of normotensive animals, while implantation of a normotensive kidney reduced the BP of hypertensive animals. This general finding has also been supported by transplantation studies in humans (46,47).

Role of Pressure–Natriuresis in Renovascular Hypertension

The kidney is directly implicated in many well-known forms of acquired hypertension including that associated with ureteral obstruction, renal wrap hypertension, reduced renal mass, infusion of various substances into the renal artery (48) or the renal medulla (49), and a variety of renal pathologies. Most interesting is the pathogenesis of hypertension that results from renal stenosis (Goldblatt hypertension), which represents a beautiful demonstration of the role of pressure–natriuresis in establishing sodium balance at the cost of a higher BP. However, the pathways by which hypertension develops depend on the type of stenosis, which can be studied experimentally as follows.

1. *One-kidney one-clip (1K1C) hypertension.* Experimentally, a stenotic clip is placed on the renal artery of one kidney whereas the contralateral kidney is removed. The renal artery stenosis reduces RPP, which may explain many of the initial events, including sodium retention and stimulation of the RAS. However, as the animal retains volume over time and becomes hypertensive, the glomerular pressure tends to return toward normal and there is no longer a strong stimulus for renin release. At this stage, administration of an ACE inhibitor has little effect on BP. The hypertension is volume dependent but no longer renin dependent. The clinical equivalent of 1K1C is renal artery stenosis in a patient with a solitary kidney, or bilateral renal artery stenoses (2K2C) or stenosis of the aorta above the origin of the renal arteries.
2. *Two-kidney one-clip (2K1C) hypertension.* The pathogenesis of hypertension in this model is more complex. The stenotic kidney is underperfused and thus secretes large amounts of renin. The resulting higher plasma Ang II levels act on the intact controlateral kidney, both by a direct effect and via stimulation of aldosterone secretion to promote enhanced sodium reabsorption. Although the exact time course in sodium excretion by each separate kidney has not been determined experimentally during 2K1C, the experimental setup used by Mizelle et al. (50) to servo-control renal arterial pressure (RAP) to one kidney in a split-bladder preparation would predict the following sequence. Initially, both kidneys may retain salt, but the stenotic kidney with its lower distal renal artery pressure and its locally stimulated RAS retains much more salt than the controlateral kidney. As BP rises due to volume expansion, systemic BP increases high enough to achieve sodium balance by the pressure–natriuresis mechanism, sodium excretion being now slightly elevated in the intact kidney and slightly decreased in the stenotic kidney. Because there is a continuing stimulus for renin release from the stenotic kidney and possible accumulation of intrarenal Ang II in the nonstenotic kidney (51), this hypertension is highly angiotensin dependent and responds well to blockers of the RAS.

Preventing Increases in RAP Worsens Hormone-Induced Hypertension

Various hormones have been implicated in the pathogenesis of hypertension. When aldosterone or other mineralocorticoids are administered to experimental animals, they induce sodium retention and a progressive rise in BP. Similar observations are found with infusions of relatively low doses of Ang II [higher doses of angiotensin are acutely natriuretic as the vasoconstriction-induced acute increase in BP promotes pressure–natriuresis and offsets the antinatriuretic properties of angiotensin (52)]. Since antinatriuretic hormones cause volume retention which in turn raises BP to a sufficient level to restore the rate of sodium excretion to normal levels, angiotensin- and aldosterone-induced hypertension may be viewed as a homeostatic mechanism to increase the kidney's ability to excrete salt and water in order to achieve sodium balance.

In line with the renal body fluid feedback theory, if one prevents RAP from rising during aldosterone (12) or angiotensin infusion (53) (this is achieved by placing a constricting cuff above the origin of the renal arteries, and servo-controlling RAP at its normal preinfusion level), the animals exhibit a marked sodium retention that persists throughout the infusion period despite large increases in ECFV and BP, which should normally favor sodium excretion. Similar observations have been made with other hypertensive hormones such as vasopressin (54) or NE (55). When infused in intact animals, vasopressin leads to water retention and urine concentration which last for a few days. BP increases during the first few days (which can even induce a small natriuresis) and then tends to return slowly toward baseline on the following days. However, when RAP is prevented from increasing via the same servo-control device, water retention and urine concentration do not escape, and ECFV and BP increase dramatically. Finally, the time course of the response to NE infusion adds interesting insights into the renal body fluid feedback system as hypertension develops despite a decrease in blood volume. In intact animals, the first few days of NE infusion are characterized by a marked increase in BP (due to the direct vasoconstrictor properties of NE), which results in a transient natriuresis. Consequently, blood volume decreases and the initial increase in BP are attenuated over the next few days. In the steady state, NE infusion is thus characterized by a low blood volume and only a mildly elevated BP. However, here again, when RAP is servo-controlled at its preinfusion level, the initial natriuresis is not observed. On the contrary, NE immediately induces sodium retention, leading to hypervolemia and severe hypertension.

Altogether, the servo-control experiments in the various models of hormone-induced hypertension (aldosterone, angiotensin, vasopressin and NE infusions) underscore the importance of RPP in achieving sodium balance. In all cases, when RPP is not allowed to increase to oppose the sodium-retaining properties of the hormones, there is marked and sustained sodium retention leading to dramatic increases in ECFV and severe systemic hypertension.

The Pressure–Natriuresis Relationship Remains Valid in Special Circumstances

The importance of the pressure–natriuresis relationship in the control of sodium balance has been challenged for two major reasons. Firstly, the chronic relationship between salt intake and BP is relatively salt insensitive, i.e., with no clear changes in BP despite wide fluctuations in salt intake. In some cases, there may even be an inverse relationship, with a small decrease in BP at high salt intake and a relatively larger increase in BP at low salt intake (a chronic renal function curve with negative slope). However, as illustrated in Figure 4D, these observations do not invalidate the pressure–natriuresis concept because the chronic renal function curve reflects the intersection of the various acute PNCs with

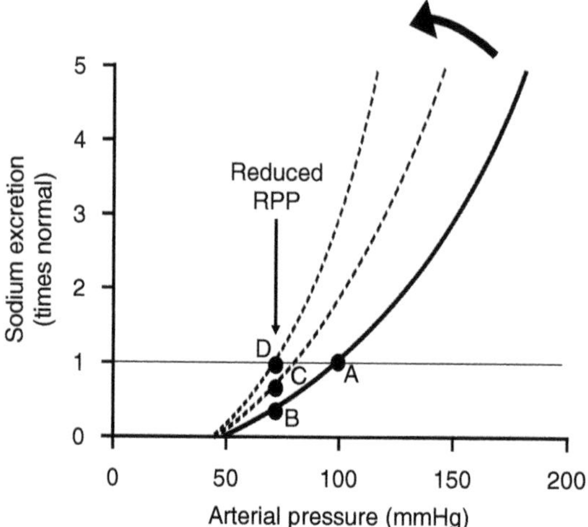

Figure 8 Achieving sodium balance during a step decrease in renal perfusion pressure: role of a progressive left shift of the acute PNC. *Abbreviations*: PNC, pressure–natriuresis curve; RPP, renal perfusion pressure.

the corresponding levels of salt intake. In other words, if a low salt intake shifts the acute PNC too much to the right along with a decreased slope, the equilibrium point will be moved too far to the right, so that a BP level higher than normal is now required to achieve sodium balance. Such a situation may be encountered in uninephrectomized sodium-restricted rats (56).

A second challenge to the importance of the pressure–natriuresis relationship in the control of sodium balance comes from experiments in dogs in which RPP is servo-controlled during four consecutive days at lower than normal values (57) and yet the sodium-retaining effect of low RPP does seem to escape despite the sustained reduction of RPP (pressure escape). Indeed, in these experiments sodium balance was achieved after two days despite RPP being held at about 80% of its normal value. However, the reestablishment of sodium balance occurred at the cost of cumulative sodium and water retention (and thus ECFV expansion) along with marked systemic hypertension and a reduction in heart rate. In addition, ANP levels were elevated more than 2.5-fold whereas plasma aldosterone concentration, initially increased, tended to decrease rapidly below control levels despite sustained high levels of plasma renin activity. Those experiments do not necessarily invalidate the role of PNC in sodium balance as they allow neurohormonal factors to fluctuate freely according to feedback regulation. As shown in Figure 8, the initial reduction in RPP will lead to marked sodium retention (point B) and an increase in ECFV and systemic BP, which may lead, via stimulation of the various natriuretic factors, to a progressive left shift and increased slope of the acute PNC, allowing the body to reach sodium balance (point D) although RPP remains low. Several factors may contribute to this profound left shift of the PNC during servo-controlled reduction in RPP.

1. *Downregulation in plasma aldosterone concentration.* In the experiments of Reinhardt et al. with servo-controlled reduction in RPP (57), plasma aldosterone concentration was increased only on the first day of reduced RPP and tended to be lower than control values on the subsequent days despite sustained elevation in plasma renin activity. This downregulation of plasma aldosterone concentration, possibly related to the high ANP levels, could contribute to

the pressure escape. Indeed, in the same model of reduced RPP, when plasma aldosterone levels were clamped at about four times the control level with an exogenous infusion of aldosterone, sodium excretion remained significantly lower than control throughout all four days of reduced RPP with no evidence of pressure escape (58).

2. *Loading of cardiopulmonary receptors.* The severe systemic hypertension and volume retention loads cardiopulmonary receptors, as evidenced by the observed decrease in heart rate in Reinhardt's dogs (57). The resulting reflex decrease in renal sympathetic nerve activity will favor sodium excretion and a return toward sodium balance (11,59).
3. *Increase in ANP.* Although ANP is not a potent natriuretic agent at low RPP (60), it can shift the normal relationship between arterial pressure and renal excretion toward lower arterial pressure so that sodium balance would be maintained at a reduced BP (61). Indeed, when ANP was infused unilaterally directly into the renal artery of conscious dogs with the urinary bladder split to allow continuous measurement of renal excretion from each kidney separately, there was a sustained increase in sodium excretion from the ANP-infused kidney for as long as the ANP infusion was maintained (seven days) without any evidence of attenuation of the natriuresis with time (61). The controlateral kidney showed some degree of sodium retention so that total sodium excretion remained normal. In this study, significant natriuresis was observed at an ANP infusion rate that would yield an estimated renal ANP concentration of about 260 pg/mL that is similar to levels observed with chronic volume expansion in dogs (15). ANP's effects to increase renal excretory capability could thus play an important role in body fluid homeostasis during sustained reductions in RPP, particularly because of the apparent nonadaptive nature of stretch receptor mechanisms of atrial myocytes (62).
4. *Release of other natriuretic factors.* Besides ANP, various natriuretic factors exhibit increased circulating levels with a high salt intake, such as bradykinin (63) and endogenous ouabain (64). Additional natriuretic substances have also been found in high concentrations in the urine during a high salt intake. These including urodilatin (36) and uroguanilyn (65), which are both potent natriuretic substances. As all these substances may increase sodium excretion without raising BP, they can contribute to a left shift of the PNC.
5. *Enteral versus parenteral salt loading.* Finally, the route of administration of the salt load may have an important effect on sodium excretion. In Reinhardt's dogs (57), all the daily food (with salt) and water was given as a single load over 20 to 30 minutes with no access to food and water for the rest of the day whereas in most other experiments in which RAP is servo-controlled (12,53–55) salt is provided evenly throughout 24 hours with a continuous intravenous infusion of saline. It is long known since the early studies of Carey et al. in both humans (66) and rabbits (67) that an oral salt load increases urinary sodium excretion to a far greater extent than the same load given intravenously, with the postulation that an intestinal natriuretic hormone delivers a signal from the gastrointestinal tract to the kidney in response to increased NaCl intake. Recently, it has been suggested that uroguanylin could be that signal as it is a highly effective natriuretic peptide produced by the intestinal mucosa and found in the circulation (68). The role of uroguanylin in promoting sodium excretion during enteral load is further supported by the observation that uroguanylin knockout mice have increased BP and impaired natriuretic response to enteral NaCl load (69).

Intriguingly, the natriuretic mechanisms listed above are not sufficient to allow sodium balance to be reached during hormone-induced hypertension unless RPP is permitted to rise [e.g., aldosterone (12), angiotensin II (53), NE (55)]. However, one explanation is that the natural feedback-induced fluctuations of all neurohormonal systems that contribute to sodium balance are not allowed to operate fully in those experiments. In particular, the expected suppression of the renin–angiotensin–aldosterone system cannot occur because of the clamped levels of aldosterone (12), angiotensin II (53) or NE (55) (this last model is characterized by elevated renin and aldosterone levels). When suppressions of renin and aldosterone are allowed, for example in the model of reduced renal mass—high salt hypertension—sodium balance is achieved despite servo-control of RAP at its normal level (70). By contrast, in hormone-induced hypertension, the PNC is primarily shifted to the right and natriuretic factors, such as ANP or renal sympathetic inhibition, do not seem to be strong enough to bring the PNC all the way back to its normal position. In these circumstances, sodium balance can only be achieved by the natriuresis induced by the elevated BP level.

Long-Term Effects of RPP on Salt Excretion

An elegant experiment that demonstrates the long-term effect of RAP on sodium excretion was conducted by Mizelle et al. (50) in dogs instrumented for separate monitoring of the function of the left and right kidneys using the split-bladder preparation described above. In addition, RAP was measured in both renal arteries using nonocclusive catheters and, on one side, a cuff was placed around the renal artery proximally to the catheter to servo-control RAP at a lower value. As shown in Figure 9, when RAP was lowered to a value between 75 and 80 mmHg sodium excretion decreased and remained low for as long as RAP was below normal. Interestingly the reduced sodium excretion in the servo-control kidney was compensated by an increased sodium excretion in the controlateral kidney, presumably in response to the slight elevation in systemic arterial pressure, so that total sodium excretion was normal. Those experiments suggest that the acute PNC does not reset to long-term changes in arterial pressure and may thus play a key role in achieving sodium balance.

Genetic Defects Affecting Sodium Handling

The final strong support for the role of BP in the control of sodium balance comes from genetic studies. In the last decades, over 20 genes have been identified to be associated with essential hypertension or responsible for rare monogenic diseases that are characterized by low or high BP (71,72). Intriguingly, most of these genes encode proteins that are involved with renal sodium handling. Mutations that favor renal sodium reabsorption increase BP whereas mutations that diminish tubular sodium reabsorption tend to decrease BP.

Several monogenic forms of hypertension have been described in humans. They include syndromes characterized by mineralocorticoid-independent excessive sodium uptake in the distal convoluted tubulus (Gordon syndrome) and the collecting duct (Liddle's syndrome, with gain-of-function mutation of the amiloride-sensitive epithelium Na channel) and various syndromes characterized by excess mineralocorticoid action in the later parts of the nephron, such as apparent mineralocorticoid excess (deficiency in 11β-hydroxysteroid dehydrogenase no longer protects the kidney from the mineralocorticoid effects of cortisol), congenital adrenal hyperplasia due to

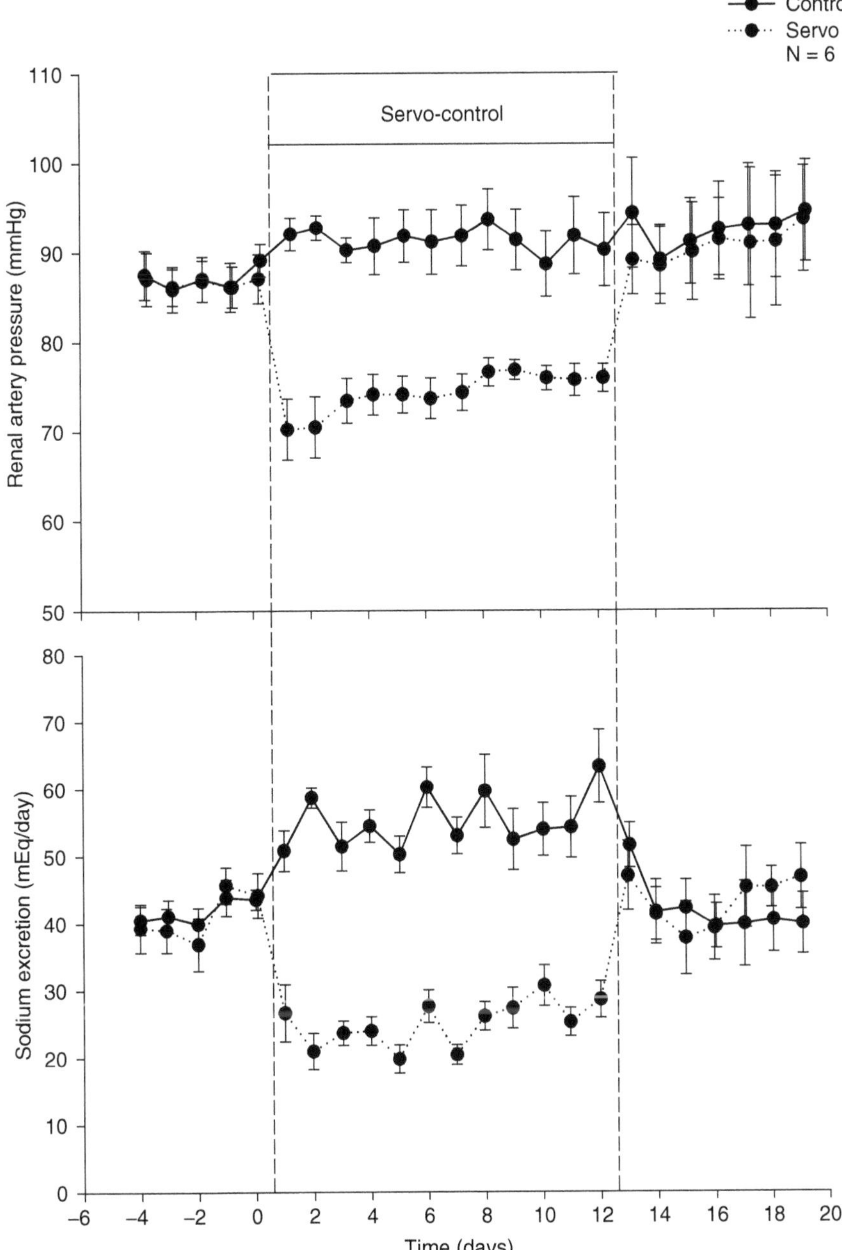

Figure 9 Twelve-day unilateral servo-controlled reduction in renal perfusion pressure in dogs with a split-bladder preparation: effects on renal artery pressure and sodium excretion in servo-controlled (dashed lines) and controlateral control (solid lines) kidneys. *Source*: From Ref. 50.

17α-hydroxylase or 11β-hydroxylase deficiency (which leads to enhanced concentrations of the potent mineralocorticoid deoxycorticosterone), glucocorticoid remediable aldosteronism (aldosterone synthesis is now under the control of adrenocorticotropic hormone) and a rare form of hypertension exacerbated by pregnancy (and due to an activating mutation of the mineralocorticoid receptor).

On the other hand, mutations that lead to salt wasting decrease BP, particularly when sodium intake is low. These include syndromes with deficient transport proteins in the thick ascending limb of Henle's loop (Barrter syndromes types 1, 2 and 3, respectively, due to a defect in the Na–K–2Cl cotransport, the apical K channel and the basolateral Cl channel), the distal convoluted tubulus (Gitelman syndrome, due to a defect of the apical thiazide-sensitive Na–Cl cotransport) as well as in the collecting duct (recessive pseudohypoaldosteronism type 1, by loss of function of the epithelium Na channel). Other salt-wasting syndromes are related to mineralocorticoid deficiency in renal tubular cells due to insufficient production of aldosterone (aldosterone synthase deficiency, congenital adrenal hyperplasia due to 21-hydroxylase deficiency) or loss-of-function mutation in the mineralocorticoid receptor (dominant pseudohypoaldosteronism type 1).

In addition to these various mutations that can alter BP in humans, numerous experimental genetic manipulations in the mouse, affecting either the transporter proteins of salt reabsorption directly or indirectly by acting on the various regulators of those proteins, all point to the same conclusions. Mutations that favor excessive sodium reabsorption increase BP whereas mutations characterized by impaired renal sodium retention tend to decrease BP, particularly under conditions of a low salt intake. Changes in BP seem thus to be a homeostatic mechanism to achieve sodium balance in the face of excessive or deficient salt reabsorption.

THE ROLE OF WHOLE-BODY BLOOD FLOW AUTOREGULATION IN THE CONTROL OF SODIUM BALANCE

The achievement of sodium balance requires the complex interaction of many control systems. One of those systems that has often been neglected in the study of sodium balance is whole body blood flow autoregulation, an important concept of cardiovascular control. The concept of autoregulation is most widely understood in the context of the local or regional circulations whereby mechanisms intrinsic to the tissue or organ make adjustments to the local vascular resistance such that: (*i*) blood flow occurs at a level that is appropriate for the metabolic or other needs of the organ/tissue and (*ii*) this level of blood flow is held relatively constant despite changes in the perfusion pressure. The mechanisms contributing to blood flow autoregulation vary from tissue to tissue and remain incompletely understood. For most organs, they involve myogenic control of the vascular smooth muscle in combination with feedback provided by local metabolism, metabolites, or oxygen delivery (73). In the kidney, blood flow is related to the control of glomerular filtration rate, itself determined by the tubuloglomerular feedback.

Since autoregulation influences the control of vascular resistance in virtually all tissues within the systemic circulation (it is absent in the pulmonary circulation), it is not surprising that autoregulation should be evident in the pressure–resistance and flow–resistance relationships of the entire circulation. Thus, by extrapolating to the whole organism, whole body autoregulation represents the ability of the body to adjust CO, i.e., whole body blood flow, to the body's needs by adjusting total peripheral resistance (TPR). Because an increase in blood volume elevates CO and leads then to secondary autoregulatory changes in vascular resistance, the concept of whole body autoregulation is often misinterpreted as the cause of systemic hypertension during volume loading. However, TPR (and therefore autoregulation) lies outside of the main feedback loop of the renal body fluid feedback mechanism, as shown in Figure 5. Consequently, the renal body fluid feedback mechanism is expected to act to regulate the long-term BP level in order to achieve sodium balance irrespective of the level of TPR. In other words, the renal body fluid feedback mechanism sets the long-term level of BP, i.e., the product of CO and TPR; whole body autoregulation is simply responsible for adjusting the balance of CO and TPR in a manner that provides an appropriate level of tissue perfusion.

Autoregulatory changes in CO and TPR have been clearly demonstrated in various models of volume-loading hypertension. In studies of conscious, chronically instrumented dogs in which salt sensitivity was induced by reducing renal mass to 30% of normal (74,75), "whole body autoregulation" of CO slowly became apparent over several days of saline infusion. A sustained infusion of saline resulted in a prompt rise in BP that was initially mediated by an increase in CO (74). Subsequently, peripheral resistance slowly rose (whole body autoregulation) and CO progressively fell [the predicted effect of increased TPR to decrease venous return and CO (26)], such that the increase in BP was eventually sustained by the increase in TPR. Similarly, in the Dahl strain of genetically salt-sensitive rats, salt loading led to hypertension that was initially caused by an increase in CO but eventually sustained by slow increases in TPR (76–78). Slow increases in TPR were also observed to occur during salt loading in dogs made salt sensitive by a chronic infusion of angiotensin II (79) or in dogs receiving a continuous infusion of aldosterone (13). In regular (i.e., salt insensitive) dogs and in the Dahl strain of salt-resistant rats, while salt loading does not lead to an increase in BP, it does produce an initial rise in CO counterbalanced by a fall in TPR (32,77,78). In time, CO and TPR returned to normal levels (76,77) as one might expect to occur in the presence of whole body autoregulation but a normal (salt insensitive) pressure–natriuresis relationship. It is also worth noting that a very slow transition from elevated CO to elevated peripheral resistance has been described in a number of longitudinal hemodynamic studies of patients with essential hypertension (Table 1 of Ref. 80). Thus, one view of the increased TPR that accompanies volume-loading hypertension is that it is an essential response to the elevated BP in order to prevent the overperfusion of the tissues that would otherwise occur.

What Are the Implications of Whole-Body Autoregulation in the Regulation of Blood Volume and Sodium Balance?

Autoregulation strongly influences which combination of TPR and CO will be used to achieve a given BP level, and the extent of fluid accumulation required to achieve the increase in CO. As such, autoregulation prevents the large changes in ECFV, blood volume, and CO which would otherwise be required to increase BP in order to achieve sodium balance. To illustrate this role of whole body autoregulation, we have used the most recent version (81) of Guyton's large circulatory model (23) to simulate the response to volume loading caused by a sixfold increase in salt intake in a salt-sensitive individual (caused by 70% reduction in renal mass) in the presence and absence of blood flow autoregulation (Fig. 10). The simulation demonstrates a valuable benefit of mathematical modeling: the ability to conduct experiments on the model that we (so far) have no way of conducting in real life.

In the presence of normal autoregulation (solid line in Fig. 10), a high level of salt intake leads to an increase in fluid volumes (blood volume and ECFV) associated with a rise in CO and BP, and an initial fall in TPR (pressure-induced distension of the vasculature). In time, however, the progressive increase in TPR (due to whole body autoregulation) slowly reduces the volume loading and CO required to sustain BP at the new equilibrium level. Thus, in the long term, the increase in salt intake leads to salt-sensitive hypertension with rather minor changes in fluid volumes or CO.

In contrast, when the same simulation is repeated with blood flow autoregulation removed (dashed line in Fig. 10), increases in fluid volumes, CO, and BP occur without

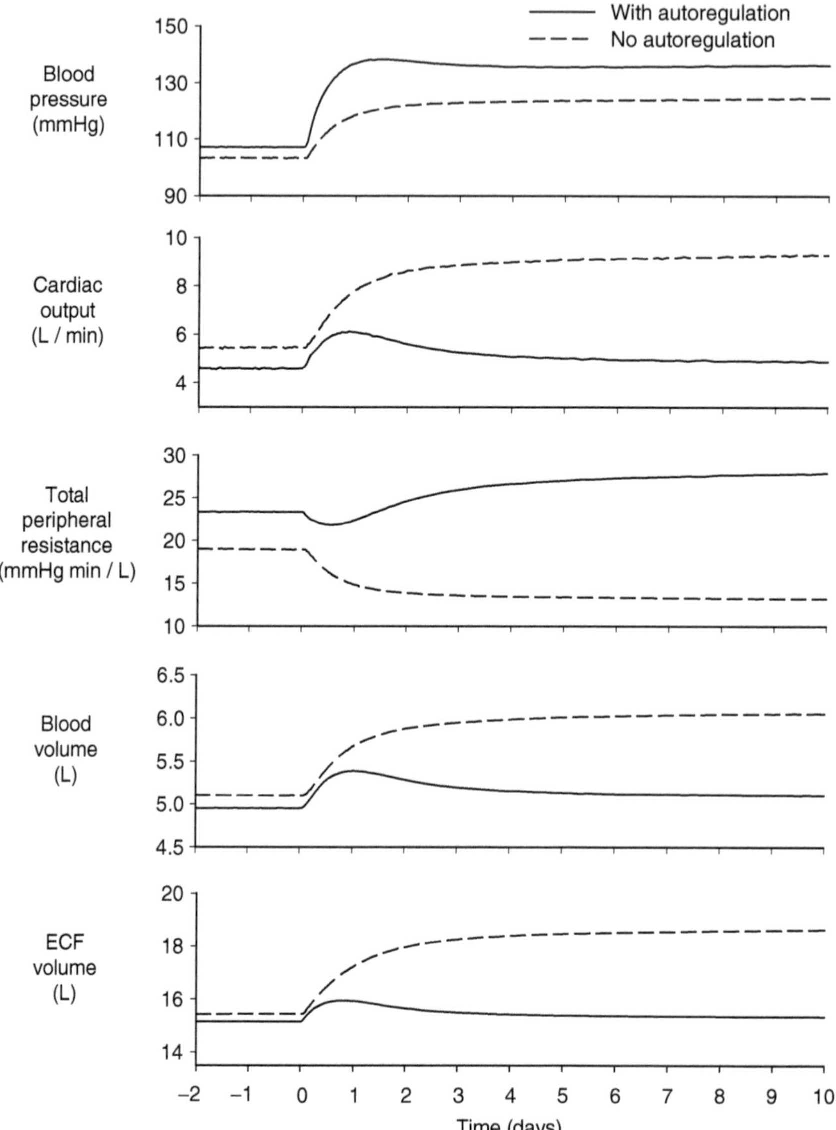

Figure 10 Computer simulation with Guyton's large circulatory model of the hemodynamic response to volume loading in salt-sensitive subjects with blood flow autoregulation intact (solid line) and after disabling mechanisms of blood flow autoregulation (dashed line). Baseline data (days −2 to 0) represent steady-state data after having reduced renal mass to 30% of normal. Volume loading was commenced at time 0 by increasing salt intake to 6×normal levels.

any increase in TPR (which in fact falls, largely due to unopposed pressure-induced distension of the vasculature). Actually, in the absence of an increase in TPR, marked increases in fluid volumes and CO are required to elevate the BP toward the equilibrium level. Indeed, equilibrium is not achieved within the time course of this simulation: by the end of 10 days of salt, fluid volumes, CO, and BP continue to rise slightly. Intriguingly, in the simulation of Figure 10, BP is lower in the absence of autoregulation both during baseline and after salt loading. However, these results can be explained almost entirely in the model by the higher levels of ANP caused by higher blood volumes. Indeed, if the simulation is repeated with ANP levels clamped at its normal level, BP is almost identical with and without autoregulation, both at baseline and after salt loading. This simulation reinforces the concept illustrated in Figure 8 that the acute PNC can be progressively shifted to the left due to volume retention, requiring thus a lower BP than expected to achieve sodium balance.

The simulations of Figure 10 illustrate that whole body autoregulation does more than just to ensure that regional blood flow occurs at a rate that meets the metabolic needs of the tissues. When fluid volumes are changed, it also serves to minimize the changes in fluid volume and CO, which are required to affect the long-term BP level. Because the ability of changes in fluid volumes to affect BP lies at the heart of the renal body fluid feedback mechanism (Fig. 5), one can readily appreciate the importance of whole body autoregulation in allowing the renal body fluid feedback mechanism to regulate the long-term BP level in a highly effective manner without the need for the large changes in fluid volumes that would otherwise be necessary.

CONCLUSIONS

Precise adjustments in renal sodium excretion are required to achieve salt balance in the face of wide fluctuations in salt intake. Any imbalance between input and output, if maintained in the long term, will result in a potentially damaging accumulation or depletion of ECFV and a resulting change in BP. Despite large possible fluctuations in salt intake, salt balance is usually achieved within a few days, making salt intake in the healthy individual the sole long-term determinant of salt excretion. The control of sodium excretion is tightly linked to the control of blood volume and arterial pressure via the pressure–natriuresis relationship that lies at the center of the renal body fluid feedback mechanism. If salt intake increases, the body gains fluid volume, raising BP and favoring sodium excretion. The increase in BP is, however, very small due to a concomitant increased ability of the kidney to excrete salt and water following a suppression of antinatriuretic mechanisms (such as Ang II and aldosterone) and a stimulation of natriuretic mechanisms (such as ANP). Any impairment in the pressure–natriuresis relationship, due to intrinsic renal defects or a lack of neurohormonal modulation with varying salt intakes, will require greater changes in blood volume and BP in order to achieve salt balance for any given salt intake. Finally, the efficiency of the renal body fluid feedback mechanism to achieve sodium balance can be greatly improved by whole-body autoregulation, which serves to minimize the changes in fluid volume and CO that are required to affect the long-term BP level.

REFERENCES

1. Eaton SB, Konner M. Paleolithic nutrition. A consideration of its nature and current implications. N Engl J Med 1985; 312:283–9.
2. Blackburn H, Prineas R. Diet and hypertension: anthropology, epidemiology, and public health implications. Prog Biochem Pharmacol 1983; 19:31–79.
3. McBurnie MI, Blair-West JR, Denton DA, Weisinger RS. Sodium intake and reproduction in BALB/C mice. Physiol Behav 1999; 66:873–9.
4. Sasaki N. High blood pressure and the salt intake of the Japanese. Jpn Heart J 1962; 3:313–24.

5. Elliott P, Dyer A, Stamler R. The INTERSALT study: results for 24 hour sodium and potassium, by age and sex. INTERSALT Cooperative Research Group. J Hum Hypertens 1989; 3:323–30.
6. Elliott P, Stamler J, Nichols R, et al. INTERSALT revisited: further analyses of 24 hour sodium excretion and blood pressure within and across populations. INTERSALT Cooperative Research Group. BMJ 1996; 312:1249–53.
7. Siani A, Iacoviello L, Giorgione N, Iacone R, Strazzullo P. Comparison of variability of urinary sodium, potassium, and calcium in free-living men. Hypertension 1989; 13:38–42.
8. Ellison DH. Disorders of sodium balance. In: Schrier RW, Berl T, Bonventre JV, eds. Atlas of Diseases of the Kidney. Disorders of Water, Electrolytes, and Acid–Base. Vol. 1. Oxford: Blackwell Science, 1999:2.1–2.22.
9. Mitch WE, Wilcox CS. Disorders of body fluids, sodium and potassium in chronic renal failure. Am J Med 1982; 72:536–50.
10. Greenberg SG, Tershner S, Osborn JL. Neurogenic regulation of rate of achieving sodium balance after increasing sodium intake. Am J Physiol 1991; 261:F300–7.
11. DiBona GF, Sawin LL. Effect of arterial baroreceptor denervation on sodium balance. Hypertension 2002; 40:547–51.
12. Hall JE, Granger JP, Smith MJ, Jr., Premen AJ. Role of renal hemodynamics and arterial pressure in aldosterone "escape". Hypertension 1984; 6:I183–92.
13. Montani JP, Mizelle HL, Adair TH, Guyton AC. Regulation of cardiac output during aldosterone-induced hypertension. J Hypertens Suppl 1989; 7:S206–7.
14. Schrier RW, Fassett RG. Pathogenesis of sodium and water retention in cardiac failure. Ren Fail 1998; 20:773–81.
15. Krieger JE, Roman RJ, Cowley AW, Jr. Hemodynamics and blood volume in angiotensin II salt-dependent hypertension in dogs. Am J Physiol 1989; 257:H1402–12.
16. Guyton AC. Circulatory Physiology III. Arterial Pressure and Hypertension. Philadelphia/London/Toronto: W.B. Saunders, 1980.
17. Starling EH, Verney EB. The excretion of urine as studied in the isolated kidney. Proc R Soc Lond 1924; 97:321–63.
18. Selkurt EE. Effect of pulse pressure and mean arterial pressure modification on renal hemodynamics and electrolyte and water excretion. Circulation 1951; 4:541–51.
19. Evans RG, Szenasi G, Anderson WP. Effects of NG-nitro-L-arginine on pressure natriuresis in anaesthetized rabbits. Clin Exp Pharmacol Physiol 1995; 22:94–101.
20. Nafz B, Ehmke H, Wagner CD, Kirchheim HR, Persson PB. Blood pressure variability and urine flow in the conscious dog. Am J Physiol 1998; 274:F680–6.
21. Cowley AW, Jr. Long-term control of arterial blood pressure. Physiol Rev 1992; 72:231–300.
22. Granger JP, Alexander BT, Llinas M. Mechanisms of pressure natriuresis. Curr Hypertens Rep 2002; 4:152–9.
23. Guyton AC, Coleman TG, Granger HJ. Circulation: overall regulation. Annu Rev Physiol 1972; 34:13–46.
24. Guyton AC. Long-term arterial pressure control: an analysis from animal experiments and computer and graphic models. Am J Physiol 1990; 259:R865–77.
25. Hall JE, Granger JP, Hester RL, Montani JP. Mechanisms of sodium balance in hypertension: role of pressure natriuresis. J Hypertens Suppl 1986; 4:S57–65.
26. Guyton AC, Jones CE, Coleman TG. Circulatory Physiology: Cardiac Output and Its Regulation. Philadelphia/London/Toronto: W.B. Saunders, 1973.
27. Hall JE, Guyton AC, Smith MJ, Jr., Coleman TG. Blood pressure and renal function during chronic changes in sodium intake: role of angiotensin. Am J Physiol 1980; 239:F271–80.
28. Luft FC, Rankin LI, Bloch R, et al. Cardiovascular and humoral responses to extremes of sodium intake in normal black and white men. Circulation 1979; 60:697–706.
29. Montani JP, Van Vliet BN. General physiology and pathophysiology of the renin–angiotensin system. In: Unger T, Scholkens BA, eds. Handbook of Experimental Pharmacology. Vol. 163/1. Angiotensin. Berlin: Springer, 2004:3–29.

30. Nashat FS, Tappin JW, Wilcox CS. Plasma sodium concentration and sodium excretion in the anaesthetized dog. J Physiol 1976; 254:183–202.
31. Fang Z, Carlson SH, Peng N, Wyss JM. Circadian rhythm of plasma sodium is disrupted in spontaneously hypertensive rats fed a high-NaCl diet. Am J Physiol Regul Integr Comp Physiol 2000; 278:R1490–5.
32. Krieger JE, Liard JF, Cowley AW, Jr. Hemodynamics, fluid volume, and hormonal responses to chronic high-salt intake in dogs. Am J Physiol 1990; 259:H1629–36.
33. Seeliger E, Lohmann K, Nafz B, Persson PB, Reinhardt HW. Pressure-dependent renin release: effects of sodium intake and changes of total body sodium. Am J Physiol 1999; 277:R548–55.
34. Johnson AG, Nguyen TV, Davis D. Blood pressure is linked to salt intake and modulated by the angiotensinogen gene in normotensive and hypertensive elderly subjects. J Hypertens 2001; 19:1053–60.
35. He FJ, Markandu ND, Sagnella GA, de Wardener HE, MacGregor GA. Plasma sodium: ignored and underestimated. Hypertension 2005; 45:98–102.
36. Drummer C, Franck W, Heer M, Forssmann WG, Gerzer R, Goetz K. Postprandial natriuresis in humans: further evidence that urodilatin, not ANP, modulates sodium excretion. Am J Physiol 1996; 270:F301–10.
37. Cowley AW, Jr., Skelton MM. Dominance of colloid osmotic pressure in renal excretion after isotonic volume expansion. Am J Physiol 1991; 261:H1214–25.
38. Weidmann P, Myttenaere-Bursztein S, Maxwell MH, de Lima J. Effect on aging on plasma renin and aldosterone in normal man. Kidney Int 1975; 8:325–33.
39. Nyengaard JR, Bendtsen TF. Glomerular number and size in relation to age, kidney weight, and body surface in normal man. Anat Rec 1992; 232:194–201.
40. Luft FC, Fineberg NS, Weinberger MH. The influence of age on renal function and renin and aldosterone responses to sodium-volume expansion and contraction in normotensive and mildly hypertensive humans. Am J Hypertens 1992; 5:520–8.
41. Fisher ND, Hurwitz S, Jeunemaitre X, Hopkins PN, Hollenberg NK, Williams GH. Familial aggregation of low-renin hypertension. Hypertension 2002; 39:914–8.
42. Rettig R. Does the kidney play a role in the aetiology of primary hypertension? Evidence from renal transplantation studies in rats and humans J Hum Hypertens 1993; 7:177–80.
43. Rettig R, Bandelow N, Patschan O, Kuttler B, Frey B, Uber A. The importance of the kidney in primary hypertension: insights from cross-transplantation. J Hum Hypertens 1996; 10:641–4.
44. Grisk O, Rettig R. Renal transplantation studies in genetic hypertension. News Physiol Sci 2001; 16:262–5.
45. Grisk O, Kloting I, Exner J, et al. Long-term arterial pressure in spontaneously hypertensive rats is set by the kidney. J Hypertens 2002; 20:131–8.
46. Botero-Velez M, Curtis JJ, Warnock DG. Brief report: Liddle's syndrome revisited—a disorder of sodium reabsorption in the distal tubule. N Engl J Med 1994; 330:178–81.
47. Guidi E, Menghetti D, Milani S, Montagnino G, Palazzi P, Bianchi G. Hypertension may be transplanted with the kidney in humans: a long-term historical prospective follow-up of recipients grafted with kidneys coming from donors with or without hypertension in their families. J Am Soc Nephrol 1996; 7:1131–8.
48. Reinhart GA, Lohmeier TE, Hord CE, Jr. Hypertension induced by chronic renal adrenergic stimulation is angiotensin dependent. Hypertension 1995; 25:940–9.
49. Mattson DL, Lu S, Nakanishi K, Papanek PE, Cowley AW, Jr. Effect of chronic renal medullary nitric oxide inhibition on blood pressure. Am J Physiol 1994; 266:H1918–26.
50. Mizelle HL, Montani JP, Hester RL, Didlake RH, Hall JE. Role of pressure natriuresis in long-term control of renal electrolyte excretion. Hypertension 1993; 22:102–10.
51. Navar LG, Zou L, Von Thun A, Tarng WC, Imig JD, Mitchell KD. Unraveling the mystery of Goldblatt hypertension. News Physiol Sci 1998; 13:170–6.
52. Olsen ME, Hall JE, Montani JP, Guyton AC, Langford HG, Cornell JE. Mechanisms of angiotensin II natriuresis and antinatriuresis. Am J Physiol 1985; 249:F299–307.
53. Hall JE, Granger JP, Hester RL, Coleman TG, Smith MJ, Jr., Cross RB. Mechanisms of escape from sodium retention during angiotensin II hypertension. Am J Physiol 1984; 246:F627–34.

54. Hall JE, Montani JP, Woods LL, Mizelle HL. Renal escape from vasopressin: role of pressure diuresis. Am J Physiol 1986; 250:F907–16.
55. Hall JE, Mizelle HL, Woods LL, Montani JP. Pressure natriuresis and control of arterial pressure during chronic norepinephrine infusion. J Hypertens 1988; 6:723–31.
56. Seymour AA, Davis JO, Freeman RH, et al. Hypertension produced by sodium depletion and unilateral nephrectomy: a new experimental model. Hypertension 1980; 2:125–9.
57. Reinhardt HW, Corea M, Boemke W, et al. Resetting of 24-h sodium and water balance during 4 days of servo-controlled reduction of renal perfusion pressure. Am J Physiol 1994; 266:H650–7.
58. Seeliger E, Boemke W, Corea M, Encke T, Reinhardt HW. Mechanisms compensating Na and water retention induced by long-term reduction of renal perfusion pressure. Am J Physiol 1997; 273:R646–54.
59. Lohmeier TE, Hildebrandt DA, Warren S, May PJ, Cunningham JT. Recent insights into the interactions between the baroreflex and the kidneys in hypertension. Am J Physiol Regul Integr Comp Physiol 2005; 288:R828–36.
60. Mizelle HL, Hall JE, Hildebrandt DA. Atrial natriuretic peptide and pressure natriuresis: interactions with the renin–angiotensin system. Am J Physiol 1989; 257:R1169–74.
61. Mizelle HL, Hildebrandt DA, Gaillard CA, et al. Atrial natriuretic peptide induces sustained natriuresis in conscious dogs. Am J Physiol 1990; 258:R1445–52.
62. Shin Y, Lohmeier TE, Hester RL, Kivlighn SD, Smith MJ, Jr. Hormonal and circulatory responses to chronically controlled increments in right atrial pressure. Am J Physiol 1991; 261:R1176–87.
63. Murphey LJ, Eccles WK, Williams GH, Brown NJ. Loss of sodium modulation of plasma kinins in human hypertension. J Pharmacol Exp Ther 2004; 308:1046–52.
64. Manunta P, Hamilton BP, Hamlyn JM. Salt intake and depletion increase circulating levels of endogenous ouabain in normal men. Am J Physiol Regul Integr Comp Physiol 2006; 290:R553–9.
65. Fukae H, Kinoshita H, Fujimoto S, Kita T, Nakazato M, Eto T. Changes in urinary levels and renal expression of uroguanylin on low or high salt diets in rats. Nephron 2002; 92:373–8.
66. Lennane RJ, Carey RM, Goodwin TJ, Peart WS. A comparison of natriuresis after oral and intravenous sodium loading in sodium-depleted man: evidence for a gastrointestinal or portal monitor of sodium intake. Clin Sci Mol Med 1975; 49:437–40.
67. Carey RM, Smith JR, Ortt EM. Gastrointestinal control of sodium excretion in sodium-depleted conscious rabbits. Am J Physiol 1976; 230:1504–8.
68. Forte LR, Fan X, Hamra FK. Salt and water homeostasis: uroguanylin is a circulating peptide hormone with natriuretic activity. Am J Kidney Dis 1996; 28:296–304.
69. Lorenz JN, Nieman M, Sabo J, et al. Uroguanylin knockout mice have increased blood pressure and impaired natriuretic response to enteral NaCl load. J Clin Invest 2003; 112:1244–54.
70. Hall JE, Mizelle HL, Brands MW, Hildebrandt DA. Pressure natriuresis and angiotensin II in reduced kidney mass, salt-induced hypertension. Am J Physiol 1992; 262:R61–71.
71. Lifton RP, Gharavi AG, Geller DS. Molecular mechanisms of human hypertension. Cell 2001; 104:545–56.
72. Mullins LJ, Bailey MA, Mullins JJ. Hypertension, kidney, and transgenics: a fresh perspective. Physiol Rev 2006; 86:709–46.
73. Borgstrom P, Grande PO, Mellander S. An evaluation of the metabolic interaction with myogenic vascular reactivity during blood flow autoregulation. Acta Physiol Scand 1984; 122:275–84.
74. Coleman TG, Guyton AC. Hypertension caused by salt loading in the dog 3. Onset transients of cardiac output and other circulatory variables. Circ Res 1969; 25:153–60.
75. Manning RD, Jr., Coleman TG, Guyton AC, Norman RA, Jr., McCaa RE. Essential role of mean circulatory filling pressure in salt-induced hypertension. Am J Physiol 1979; 236:R40–7.
76. Simchon S, Manger WM, Brown TW. Dual hemodynamic mechanisms for salt-induced hypertension in Dahl salt-sensitive rats. Hypertension 1991; 17:1063–71.

77. Ganguli M, Tobian L, Iwai J. Cardiac output and peripheral resistance in strains of rats sensitive and resistant to NaCl hypertension. Hypertension 1979; 1:3–7.
78. Greene AS, Yu ZY, Roman RJ, Cowley AW, Jr. Role of blood volume expansion in Dahl rat model of hypertension. Am J Physiol 1990; 258:H508–14.
79. Krieger JE, Cowley AW, Jr. Prevention of salt angiotensin II hypertension by servo control of body water. Am J Physiol 1990; 258:H994–1003.
80. Lund-Johansen P. Hemodynamic patterns in the natural history of borderline hypertension. J Cardiovasc Pharmacol 1986; 8(Suppl. 5):S8–14.
81. Montani JP, Adair TH, Summers RL, Coleman TG, Guyton AC. A simulation support system for solving large physiological models on microcomputers. Int J Biomed Comput 1989; 24:41–54.

10

Animal Models of Abnormal Sodium Handling

Pierre Meneton
Department of Public Health and Medical Information, Paris Descartes University, Paris, France

INTRODUCTION

Animal models are major tools for exploring complex physiological and pathological processes offering experimental approaches that are inapplicable in humans and providing the opportunity to perform studies in which all factors are kept constant, except those that are evaluated (1). This latter possibility is critical for analyzing processes that arise from the combined action of many genetic and environmental factors, each typically exerting small effects on the overall processes (2). In practice however, investigators do not always take full advantage of this opportunity. For example, the phenotype resulting from a specific mutation is frequently different from one study to another due to the lack of control of the genetic background (3–5). A large phenotypic variability can also arise from the environment of the animals that can widely differ from one laboratory to another with respect to the microbiological, viral and parasitic status of the breeding facility, the physical housing conditions (temperature, humidity, light/dark cycle) and/or the diet. Despite these inconsistencies, the investigations conducted in animal models during the last decades have provided valuable insights concerning the mechanisms by which the kidneys match urinary sodium excretion to dietary intake and the pathological phenotypes linked to an abnormal renal sodium handling. This chapter briefly describes the large body of data, which has been mostly gained in rodents, on the relationships between altered renal capacity to excrete sodium and long-term control of blood pressure (6,7).

SURGICALLY ALTERED ANIMALS WITH A REDUCED RENAL CAPACITY TO EXCRETE SODIUM

Animal models with an abnormal renal sodium handling can be obtained by surgical procedures that perturb the overall renal function. These models that often show an increased blood pressure have been created in different species, including large animals possibly comparable to humans. The pioneering work of Goldblatt in 1934 introduced the first model of hypertension induced by unilateral constriction of the renal artery (two-kidneys, one-clip model) in dogs (8). Partial occlusion of the renal artery has subsequently been shown to also lead to the development of hypertension in rats, rabbits, pigs, monkeys, and mice (9–13). Depending on the species, the increase in blood pressure is more or less rapid and can be sustained for a variable number of weeks. These differences could result from variable renal regulatory abilities and from the higher capacity of small animals to maintain sodium and fluid balance (14). The immediate increase in blood pressure results from the release of renin from the stenotic kidney and the subsequent formation of angiotensin II and aldosterone (15). The interplay between plasma renin and the extracellular volume is complex: the contralateral kidney suppresses renin synthesis and increases sodium excretion through an inhibition of the sympathetic system, which tends to decrease blood pressure. The resulting decrease of the perfusion pressure in the stenotic kidney tends to resume renin release, which in turn elevates blood pressure (16–18). As expected from the increased pressure natriuresis in the contralateral kidney and higher angiotensin II and aldosterone plasma levels, the sodium balance is perturbed in two-kidneys, one-clip animals with an overall tendency to retain sodium (19). Not surprisingly, a sodium restriction attenuates the development of hypertension while a high sodium diet favors its development in moderately hypertensive animals (20,21).

SPONTANEOUS OR SELECTED RAT STRAINS WITH A REDUCED RENAL CAPACITY TO EXCRETE SODIUM

In several spontaneous or selected strains of hypertensive rats, renal cross transplantation experiments with normotensive strains have demonstrated that the rise in blood pressure is due to abnormal kidneys (22–28). When a kidney from a normotensive rat is inserted into a young bilaterally nephrectomized hypertensive rat, the blood pressure of the hypertensive rat does not rise, and conversely when a kidney from a young hypertensive rat (before it has developed hypertension) is inserted into a bilaterally nephrectomized normotensive rat, the blood pressure of the normotensive rat will rise. This indicates that whatever functional abnormalities may occur at other sites, the primary disturbances that initiate the rise in blood pressure in these hereditary forms of hypertension reside in the kidneys. Thus, the kidneys of the hypertensive strains of rats have a reduced ability to excrete salt. In the spontaneously hypertensive rat (SHR), sodium is retained between four and six weeks of age, when the sodium excretion of the SHR is significantly less than that of the control Wistar–Kyoto (WKY) rat (29,30). Urinary sodium excretion has also been monitored during the development of hypertension in the Milan hypertensive rat. At 24 days, there is a statistically significant retention of sodium associated with a transient fall in urinary excretion of sodium but accompanied by an increased fecal content of sodium. The overall result, however, is an average retention of a few millimoles of sodium (31,32).

The reduced capacity of the kidneys in hypertensive rat strains to excrete sodium has been linked to several structural and functional renal abnormalities. In the SHR, the number of glomeruli (and therefore of nephrons) is significantly lower than in the normotensive WKY control (33). Furthermore, the number and diameter of glomerular fenestrated capillaries in the six-week-old SHR are significantly smaller than in the WKY rat, while the number of cytoplasmic ridges that course across the surface of the capillary endothelium, and thus influence its filtering surface, is increased. These changes may explain the SHR's lower glomerular capillary coefficient and filtration rate (34). A decrease in glomerular filtration rate reduces the rate of delivery of tubular fluid to the macula densa, the cells of which then signal the adjoining afferent arteriole to dilate.

This vascular dilatation increases the filtration rate and the delivery of tubular fluid to the macula densa and elevates urinary sodium excretion, the so-called tubuloglomerular feedback (35). In the normal animal, the sensitivity and reactivity of tubuloglomerular feedback increases when there is a need to conserve sodium, as in hemorrhage and dehydration (36,37) and diminishes when there is a prolonged need to increase sodium excretion, as in chronic salt loading (38,39) and deoxycorticosterone acetate administration (40,41). In the six-week-old SHR, when there is most evidence of sodium retention, tubuloglomerular feedback is increased (42,43). This paradoxical increase that should enhance sodium reabsorption is independent of the associated rise in blood pressure. Conversely, if the SHR is chronically loaded with salt, the resultant fall in tubuloglomerular feedback is less than in the salt loaded control WKY rat. By measuring tubuloglomerular feedback activity while perfusing the tubule with harvested tubular fluid from SHR and control rats, it has been demonstrated that the increase in tubuloglomerular feedback activity in the SHR is due to the defective action of a feedback inhibitory substance in the tubule fluid (44). The situation is similar in the Milan hypertensive strain rat. At 3.5 to 5 weeks when the Milan hypertensive strain rat is in a state of slight volume expansion, tubuloglomerular feedback activity is appropriately absent. Two weeks later, however, when the blood pressure starts to rise, tubuloglomerular feedback increases inappropriately to high levels, in turn diminishing the kidney's ability to excrete sodium (45).

Renal circulation is also perturbed in hereditary strains of hypertensive rats and may participate to the impaired renal capacity to excrete sodium. In the SHR, renal blood flow is reduced, like glomerular filtration rate, before the rise in blood pressure (46). The kidneys of immature pre-hypertensive SHR demonstrate a blunted pressure-natriuresis which worsens with maturity so that by the age of 10 to 20 weeks an increase in perfusion pressure of about 50 mmHg gives rise to only a fourfold rise in sodium excretion compared to a nine-fold increase in controls (47). In the SHR, this decrease seems to concern more specifically the medullary circulation. Measurements from the third to the sixteenth week show that whereas cortical and total blood flow in the SHR and WKY rat are similar, papillary blood flow in the SHR, at six and nine weeks onwards, is consistently less than in the WKY rat (48). It has been suggested that the increased medullary vascular tone prevents the normal increase in renal interstitial pressure upon which the mechanism of pressure-natriuresis depends and that the decreased papillary blood flow in the six and nine-week-old rat would enhance sodium reabsorption (49). There is evidence in the SHR that the circulatory abnormalities are related to local disturbances of arachidonic acid metabolism, particularly cytochrome P-450 dependent monooxygenase activity. Thus, higher levels of both cytochrome P-450 and its products are detected in renal microsomal fractions from 5 to 13 week-old SHR compared with WKY rat (50). Treatment with stannous chloride (which stimulates renal heme oxygenase production and so reduces the availability of heme for the formation of other hemoproteins including cytochrome P-450 monooxygenases) for four days causes a reduction of the blood pressure in seven-week-old SHR that is maintained for at least seven weeks and is associated with a natriuresis and a reduction in the renal content of cytochrome P-450 and its arachidonic acid metabolites (50). Stannous chloride does not affect the blood pressure of 20-week-old hypertensive SHR or WKY rats. The administration of stannous chloride to SHR from 5 to 13 weeks of age prevents the development of hypertension during this period and for seven weeks thereafter (51). There is also evidence of enhanced renal vascular tone and reactivity in Dahl salt sensitive rats, which both precede and accompany the rise in arterial pressure. The impaired pressure-natriuresis is due principally to a defect in the sensitivity of the tubule to alter sodium reabsorption in response to changes in interstitial pressure (52,53).

In the Dahl salt sensitive rat however, in contrast to the SHR, one factor responsible for the development of salt induced hypertension is an inability to increase vasodilatory nitric oxide production (54). In addition, there is an absence of vasodilatation to atrial natriuretic peptide and nitroprusside and an increased vasoconstrictive response to norepinephrine and angiotensin II (55).

Several abnormalities in trans-epithelial sodium reabsorption along the nephron have been described in hereditary strains of hypertensive rats, which may explain part of their reduced renal capacity to excrete sodium. In the SHR, there is an increase of the plasma's capacity to inhibit the Na-K-ATPase, which has a tendency to raise blood pressure by inhibiting the sodium–calcium exchange pump in vascular smooth muscle (56,57). It has been shown that acute volume expansion increases this plasma's capacity to inhibit the Na–K-ATPase in both the SHR and the Milan hypertensive rat. However, the nature of the plasma substance responsible for the Na–K-ATPase inhibition has been difficult to elucidate. In the Milan hypertensive rat strain, there is also an increase in the Na–K-ATPase activity which may be related to an abnormality of adducin, a cytoskeletal protein that modulates the activity of ion transport system in epithelial cells (58). Indeed, a mutation was found in this rat strain in two of the genes which code for adducin (59). The interaction of these missense mutations could explain up to 50% of blood pressure differences between the Milan hypertensive and its normotensive control. In the SHR, the activity of the Na–K-ATPase in five and eight-week-old rats is significantly higher in proximal tubules but significantly lower in the thick ascending limb of the loop of Henle compared to the WKY control rat, although these differences are no longer present at 20 weeks (60). An abnormality has also demonstrated in G-protein control of the Na–K-ATPase in suspensions of SHR renal proximal tubules, which may increase sodium reabsorption (61). In the Dahl salt sensitive hypertensive male rat, there is a significant mutation in the Na–K-ATPase α_1 catalytic subunit in the form of a leucine substitution for glutamine leading to a 3:1 sodium–potassium transport ratio instead of the normal 3:2 ratio in the normotensive salt resistant rat (62). This change would lead to an excess of sodium ions reabsorbed by the renal tubule for each potassium ion transported.

Associated with the upregulation of the Na–K-ATPase which mediates Na reabsorption across the basolateral membrane, there is an increase in the activity of the ion transport systems that allow entry of luminal sodium into the epithelial cells. Thus, apical membrane vesicles from young pre-hypertensive Milan hypertensive rats and SHR demonstrate an increased sodium uptake via sodium/proton exchange (63–65). The regulatory systems of tubular sodium reabsorption are also perturbed in the hypertensive rat strains. In the SHR, basal urinary dopamine production is normal but the rise following salt loading is greater in the SHR than in the WKY control rat (66). Nevertheless, the SHR is unable to eliminate an acute sodium load as efficiently as the WKY rat, and also exhibits a poor response to exogenous L-3,4 dihydroxyphenylalanine, dopamine or fenoldam, a D_{1A} receptor agonist (67,68). The fact that there is no evidence of defective binding of dopamine to the D_{1A} receptor in the proximal tubule of the SHR compared to the WKY rat (69,70) suggests that the abnormal dopamine response to salt loading in the SHR may be related to a post-translocation modification of the D_{1A} receptor, such as glycosylation, or that there is a defect distal to the D_{1A} receptor. In both the Dahl salt sensitive and salt resistant rats, salt loading increases urinary dopamine excretion, and, also in both, there is a blunted natriuretic response to exogenous dopamine compared with the Sprague–Dawley rat. In the Dahl salt sensitive rat, however, the impaired natriuretic response to salt loading is accompanied by evidence of defective coupling between the D_{1A} receptor and adenylcyclase (71,72).

The reduced capacity of the kidneys from hereditary hypertensive rats to excrete sodium leads to an elevation of blood pressure when dietary salt intake is high. This would involve both a rise in plasma sodium and an increase in extracellular fluid volume. It has been shown that an acute experimental increase in plasma sodium in rats can raise the blood pressure, in spite of a fall in extracellular volume (73). And in dogs a substantial acute increase in cerebrospinal fluid sodium (15 mmols/L) obtained by infusing hypertonic saline into the third ventricle raises the blood pressure within minutes (74), whereas a prolonged infusion which only raises cerebrospinal fluid sodium by about 4 to 5 mmols/L may take 6 to 10 days to raise the blood pressure (75). But it is possible that in normal circumstances it may be difficult to detect such a modest rise in plasma osmolarity (which is equivalent to a change in plasma sodium of less than 1%) that will still stimulate the thirst centre in the hypothalamus (76). The suggestion that in the SHR there is a rise in plasma osmolarity (sufficient to affect the hypothalamus) is also consistent with the finding that, though it suggests a state of continuous correction of a slightly expanded extracellular fluid volume that would tend to lower vasopressin secretion, yet both plasma and urinary arginine vasopressin are raised (77). There is one study in the SHR and WKY control rat in which plasma sodium was measured at one and two hour intervals throughout the 24 hours (78). Plasma sodium was about 1 to 3 mmols/L greater in the SHR than in the WKY rat throughout the 24 hours. Overall therefore acute experimental increases in plasma or cerebrospinal fluid sodium concentration greater than 5 mmols/L can raise the blood pressure, independent of the extracellular fluid volume. The rate of rise in the blood pressure in such experiments is related to the extent of the rise in sodium concentration. It is proposed that with the 1 to 3 mmols/L rise in sodium concentration that appear to occur in hypertension the delay is likely to be considerably longer and that such an increase in plasma sodium not only tends to increase the extracellular fluid volume but may itself be a primary factor in the pressor effect of dietary salt (79). Measurement of the extracellular volume expansion in hypertensive animals is also difficult due to its modest magnitude. In the SHR, the extracellular volume or exchangeable sodium are significantly greater than in the WKY control rat (29,30,32). In the Milan hypertensive rat however, exchangeable sodium is not significantly different from that of the Milan normotensive rat (31,32). Perhaps the most striking evidence in favor of the proposition that in hypertension there is a state of continuous correction of a slightly expanded extracellular fluid volume is the exaggerated natriuretic response of SHR to a rapid saline infusion, which does not occur in control rats (80). Such a response is well-documented in circumstances in which there is a tightly controlled state of volume expansion and in normal animals given aldosterone, even when it may not be possible to detect an increase in extracellular volume (81).

GENETICALLY ENGINEERED MOUSE STRAINS WITH A PRIMARY DEFECT IN RENAL SODIUM HANDLING

During the last decade, the use of gene targeting techniques in the mouse has made it possible to assess the effect of a primary defect in the genes encoding renal sodium transport systems or their regulatory pathways. Their individual participation and their integration into the overall renal function can thus be directly investigated. In the majority of cases, these mutations trigger a chronic change of blood pressure in adult mice (7). Mutations increasing renal sodium reabsorption raise blood pressure whereas those diminishing sodium reabsorption lower blood pressure. Of interest, all the genes identified as being directly involved in renal sodium handling and blood pressure control in mice are also found to regulate the same processes in humans, indicating a high evolutionary conservation of the underlying molecular mechanisms (6). Like in humans, renal sodium handling and blood pressure levels appear not to be determined by the preponderant action of a few genes but rather by a large number of genes each having a relatively small effect. Overall, the currently available genetic data strongly reinforce the concept that regulation of extracellular fluid volume by the kidneys is the major blood pressure control mechanism in the long term (82).

Epithelial Sodium Channel

The amiloride-sensitive epithelial sodium channel (ENaC) is the rate-limiting step in salt reabsorption in the terminal part of the nephron. The three genes encoding the ENaC subunits (α,β,γ) have been found in humans to harbor mutations or polymorphisms related to gain or loss of function of the channel, increased or decreased renal sodium reabsorption and high or low blood pressure (83). The truncation of the β subunit deleting a critical proline-rich region of the cytosolic tail that interacts with a regulatory protein called Nedd4 (84), thus resulting in an accumulation of ENaC in the luminal membrane and an increased sodium reabsorption, has been reproduced in the mouse using gene targeting and Cre/loxP techniques (85). Under low-salt diet, the homozygous mutated mice have a blood pressure not different from wild-type mice despite evidence for chronic hypervolemia such as increased sodium reabsorption in distal colon and low plasma aldosterone. Under high-salt diet, the mice develop hypokalemic metabolic alkalosis, high blood pressure with suppressed aldosterone secretion thus reproducing to a large extent the human Liddle's syndrome. A mouse model for pseudohypoaldosteronism type 1 has also been generated by disrupting the gene encoding the β subunit (86). On a high salt intake, homozygous β subunit-deficient mice exhibit elevated plasma aldosterone level and compensated metabolic acidosis compared to wild-type mice, but no change in blood pressure. When fed a low-salt diet, these mice develop features of an acute pseudohypoaldosteronism type 1 with weight loss, salt wasting in the urine, hyperkalemia, decreased blood pressure, and they are unable to survive more than a few weeks after the dietary switch. Recently, a selective inactivation of the gene encoding the β subunit has been achieved by using Cre-loxP technology and a tissue-specific promoter (Hoxb7) expressed along the collecting duct but not in the upstream late distal convoluted tubule and connecting tubule where ENaC expression is left intact (87). In these conditions, the mice subjected to a low sodium intake are still able to maintain their sodium balance, despite the fact that the apical accumulation of ENaC is strictly limited to the late distal convoluted tubule and connecting tubule. This shows that the expression of ENaC in the collecting duct is not critical for achieving sodium balance and that more proximal ENaC containing segments (i.e., late distal convoluted tubule and connecting tubule) are probably sufficient for maintaining the balance (88). This point is consistent with the variation of the distribution pattern of ENaC from the late portion of the distal convoluted tubule down to the collecting duct in response to changes in dietary salt intake. Indeed, when wild-type mice are fed a low-salt diet in the physiological range, the translocation of the β and γ subunits from intracellular membranous dispersed sites to the apical plasma membrane takes place mainly in the late part of the distal convoluted tubule and in the connecting tubule, the collecting duct being practically not affected (89).

Sodium–Chloride Cotransport

Homozygous Sodium–Chloride Cotransport (NCC) deficient mouse strain with a phenotype similar to the human Gitelman's syndrome have been generated (90). These mice exhibit low rates of urinary calcium excretion and low plasma magnesium concentrations together with some evidence of salt wasting (increased plasma aldosterone and low blood pressure under dietary sodium restriction) and compensated metabolic alkalosis (91). In contrast to the human syndrome, the NCC-deficient mice do not manifest hypokalemia. This discrepancy may be explained by species differences, but may be also related to ascertainment bias in identifying patients with Gitelman's syndrome. Indeed, hypokalemia is among the inclusion criteria used to diagnose the syndrome and it is therefore not surprising to find these features in all clinically defined patients. It is possible that in other individuals, mutations in the NCC gene provoke only hypomagnesemia and hypocalciuria without hypokalemia due to a different genetic background. This hypothesis could be tested both by searching for subsets of patients without hypokalemia and by looking at the phenotype of NCC-deficient mice in different genetic inbred backgrounds. Immunocytochemistry studies show that the initial part of the distal convoluted tubule is completely missing in the NCC-deficient mice, so that the cortical thick ascending limb characterized by the expression of the sodium/potassium/chloride cotransport (NKCC2) is directly in continuity with the late distal convoluted tubule that expresses ENaC (92). Given that NCC normally reabsorbs about 7% of the filtered sodium load along the distal convoluted tubule, the loss of function of the transporter significantly increases sodium delivery to the connecting tubule and collecting duct. As expected according to the increased plasma aldosterone, the amount of ENaC is upregulated in the apical membrane of principal cells along the connecting tubule (92). This compensatory phenomenon is not observed in the collecting duct suggesting that the increased ENaC-mediated sodium reabsorption in the late distal tubule and connecting tubule is sufficient to compensate for NCC inactivation (88).

NKCC2 and Potassium Channel (ROMK1)

Loss of function mutations in NKCC2 and ROMK1 have been associated to Bartter's syndrome in humans (93,94), a disorder characterized by severe salt wasting and low blood pressure despite elevated plasma renin and aldosterone levels (95). These two genes are expressed in the thick ascending limb of Henle's loop where they are involved either directly (NKCC2) or indirectly (ROMK1) in sodium reabsorption. Homozygous NKCC2 deficient mice have many similarities with patients with Bartter's syndrome. These mice display signs of dehydration (increased hematocrit) as early as one day after birth. They fail to thrive and usually die before weaning. After one week, they exhibit hyperkalemic metabolic acidosis, hydronephrosis and an upregulation of the renin–angiotensin system as observed in some human perinatal cases of Bartter's syndrome. When treated with indomethacin, some mice can survive to the adult stage but then exhibit severe polyuria and hydronephrosis, hypokalemic metabolic alkalosis and hypercalciuria (96). In addition, they are hypotensive on a high-salt diet and do not survive on a low-salt diet. Thus, the complete absence of NKCC2 causes polyuria and low blood pressure that cannot be compensated elsewhere along the nephron. In contrast, heterozygous mutant mice can compensate entirely for the loss of one copy of the gene and the resulting 50% reduction in renal mRNA expression of NKCC2, apparently by restoring the protein level to near normal in the apical membrane; these mutant mice are identical to wild-type mice considering blood pressure, blood gas, electrolytes, creatinine, plasma renin concentration, urine volume and osmolality, ability to concentrate and dilute urine and response to furosemide (97). Homozygous ROMK1 deficient mice also develop hydronephrosis and are severely dehydrated; most of them die before three weeks of age. The mice that survived beyond weaning grow to adulthood and show features of Bartter's syndrome such as metabolic acidosis, elevated blood concentrations of sodium and chloride, reduced blood pressure, polydipsia, polyuria and poor urinary concentrating ability. Whole kidney glomerular filtration rate is sharply reduced, apparently as a result of hydronephrosis, and fractional excretion of electrolytes is elevated. Single nephron glomerular filtration rate is relatively normal, absorption of sodium in the thick ascending limb of Henle's loop is reduced but not eliminated, and tubuloglomerular feedback is severely impaired (98).

Sodium/Proton Exchanger 3

Most of the filtered sodium load is reabsorbed in the proximal convoluted tubule and mutations or polymorphisms in genes encoding proximal sodium transport systems have the potential to significantly alter extracellular fluid volume and blood pressure. A mouse model with a targeted disruption of the Sodium/Proton Exchanger 3 (NHE3) gene demonstrates the importance of proximal sodium reabsorption in the long-term control of blood pressure. On a high-salt diet, homozygous NHE3 deficient mice are hypotensive, hyperkalemic, and acidotic (99). The large reduction of fluid reabsorption in the proximal convoluted tubule overloads downstream segments of the nephron, which develop compensatory responses for increasing distal sodium and bicarbonate reabsorption (100). Thus, in parallel to a strong activation of the renin–angiotensin–aldosterone axis, ENaC γ subunit abundance is higher in the kidneys of these mice (101). The main renal compensatory mechanism seems to be the decrease in single-nephron glomerular filtration rate, which is mediated in part by the activation of tubuloglomerular feedback (102,103). Nevertheless, these adaptive processes are insufficient to fully compensate for the large reduction of proximal sodium reabsorption, and NHE3 deficient mice display significant urinary salt wasting and cannot survive on a low-salt diet (104). It can be also mentioned that in contrast to NCC and NKCC2 which are specifically expressed in the kidneys, NHE3 is strongly expressed along the intestine where the exchanger normally mediates sodium and bicarbonate reabsorption (105). It is therefore not surprising that NHE3 deficient mice have intestinal defects resulting in diarrhea and a marked increase in the volume content of the distal segments of the intestine despite the presence of a number of compensatory mechanisms occurring to limit fluid wasting in the feces (99). For example, mRNAs encoding ENaC β and γ subunits are upregulated and trans-epithelial amiloride-sensitive sodium current is sharply increased in the distal colon in parallel to the high plasma aldosterone level. The recent development of homozygous NHE3 deficient mice with transgenic expression of NHE3 in the small intestine has allowed the assessment of the specific role of the renal NHE3 in overall maintenance of blood pressure and pressure natriuresis (106). Blood pressure is lower in transgenic homozygous NHE3 deficient mice than in transgenic wild-type controls when the mice are maintained on a relatively low-sodium diet but is normalized when they are provided with a high sodium intake. Administration of an AT1-receptor blocker shows that angiotensin II plays a major role in maintaining blood pressure in transgenic homozygous NHE3 deficient mice fed a low-sodium diet but not in those receiving a high-sodium diet. Clearance studies reveal a blunted pressure natriuresis response at lower blood pressures but a robust response at higher blood pressures. These data show that NHE3 has an important role in the diuretic and natriuretic responses to increases in blood pressure but also show that mechanisms not involving NHE3 mediate pressure natriuresis in the higher range of blood pressure.

Regulatory Systems

Several regulatory systems are involved in the complex physiological scheme that has evolved to regulate urinary excretion of salt, sodium balance and blood pressure. Aldosterone synthesis and signaling pathways play a major role in the control of sodium reabsorption in the distal parts of the nephron (107). Homozygous mineralocorticoid receptor deficient mice die in the second week after birth, showing symptoms of pseudohypoaldosteronism with hyponatremia, hyperkalemia, marked renal salt wasting and a strongly activated renin–angiotensin–aldosterone system (108). The activity of ENaC is strongly reduced in colon and kidneys. Daily subcutaneous injections of isotonic salt solution until weaning and continued oral NaCl supply lead to survival of the homozygous mice. The salt-rescued mice display almost no renal ENaC activity, a strongly enhanced fractional renal excretion of sodium, hyperkalemia and a persistently activated renin–angiotensin–aldosterone system. Homozygous mice deficient in the 11β-hydroxysteroid dehydrogenase type II (11β-HSD2), which insures the specificity of in vivo mineralocorticoid receptor activation by aldosterone by metabolizing the excess of cortisol to cortisone, appear normal at birth although approximately half of them show motor weakness and die within 48 hours (109). Survivors are markedly hypertensive and exhibit hypokalemia, hypotonic polyuria and apparent mineralocorticoid activity of corticosterone. The epithelium of the distal parts of the nephron shows striking hypertrophy and hyperplasia that do not readily reverse with mineralocorticoid receptor antagonism. Thus, 11β-HSD2 deficient mice display a phenotype directly comparable to the syndrome of apparent mineralocorticoid excess in humans carrying inactivating mutations of the 11β-HSD2 gene (107). The effects of aldosterone and other hormonal (insulin) and non-hormonal (osmolarity) regulators on sodium transport in the colon and distal nephron are mediated in part by a serine/threonine serum and glucocorticoid-regulated kinase (SGK1). In particular, aldosterone-activated mineralocorticoid receptor induces the synthesis of SGK1 that in turn modulates the activity of channels such as ENaC (110). Homozygous SGK1 deficient mice display renal water and electrolyte excretion indistinguishable from that of wild-type mice on a high salt intake. However, dietary salt restriction reveals an impaired ability of these mice to adequately decrease sodium excretion despite increased plasma aldosterone levels and proximal tubular sodium and fluid reabsorption and decreased blood pressure and glomerular filtration rate (111). Angiotensin II is one of the main controllers of aldosterone release from the adrenals and it also stimulates directly renal sodium reabsorption in the proximal and distal tubules through type 1 angiotensin II receptor (AT1R). Mouse strains with one, two, three or four functional copies of the AT1R gene demonstrate a causal link between angiotensin II and blood pressure (112,113). Interestingly, compared to wild-type mice, blood pressure of homozygous AT1R deficient mice is very sensitive to changes in dietary salt intake whereas the hypertension displayed by homozygous type 2 angiotensin II receptor (AT2R) deficient mice is not salt-sensitive (114,115). The role of the AT2R remains unclear although it is possible that this receptor type may have an hypotensive effect antagonist to the hypertensive effect of AT1R as suggested by the observed hypertension in homozygous AT2R deficient mice (115).

The dopaminergic and renin–angiotensin systems counter-regulate renal sodium reabsorption. The inhibitory effect of dopamine is most evident under conditions of moderate sodium excess while the stimulatory effect of angiotensin II is prominent during sodium deficit. Dopamine is synthesized within the proximal tubule and exerts its effects through at least three receptor subtypes (116). The D_1 receptor inhibits the Na–K-ATPase and NHE3. Thus, activation of the D_1 receptor results in an increase of natriuresis and diuresis and a stimulation of renal renin release. In contrast, inhibition of the D_1 receptor leads to sodium retention and simultaneously produces a low renin state. The effect of D_{1A} receptor loss on blood pressure is evident in heterozygous and homozygous null mice which both develop hypertension (117). The D_3 receptor, which is located in juxtaglomerular cells, also seems to be an important regulator of sodium transport and blood pressure. Homozygous or heterozygous D_3 deficient mice exhibit a decrease in urinary sodium excretion rate when they are volume expanded. These mice also have elevated blood pressure and high plasma renin, suggesting an inhibitory role of the D_3 receptor on renin release (118). Recently, the generation of mice lacking the D_2 receptor has produced evidence for the involvement of this receptor subtype in sodium handling and blood pressure control. A high-salt diet causes a significant increase in systolic blood pressure in homozygous D_2 deficient mice but not in wild-type mice (119). The absence of a functional D_2 receptor is also associated to a state of sodium retention when the animals are fed a high-salt diet. These results suggest that the D_2 receptor promotes urinary sodium excretion and may participate to sodium-dependent blood pressure elevation. A G protein-coupled receptor kinase has been shown to be a major regulator of dopamine receptors in the kidney (120). Mice overexpressing a variant with an increased enzymatic activity resulting in the phosphorylation and uncoupling of the D_1 dopamine receptor from its G protein and effector complexes in the proximal tubule, develop hypertension and impaired diuretic and natriuretic responses to D_1-like agonist stimulation (121).

Several peptides synthesized in the heart, the gastrointestinal tract, the kidneys and/or the central nervous system induce a natriuretic effect associated to a decrease in blood pressure (122). This is the case for atriopeptin-A, atriopeptin-B, and uroguanylin, which are respectively formed in the myocardium and the gastrointestinal tract. These peptides are also produced locally in the kidneys where they could participate in intra-renal mechanisms controlling tubular sodium transport and thus contribute to the natriuresis elicited by high dietary salt intake. Among the receptor subtypes that implement the effect of atriopeptins, the guanylcyclase natriuretic peptide receptor A (NPRA) seems to be directly involved in blood pressure control. The existence of a linear relationship between the number of functional NPRA gene copies and blood pressure has been demonstrated in mice (123). Homozygous mice lacking atriopeptin-A have slightly increased blood pressure and develop a marked hypertension on a moderately elevated salt diet, similar to that observed in heterozygous deficient mice fed a high-salt diet (124,125). The targeted disruption of the NPRA gene also leads to the development of hypertension in homozygous mice but the elevation of blood pressure is not sensitive to dietary salt intake (126). Recently, homozygous mice lacking uroguanylin have been generated; these mice have an impaired capacity to excrete salt in urine when subjected to oral salt loads and display an increased blood pressure that is independent of the level of dietary salt intake (127). These findings establish the existence of an endocrine axis linking together the gastrointestinal tract and the kidneys via uroguanylin serving as a natriuretic hormone produced by the stomach and/or intestine and released into the circulatory system when excess salt is ingested. Another important natriuretic system is based on the γ-melanocyte-stimulating hormone (γ-MSH) produced from proopiomelanocortin (POMC) by the prohormone convertase 2 (PC2) in the pituitary gland (128). The synthesis of POMC and PC2 is induced by a high dietary salt intake, thus increasing the release of γ-MSH into the circulation; γ-MSH promotes urinary salt excretion via the melanocortin receptor type 3 (MC3R) expressed in the kidneys. The natriuretic role of γ-MSH has been demonstrated in homozygous mice lacking either PC2 or MC3R, which develop a marked hypertension when fed a high-salt diet (129).

CONCLUSION

Our understanding of renal sodium handling abnormalities has greatly expanded since the early experiments in the 1930s using surgically altered animals. During the last decades, the analysis of spontaneous, selected or genetically engineered animal strains has provided a large body of data concerning the role of the different renal sodium transport systems and of their regulatory pathways. In particular, these approaches have unequivocally established that abnormal renal sodium handling directly affects long-term regulation of extracellular volume and blood pressure. The last technical development, i.e., gene targeting in the mouse, gives in theory the opportunity to systematically apply a single-factor strategy that should help decipher the integration of each sodium transport or regulatory system into renal and whole-body physiology. In practice, this will necessitate a better control of the experimental conditions (both environmental and genetic) that could be only attained by significantly increasing the scale of the experiments. The data obtained in animal models are until now remarkably consistent with those gained in humans by genetic analysis of candidate genes, linkage studies, and positional cloning in clinically characterized pedigrees (6). However, some species differences will remain as an inescapable limit of these approaches. For example, it is obvious that the efficiency of the homeostatic mechanisms that maintain sodium balance is very different in animals in which the entire extracellular fluid volume is filtered through renal glomeruli 15 times per day (humans), 50 times per day (rats) or 100 times per day (mice) (14).

REFERENCES

1. Williams SM, Haines JL, Moore JH. The use of animal models in the study of complex disease: all else is never equal or why do so many human studies fail to replicate animal findings? Bioessays 2004; 26:170–9.
2. Kiberstis P, Roberts L. It's not just the genes. Science 2002; 296:685.
3. Montagutelli X. Effect of the genetic background on the phenotype of mouse mutations. J Am Soc Nephrol 2000; 11(Suppl. 16):S101–5.
4. Pearson H. Surviving a knockout blow. Nature 2002; 415:8–9.
5. Sanford LP, Kallapur S, Ormsby I, et al. Influence of genetic background on knockout mouse phenotypes. Methods Mol Biol 2001; 158:217–25.
6. Meneton P, Jeunemaitre X, de Wardener HE, et al. Links between dietary salt intake, renal salt handling, blood pressure, and cardiovascular diseases. Physiol Rev 2005; 85:679–715.
7. Meneton P, Warnock DG. Involvement of renal apical Na transport systems in the control of blood pressure. Am J Kidney Dis 2001; 37:S39–47.
8. Goldblatt H, Lynch J, Hanzal RF, et al. Studies of experimental hypertension. I. Production of persistent elevation of systolic blood pressure by means of renal ischemia. J Exp Med 1934; 59:347–79.
9. Lerman LO, Schwartz RS, Grande JP, et al. Noninvasive evaluation of a novel swine model of renal artery stenosis. J Am Soc Nephrol 1999; 10:1455–65.
10. Panek RL, Ryan MJ, Weishaar RE, et al. Development of a high renin model of hypertension in the cynomolgus monkey. Clin Exp Hypertens A 1991; 13:1395–414.
11. Pickering GW, Prinzmetal M. Experimental hypertension of renal origin in the rabbit. Clin Sci 1937; 3:357–68.
12. Wiesel P, Mazzolai L, Nussberger J, et al. Two-kidney, one clip and one-kidney, one clip hypertension in mice. Hypertension 1997; 29:1025–30.
13. Wilson C, Byrom FB. Renal changes in malignant hypertension. Lancet 1939; 1:136–9.
14. Schnermann J, Briggs JP. The macula densa is worth its salt. J Clin Invest 1999; 104:1007–9.
15. Romero JC, Fiksen-Olsen MJ, Schryver S. Pathophysiology of hypertension: the use of experimental models to understand the clinical features of the hypertensive disease. In: Spittel JA, Jr., ed. Clinical Medicine. Vol. 7. Philadelphia, PA: Harper & Row, 1981:1–51.
16. Della Bruna R, Bernhard I, Gess B, et al. Renin gene and angiotensin II AT1 receptor gene expression in the kidneys of normal and of two-kidney/one-clip rats. Pflugers Arch 1995; 430:265–72.

17. Romero JC, Knox FG. Mechanisms underlying pressure-related natriuresis: the role of the renin–angiotensin and prostaglandin systems. State of the art lecture. Hypertension 1988; 11:724–38.
18. Stella A, Zanchetti A. Interactions between the sympathetic nervous system and the kidney: experimental observations. J Hypertens Suppl 1985; 3:S19–25.
19. Mohring J, Mohring B, Naumann HJ, et al. Salt and water balance and renin activity in renal hypertension of rats. Am J Physiol 1975; 228:1847–55.
20. Machida J, Ueda S, Yoshida M, et al. Role of sodium and renal prostaglandin E2 in the maintenance of hypertension in the chronic phase of two-kidney one-clip renovascular hypertension in rabbits. Nephron 1988; 49:74–80.
21. Miksche LW, Miksche U, Gross F. Effect of sodium restriction on renal hypertension and on renin activity in the rat. Circ Res 1970; 27:973–84.
22. Bianchi G, Fox U, Di Francesco GF, et al. The hypertensive role of the kidney in spontaneously hypertensive rats. Clin Sci Mol Med Suppl 1973; 45(Suppl. 1):135S–9.
23. Dahl LK, Heine M, Thompson K. Genetic influence of renal homografts on the blood pressure of rats from different strains. Proc Soc Exp Biol Med 1972; 140:852–6.
24. Dahl LK, Heine M, Thompson K. Genetic influence of the kidneys on blood pressure. Evidence from chronic renal homografts in rats with opposite predispositions to hypertension. Circ Res 1974; 40:94–101.
25. Greene AS, Yu ZY, Roman RJ, et al. Role of blood volume expansion in Dahl rat model of hypertension. Am J Physiol 1990; 258:H508–14.
26. Morgan DA, DiBona GF, Mark AL. Effects of interstrain renal transplantation on NaCl-induced hypertension in Dahl rats. Hypertension 1990; 15:436–42.
27. Rettig R, Folberth C, Stauss H, et al. Role of the kidney in primary hypertension: a renal transplantation study in rats. Am J Physiol 1990; 258:F606–11.
28. Heller J, Schubert G, Havlickova J, et al. The role of the kidney in the development of hypertension: a transplantation study in the Prague hypertensive rat. Pflugers Arch 1993; 425:208–12.
29. Mullins MM. Body fluid volumes in prehypertensive spontaneously hypertensive rats. Am J Physiol 1983; 244:H652–5.
30. Toal CB, Leenen FH. Body fluid volumes during development of hypertension in the spontaneously hypertensive rat. J Hypertens 1983; 1:345–50.
31. Bianchi G, Baer PG, Fox U, et al. Changes in renin, water balance, and sodium balance during development of high blood pressure in genetically hypertensive rats. Circ Res 1975; 36:153–61.
32. Harrap SB. Genetic analysis of blood pressure and sodium balance in spontaneously hypertensive rats. Hypertension 1986; 8:572–82.
33. Skov K, Nyengaard JR, Korsgaard N, et al. Number and size of renal glomeruli in spontaneously hypertensive rats. J Hypertens 1994; 12:1373–6.
34. Gebremedhin D, Fenoy FJ, Harder DR, et al. Enhanced vascular tone in the renal vasculature of spontaneously hypertensive rats. Hypertension 1990; 16:648–54.
35. Haberle DA, von Baeyer H. Characteristics of glomerulotubular balance. Am J Physiol 1983; 244:F355–66.
36. Kaufman JS, Hamburger RJ, Flamenbaum W. Tubuloglomerular feedback response after hypotensive hemorrhage. Ren Physiol 1982; 5:173–81.
37. Persson AE, Boberg U, Hahne B, et al. Interstitial pressure as a modulator of tubuloglomerular feedback control. Kidney Int Suppl 1982; 12:S122–8.
38. Haberle DA, Davis JM. Resetting of tubuloglomerular feedback: evidence for a humoral factor in tubular fluid. Am J Physiol 1984; 246:F495–500.
39. Schnermann J, Schubert G, Briggs J. Tubuloglomerular feedback responses with native and artificial tubular fluid. Am J Physiol 1986; 250:F16–21.
40. Moore LC, Mason J. Tubuloglomerular feedback control of distal fluid delivery: effect of extracellular volume. Am J Physiol 1986; 250:F1024–32.

41. Schnermann J, Hermle M, Schmidmeier E, et al. Impaired potency for feedback regulation of glomerular filtration rate in DOCA escaped rats. Pflugers Arch 1975; 358:325–38.
42. Dilley JR, Arendshorst WJ. Enhanced tubuloglomerular feedback activity in rats developing spontaneous hypertension. Am J Physiol 1984; 247:F672–9.
43. Ploth DW, Dahlheim H, Schmidmeier E, et al. Tubuloglomerular feedback and autoregulation of glomerular filtration rate in Wistar–Kyoto spontaneously hypertensive rats. Pflugers Arch 1978; 375:261–7.
44. Ushiogi Y, Takabatake T, Haberle DA. Blood pressure and tubuloglomerular feedback mechanism in chronically salt-loaded spontaneously hypertensive rats. Kidney Int 1991; 39:1184–92.
45. McDonald SJ, de Wardener HE. The relationship between the renal arterial perfusion pressure and the increase in sodium excretion which occurs during an infusion of saline. Nephron 1965; 10:1–14.
46. Dilley JR, Stier CT, Jr., Arendshorst WJ. Abnormalities in glomerular function in rats developing spontaneous hypertension. Am J Physiol 1984; 246:F12–20.
47. Roman RJ, Cowley AW, Jr. Abnormal pressure-diuresis–natriuresis response in spontaneously hypertensive rats. Am J Physiol 1985; 248:F199–205.
48. Cowley AW, Jr., Mattson DL, Lu S, et al. The renal medulla and hypertension. Hypertension 1995; 25:663–73.
49. Roman RJ, Kaldunski ML. Renal cortical and papillary blood flow in spontaneously hypertensive rats. Hypertension 1988; 11:657–63.
50. Sacerdoti D, Abraham NG, McGiff JC, et al. Renal cytochrome P-450-dependent metabolism of arachidonic acid in spontaneously hypertensive rats. Biochem Pharmacol 1988; 37:521–7.
51. Escalante B, Sacerdoti D, Davidian MM, et al. Chronic treatment with tin normalizes blood pressure in spontaneously hypertensive rats. Hypertension 1991; 17:776–9.
52. Roman RJ. Abnormal renal hemodynamics and pressure–natriuresis relationship in Dahl salt-sensitive rats. Am J Physiol 1986; 251:F57–65.
53. Roman RJ. Alterations in renal medullary hemodynamics and the pressure–natriuretic response in genetic hypertension. Am J Hypertens 1990; 3:893–900.
54. Chen PY, Sanders PW. L-Arginine abrogates salt-sensitive hypertension in Dahl/Rapp rats. J Clin Invest 1991; 88:1559–67.
55. Simchon S, Manger WM, Shi GS, et al. Impaired renal vascular reactivity in prehypertensive Dahl salt-sensitive rats. Hypertension 1992; 20:524–32.
56. de Wardener HE, MacGregor GA. The relation of a circulating sodium transport inhibitor (the natriuretic hormone?) to hypertension Medicine (Baltimore) 1983; 62:310–26.
57. Blaustein MP. Sodium ions, calcium ions, blood pressure regulation, and hypertension: a reassessment and a hypothesis. Am J Physiol 1977; 232:C165–73.
58. Bianchi G, Tripodi G, Casari G, et al. Two point mutations within the adducin genes are involved in blood pressure variation. Proc Natl Acad Sci USA 1994; 91:3999–4003.
59. Bianchi G, Tripodi G. Genetics of hypertension: the adducin paradigm. Ann NY Acad Sci 2003; 986:660–8.
60. Garg LC, Narang N, McArdle S. Na–K-ATPase in nephron segments of rats developing spontaneous hypertension. Am J Physiol 1985; 249:F863–9.
61. Gurich RW, Beach RE. Abnormal regulation of renal proximal tubule Na–K-ATPase by G proteins in spontaneously hypertensive rats. Am J Physiol 1994; 267:F1069–75.
62. Herrera VL, Xie HX, Lopez LV, et al. The alpha1 Na, K-ATPase gene is a susceptibility hypertension gene in the Dahl salt-sensitive HSD rat. J Clin Invest 1998; 102:1102–11.
63. Morduchowicz GA, Sheikh-Hamad D, Jo OD, et al. Increased Na/H antiport activity in the renal brush border membrane of SHR. Kidney Int 1989; 36:576–81.
64. Lewis JL, Warnock DG. Renal apical membrane sodium–hydrogen exchange in genetic salt-sensitive hypertension. Hypertension 1994; 24:491–8.
65. Parenti P, Hanozet GM, Bianchi G. Sodium and glucose transport across renal brush border membranes of Milan hypertensive rats. Hypertension 1986; 8:932–9.

66. Stier CT, Itskovitz HD, Chen YH. Urinary dopamine and sodium excretion in spontaneously hypertensive rats. Clin Exp Hypertens 1993; 15:105–23.
67. Chen CJ, Lokhandwala MF. An impairment of renal tubular DA-1 receptor function as the causative factor for diminished natriuresis to volume expansion in spontaneously hypertensive rats. Clin Exp Hypertens A 1992; 14:615–28.
68. Felder RA, Seikaly MG, Cody P, et al. Attenuated renal response to dopaminergic drugs in spontaneously hypertensive rats. Hypertension 1990; 15:560–9.
69. Kinoshita S, Sidhu A, Felder RA. Defective dopamine-1 receptor adenylate cyclase coupling in the proximal convoluted tubule from the spontaneously hypertensive rat. J Clin Invest 1989; 84:1849–56.
70. Sidhu A, Vachvanichsanong P, Jose PA, et al. Persistent defective coupling of dopamine-1 receptors to G proteins after solubilization from kidney proximal tubules of hypertensive rats. J Clin Invest 1992; 89:789–93.
71. Felder RA, Kinoshita S, Sidhu A, et al. A renal dopamine-1 receptor defect in two genetic models of hypertension. Am J Hypertens 1990; 3:96S–9.
72. Nishi A, Eklof AC, Bertorello AM, et al. Dopamine regulation of renal Na, K-ATPase activity is lacking in Dahl salt-sensitive rats. Hypertension 1993; 21:767–71.
73. Friedman SM, McIndoe RA, Tanaka M. The relation of blood sodium concentration to blood pressure in the rat. J Hypertens 1990; 8:61–6.
74. Andersson B, Eriksson L, Fernandez O, et al. Centrally mediated effects of sodium and angiotensin II on arterial blood pressure and fluid balance. Acta Physiol Scand 1972; 85:398–407.
75. Seshiah PN, Weber DS, Rocic P, et al. Angiotensin II stimulation of NAD(P)H oxidase activity: upstream mediators. Circ Res 2002; 91:406–13.
76. Fitzsimons JT. The effects of slow infusions of hypertonic solutions on drinking and drinking thresholds in rats. J Physiol 1963; 167:344–54.
77. de Wardener HE. The hypothalamus and hypertension. Physiol Rev 2001; 81:1599–658.
78. Fang Z, Carlson SH, Peng N, et al. Circadian rhythm of plasma sodium is disrupted in spontaneously hypertensive rats fed a high-NaCl diet. Am J Physiol Regul Integr Comp Physiol 2000; 278:R1490–5.
79. He FJ, Markandu ND, Sagnella GA, et al. Plasma sodium: ignored and underestimated. Hypertension 2005; 45:98–102.
80. Ben-Ishay D, Knudsen KD, Dahl LK. Exaggerated response to isotonic saline loading in genetically hypertension-prone rats. J Lab Clin Med 1973; 82:597–604.
81. Willis LR, Bauer JH. Aldosterone in the exaggerated natriuresis of spontaneously hypertensive rats. Am J Physiol 1978; 234:F29–35.
82. Guyton AC. Blood pressure control-special role of the kidneys and body fluids. Science 1991; 252:1813–6.
83. Rossier BC, Pradervand S, Schild L, et al. Epithelial sodium channel and the control of sodium balance: interaction between genetic and environmental factors. Annu Rev Physiol 2002; 64:877–97.
84. Abriel H, Loffing J, Rebhun JF, et al. Defective regulation of the epithelial Na channel by Nedd4 in Liddle's syndrome. J Clin Invest 1999; 103:667–73.
85. Pradervand S, Wang Q, Burnier M, et al. A mouse model for Liddle's syndrome. J Am Soc Nephrol 1999; 10:2527–33.
86. Pradervand S, Barker PM, Wang Q, et al. Salt restriction induces pseudohypoaldosteronism type 1 in mice expressing low levels of the beta-subunit of the amiloride-sensitive epithelial sodium channel. Proc Natl Acad Sci USA 1999; 96:1732–7.
87. Rubera I, Loffing J, Palmer LG, et al. Collecting duct-specific gene inactivation of alphaENaC in the mouse kidney does not impair sodium and potassium balance. J Clin Invest 2003; 112:554–65.
88. Meneton P, Loffing J, Warnock DG. Sodium and potassium handling by the aldosterone-sensitive distal nephron: the pivotal role of the distal and connecting tubule. Am J Physiol Renal Physiol 2004; 287:F593–601.

89. Loffing J, Pietri L, Aregger F, et al. Differential subcellular localization of ENaC subunits in mouse kidney in response to high- and low-Na diets. Am J Physiol Renal Physiol 2000; 279:F252–8.
90. Schultheis PJ, Lorenz JN, Meneton P, et al. Phenotype resembling Gitelman's syndrome in mice lacking the apical Na–Cl cotransporter of the distal convoluted tubule. J Biol Chem 1998; 273:29150–5.
91. Nicolet-Barousse L, Blanchard A, Roux C, et al. Inactivation of the Na–Cl co-transporter (NCC) gene is associated with high BMD through both renal and bone mechanisms: analysis of patients with Gitelman syndrome and NCC null mice. J Bone Miner Res 2005; 20:799–808.
92. Loffing J, Vallon V, Loffing-Cueni D, et al. Altered renal distal tubule structure and renal Na and Ca handling in a mouse model for Gitelman's syndrome. J Am Soc Nephrol 2004; 15:2276–88.
93. Simon DB, Karet FE, Hamdan JM, et al. Bartter's syndrome, hypokalaemic alkalosis with hypercalciuria, is caused by mutations in the Na–K–2Cl cotransporter NKCC2. Nat Genet 1996; 13:183–8.
94. Simon DB, Karet FE, Rodriguez-Soriano J, et al. Genetic heterogeneity of Bartter's syndrome revealed by mutations in the K channel, ROMK. Nat Genet 1996; 14:152–6.
95. Bartter FC, Pronove P, Gill J, et al. Hyperplasia of the juxtaglomerular complex with hyperaldosteronism and hypokalemic alkalosis: a new syndrome. Am J Med 1962; 33:811–28.
96. Takahashi N, Chernavvsky DR, Gomez RA, et al. Uncompensated polyuria in a mouse model of Bartter's syndrome. Proc Natl Acad Sci USA 2000; 97:5434–9.
97. Takahashi N, Brooks HL, Wade JB, et al. Posttranscriptional compensation for heterozygous disruption of the kidney-specific NaK2Cl cotransporter gene. J Am Soc Nephrol 2002; 13:604–10.
98. Lorenz JN, Baird NR, Judd LM, et al. Impaired renal NaCl absorption in mice lacking the ROMK potassium channel, a model for type II Bartter's syndrome. J Biol Chem 2002; 277:37871–80.
99. Schultheis PJ, Clarke LL, Meneton P, et al. Renal and intestinal absorptive defects in mice lacking the NHE3 Na/H exchanger. Nat Genet 1998; 19:282–5.
100. Wang T, Yang CL, Abbiati T, et al. Mechanism of proximal tubule bicarbonate absorption in NHE3 null mice. Am J Physiol 1999; 277:F298–302.
101. Brooks HL, Sorensen AM, Terris J, et al. Profiling of renal tubule Na transporter abundances in NHE3 and NCC null mice using targeted proteomics. J Physiol 2001; 530:359–66.
102. Lorenz JN, Schultheis PJ, Traynor T, et al. Micropuncture analysis of single-nephron function in NHE3-deficient mice. Am J Physiol 1999; 277:F447–53.
103. Woo AL, Noonan WT, Schultheis PJ, et al. Renal function in NHE3-deficient mice with transgenic rescue of small intestinal absorptive defect. Am J Physiol Renal Physiol 2003; 284:F1190–8.
104. Ledoussal C, Lorenz JN, Nieman ML, et al. Renal salt wasting in mice lacking NHE3 Na/H exchanger but not in mice lacking NHE2. Am J Physiol Renal Physiol 2001; 281:F718–27.
105. Shull GE, Miller ML, Schultheis PJ. Lessons from genetically engineered animal models VIII. Absorption and secretion of ions in the gastrointestinal tract. Am J Physiol Gastrointest Liver Physiol 2000; 278:G185–90.
106. Noonan WT, Woo AL, Nieman ML, et al. Blood pressure maintenance in NHE3-deficient mice with transgenic expression of NHE3 in small intestine. Am J Physiol Regul Integr Comp Physiol 2005; 288:R685–91.
107. Lifton RP, Gharavi AG, Geller DS. Molecular mechanisms of human hypertension. Cell 2001; 104:545–56.
108. Berger S, Bleich M, Schmid W, et al. Mineralocorticoid receptor knockout mice: lessons on Na metabolism. Kidney Int 2000; 57:1295–8.
109. Kotelevtsev Y, Brown RW, Fleming S, et al. Hypertension in mice lacking 11beta-hydroxysteroid dehydrogenase type 2. J Clin Invest 1999; 103:683–9.
110. Pearce D. The role of SGK1 in hormone-regulated sodium transport. Trends Endocrinol Metab 2001; 12:341–7.

111. Wulff P, Vallon V, Huang DY, et al. Impaired renal Na retention in the sgk1-knockout mouse. J Clin Invest 2002; 110:1263–8.
112. Le TH, Kim HS, Allen AM, et al. Physiological impact of increased expression of the AT1 angiotensin receptor. Hypertension 2003; 42:507–14.
113. Ito M, Oliverio MI, Mannon PJ, et al. Regulation of blood pressure by the type 1A angiotensin II receptor gene. Proc Natl Acad Sci USA 1995; 92:3521–5.
114. Mangrum AJ, Gomez RA, Norwood VF. Effects of AT(1A) receptor deletion on blood pressure and sodium excretion during altered dietary salt intake. Am J Physiol Renal Physiol 2002; 283:F447–53.
115. Gross V, Milia AF, Plehm R, et al. Long-term blood pressure telemetry in AT2 receptor-disrupted mice. J Hypertens 2000; 18:955–61.
116. Hussain T, Lokhandwala MF. Renal dopamine receptors and hypertension. Exp Biol Med (Maywood) 2003; 228:134–42.
117. Albrecht FE, Drago J, Felder RA, et al. Role of the D1A dopamine receptor in the pathogenesis of genetic hypertension. J Clin Invest 1996; 97:2283–8.
118. Asico LD, Ladines C, Fuchs S, et al. Disruption of the dopamine D3 receptor gene produces renin-dependent hypertension. J Clin Invest 1998; 102:493–8.
119. Ueda A, Ozono R, Oshima T, et al. Disruption of the type 2 dopamine receptor gene causes a sodium-dependent increase in blood pressure in mice. Am J Hypertens 2003; 16:853–8.
120. Watanabe H, Xu J, Bengra C, et al. Desensitization of human renal D1 dopamine receptors by G protein-coupled receptor kinase 4. Kidney Int 2002; 62:790–8.
121. Felder RA, Sanada H, Xu J, et al. G protein-coupled receptor kinase 4 gene variants in human essential hypertension. Proc Natl Acad Sci USA 2002; 99:3872–7.
122. Forte LR. A novel role for uroguanylin in the regulation of sodium balance. J Clin Invest 2003; 112:1138–41.
123. Oliver PM, John SW, Purdy KE, et al. Natriuretic peptide receptor 1 expression influences blood pressures of mice in a dose-dependent manner. Proc Natl Acad Sci USA 1998; 95:2547–51.
124. John SW, Krege JH, Oliver PM, et al. Genetic decreases in atrial natriuretic peptide and salt-sensitive hypertension. Science 1995; 267:679–81.
125. Melo LG, Veress AT, Chong CK, et al. Salt-sensitive hypertension in ANP knockout mice: potential role of abnormal plasma renin activity. Am J Physiol 1998; 274:R255–61.
126. Lopez MJ, Wong SK, Kishimoto I, et al. Salt-resistant hypertension in mice lacking the guanylyl cyclase-A receptor for atrial natriuretic peptide. Nature 1995; 378:65–8.
127. Lorenz JN, Nieman M, Sabo J, et al. Uroguanylin knockout mice have increased blood pressure and impaired natriuretic response to enteral NaCl load. J Clin Invest 2003; 112:1244–54.
128. Humphreys MH. Gamma-MSH, sodium metabolism, and salt-sensitive hypertension. Am J Physiol Regul Integr Comp Physiol 2004; 286:R417–30.
129. Ni XP, Pearce D, Butler AA, et al. Genetic disruption of gamma-melanocyte-stimulating hormone signaling leads to salt-sensitive hypertension in the mouse. J Clin Invest 2003; 111:1251–8.

11

Sodium and the Development of Hypertension: Experimental Evidence

Trefor Owen Morgan and Robert Di Nicolantonio
Department of Physiology, The University of Melbourne, Victoria, Australia

INTRODUCTION

A key question is whether an excess intake of sodium—or more correctly sodium chloride—is the major cause of hypertension in the population. Such a finding would have extremely important public health implications. Absolute experimental proof is not available and the required experiments to satisfy skeptics will probably never be undertaken. The circumstantial and epidemiological evidence discussed in Chapter 12 (1), together with the experimental data, provides overwhelming evidence in favor of such a proposition.

There has been no definitive experimental proof that excess sodium chloride is the primary cause of essential hypertension in humans but accumulated evidence from many experiments indicate that in most circumstances a rise in blood pressure (BP) will only occur when sodium intake is above a critical level and that the accompanying rises in BP with these manipulations are prevented by a low sodium intake. The concept that a high sodium intake is the sole or primary cause of hypertension in every individual is naïve as the effect of a high salt intake is clearly modified by inheritance (2), other dietary components, physical activity, and as yet unidentified factors.

This review discusses the following:

1. Increased sodium chloride intake in human and animals almost always causes an elevation in BP but the amount required to cause hypertension may be extremely large.
2. When sodium chloride excretion is impaired by either renal damage or by endocrine disorders BP is highly dependent on sodium intake and the body balance of sodium.
3. The relationship between sodium chloride intake and BP is multifactorial in that factors such as age, exercise, obesity, alcohol intake, potassium intake, genetic make and other variables alter the relationship and may negate the effect.

EXCESS SALT INTAKE

Studies in the Rat

Increasing the sodium chloride intake in rats usually causes an increase in BP. In the 1950s, Ball and Meneely (3) demonstrated that when rats were fed diets containing between

0.15% and 9.8% NaCl for nine months, the average BP correlated with the level of sodium intake. However the effect of increased sodium intake was not consistent. Certain strains such as the Dahl (4), Milan (5) and stroke prone spontaneously hypertensive rat (SHR) (6) increase BP when sodium intake is altered. In the SHR, studies have been contradictory. Some investigations reported sodium chloride dependency while others failed to do so (7). This effect may depend upon the stage of development at which rats are exposed to extra sodium chloride (8). In non-hypertensive strains it may be difficult to show a BP increase with a high sodium chloride intake but it may still cause cardiac hypertrophy (9). However, most studies have used tail-cuff BP measurements which are insensitive to small BP changes and therefore these studies should be repeated with telemetric recording of BP. This may confirm and detect small, but important changes and might also show that increased sodium chloride elevates nocturnal BP which is an important determinant of cardiac hypertrophy (10).

In the one kidney, one clip Goldblat hypertensive rat blockade of the renin-angiotensin system has little effect on the elevated BP or cardiac hypertrophy. However, if such a model is placed on a low sodium intake and the renin system inhibited, BP and cardiac hypertrophy are normalized (11). If normal rats are treated with large doses of an angiotensin converting enzyme (ACE) inhibitor combined with an angiotensin receptor blocking drug it is found that BP falls markedly, the heart involutes and rats die within two weeks (12,13). This effect is seen in Sprague–Dawley rats and the SHR. Most of the above features are reversed by placing the rats on a high sodium chloride intake (Table 1).

Studies by Di Nicolantonio (8) indicate that the time at which the animals are exposed to different salt intake may be of importance. The SHR were placed on different salt intakes until eight weeks of age and then all continued on the same salt intake and diet thereafter. The rats that were on the lower salt intake during the initial phase had a lower BP throughout the rest of their life and lived longer than those on the higher intake. This effect is similar to that achieved by treating rats with an ACE I at a similar stage of growth (14).

While these studies are of interest and indicate that BP can be modified by sodium chloride, the opponents of the hypothesis "that excess sodium chloride causes essential hypertension" reject these data as irrelevant to the human. However such animal studies clearly indicate that sodium chloride intake alters BP and there are important interactions between sodium chloride intake and the renin-angiotensin system.

Table 1 Reversal of Effects of Combined Blockade (ACEI + ARB) of the Renin-Angiotensin System by a High Salt Intake in Sprague–Dawley Rats

		Combined blockade	
	Control	0.2% NaCl	4% NaCl
Systolic BP (mmHg)	122	75	110
Diastolic BP (mmHg)	88	45	77
Weight gain (g)	30	−34	−30
Cardiac weight gain (g)	120	−281	−100
Cardiac index	3.23	2.96	3.37
Cardiac weight (g)	1214	933	1118

Abbreviations: ACE, angiotensin-converting enzyme; ARB, angiotensin receptor-blocking drug; BP, blood pressure.
Source: From Ref. 11.

Nonhuman Primates

Sodium chloride intake was increased in Baboons by adding 4% salt to the diet (15). BP rose whether this was given during the growing period or in adults. The effect was greater the longer the time of exposure to sodium chloride. When sodium chloride was stopped the BP returned towards its prestudy level. A further important study was undertaken in chimpanzees by Denton et al. (16) In this study the salt intake was increased by up to 16 g/day and importantly, this was the only difference in diet and activity between the control and experimental group. BP rose when the chimpanzees were on the higher salt intake and fell when they returned to a low salt intake (Table 2). Of note, not all chimpanzees became hypertensive, which mimics the situation in humans. This study is of major importance but presentation of BP data before, during and after cessation of salt intake for individual animals would allow better interpretation of the data. Thus the genetic background of an individual chimpanzees or person is one of the important factors that determine the amount of sodium chloride that can be handled without the development of hypertension. This study implies that the major reason that hypertension develops when a hunter–gatherer community moves to an urban society is due to the increase sodium chloride intake rather than alteration in other dietary components or activity.

Human

Humans Normotensive

Numerous studies have been performed examining the effects of salt on BP in humans. The subjects have been either hypertensive or normotensive though it should be noted that the definition of hypertension has altered over the years.

In normotensive people restriction of salt intake has produced conflicting results with either no change in BP or a small fall. However in a meta analysis (17) of 10 randomized trials in normotensive individuals, BP fell by $1.6 \pm 0.3/0.6 \pm 0.2$ mmHg. A small or no change in BP in normotensive people is not unexpected because the normal BP in this group indicates that the person can handle their present sodium load. The studies that need to be performed in young normotensive patients are to increase sodium chloride intake. This has been undertaken by Luft et al. (18), who gave increasing amounts of sodium chloride to young males with normal renal function. The BP rose in all subjects though the amount to achieve a significant rise was highly variable (Table 3). This indicates that genetic and other factors determine the level at which the rise becomes

Table 2 Systolic BP (mmHg) in Chimpanzees Fed a High Salt Intake

	Control	Experimental
n	12	10
Pretreatment	119	110
Treat 6 months	123	120*
Treat 15 months	122	136*
Treat 21 months	121	141*
Post 3 months	122	118
Post 7 months	115	112

*$p < 0.05$ compared with baseline.
Abbreviation: BP, blood pressure.
Source: From Ref. 16.

Table 3 Systolic and Diastolic BP on Different Levels of NaCl Intake in Young Normotensive Males

Sodium intake (mmol/day)	n	BP (mmHg)	
		Systolic	Diastolic
10	14	113±2	69±2
300	14	117±2	70±2
600	6	119±3	71±3
800	8	121±3	76±3
1200	6	125±3	78±3
1500	8	131±4	85±3

$p<0.001$ for association between sodium intake and BP.
Abbreviation: BP, blood pressure.
Source: From Ref. 18.

significant, or possibly more correctly the level of sodium chloride intake that cannot be handled by the usual endocrine systems of that patient.

Myers and Morgan (19) performed a study in 201 normotensive people of different ages and gender (Table 4). After a run in period of two weeks they were randomized to a high (> 200 mmol/day) or low (<70 mmol/day) diet for two weeks. BP was measured, urine collected and the subjects were crossed over to the other diet for two weeks. Diastolic BP was found to be 4.5±0.5 mmHg higher while on the high salt intake.

The changes in BP were more pronounced in the older age group and all except 2 of the 21 patients >60 year had a rise in BP (mean rise 17±3.1/10±3.0 mmHg). In people less than 50 years the rise in mean BP was 2.8±0.6 mmHg. The response depended on the age of the patient and the initial BP, which also correlated with age. In the younger age groups some patients had no significant change in BP but the number who had a rise in BP increased in each succeeding decade. On the low salt intake 21 of 154 patients had a diastolic BP >90 mmHg while on the higher salt intake 42 of 154 patients who were compliant with the diets had a diastolic BP >90 mmHg. Thus alteration of dietary salt intake would have decreased the number of patients requiring treatment by 50% using criteria prevalent in 1983.

Recent studies have shown significant falls in "normotensive" patients following a reduced sodium intake. In an important study from the U.S.A., when compared to controls, the dietary approaches to stop hypertension (DASH) diet lowered BP by 5.5/3.0 mmHg (20).

Table 4 Rise in Supine Systolic and Diastolic BP mmHg with a Change in Sodium Intake from 70 to 200 mmol/day in Normotensive People

Age	Males BP (mmHg)		Females BP (mmHg)	
	Systolic	Diastolic	Systolic	Diastolic
10–19	−0.5	1.5	−1.0	4.7
20–29	2.7	0.6	46	3.4
30–39	2.4	1.2	1.0	2.4
40–49	5.1*	1.4	4.8*	3.9*
50–59	15.4*	7.4*	6.4*	5.8*
>60	14.6*	6.9*	20.2*	16.0*

*$p<0.05$ $n=6$ to 19 in each group.
Source: From Ref. 19.

Table 5 Fall in BP (mmHg) with Variation in Sodium Chloride Intake Related to the K^+ Content of the Diet in the DASH Study

Potassium intake (mmol/day)	Sodium change (mmol/day)	BP change (mmHg)	
		Sys	Dias
40	144–107	2.1	0.6
	144–67	6.7	1.7
75	141–106	1.3	1.0
	141–67	3.0	1.2

Abbreviations: BP, blood pressure; DASH, dietary approaches to stop hypertension.
Source: From Ref. 21.

It was estimated that 2.7/1.9 mmHg of this fall was attributable to a diet high in fruit and vegetables while the remaining 2.8/1.1 mmHg by the extra additions of nuts and diary products included in the DASH diet. Sodium intake in the three diet groups studied was similar, but potassium intake doubled in both intervention diets. An extension of the DASH Study (21) examined the effect of varying sodium intake in people on a control or DASH diet (Table 5). Restriction of sodium intake from 140 to 105 to 65 mmol/day lowered BP in both groups but the fall in BP (6.7/3.5 mmHg) was greater in the patients on control diet compared with those on the DASH diet (3.0/3.4 mmHg). The BP in people on the reduced sodium intake was 2.2/1.0 mmHg lower on the DASH compared to the control diet.

In Australia, Nowson (22) conducted a similar though community-based study. In this study the "DASH" type diet (Oz DASH), when compared with the "usual diet" of subjects, had a smaller effect on BP compared with the American study possibly because the K^+ intake of the usual Australian diet was approximately 67 mmol/day, compared with 40 mmol/day on the controlled American diet. The fall in BP with a diet that restricted sodium chloride and increased potassium intake caused a greater fall in BP than the holistic diet (Oz DASH) (Table 6).

The results of the American and Australian Studies infer that sodium restriction has a greater effect when people are on a low potassium intake or conversely that a high potassium intake has more effect when people are on a high sodium intake. While the American and Australian studies used so called normotensive patients, they deliberately studied people in the "high-end" of the normal range.

Table 6 Urine Sodium and Potassium and BP in the Australian Oz DASH Study

	Urine Na (mmol/day)	Urine K (mmol/day)	BP (mmHg)	
			Systolic	Diastolic
Control	143	67	127	80
Oz DASH	116	100	125*	79
Low Na high K	59	106	123*	78*
High calcium	152	85	128	80

*$p<0.05$ Compared with control and high calcium.
**$p<0.05$ Compared with control, high calcium and Oz DASH.
Abbreviations: BP, blood pressure; DASH, dietary approaches to stop hypertension.

Humans—Hypertensive

A randomized study in mildly hypertensive patients performed in 1978 (23) showed that reduced sodium chloride intake and increased potassium intake caused a significant fall in BP. This result was confirmed by MacGregor (24) in double blind studies in a relatively small number of patients. It was extended in a larger number of patients in two major Australian salt studies (25–27). In these studies performed in older people with elevated diastolic BP (>90 mmHg), BP fell significantly. There were multiple measurements on each subject and only 4 of 52 subjects had a higher BP (all less than 5 mmHg) when on sodium chloride placebo (27). It should be noted that to achieve a fall in BP in patients with hypertension does not require severe restriction of sodium chloride. Modest reduction in sodium chloride appears to be sufficient (28). This implies that in an individual there may be a threshold which activates a rise in BP to excrete the extra sodium chloride (28). There is however, a dose dependency of the effect of sodium chloride demonstrated both in hypertensive patients (29) and in normotensive patients in the DASH Study (20).

IMPAIRED CAPACITY TO EXCRETE SODIUM

While in rats excess sodium chloride intake does increase BP, hypertension with end organ damage frequently does not result. To obtain a BP level that leads to hypertensive complications up to 2/3 or more of the renal tissue needs to be removed (30). In this remnant kidney model important interactions between sodium chloride intake and ACE inhibitors are also observed. Thus, in rat's studies on a normal sodium intake, the administration of an ACE inhibitor alone had little effect on BP, proteinuria and progression of renal damage. However, if place on a reduced sodium chloride intake (0.25% compared to control of 0.5%), hypertension was prevented by a variety of different drugs and ACE inhibitors provided dramatic protection against the progression of renal damage. Interestingly, the renal protective effect was not seen with calcium channel blocking drugs despite similar BP control.

This impaired capacity to excrete sodium chloride with a resultant increased BP is observed in humans with renal failure and even more markedly in humans on dialysis. In both situations the BP is highly dependent on sodium chloride intake (31). Administration of aldosterone or other mineralocorticoids cause retention of sodium chloride. If administered to animals or humans on low sodium intake BP may not increase. It is likely that the major reason that aldosterone causes alteration in BP and other cardiovascular complications is by its effects fundamentally on the kidney causing retention of sodium and loss of potassium (32).

INFLUENCE OF OTHER LIFESTYLE VARIABLES

The pressure effects of sodium chloride should not be considered in isolation. As sodium chloride intake increases in the community there are frequently accompanying changes in activity, in caloric intake leading to obesity and these are important contributors to hypertension and vascular disease. Epidemiological evidence suggests that vigorous physical activity can offset the rise in BP usually caused by a high sodium chloride intake (33). The most common alteration in dietary constituents associated with a rise in sodium intake is an accompanying fall in K^+ intake and a rise in chloride intake. In a "hunter–gatherer" diet, the K^+ intake is usually high (200–400 mmol/day) and most of this is in the form of an alkaline salt of potassium (e.g., potassium tartrate, citrate etc). When

Table 7 Effect of NaCl, $NaHCO_3$, and NaCl + KCL on BP in Patients with Salt-Sensitive Hypertension

	BP (mmHg)		
	Systolic	Diastolic	Urine Na^+ (mmol/day)
Pretreatment	161	105	204
Reduced salt diet	142*	89*	95
Placebo	139*	87*	84
NaCl 70 mmol/day	158	101	157
$NaHCO_3$ 70 mmol/day	147*	92*	149
NaCl 70 mmol/day + KCl 70 mmol/day	148*	93*	156

*$p < 0.05$ compared with the addition of NaCl 70 mmol/day and pretreatment.
Abbreviation: BP, blood pressure.
Source: From Ref. 34.

metabolized these salts form bicarbonate, equating their intake to ingesting potassium bicarbonate. Furthermore, when food is commercially processed, the potassium salts tend to be removed and are replaced by sodium chloride.

When patients with hypertension who had a fall in BP with dietary restriction of sodium were given sodium chloride, the BP returned towards its previous level (34). When given the same amount of sodium but as sodium bicarbonate the rise in BP was significantly less (Table 7) (34). If given the same amount of sodium chloride and the potassium intake increased through use of potassium chloride tablets, the rise in BP was also blunted (Table 7). The effect of potassium chloride on BP was investigated in a further study (35) in which it was shown that potassium chloride supplementation reduced BP and the effect appeared to be greater in patients on a higher salt intake. These studies were later confirmed by MacGregor and colleagues (36).

Kurtz et al. (37,38) extended these studies by examining the effects of alkaline salts of potassium. They demonstrated significant fall in BP. Experimentally, in stroke prone rats Tobian (39) has shown similar effects. They also showed a marked reduction in stroke mortality independent of the BP lowering effect. Epidemiological studies (40) indicate that strokes occur in populations on lower levels of potassium intake. Analysis of the Systolic Hypertension in the Elderly Program study (41,42) showed that strokes and sudden deaths were more common in people who developed a low K^+. Thus the pressure effects of sodium intake should not be considered in isolation as it is related to potassium and anion intake.

CONCLUSION

Increased sodium chloride increases BP. The rise in BP is greatest if a person has impaired ability to excrete sodium chloride. This occurs with reduction in renal function due either to age or disease or with impaired ability to excrete sodium chloride caused by endocrine or inherited disorder. The effect of sodium chloride on BP elevation may be reduced by several factors, the principal ones are high potassium intake (preferably as an alkaline salt) and physical activity. Definitive evidence obtained in double-blind studies that sodium chloride causes essential hypertension is however lacking but it should be noted that in persons on a restricted sodium chloride intake (<50 mmol/day) hypertension of any form is uncommon.

REFERENCES

1. McGregor GA, He FJ. Sodium and hypertension: epidemiological and clinical evidence for a link. In: Burnier M, ed. Sodium in Health and Disease. Informa 2008:217–26.
2. Bochud M, Burnier M. Salt and Blood Pressure. In: Burnier M, ed. Sodium in Health and Disease. Informa 2008:267–92.
3. Ball O, Meneely G. Observations on dietary sodium chloride. J Am Diet Assoc 1957; 33:366–70.
4. Rapp J. Dahl salt-susceptible and salt-resistant rats. A review. Hypertension 1982; 4:753–63.
5. Pontremoli T, Spalvins A, Menachery A, et al. Red cell sodium–proton exchange is increased in Dahl salt-sensitive hypertensive rats. Kidney Int 1992; 42(6):1355–62.
6. Tobian L, Lange J, Ulm K, et al. Potassium reduces cerebral hemorrhage and death rate in hypertensive rats, even when blood pressure is not lowered. Hypertension 1985; 7(3 Pt 2):1110–4.
7. Toal C, Leenan F. Dietary sodium restriction and development of hypertension in spontaneously hypertensive rats. Am J Physiol 1983; 245:H1081–4.
8. Di Nicolantonio R, Hoy K, Spargo S, et al. Perinatal salt intake alters blood pressure and salt balance in hypertensive rats. Hypertension 1990; 15(2):177–82.
9. Yuan B, Leenen F. Dietary sodium intake and left ventricular hypertrophy in nomotensive rats. Am J Physiol 1991; 261:H1397–401.
10. Morgan T, Brunner H, Aubert J, et al. Cardiac hypertrophy depends upon sleep blood pressure: a study in rats. J Hypertens 2000; 18:445–51.
11. Morgan T, Aubert J, Brunner H. Interaction between sodium intake, angiotensin II and blood pressure as a cause of cardiac hypertrophy. Am J Hypertens 2001; 14(9):914–20.
12. Abro E, Griffiths C, Morgan T, et al. Regression of cardiac hypertrophy in the SHR by combined renin–angiotensin system blockade and dietary sodium restriction. JRAAS 2001; 2(Suppl. 1):S148–53.
13. Griffiths C, Morgan T, Delbridge L. Effects of combined administration of ACE inhibitor and angiotensin II receptor antagonist are prevented by a high NaCl intake. J Hypertens 2001; 19(11):2087–95.
14. Harrap S, Nicolaci J, Doyle A. Persistent effects on blood pressure and renal haemodynamics following chronic angiotensin converting enzyme inhibition with perindopril. Clin Exp Pharmacol Physiol 1985; 13:753–65.
15. Cherchovich G, Capek K, Jefremova Z, et al. High salt intake and blood pressure in lower primates (*Papio hamadryas*). J Appl Physiol 1976; 40:601–4.
16. Denton D, Weisinger R, Mundy N, et al. The effect of increased salt intake on blood pressure of chimpanzees. Nat Med 1995; 1:1009–16.
17. He F, MacGregor G. Effect of modest salt reduction on blood pressure: a meta-analysis of randomized trials. Implications for public health. J Hum Hypertens 2002; 16:761–70.
18. Luft F, Rankin L, Bloch R, et al. Cardiovascular and humoral responses to extremes of sodium intake in normal black and white men. Circulation 1979; 60:697–706.
19. Myers J, Morgan T. The effect of sodium intake on the blood pressure related to age and sex. Clin Exp Hypertens 1983; A5(1):99–118.
20. Appel L, Moore T, Obarzanek E, et al. A clinical trial of the effects of dietary patterns on blood pressure. DASH Collaborative Research Group. N Engl J Med 1997; 336:1117–24.
21. Sacks F, Svetkey L, Vollmer W, et al. Effects on blood pressure of reduced dietary sodium and the Dietary Approaches to Stop Hypertension (DASH) diet. DASH-Sodium Collaborative Research Group. N Eng J Med 2001; 344:3–10.
22. Nowson C, Worsley A, Margerison C, et al. Human nutrition and metabolism. Blood pressure response to dietary modifications in free-living individuals. Am Soc Nutr Sci 2004; 134:2322–8.
23. Morgan T, Gillies A, Morgan G, et al. Hypertension treated by salt restriction. Lancet 1978; 1:227–30.
24. MacGregor G, Markandu N, Best F, et al. Double-blind randomised crossover trial of moderate sodium restriction in essential hypertension. Lancet 1982; 1:351–5.

25. Chalmers J, Morgan T, Doyle A, et al. Australian National Health and Medical Research Council dietary salt study in mild hypertension. J Hypertens 1986; 4(Suppl. 6):S629–37.
26. Australian National Health & Medical Research Council Dietary Salt Study Management Committee. Modest reduction in dietary salt intake reduces blood pressure. Lancet 1989; 1:399–402.
27. Morgan T, Nowson C. The Australian sodium potassium study in untreated mild hypertension. In: Rettig R, Ganten D, Luft F, eds. Salt and Hypertension. Heidelberg: Springer, 1988:309–18.
28. Morgan T, Nowson C. The role of sodium restriction in the management of hypertension. Can J Physiol Pharm 1986; 64:786–92.
29. MacGregor G, Markandu N, Sagnella G, et al. Double-blind study of three sodium intakes and long-term effects of sodium restriction in essential hypertension. Lancet 1989; 2:1244–7.
30. Terzi F, Beautils H, Laouari D, et al. Renal effect of antihypertensive drugs depends on sodium diet in the excision remnant kidney model. Kidney Int 1992; 42:354–63.
31. Weinberger M, Miller J, Luft F, et al. Definitions and characteristics of sodium sensitivity and blood pressure resistance. Curr Opin Nephrol Hypertens 1993; 2:341–9.
32. Horton R. Aldosterone: review of its physiology and diagnostic aspects of primary aldosteronism. Metabolism 1973; 22(12):1525–45.
33. Connor WE, Cerqueria M, Connor R. The plasma lipids, lipoproteins and diet of the Tarahumara Indians of Mexico. Am J Clin Nutr 1978; 31:1131–42.
34. Morgan T. The effect of potassium and bicarbonate ions on the rise in blood pressure caused by sodium chloride. Clin Sci 1982; 63:S407–9.
35. Morgan T, Myers J, Teow B, et al. The effect of low sodium and high potassium diets on blood pressure. In: Proceedings April 22–23, Potassium, Blood Pressure and Cardiovascular Disease. Amsterdam: Excerpta Medica, 1983:114–22.
36. MacGregor G, Markandu N, Best F, et al. Moderate potassium supplementation in essential hypertension. Lancet 1982; I:351–5.
37. Kurtz T, Morris R. Dietary chloride as a determinant of dosordered calcium and sodium metabolism in salt dependent hypertension. Life Sci 1985; 36:921–9.
38. Kurtz T, Al-Bander H, Morris R. "Salt-sensitive" hypertension in men: is the sodium ion alone important? N Engl J Med 1987; 317:1043–8.
39. Tobian L, Lange J, Johnson M, et al. High-K diets reduce brain haemorrhage and infarcts, death rate and mesenteric arteriolar hypertrophy in stroke-prone spontaneously hypertensive rats. Hypertens Suppl 1986; 4(5):S205–7.
40. Khaw K, Barrett-Connor E. Dietary potassium and stroke-associated mortality. A 12-year prospective population study. N Engl J Med 1987; 316(5):235–40.
41. SHEP and Coperative Research Group. Prevention of stroke by antihypertensive drug treatment in older persons with isolated systolic hypertension. Final results of the Systolic Hypertension in the Elderly Program (SHEP). J Am Med Assoc 1991; 265:3255–64.
42. Franse L, Pahor M, De Bari M, et al. Hypokalemia Associated with diuretic use and cardiovascular events in the Systolic Hypertension in the Elderly Program. Hypertension 2000; 35:1025–30.

12

Salt and Hypertension: Epidemiological and Clinical Evidence for a Link

Feng J. He and Graham A. MacGregor
Blood Pressure Unit, Cardiac and Vascular Sciences, St. George's University of London, London, U.K.

INTRODUCTION

Salt is a chemical that consists of sodium and chloride and, as something added to food, is not a normal constituent of a human's or any mammal's diet. For several million years the evolutionary ancestors of humans ate a diet that contained less than 0.25 g/day of salt (1). Sufficient sodium exists in natural foods to ensure that mammals could develop away from the sea. However, chemical salt has played an important role in the development of civilization (2). It was first found to have the magical property of preserving foods, probably by the Chinese around 5000 years ago, when they found that meat or fish could be preserved for a long time when they were soaked in saline solutions. This ability to preserve food allowed the development of settled communities. Salt became one of the most traded commodities in the world, as well as one of the most taxed. Salt was initially expensive to produce and was regarded as a luxury, but with the mining of salt it became much more plentiful and was added to fresh food as this food tasted bland compared to the highly salted preserved foods that most people were used to eating. It was also found that when salt was added to food that was going putrid, the bitter flavors were removed and the food became edible. Salt was seen as almost magical and became a symbol of purity in most religions. In the late nineteenth century deep freezers and refrigerators were invented and salt lost its importance as a preservative. Since that time salt intake has been gradually falling. However, with the increased consumption of processed, restaurant, and fast foods, which contain large amounts of hidden salt, salt intake is now increasing. More than three-quarters of salt intake in most developed countries now comes from salt added to processed foods (3).

Evolving on a low-salt diet of no more than 0.25 g/day, humans are genetically programmed to this amount of salt, and have exquisite mechanisms to conserve sodium within the body, i.e., they are able to reduce sodium excretion in the urine and sweat to almost zero. The recent change, in evolutionary terms, to the current very high salt intake of 9 to 12 g/day (4,5) (40 times more than previously consumed) presents a major challenge to the physiological systems in the body to excrete these very large amounts of salt through the kidney into the urine. Thus, there has been little time for physiological systems to adapt. The consequence of this is that our current high salt intake increases blood pressure, cardiovascular disease, renal disease, and bone demineralization (6).

In this chapter, the evidence that relates salt to raised blood pressure is reviewed. Also discussed are other harmful effects of salt on health that may be independent of salt's effect on blood pressure.

DEFINITION OF HYPERTENSION (HIGH BLOOD PRESSURE)

Blood pressure throughout the range seen in Western populations is an important risk factor for cardiovascular disease. The relationship between blood pressure and cardiovascular disease displays a continuous graded relationship, and there is no evidence of any threshold level of blood pressure below which lower levels of blood pressure are not associated with lower risks of cardiovascular disease (7). Thus, any classification of people into dichotomous categories ("normotensive" and "hypertensive") is inherently arbitrary. Nevertheless, it is useful to provide a classification of blood pressure for the purpose of identifying high-risk individuals and providing guidelines for treatment with tablets and follow-up.

Geoffrey Rose suggested that "the operational definition of hypertension is the level at which the benefits… of action exceed those of inaction." The criteria for the classification of hypertension have changed over the past 40 years as more recent studies have shown benefit at lower levels of blood pressure (8). The recent Seventh Joint National Committee (JNC VII) (9) defined individuals with blood pressure less than 120/80 mmHg as "normal" and those with blood pressure $\geq$140 mmHg systolic or $\geq$90 mmHg diastolic as "hypertension," whereas for those with blood pressure ranging from 120 to 139 mmHg systolic and/or 80 to 89 mmHg diastolic, the JNC VII report has introduced a new term "prehypertension." This new designation is intended to identify those individuals in whom early intervention by adoption of healthy lifestyles could reduce blood pressure, decrease the rate of progression of blood pressure to hypertensive levels with age, or prevent hypertension entirely.

Hypertension is extremely common in Western countries. For instance, in England, just under 40% of the entire adult population have hypertension (systolic $\geq$140 mmHg and/or diastolic $\geq$90 mmHg) (10). The prevalence of hypertension increases with age, e.g., at the age of 50 to 59 years, approximately 50% have high blood pressure, and at the age of 60 to 79 years, 70% have high blood pressure. Worldwide, 26.4% of the adult population had high blood pressure (greater than 140/90 mmHg) and the estimated total number of adults with high blood pressure was 972 million in 2000. This number is predicted to increase to a total of 1.56 billion in 2025 (11).

Many treatment trials in hypertensive individuals have demonstrated a clear benefit of lowering blood pressure in reducing strokes, heart attacks and heart failure (12). On average, antihypertensive treatment is associated with reductions in strokes of 35% to 40%, myocardial infarction 20% to 25%, and heart failure over 50% (13).

BENEFITS OF LOWERING BLOOD PRESSURE IN THE "NORMAL" RANGE

In the general population, blood pressure is distributed in a roughly normal or Gaussian manner in a bell-shaped curve with a slight skew toward higher readings. Although the risk of cardiovascular mortality increases progressively with increasing blood pressure, for the population at large the greatest number of strokes, heart attacks, and heart failure attributable to blood pressure occur in the upper range of average (i.e., systolic between 130 and 140 mmHg and diastolic between 80 and 90 mmHg) because there are so many individuals who have blood pressure at these levels in the population (14). Therefore, a population-based approach aimed at achieving a downward shift in the distribution of blood pressure in the whole population, even by a small amount, will have a large impact on reducing the number of strokes, heart attacks and heart failure (15).

SALT AND BLOOD PRESSURE—EVIDENCE FOR A LINK

The earliest comment that relates dietary salt to blood pressure was recorded in the ancient Chinese medical literature—the Yellow Emperor's classic on internal medicine, Huang Ti Nei Ching Su Wein, 2698–2598 BC. It is stated that "If too much salt is used for food, the pulse hardens…." However, the first meaningful scientific evidence for a link between salt intake and blood pressure only emerged in the early 1900s. There is now overwhelming evidence for a causal relationship between salt intake and blood pressure. The evidence comes from epidemiological studies, migration studies, population-based intervention studies, treatment trials, animal and genetic studies.

Epidemiological Studies

In 1960, Dahl reported a strong relationship between average salt intake and prevalence of hypertension in an ecological study of five geographically diverse populations (16). Subsequently, several other authors have confirmed Dahl's findings. The limitations of these across-population studies are that the data were from several different studies that used unstandardized methods, and few collected data on potential confounding factors and the multiple social and environmental differences among populations around the world may affect the relationship between salt intake and blood pressure.

Within-population studies have been hampered by a number of methodological challenges including measurement difficulties caused by variations in day-to-day salt intake, and a wide range of blood pressure values at any level of salt intake caused by the multifactorial nature of environmental and genetic influence on blood pressure. As such, a large number of individuals would be required to demonstrate a significant association between habitual salt intake and blood pressure. The INTERSALT (5) is one of the largest cross-sectional epidemiological studies that have looked at the relationship between salt intake and blood pressure. Over 10,000 individuals from 52 centers around the world were studied using standardized methods of measuring blood pressure and 24-hour urinary sodium excretion. Within-center analysis showed that 24-hour urinary sodium excretion was significantly associated with both systolic and diastolic blood pressure in individual subjects, i.e., the higher the salt intake, the higher the blood pressure. Cross-center analysis showed a positive linear relation between median 24-hour sodium excretion and slope of both systolic and diastolic blood pressure with age, indicating the higher the salt intake the greater the rise in blood pressure with age (Fig. 1). It was estimated that an increase of 6 g/day in salt intake is related to a rise of 10/6 mmHg in blood pressure over 30 years (e.g., from age of 25 to 55 years), which represents a large increase in population blood pressure.

In the INTERSALT study, when the analyses were restricted to 48 population samples (excluding four communities consuming less than 3 g of salt per day), cross-center

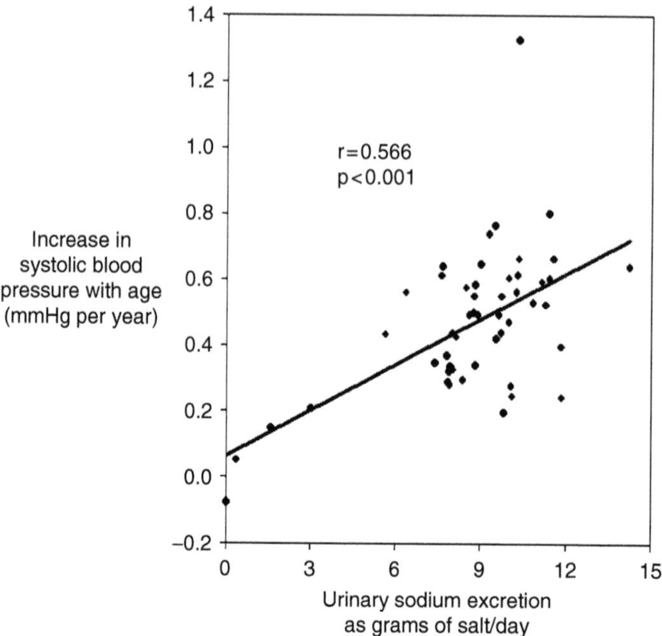

Figure 1 The relationship between salt intake and the slope of the rise in systolic blood pressure with age in 52 centers in the INTERSALT study. *Source*: From Ref. 5.

analysis showed no association between urinary sodium excretion and blood pressure. This is due to the fact that the truncated analyses of 48 samples were lower in statistical power than those of 52 samples, both because of the smaller number of populations and because much of the variation in sodium excretion (designed at outset to be as wide as possible) was removed (17). However, the highly significant within-population association between urinary sodium excretion and systolic blood pressure across all 52 population samples was virtually unchanged when the four low-salt populations were excluded, and the association between sodium excretion and the rise in blood pressure with age found across 52 population samples persisted across 48 samples (18).

Many of the INTERSALT investigators have collaborated in another major nutrition–blood pressure study, the INTERMAP study, which shed additional light on the salt–blood pressure relationship. One article from the INTERMAP group reports nutrient intakes in four countries: China, Japan, U.K., and U.S.A. (19). The results confirm findings from INTERSALT that China and Japan where both the prevalence of hypertension and stroke mortality are very high, have a higher salt intake, lower potassium intake, and therefore, a higher salt/potassium ratio, compared with the U.K. and the U.S.A. Another INTERMAP article (20) demonstrates that most of the adverse effect of a low education level which is known to be inversely related to blood pressure, is attributable to dietary variables, including a higher salt intake in those with a lower education level.

In a recently published paper, Khaw et al. examined the relationship between salt intake and blood pressure in 23,104 individuals who participated in the Norfolk Cohort of the European Prospective Investigation into Cancer (EPIC-Norfolk) study (21). They found that a difference of 8.2 g/day in salt intake was associated with a difference of

7.2/3.0 mmHg in blood pressure ($p < 0.0001$). The prevalence of individuals with systolic blood pressure greater than or equal to 160 mmHg was 12% in those with a salt intake of 12.9 g/day, whereas it was only 6% in those with a salt intake of 4.7 g/day.

In the INTERSALT study, only four communities had salt intake less than 3 g/day. A number of other studies have studied the nonacculturated tribes which have a low salt intake (less than 3 g/day). Individuals in these tribes have lower levels of blood pressure and more importantly, their blood pressure does not rise with age. The most striking example is the Yanomamo Indians on the border between Venezuela and Brazil (22,23). They have a salt intake of 0.05 g/day. The average blood pressure for adults is only 96/61 mmHg, and there is no rise in blood pressure with age and no evidence of cardiovascular disease. Whilst there may be other factors that also account for the lower blood pressure, several studies have clearly demonstrated the profound importance of salt. A study in the Pacific Islands where one undeveloped community used salt water in their food and the other did not, showed that the community using salt had higher blood pressure (24). Another study in Nigeria of two rural communities, one of which had access to salt from a salt lake and the other did not, showed differences in salt intake and differences in blood pressure, and yet in all other aspects of lifestyle and diet the two communities were similar. The Qash'qai, an undeveloped tribe living in Iran who have access to salt deposits on the ground, develop high blood pressure and a rise in blood pressure with age similar to that which occurs in Western communities, but they live a lifestyle similar to nonacculturated societies (25).

Migration Studies

A number of studies have shown that migration from isolated low-salt societies to Westernized environment with a high salt intake is associated with an increase in blood pressure, a rise in blood pressure with age, and a higher prevalence of hypertension. For instance, a well-controlled migration study of a rural tribe in Kenya showed that on migration to an urban environment, there was an increase in salt intake and a reduction in potassium intake, and blood pressure rose after a few months, compared to those in the control group who remained in the rural environment (26). The blood pressure difference became more marked by two years after migration.

Another example of migration study is that of the Yi people, an ethnic minority living in southwestern China (27,28). Blood pressure rose very little with increasing age (0.13/0.23 mmHg/yr) in the Yi farmers who lived in their natural remote mountainous environment and consumed a low-salt diet. In contrast, Yi migrants and Han people who lived in urban areas consumed a high-salt diet and experienced a much greater increase in blood pressure with increasing age (0.33/0.33 mmHg/yr) (27). In a sample of 417 recent migrants (Yi) or native (Han) men living in the urban areas, there was a significant positive relationship between salt intake and blood pressure. An increase of 6 g/day in salt intake is associated with an increase of 2.3 mmHg in systolic blood pressure and 1.8 mmHg in diastolic pressure after adjusting for age, body mass index, heart rate, alcohol, and total energy intakes. These findings suggest that changes in lifestyle, e.g., higher salt intake, contribute to the higher blood pressure among Yi migrants (28).

Population-Based Intervention Studies

In the late 1950s the Japanese became aware that certain parts of Japan, particularly the north, had a high salt consumption and deaths from stroke were amongst the highest in the world. It was then found that the number of strokes in different parts of Japan was directly related to the levels of salt intake. In view of these findings, there was a Government campaign to reduce salt intake, which was successful in reducing salt intake over the following decade from an average of 13.5 to 12.1 g/day. However, in the north of Japan the salt intake fell from 18 to 14 g/day. This resulted in a gradual fall in blood pressure both in adults and children, and an 80% reduction in stroke mortality (29–31).

Several population-based well-controlled intervention studies have been carried out. One was conducted in two similar villages in Portugal (32). Each village had approximately 800 inhabitants who had salt intakes of 21 g/day and the prevalence of hypertension and stroke mortality are very high. During the two year intervention period, there was a vigorous, widespread health education effort to reduce salt intake especially from those foods that had previously been identified as the major sources of salt in the intervention village. Whereas, in the control village, no dietary advice was given. The intervention was successful in achieving a difference of approximately 50% in salt intake between the two villages. This caused a significant difference in blood pressure at one year and a more pronounced difference at two years (a difference of 13/6 mmHg in blood pressure between the two villages; Fig. 2).

Another population-based intervention study was carried out in Tianjin, China, where the salt intake, as well as the prevalence of hypertension and stroke mortality are also very high. The intervention was based on examinations of independent cross-sectional population samples in 1989 (1719 persons) and 1992 (2304 persons) (33). During the intervention period, there was a small reduction in salt intake in the intervention area, whereas in the control area there was a small increase in salt intake, so that the net difference in the change in salt intake between the intervention and control area was 2.4 g/day in men and 0.9 g/day in women. This was associated with a difference in systolic blood pressure of 5 mmHg in men and 4 mmHg in women.

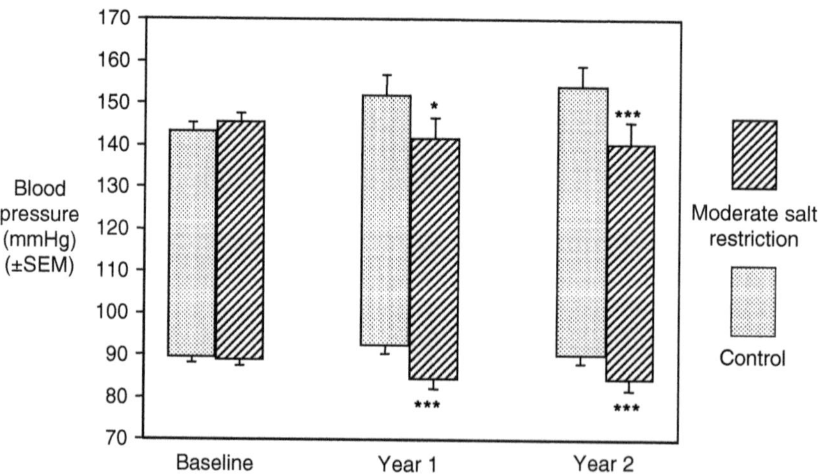

Figure 2 Blood pressure changes with time in two Portuguese villages, one of which had salt intake reduced. The other had similar measurements of blood pressure but no advice on diet. Note the significant differences in blood pressure at one year and continuing differences at two years. *Source*: From Ref. 32.

The above two population-based intervention studies clearly demonstrate that a reduction in population salt intake lowers population blood pressure. A reduction in population blood pressure, even by a small amount, will have a large impact on reducing cardiovascular morbidity and mortality (15).

Two other intervention studies (one in Belgium, and the other in North Karelia) are often quoted as being negative (34,35). However, neither was successful in reducing salt intake and it is not surprising that there was no difference in blood pressure in these studies between the community that was instructed on reducing salt, but failed to do so, and the community that was not given such instructions.

Treatment Trials

Effect of Salt Reduction on Blood Pressure

Ambard and Beaujard were the first to show that reducing salt intake lowered blood pressure in 1904. These results were confirmed over the next 30 years by several workers, but it was not until Kempner (1948) resuscitated the idea of a large reduction in salt intake that salt restriction became widely used in the treatment of hypertension.

The first double-blind placebo-controlled trial of a more modest reduction in salt intake was performed in the early 1980s (36). Nineteen patients with untreated mild to moderate essential hypertension were advised not to add salt to food and to avoid salt-laden foods. After two weeks of salt restriction patients were entered into an eight-week double-blind randomized crossover study of "Slow Sodium" versus "Slow Sodium Placebo," while remaining on the low-salt diet throughout the study. Urinary sodium excretion in the fourth week of slow sodium was 162 mmol/24 hr (equivalent to 9.5 g of salt per day) and that in the fourth week of placebo was 86 mmol/24 hr (5.1 g of salt; $p < 0.001$). The mean supine blood pressure was 7.1 mmHg (6.1%) lower in the fourth week of placebo than that in the fourth week of slow sodium ($p < 0.001$). The fall in blood pressure observed in this study was equivalent to that seen with a diuretic.

Since the first double-blind trial of a modest reduction in salt intake published in 1982 (36), there have been a large number of salt reduction trials carried out not only in hypertensive individuals, but also in normotensive subjects. Several meta-analyses of salt reduction trials have been performed (37–41). In two meta-analyses (38,40), it was claimed that the results showed that salt reduction had no or very little effect on blood pressure in individuals with normal blood pressure. The authors concluded that a reduction in population salt intake is not warranted. Furthermore, these papers were used as the basis of a commentary in Science (42) casting doubt on the link between salt intake and blood pressure, and have also been used to oppose public health recommendations for a reduction in salt intake (43). However, detailed examination of these two meta-analyses (38,40) shows that they are flawed. Both meta-analyses included trials of very short duration of salt restriction, many for only five days. On average, the median duration of salt reduction in individuals with normal blood pressure was only eight days in one meta-analysis and 14 days in the other. Furthermore, around half of these trials compared the effects of acute salt loading to abrupt and severe salt restriction, e.g., from 20 to less than 1 g/day of salt for only a few days. It is known that these acute and large changes in salt intake cause an increase in sympathetic activity, plasma renin activity and angiotensin II concentration (44), which would counteract the effects on blood pressure. It is also known that most blood pressure-lowering drugs do not exert their maximal effect within five days; this is particularly true with diuretics which are likely to work by a similar mechanism to that of a reduction in salt intake. For these reasons it is inappropriate to include the acute salt restriction trials in a meta-analysis that attempts to apply them to public health recommendations for a longer-term modest reduction in salt intake.

A recent meta-analysis by Hooper et al. (41) is an important attempt to look at whether long-term salt reduction (i.e., more than six months) in randomized trials causes a fall in blood pressure. However, most trials included in this meta-analysis only achieved a very small reduction in salt intake and, on average, salt intake was only reduced by 2 g/day. It is, therefore, not surprising that there was only a small, but still highly significant fall in blood pressure.

More recently, we carried out a meta-analysis of randomized trials. We only included trials of modest reductions in salt intake and with duration of one month or longer (45). Seventeen trials in hypertensives ($n=734$) and 11 trials in normotensives ($n=2220$) met the inclusion criteria. The median reduction in 24-hour urinary sodium excretion was 78 mmol (equivalent to 4.6 g of salt per day) in hypertensives and 74 mmol (4.4 g of salt per day) in normotensives. This modest reduction in salt intake was associated with a significant fall in blood pressure not only in hypertensive individuals, but also in those with normal blood pressure (Fig. 3). The pooled estimates of blood pressure fall were 4.96/2.73 mmHg in hypertensives ($p<0.001$ for both systolic and diastolic) and 2.03/0.97 mmHg in normotensives ($p<0.001$ for both systolic and diastolic). Furthermore, this meta-analysis demonstrated a dose–response relationship between the change in urinary sodium and the change in blood pressure, i.e., the greater the reduction in salt intake, the greater the fall in blood pressure.

Although the recent dietary approaches to stop hypertension (DASH)—sodium trial (46) was included in the above meta-analysis, it is still worth mentioning. It is a well-controlled feeding trial studying three levels of salt intake (8, 6, and 4 g/day) on two different diets (i.e., the normal American diet and the DASH diet, which is rich in fruits, vegetables, and low-fat dairy products). This study demonstrates that salt reduction lowers blood pressure in both hypertensive and normotensive individuals, and there is a dose–response relationship to salt reduction. Furthermore, salt reduction causes a further fall in blood pressure in individuals who consume the DASH diet. This is of importance in that it demonstrates that not only would there be benefit from reducing salt intake on the diet we currently consume, but there would be additional benefits if salt reduction is combined with an increase in fruit and vegetable consumption (Fig. 4).

Differences in Blood Pressure Response to Salt Reduction

Treatment trials have shown that, for a given reduction in salt intake, the falls in blood pressure are larger in individuals of African origin, in the older subjects, and in those with raised blood pressure (46,47). For instance, in the DASH-sodium study, when salt intake was reduced from 8 to 4 g/day, blood pressure fell by 8.0/4.5 mmHg in African Americans, whereas in non-African Americans blood pressure fell by 5.1/2.2 mmHg. In individuals with age of over 45 years, blood pressure fell by 7.5/3.8 mmHg, whereas in those ≤ 45 years blood pressure fell by 5.3/2.8 mmHg. In individuals with hypertension ($\geq 140/90$ mmHg), blood pressure fell by 8.3/4.4 mmHg, whereas in normotensive individuals blood pressure fell by 5.6/2.8 mmHg. Meta-analyses of randomized salt reduction trials have also shown that the falls in blood pressure are greater in hypertensives than normotensives (45). It has been shown that the difference in blood pressure responses to salt reduction is, at least in part, due to the difference in the levels of plasma renin activity and, thereby, angiotensin II, as well as the responsiveness of the renin-angiotensin system (48,49).

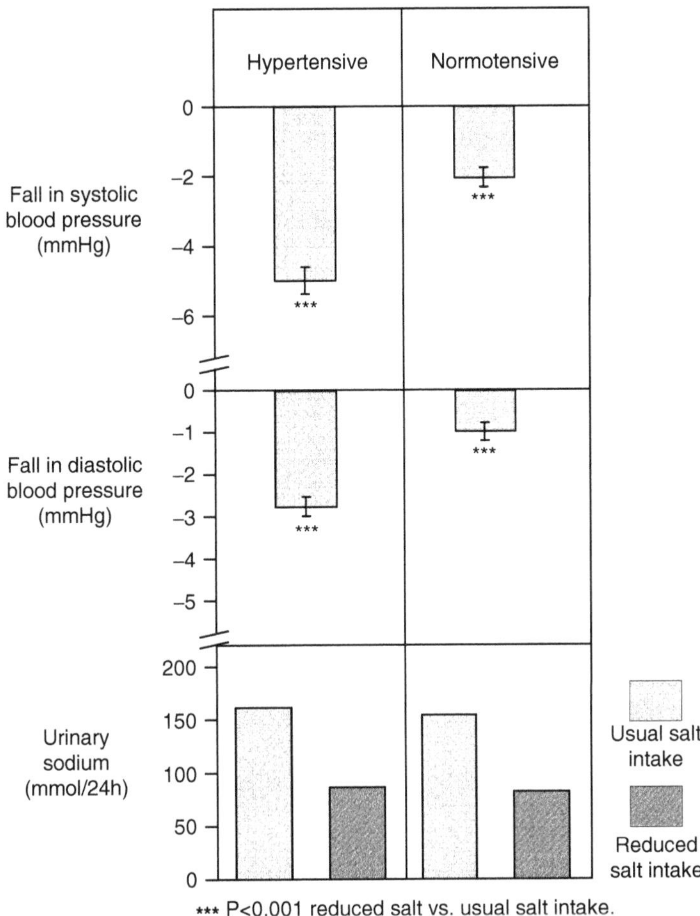

Figure 3 Effect of modest salt reduction on blood pressure in hypertensive and normotensive individuals in a meta-analysis of 28 randomized controlled trials of one month or longer.

Salt Reduction is Additive to Antihypertensive Drug Treatments and Reduces the Need for Antihypertensive Drug Therapy

The renin-angiotensin system is an important mechanism in maintaining blood pressure during the changes in salt intake. In other words, the reactive rise in plasma renin activity, and thereby, angiotensin II, with a reduction in salt intake offsets the fall in blood pressure that occurs with a low-salt diet (49). Salt reduction is therefore more effective in lowering blood pressure when the renin-angiotensin system is blocked by an angiotensin converting enzyme (ACE) inhibitor or angiotensin II antagonist. A randomized double-blind trial showed that a modest reduction in salt intake reduced blood pressure by 13/9 mmHg in hypertensive patients who were already on Captopril (50), whereas a similar reduction in salt intake lowered blood pressure by 8/5 mmHg in patients with a similar level of high blood pressure but who were not on any drugs (36,51).

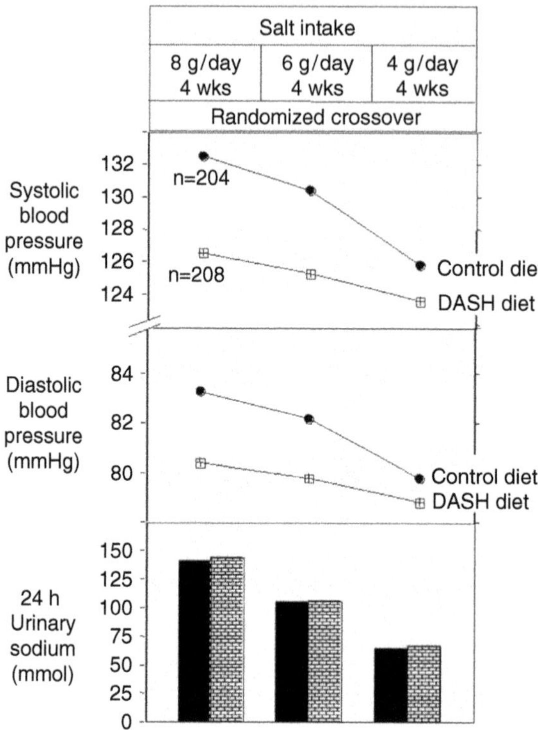

Figure 4 Changes in blood pressure and 24-hour urinary sodium excretion with the reduction in salt intake in all participants (hypertensives: $n=169$; normotensives: $n=243$) on the normal American diet (i.e., control diet) and on DASH diet. *Abbreviation*: DASH, dietary approaches to stop hypertension. *Source*: From Ref. 46.

Treatment trials have also shown that salt reduction enhances blood pressure control and reduces the need for antihypertensive drug therapy (52,53). The Trial of Nonpharmacologic Interventions in the Elderly evaluated the effects of salt reduction on blood pressure and hypertension control in 681 hypertensive patients, aged 60 to 80 years. Participants who had systolic blood pressure less than 145 mmHg and diastolic blood pressure less than 85 mmHg while taking one antihypertensive medication, were randomly assigned to a reduced salt or control group. Three months after the start of intervention, medication was withdrawn. The results showed that salt intake was reduced by an average of 2.4 g/day and this was associated with a significant reduction in trial end point (i.e., elevated blood pressure, resumption of medication, and cardiovascular events). The relative hazard ratios (HRs) for the reduced salt compared with usual salt was 0.68 ($p<0.001$), indicating a reduction of 32% in trial end point. At the end of follow-up (i.e., 30 months after drug withdrawal), 36% in the reduced salt group remained end point free, whereas in the usual salt group only 21% were free of end point (53).

Animal Studies

There are numerous studies in the rat, dog, chicken, rabbit, baboon, and chimpanzee, all of which have shown that when there is a prolonged increase in salt intake there is an increase in blood pressure. Furthermore, in all forms of experimental hypertension, whatever the animal model, a high salt intake is essential for blood pressure to rise.

A recent study was carried out in chimpanzees (98.8% genetic homology with man) (54). In a randomized parallel study, one group of chimpanzees was maintained on their normal diet of around half a gram of salt per day ($N=12$), and the other had salt intake increased to 5, 10, and 15 g/day ($N=10$). During the study there was no significant change in blood pressure in the control group. However, in the 10 animals assigned to the increased salt intake, mean systolic blood pressure was increased by 12 mmHg compared to the corresponding baseline level ($p<0.05$) after the first 19 weeks of supplementary salt intake (5 g/day). Following the 39 weeks of supplementation with 10 g/day of salt (three weeks) and 15 g/day of salt (36 weeks), mean systolic was increased by 26 mmHg ($p<0.001$). Following a further 26 weeks of supplementation with 15 g/day of salt (a total of 84 weeks of supplementation with salt), mean systolic was increased by 33 mmHg ($p<0.001$). Twenty weeks after the end of the salt supplementation period, the average level of blood pressure returned to its baseline level (Fig. 5). This experiment provides a direct evidence for a causal relationship between a high salt intake and a rise in blood pressure.

Human Genetic Studies

Attempts to identify the genes whose function or dysfunction have shed light on the importance of salt in regulating blood pressure. It is generally accepted that several genes may contribute to the blood pressure levels which reflects a complex network of gene–gene and gene–environment interactions. However, in some individuals, defects in a single gene cause marked abnormalities of blood pressure regulation. Genetic studies of

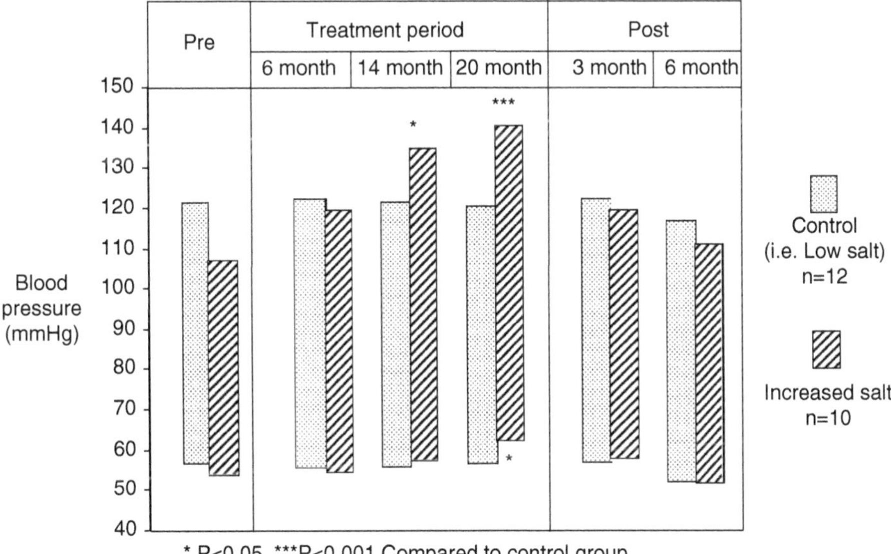

Figure 5 Blood pressure in chimpanzees that either continued on their usual low-salt diet or were given an increased salt intake. At the end of the 20-month study, the salt supplements were stopped and blood pressure declined to that of the control group. *Source*: From Ref. 54.

these rare Mendelian form of high and low blood pressure have shown an underlying common pathway: the kidney's ability to excrete or retain sodium (55,56). The monogenic causes of high blood pressure reduce the kidney's ability to excrete sodium and cause high blood pressure if salt is consumed. The monogenic causes of low blood pressure result in the kidney being unable to hold on to sodium normally, thereby causing low blood pressure. These forms of low blood pressure are ameliorated by a high salt intake. Overall these genetic studies clearly indicate the vital importance of salt in regulating blood pressure in humans.

SALT AND BLOOD PRESSURE IN CHILDREN—EPIDEMIOLOGICAL AND CLINICAL EVIDENCE FOR A LINK

A number of cross-sectional observational studies have looked at the relationship between salt intake and blood pressure in children (57–60). Most of these studies did not show a significant association. This is not surprising given the large day-to-day intra-individual variations of salt intake. However, the National Diet and Nutrition Survey for young people (aged 4 to 18 years) which measured blood pressure and salt intake using a seven-day dietary record in over 1500 children in the United Kingdom, did show that blood pressure tended to be higher in young people who usually added salt to their food at the table or added salt to their food in cooking compared to those who did not add salt (58). In another carefully-conducted study where seven consecutive 24-hour urines were collected by 73 children aged 11 to 14 years, there was a significant relationship between urinary sodium excretion and blood pressure, i.e., the higher the urinary sodium excretion, the higher the blood pressure (60). The relationship remained significant after controlling for age, sex, race, height, and body weight.

A longitudinal study of a cohort of 233 children with annual measurements blood pressure and overnight urinary sodium and potassium during an average follow-up period of seven years showed that the rise in blood pressure in childhood was significantly associated with urinary sodium/potassium ratio, i.e., the higher the sodium/potassium ratio, the greater the rise in blood pressure (61).

Several studies have looked at the effect of reducing dietary salt intake on blood pressure in children (62,63). However, most of the studies either did not achieve any reduction in salt intake, or were underpowered to detect a small fall in blood pressure with a reduction in salt intake in children. One study (the Exeter-Andover Project) was successful in reducing salt intake and did demonstrate a significant fall in blood pressure in adolescents (63). The Exeter-Andover Project was carried out in two boarding high schools with the intervention applied in each of the schools in alternate school years, with the second school serving as a control in each year. A total of 650 students (average age: 15 years old) participated in the study (341 in the intervention group and 309 in the control group). The intervention through changes in food purchasing and in preparation practices in the schools' kitchens achieved a reduction in salt intake of 15% to 20%. By the 24 weeks of the study the estimated net intervention effects were a decrease of 1.7/1.5 mmHg in blood pressure ($p<0.01$) with adjustments for sex and baseline blood pressure.

A well-controlled double-blind study in just under 500 newborn babies showed that when salt intake was reduced by about half (intervention vs. control group) for six months, as judged by spot urinary sodium concentrations, there was a progressive difference in systolic blood pressure (64). At the end of six months the babies on the lower salt intake had a 2.1 mmHg lower systolic blood pressure ($p<0.01$; Fig. 6). The study was discontinued at six months. Fifteen years later, 35% of these babies were restudied.

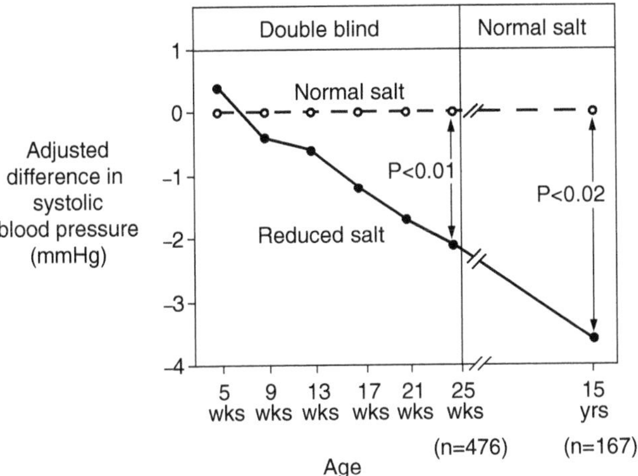

Figure 6 Difference in systolic blood pressure in newborn babies, randomized to either a normal salt intake or a reduced salt intake over the first six months of life. At six months, the study was discontinued, with all participants resuming their usual salt intake. Fifteen years later, a subgroup of those in the study had blood pressure remeasured. *Source*: From Refs. 64, 65.

There remained a significant difference in blood pressure, when adjusted for confounding factors, between those babies who in the first six months of life had a reduced salt intake compared to those that had not (65). This study suggests that there was a programming effect of salt intake in early life, which fits with several studies in animals (66).

HOW FAR SHOULD SALT INTAKE BE REDUCED?

Salt intake in many countries is between 9 and 12 g/day (4,5). The current World Health Organization recommendations for adults are to reduce salt intake to 5 g/day or less (67) and the U.K. and U.S. recommendations are to 6 g/day or less (15,68). However, these recommendations are based on what is feasible and not on what might have been the maximum impact on blood pressure and cardiovascular disease. Recent evidence suggests that these levels, whilst they may be feasible, are too high.

Studies in experimental animals have shown a clear dose–response relationship between salt intake and blood pressure, i.e., the higher the salt intake, the higher the blood pressure (66). A recent study in chimpanzees which has been referred to earlier, demonstrated a dose–response relationship when salt was increased from their usual intake of 0.5 g/day to 5, 10, and 15 g/day (54). In humans it is difficult to conduct such trials, particularly to keep individuals on a low-salt diet long term due to the widespread presence of salt in nearly all processed, restaurant, canteen, and fast foods. However, two well-controlled trials have studied three salt intakes, each for four weeks (46,51). One is our double blind study in 19 patients with untreated essential hypertension, and the other is the DASH-sodium study, where 79 untreated hypertensives and 116 normotensives were studied on the normal American diet and 81 untreated hypertensives and 121 normotensives were studied on the DASH diet. Both studies showed a clear dose–response relationship, i.e., the lower the salt intake, the lower the blood pressure (Fig. 7).

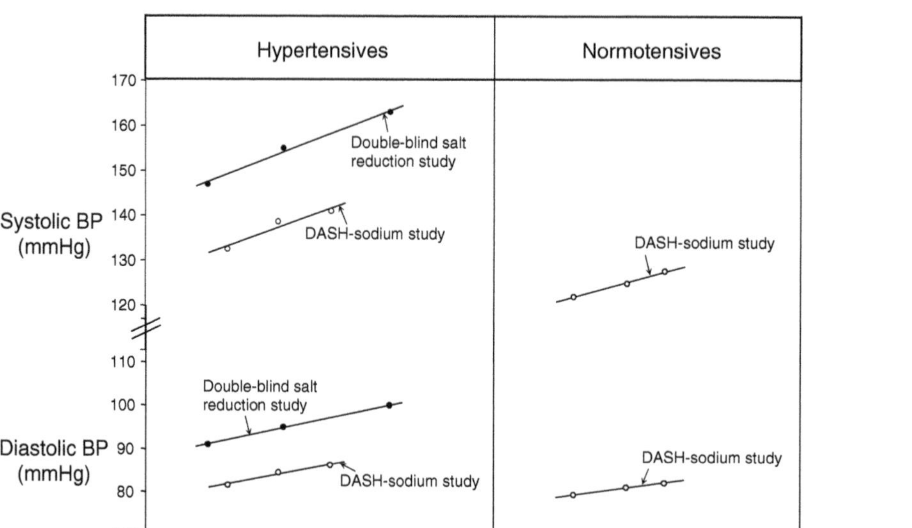

Figure 7 The dose–response relation between 24-hour urinary sodium and BP in the double-blind salt reduction study and the DASH-sodium study (individuals who were studied on the normal American diet). *Abbreviations*: BP, blood pressure; DASH, dietary approaches to stop hypertension. *Source*: From Refs. 46, 51.

In our double blind study with three salt intakes (51), the blood pressure decreased by 8/5 mmHg when salt intake, as judged by 24-hour urinary sodium, changed from 190 to 108 mmol/24 hr (11.2–6.4 g/day), and the blood pressure decreased by 8/4 mmHg when salt intake changed from 108 to 49 mmol/24 hr (6.4–2.9 g/day). The DASH-sodium study (46) showed that, in all individuals (i.e., both hypertensives and normotensives) who were studied on the normal American diet, the blood pressure decreased by 2.1/1.1 mmHg when salt intake changed from 141 to 106 mmol/24 hr (8.3–6.2 g/day), and the blood pressure decreased by 4.6/2.4 mmHg when salt intake changed from 106 to 64 mmol/24 hr (6.2–3.8 g/day). In those who were studied on the DASH diet, the blood pressure decreased by 1.3/0.6 mmHg when salt intake changed from 144 to 107 mmol/24 hr (8.5–6.3 g/day), and the blood pressure decreased by 1.7/1.0 mmHg when salt intake changed from 107 to 67 mmol/24 hr (6.3–3.9 g/day).

A recent meta-analysis of randomized trials of modest salt reduction for one month or longer demonstrates a significant relationship between the reduction in 24-hour urinary sodium and the fall in blood pressure, indicating the greater the reduction in salt intake, the greater the fall in blood pressure (Fig. 8) (45). A comparison of the dose–response relationship found in the meta-analysis with the two studies that had three levels of salt intake showed a consistent dose–response relationship to salt reduction within the range that was studied, i.e., 12 to 3 g/day, though the falls in blood pressure were greater in the better controlled studies (Fig. 9) (46,51). A reduction of 6 g/day (e.g., from the current intake of 12 g/day to the recommended level of 6 g/day) predicts a fall in blood pressure of 7 to 11/4 to 6 mmHg in hypertensives and 4 to 7/2 to 4 mmHg in

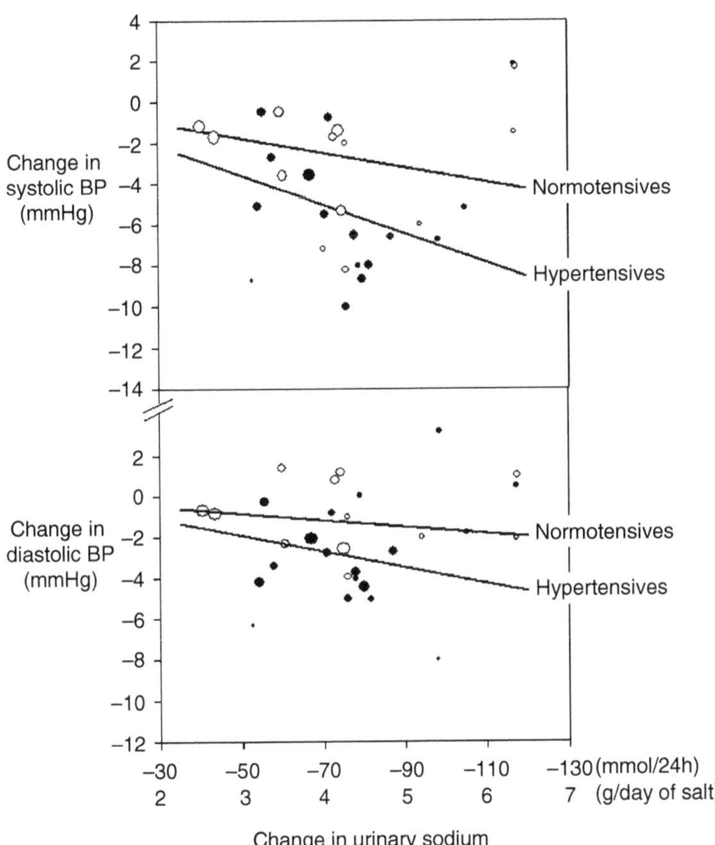

Figure 8 Relationship between the net change in urinary sodium excretion and BP in a meta-analysis of modest salt-reduction trials. The open circles represent normotensives and the solid circles represent hypertensives. The slope is weighted by the inverse of the variance of the net change in BP. The size of the circle is in proportion to the weight of the trial. *Abbreviations*: BP, blood pressure. *Source*: From Ref. 45.

normotensives depending on study. The effect would be much larger if salt intake were reduced further to 3 g/day (69).

From the evidence above, it is clear that the current public health recommendations to reduce salt intake from 9 to 12 g/day to 5 to 6 g/day will have a major effect on blood pressure, but are not ideal. A further reduction to 3 g/day will have a much greater effect and should, therefore, now become the long-term target for population salt intake worldwide.

SALT AND CARDIOVASCULAR MORTALITY

One of the difficulties of drawing conclusions about the importance of dietary or other lifestyle changes in cardiovascular disease is the gap in the evidence that relates to mortality. One has to accept that outcome studies of changing diet in the population are

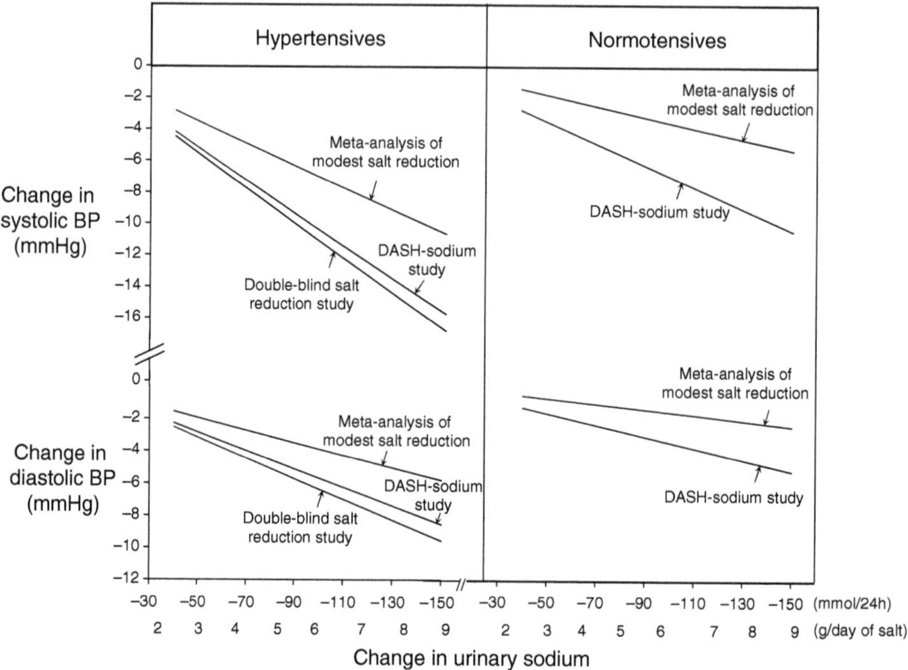

Figure 9 Comparison of the dose–response relationship among three studies: (*i*) meta-analysis of modest salt reduction trials; (*ii*) double-blind study with three levels of salt intake; and (*iii*) DASH-sodium study (individuals who were studied on the normal American diet). *Abbreviations*: BP, blood pressure; DASH, dietary approaches to stop hypertension. *Source*: From Refs. 45, 46, 51.

extremely difficult and there is unlikely to ever be outcome evidence on mortality for dietary variables, e.g., fruit and vegetables or other lifestyle changes, i.e., stopping smoking, losing weight, or taking exercise. For instance, a study on salt would need to randomize subjects at the time of conception to a lower and higher salt intake and then follow-up the two groups of offspring on a high and low salt intake for the rest of their lives. Such studies are impractical and would be unethical in the light of current knowledge.

Increasing blood pressure throughout the range is an important risk factor for cardiovascular disease. A reduction in salt intake lowers blood pressure, and would therefore be predicted to reduce cardiovascular disease. Based on falls in blood pressure from the meta-analysis of randomized salt reduction trials and the relationship between blood pressure and stroke and ischemic heart disease (IHD) from a recent meta-analysis of one million adults from 62 prospective studies, we estimated that a reduction of 3 g/day in salt intake would reduce strokes by 13% and IHD by 10% (69). In the U.K., the total number of stroke death is 60,666 a year and the total number of IHD death is 124,037 a year. Therefore, a reduction of 3 g/day in salt intake would prevent approximately 7800 stroke deaths and 11,500 IHD deaths a year. The effects on strokes and IHD would be almost doubled if salt intake were reduced by 6 g/day, and tripled with a 9 g/day reduction. A reduction of 9 g/day in salt intake (e.g., from 12 to 3 g/day) would reduce strokes by approximately a third and IHD by a quarter. In the U.K., this would prevent around 20,500 stroke deaths and 31,400 IHD deaths a year.

Approximately 50% of patients who suffer strokes or heart attacks survive, therefore, there would be a proportionate reduction in the numbers of these people. This would result in a reduction in disability and major cost savings both to individuals, their families and the Health Service. Furthermore, high blood pressure is an important risk factor for heart failure. A reduction in salt intake would therefore have a major effect on heart failure.

A reduction in salt intake not only lowers blood pressure, but also has other beneficial effect on the cardiovascular system, independent of and additive to the effect of salt reduction on blood pressure, e.g., a direct effect on stroke (70), left ventricular hypertrophy (71,72), renal disease and proteinuria. Therefore, the true effect of salt reduction on the cardiovascular outcome may be larger than those estimated from blood pressure fall alone.

Several epidemiological studies have looked at the relationship between salt intake and cardiovascular disease. A recently published prospective study of 29,079 Japanese men and women living in Takayama City and Gifu showed a significant association between salt intake and death from ischemic stroke (HR 3.22) and intracerebral hemorrhage (HR 3.85) in men and borderline associations (HR 1.70 and 2.10, respectively) in women (73). More convincingly, because avoiding potential inaccuracy of estimating the habitual salt intake from 24-hour dietary recall, a prospective Finnish cohort study conducted in 1173 men and 1263 women aged 25 to 64 years demonstrates a significant association between salt intake (judged by 24-hour urinary sodium excretion) and coronary heart disease mortality, cardiovascular disease mortality and total mortality (Fig. 10) (74). The HRs for coronary heart disease, cardiovascular disease, and all deaths associated with a 6 g increase in salt intake were 1.56, 1.36, and 1.22 respectively. In this study, the HR for cardiovascular disease mortality was 1.23 in men with normal body weight, while it was 1.44 for men who are overweight (body mass index ≥ 27 kg/m^2). This suggests that a high salt intake increased the risk of subsequent cardiovascular disease

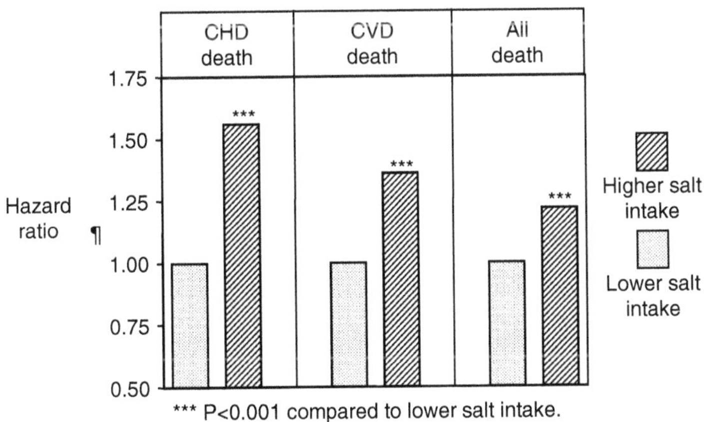

Figure 10 The hazard ratios for CHD, CVD, and all-cause mortality associated with a 6 g/day increase in salt intake as judged by 24-hour urinary sodium excretion. *Abbreviations*: CHD, coronary heart disease; CVD, cardiovascular disease. *Source*: From Ref. 74.

in both normal weight and overweight people, and the effect is larger in those who are overweight.

Alderman et al. have also attempted to look at the relationship between salt intake and cardiovascular disease in two cohort studies. The first one was in hypertensive individuals who had renin profiling performed prior to entering a study of long-term follow-up on blood pressure lowering drugs (75). In order to perform the renin profiling, all subjects had their salt intake restricted for five days to stimulate renin release. This enabled the subjects to be subgrouped into low, normal or high renin groups. Alderman found that the 24-hour urinary sodium excretion on the fifth day of a reduced salt intake was related to subsequent myocardial infarction and made the extraordinary claim that a lower salt intake led to more heart attacks. However, no measurement of salt intake had been carried out on the subjects' normal diet. Furthermore, no attempt was made to monitor salt intake during the follow-up period. Analysis of the 24-hour urinary sodium data also revealed severe methodological problems as the lowest salt quartile had a much lower 24-hour urinary creatinine excretion. This demonstrated that many of those who had been attributed to the lowest salt quartile on the fifth day of a reduced salt intake were there not because they had been successful in reducing their salt intake more, but had collected incomplete 24-hour urine samples (76).

The second study by Alderman et al. involved the National Health and Nutrition Examination Survey (NHANES 1)—a dietary survey of U.S. adults from the mid 1970s (77). However, any analysis of salt intake from this study is difficult to judge as 24-hour urinary sodium excretion was not measured and dietary salt was assessed by dietary history with no account taken of discretionary salt (i.e., salt added at the table or in cooking), which at that time would have accounted for more than half of the salt intake. Alderman claimed that salt intake was inversely related to cardiovascular disease. However, examination of the data showed major discrepancies, e.g., subjects in the lower salt group were on a calorie intake that was near starvation levels and yet weighed 4 kg more than those on the higher salt and calorie intake (78–81).

In view of the serious flaws in these two studies by Alderman et al., they cannot be used in any way to interpret the long-term effects of salt reduction. Indeed, a more appropriate analysis of the same NHANES 1 data showed a positive relationship between dietary salt intake and risk of stroke, coronary heart disease and heart failure in overweight individuals (body mass index >27 kg/m^2) (82).

OTHER HARMFUL EFFECTS OF SALT

There is increasing evidence that salt has other harmful effects on human health (6), which may be independent of and additive to the effect of salt on blood pressure, e.g., a direct effect on stroke (70), left ventricular hypertrophy (71,72), progression of renal disease and albuminuria (83–85), cancer of stomach (86,87), and bone demineralization (88).

Salt and Water Retention

When salt intake is increased, there is retention of sodium and thereby water, and this expands the extracellular fluid volume. This increase in extracellular volume is a trigger for various compensatory mechanisms to increase urinary sodium excretion but at the expense of continued retention of sodium and water. The increase in extracellular fluid exacerbates all forms of sodium and water retention, e.g., heart failure, and is a major cause of oedema in women, aggravating both cyclical and idiopathic oedema (89).

Salt and Stroke

Increasing blood pressure throughout the range is the major cause of stroke. A high salt intake causes a rise in blood pressure which will increase the risk of stroke. However, experimental studies in animals (90) and epidemiological studies in humans (70,91) have shown that a high-salt diet may have a direct effect on stroke, independent of and additive to its effect on blood pressure. Peery and Beevers performed an ecological analysis of the relationship between urinary sodium excretion (data from INTERSALT study) and stroke mortality in Western Europe. They found a significant positive correlation between urinary sodium excretion and stroke mortality (Fig. 11) (70), and this relationship is much stronger than that found when urinary sodium is plotted against blood pressure.

Salt and Left Ventricular Hypertrophy

Left ventricular hypertrophy is an important independent predictor of cardiovascular morbidity and mortality and is highly prevalent in individuals with raised blood pressure (92,93). Several cross-sectional studies have shown a positive correlation between urinary sodium excretion and left ventricular mass in both hypertensives and normotensives (Fig. 12) (71,94,95). More importantly, 24-hour urinary sodium has been shown to be

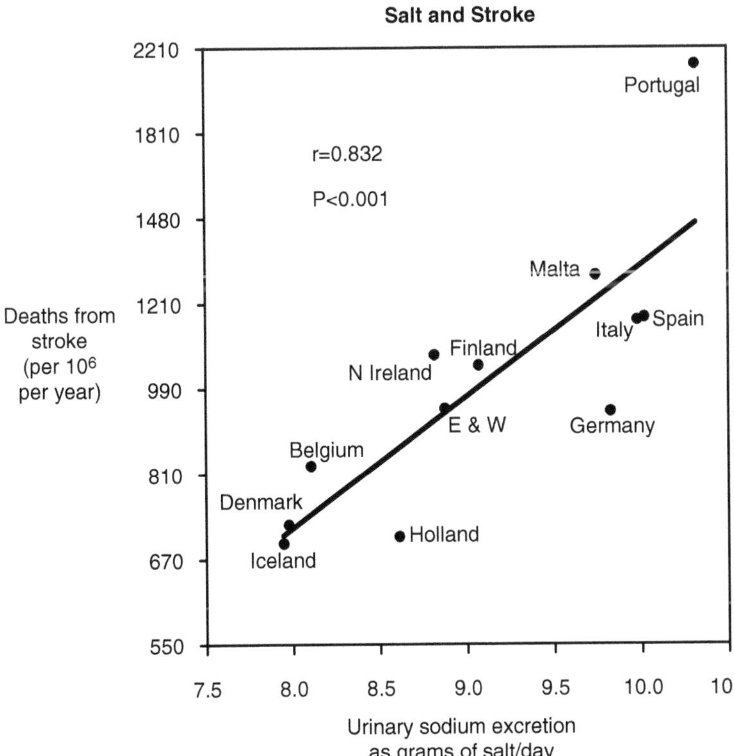

Figure 11 Relationship between salt intake and deaths from strokes in 12 European countries. *Abbreviation*: E & W, England and Wales. *Source*: From Ref. 70.

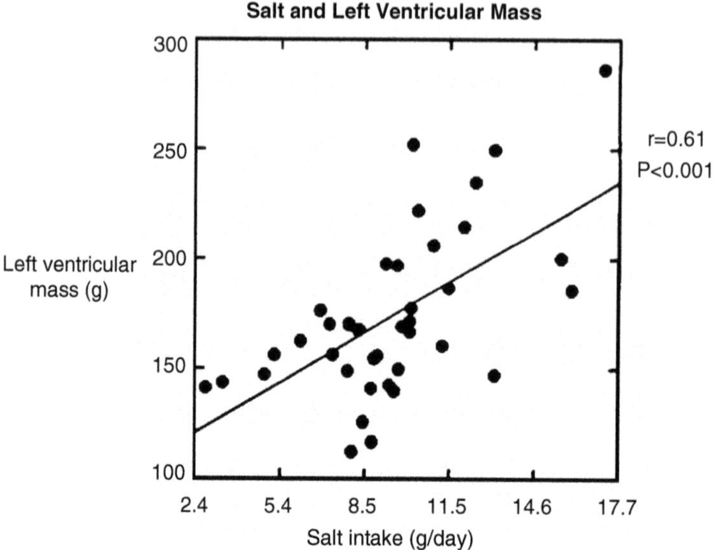

Figure 12 Relationship between salt intake and left ventricular mass in individuals with systolic blood pressure greater than 121 mmHg. *Source*: From Ref. 71.

an independent and more powerful determinant for left ventricular wall thickness than blood pressure (94). A reduction in salt intake has been shown to decrease left ventricular mass in patients with essential hypertension (96–98).

Salt and Blood Vessels

Stiffness of conduit arteries, measured as an increase in pulse wave velocity or pulse pressure, is a strong independent predictor of cardiovascular risk (99,100). Studies in both humans and experimental animals have shown that an increase in salt intake increases the stiffness of conduit arteries and the reactivity of the small resistance vessels and the wall thickness of both (101,102). In a study of two Chinese populations, the age-associated increase in pulse wave velocity was blunted in the population with a lower salt intake (103). Another study in normotensive subjects showed that a low-salt diet reduced arterial stiffness, independent of blood pressure (104). A recent randomized double-blind study shows that a modest reduction in dietary salt intake reduces pulse pressure both in individuals with isolated systolic hypertension and in those with both raised systolic and diastolic blood pressure, suggesting that salt reduction improves arterial distensibility (105). Another recently published paper by Gates et al. demonstrates that directly measured large elastic artery compliance is increased by dietary salt restriction in middle-aged and older men and women with stage one systolic hypertension (106).

Salt and Albuminuria

Urinary albumin excretion have been shown to be an independent and continuous risk factor for both renal and cardiovascular disease (107–109). Epidemiological studies have shown a direct association between salt intake and urinary albumin excretion, i.e., the higher the salt intake, the higher the urinary albumin excretion (110,111). A recent randomized double-blind trial in 40 hypertensive blacks demonstrates that a modest

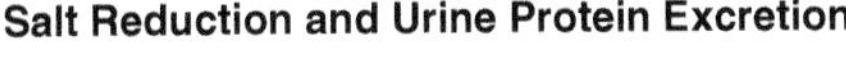

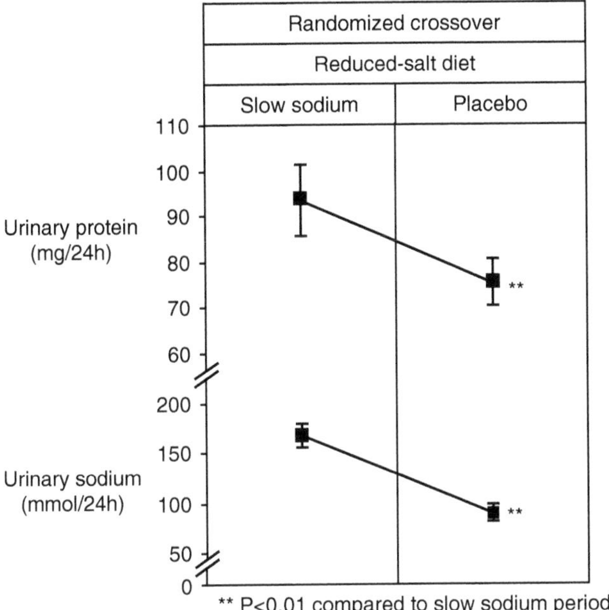

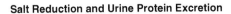

Figure 13 Change in urinary sodium and protein excretion with a modest reduction in salt intake in 40 hypertensive blacks.

reduction in salt intake from approximately 10 to 5 g/day, as currently recommended, reduces urinary protein excretion significantly (Fig. 13) (85). Other studies have shown that the antiproteinuric effect of ACE inhibitor is dependent on salt intake, i.e., a low salt intake enhances and a high salt intake abolishes the antiproteinuric effect of ACE inhibitor (84).

Salt and Stomach Cancer

Death from stomach cancer is the second commonest cause of death from cancer worldwide. An ecological analysis showed a significant direct association between salt intake (as judged by 24-hour urinary sodium excretion) and deaths from stomach cancer among 39 populations from 24 countries (Fig. 14) (86). A recent study from Japan confirms a close relationship between salt intake and stomach cancer within a single country (87). A number of studies have shown that H-pylori infection, which underlies the cause of both duodenal and gastric ulcers and stomach cancer, is also closely associated with salt intake in different countries in both women and men (112–114). Foods that contain high concentrations of salt are irritating to the delicate lining of the stomach. It is possible that this makes H-pylori infection more likely or more severe and that the H-pylori infection then leads to stomach cancer. A modest reduction in salt intake may reduce H-pylori infection and therefore lead to stomach cancer prevention.

Salt and Renal Stones and Bone Mineral Density

Salt intake is one of the major dietary determinants of urinary calcium excretion. Both epidemiological studies and randomized trials show that a reduction in salt intake causes

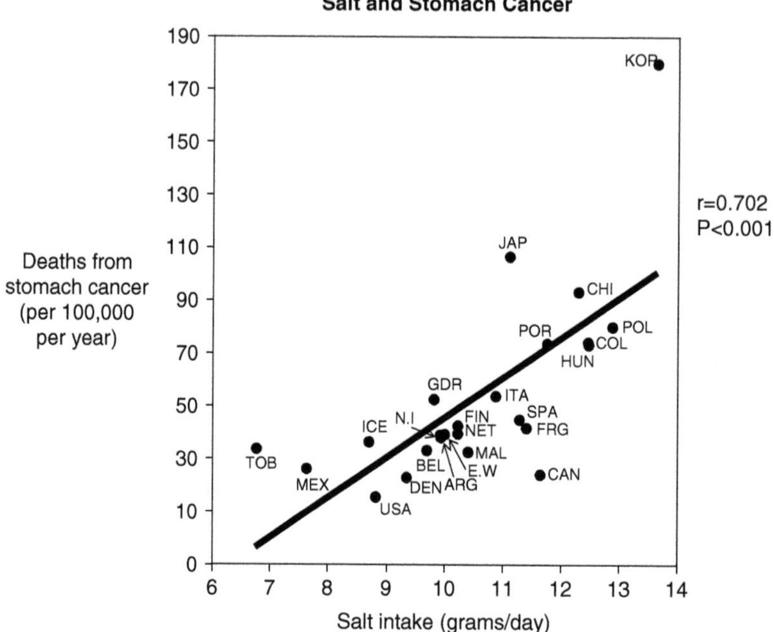

Figure 14 Relationship between salt intake and deaths from stomach cancer. *Abbreviation*: E & W, England and Wales. *Source*: From Ref. 86.

a decrease in urinary calcium excretion (115–118). As calcium is the main component of most urinary stones, salt intake is therefore an important cause of renal stones.

Until recently, it was assumed that when salt intake was increased, the increase in calcium excretion was compensated for by an increase in intestinal calcium absorption. There is now evidence to suggest that, when salt intake is increased, there is a negative calcium balance with stimulation of mechanisms not only to increase intestinal absorption of calcium, but also to mobilize calcium from bone. A study in postmenopausal women showed that the loss of hip bone density over two years was related to the 24-hour urinary sodium excretion at entry to the study and was as strong as that relating to calcium intake (88). Diuretics, through a reduction in extra cellular volume, reduce calcium excretion leading to a positive calcium balance, increase bone density and reduce bone fractures. Salt reduction is likely to do the same.

Salt and Asthma

Epidemiological evidence suggests that the severity of asthma may be related to salt intake in different countries (119). A double-blind study of modest salt reduction caused a decrease in the severity of asthma attacks and a reduction in the use of medication and an improvement in the measurement of airways' resistance (120). A more recent double-blind study illustrates the mechanism whereby a higher salt intake exacerbates asthma (121).

CONCLUSIONS

The evidence that links salt intake to blood pressure is now overwhelming. Current recommendations are to reduce salt intake from 9 to 12 g/day to 5 to 6 g/day. From the evidence reviewed in this chapter, it is clear that these reductions will have a major effect on blood pressure and cardiovascular disease, but reducing salt intake further than 3 g/day will have additional large effects. Therefore, the target of 5 to 6 g/day should be seen as an interim target and the long-term target for population salt intake worldwide should now be 3 g/day.

One important point is how to reduce salt intake to the target levels of 5 to 6 g/day. In most developed countries 75% to 80% of salt intake now comes from salt added to processed foods. The best strategy would be to have the food industry gradually reduce the salt concentration of all processed foods, starting with a 10% to 25% reduction, which is not detectable by human salt taste receptors (122) and causes no problem in the food technology, and continuing a sustained reduction over the course of the next decade. This strategy has now been adopted in the U.K. by the Department of Health and Food Standards Agency and several leading supermarkets and food manufacturers that have already started to implement such changes. Of all the dietary changes that can help to prevent cardiovascular disease, a reduction in salt intake is the easiest change to make as it can be done without the consumers' knowledge. But it requires the cooperation of the food industry. Clearly it would be helped if individuals also reduced the amount of salt they add to food prepared at home.

Some members of the food industry are reluctant to reduce the salt content of processed foods. This is because salt makes cheap, unpalatable food edible at low cost (3). If high-salt foods are consistently consumed, the salt taste receptors are suppressed and habituation to high-salt foods occurs, with greater demand for cheap but profitable high-salt processed foods (Fig. 15). Salt also has two other important properties—one is in meat products where increasing the salt concentration in conjunction with other water-binding chemicals increases the amount of water that can be bound into the meat product and the weight of the product can be increased by up to 20% with water. The other important property is that salt is a major determinant of thirst and any reduction in salt intake will

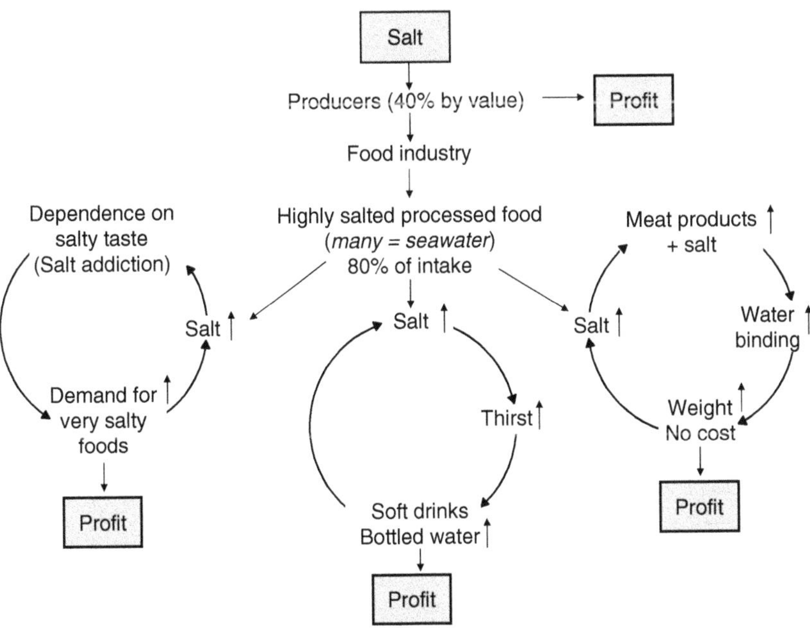

Figure 15 The commercial importance of salt in processed food.

reduce fluid consumption with a subsequent reduction in soft drink and bottled water sales (123). Some of the largest snack companies in the world are owned by companies selling soft drinks. It is therefore not surprising that the salt industry and some members of the food industry are very reluctant to see any reduction in salt intake and have been largely responsible for trying to make salt such a controversial issue relative to other dietary changes. Their strategies are identical to the techniques used by the tobacco industry and the Tobacco Manufacturers Association. The commercial reasons for this opposition need to be acknowledged. However, they should not be allowed to stand in the way of a reduction in salt intake as this reduction will be of major benefit to the future health of the whole population, particularly if it is combined with other dietary and lifestyle changes, e.g., increasing fruit and vegetable consumption, reducing saturated fat intake, and stopping smoking. The bulk of the food industry has nothing to fear for gradually reducing the very high-salt concentration of the many foods they produce. Indeed these foods are healthier. They lower blood pressure and reduce the risk of cardiovascular disease, renal disease, stomach cancer, and bone demineralization. The population will therefore live longer and there will be an increase in the number of consumers.

REFERENCES

1. Eaton SB, Konner M. Paleolithic nutrition. A consideration of its nature and current implications. N Engl J Med 1985; 312:283–9.
2. MacGregor GA, de Wardener HE. Salt, Diet and Health. Cambridge, MA: Cambridge University Press, 1998.
3. Nestle M. Food Politics—How the Food Industry Influences Nutrition and Health. London: University of California Press, 2002.
4. Henderson L, Irving K, Gregory J, et al. National Diet and Nutrition Survey: adults aged 19 to 64. Vol. 3. London: TSO, 2003:127–36.
5. INTERSALT. Intersalt: an international study of electrolyte excretion and blood pressure. Results for 24 hour urinary sodium and potassium excretion. Intersalt Cooperative Research Group. BMJ 1988; 297:319–28.
6. de Wardener HE, MacGregor GA. Harmful effects of dietary salt in addition to hypertension. J Hum Hypertens 2002; 16:213–23.
7. Lewington S, Clarke R, Qizilbash N, Peto R, Collins R. Age-specific relevance of usual blood pressure to vascular mortality: a meta-analysis of individual data for one million adults in 61 prospective studies. Lancet 2002; 360:1903–13.
8. Vasan RS, Larson MG, Leip EP, et al. Impact of high-normal blood pressure on the risk of cardiovascular disease. N Engl J Med 2001; 345:1291–7.
9. Chobanian AV, Bakris GL, Black HR, et al. Seventh Report of the Joint National Committee on Prevention, Detection, Evaluation, and Treatment of High Blood Pressure. Hypertension 2003; 42:1206–52.
10. Primatesta P, Brookes M, Poulter NR. Improved hypertension management and control: results from the health survey for England 1998. Hypertension 2001; 38:827–32.
11. Kearney PM, Whelton M, Reynolds K, Muntner P, Whelton PK, He J. Global burden of hypertension: analysis of worldwide data. Lancet 2005; 365:217–23.
12. Staessen JA, Wang JG, Thijs L. Cardiovascular protection and blood pressure reduction: a meta-analysis. Lancet 2001; 358:1305–15.
13. Neal B, MacMahon S, Chapman N. Effects of ACE inhibitors, calcium antagonists, and other blood-pressure-lowering drugs: results of prospectively designed overviews of randomised trials. Blood Pressure Lowering Treatment Trialists' Collaboration. Lancet 2000; 356:1955–64.
14. MacMahon S. Blood pressure and the prevention of stroke. J Hypertens Suppl 1996; 14:S39–46.

15. Whelton PK, He J, Appel LJ, et al. Primary prevention of hypertension: clinical and public health advisory from The National High Blood Pressure Education Program. JAMA 2002; 288:1882–8.
16. Dahl L. Possible role of salt intake in the development of essential hypertension. In: Cottier P, Bock KD, eds. Essential Hypertension—An International Symposium. Berlin: Springer, 1960:53–65.
17. Elliott P, Stamler J, Nichols R, et al. Intersalt revisited: further analyses of 24 hour sodium excretion and blood pressure within and across populations. Intersalt Cooperative Research Group. BMJ 1996; 312:1249–53.
18. Elliott P, Stamler J. Evidence on salt and blood pressure is consistent and persuasive. Int J Epidemiol 2002; 31:316–9.
19. Zhou BF, Stamler J, Dennis B, et al. Nutrient intakes of middle-aged men and women in China, Japan, United Kingdom, and United States in the late 1990s: the INTERMAP study. J Hum Hypertens 2003; 17:623–30.
20. Stamler J, Elliott P, Appel L, Chan Q, Buzzard M, Dennis B, Dyer AR, Elmer P, Greenland P, Jones D, et al. Higher blood pressure in middle-aged American adults with less education-role of multiple dietary factors: the INTERMAP study. J Hum Hypertens 2003; 17:655–775.
21. Khaw KT, Bingham S, Welch A, et al. Blood pressure and urinary sodium in men and women: the Norfolk Cohort of the European Prospective Investigation into Cancer (EPIC-Norfolk). Am J Clin Nutr 2004; 80:1397–403.
22. Mancilha-Carvalho JJ, de Oliveira R, Esposito RJ. Blood pressure and electrolyte excretion in the Yanomamo Indians, an isolated population. J Hum Hypertens 1989; 3:309–14.
23. Oliver WJ, Cohen EL, Neel JV. Blood pressure, sodium intake, and sodium related hormones in the Yanomamo Indians, a "no-salt" culture. Circulation 1975; 52:146–51.
24. Page LB, Damon A, Moellering RC, Jr. Antecedents of cardiovascular disease in six Solomon Islands societies. Circulation 1974; 49:1132–46.
25. Page LB, Vandevert DE, Nader K, Lubin NK, Page JR. Blood pressure of Qash'qai pastoral nomads in Iran in relation to culture, diet, and body form. Am J Clin Nutr 1981; 34:527–38.
26. Poulter NR, Khaw KT, Hopwood BE, et al. The Kenyan Luo migration study: observations on the initiation of a rise in blood pressure. BMJ 1990; 300:967–72.
27. He J, Klag MJ, Whelton PK, et al. Migration, blood pressure pattern, and hypertension: the Yi Migrant Study. Am J Epidemiol 1991; 134:1085–101.
28. He J, Tell GS, Tang YC, Mo PS, He GQ. Relation of electrolytes to blood pressure in men. The Yi people study. Hypertension 1991; 17:378–85.
29. Iso H, Shimamoto T, Yokota K, et al. Changes in 24-hour urinary excretion of sodium and potassium in a community-based heath education program on salt reduction. Nippon Koshu Eisei Zasshi 1999; 46:894–903.
30. Kimura N. Changing patterns of coronary heart disease, stroke, and nutrient intake in Japan. Prev Med 1983; 12:222–7.
31. Tanaka H, Tanaka Y, Hayashi M, et al. Secular trends in mortality for cerebrovascular diseases in Japan, 1960 to 1979. Stroke 1982; 13:574–81.
32. Forte JG, Miguel JM, Miguel MJ, de Padua F, Rose G. Salt and blood pressure: a community trial. J Hum Hypertens 1989; 3:179–84.
33. Tian HG, Guo ZY, Hu G, et al. Changes in sodium intake and blood pressure in a community-based intervention project in China. J Hum Hypertens 1995; 9:959–68.
34. Staessen J, Bulpitt CJ, Fagard R, Joossens JV, Lijnen P, Amery A. Salt intake and blood pressure in the general population: a controlled intervention trial in two towns. J Hypertens 1988; 6:965–73.
35. Tuomilehto J, Puska P, Nissinen A, et al. Community-based prevention of hypertension in North Karelia, Finland. Ann Clin Res 1984; 16(Suppl. 43):18–27.
36. MacGregor GA, Markandu ND, Best FE, et al. Double-blind randomised crossover trial of moderate sodium restriction in essential hypertension. Lancet 1982; 1:351–5.
37. Law MR, Frost CD, Wald NJ. By how much does dietary salt reduction lower blood pressure? III–Analysis of data from trials of salt reduction BMJ 1991; 302:819–24.

38. Midgley JP, Matthew AG, Greenwood CM, Logan AG. Effect of reduced dietary sodium on blood pressure: a meta-analysis of randomized controlled trials. JAMA 1996; 275:1590–7.
39. Cutler JA, Follmann D, Allender PS. Randomized trials of sodium reduction: an overview. Am J Clin Nutr 1997; 65:643S–51.
40. Graudal NA, Galloe AM, Garred P. Effects of sodium restriction on blood pressure, renin, aldosterone, catecholamines, cholesterols, and triglyceride: a meta-analysis. JAMA 1998; 279:1383–91.
41. Hooper L, Bartlett C, Davey Smith G, Ebrahim S. Systematic review of long term effects of advice to reduce dietary salt in adults. BMJ 2002; 325:628.
42. Taubes G. The (political) science of salt. Science 1998; 281:898–901.
43. Swales J. Population advice on salt restriction: the social issues. Am J Hypertens 2000; 13:2–7.
44. He FJ, Markandu ND, MacGregor GA. Importance of the renin system for determining blood pressure fall with acute salt restriction in hypertensive and normotensive whites. Hypertension 2001; 38:321–5.
45. He FJ, MacGregor GA. Effect of modest salt reduction on blood pressure: a meta-analysis of randomized trials. Implications for public health. J Hum Hypertens 2002; 16:761–70.
46. Sacks FM, Svetkey LP, Vollmer WM, et al. Effects on blood pressure of reduced dietary sodium and the Dietary Approaches to Stop Hypertension (DASH) diet. DASH-Sodium Collaborative Research Group. N Engl J Med 2001; 344:3–10.
47. Vollmer WM, Sacks FM, Ard J, et al. Effects of diet and sodium intake on blood pressure: subgroup analysis of the DASH-sodium trial. Ann Intern Med 2001; 135:1019–28.
48. He FJ, Markandu ND, Sagnella GA, MacGregor GA. Importance of the renin system in determining blood pressure fall with salt restriction in black and white hypertensives. Hypertension 1998; 32:820–4.
49. He FJ, MacGregor GA. Salt, blood pressure and the renin-angiotensin system. J Renin Angiotensin Aldosterone Syst 2003; 4:11–6.
50. MacGregor GA, Markandu ND, Singer DR, Cappuccio FP, Shore AC, Sagnella GA. Moderate sodium restriction with angiotensin converting enzyme inhibitor in essential hypertension: a double blind study. BMJ (Clin Res Ed) 1987; 294:531–4.
51. MacGregor GA, Markandu ND, Sagnella GA, Singer DR, Cappuccio FP. Double-blind study of three sodium intakes and long-term effects of sodium restriction in essential hypertension. Lancet 1989; 2:1244–7.
52. Whelton PK, Appel LJ, Espeland MA, et al. Sodium reduction and weight loss in the treatment of hypertension in older persons: a randomized controlled trial of nonpharmacologic interventions in the elderly (TONE). TONE Collaborative Research Group. JAMA 1998; 279:839–46.
53. Appel LJ, Espeland MA, Easter L, Wilson AC, Folmar S, Lacy CR. Effects of reduced sodium intake on hypertension control in older individuals: results from the Trial of Nonpharmacologic Interventions in the Elderly (TONE). Arch Intern Med 2001; 161:685–93.
54. Denton D, Weisinger R, Mundy NI, et al. The effect of increased salt intake on blood pressure of chimpanzees. Nat Med 1995; 1:1009–16.
55. Lifton RP. Molecular genetics of human blood pressure variation. Science 1996; 272:676–80.
56. Lifton RP, Gharavi AG, Geller DS. Molecular mechanisms of human hypertension. Cell 2001; 104:545–56.
57. Simon JA, Obarzanek E, Daniels SR, Frederick MM. Dietary cation intake and blood pressure in black girls and white girls. Am J Epidemiol 1994; 139:130–40.
58. Gregory J, Lowe S. National Diet and Nutrition Survey: young people aged 4 to 18 years. Vol 1: Report of the diet and nutrition survey. London: The stationery office, 2000.
59. Maldonado-Martin A, Garcia-Matarin L, Gil-Extremera B, et al. Blood pressure and urinary excretion of electrolytes in Spanish schoolchildren. J Hum Hypertens 2002; 16:473–8.
60. Cooper R, Soltero I, Liu K, Berkson D, Levinson S, Stamler J. The association between urinary sodium excretion and blood pressure in children. Circulation 1980; 62:97–104.

61. Geleijnse JM, Grobbee DE, Hofman A. Sodium and potassium intake and blood pressure change in childhood. BMJ 1990; 300:899–902.
62. Falkner B, Michel S. Blood pressure response to sodium in children and adolescents. Am J Clin Nutr 1997; 65:618S–21.
63. Ellison RC, Capper AL, Stephenson WP, et al. Effects on blood pressure of a decrease in sodium use in institutional food preparation: the Exeter-Andover Project. J Clin Epidemiol 1989; 42:201–8.
64. Hofman A, Hazebroek A, Valkenburg HA. A randomized trial of sodium intake and blood pressure in newborn infants. JAMA 1983; 250:370–3.
65. Geleijnse JM, Hofman A, Witteman JC, Hazebroek AA, Valkenburg HA, Grobbee DE. Long-term effects of neonatal sodium restriction on blood pressure. Hypertension 1997; 29:913–7.
66. Dahl LK, Knudsen KD, Heine MA, Leitl GJ. Effects of chronic excess salt ingestion. Modification of experimental hypertension in the rat by variations in the diet. Circ Res 1968; 22:11–8.
67. WHO. Joint WHO/FAO expert consultation on diet, nutrition and the prevention of chronic diseases. Geneva, 2003. (Accessed March 22, 2005 at http://www.who.int/hpr/NPH/docs/who_fao_experts_report.pdf)
68. SACN. Scientific Advisory Committee on Nutrition, Salt and Health. The Stationery Office, 2003. (Accessed March 22, 2005 at http://www.sacn.gov.uk/pdfs/sacn_salt_final.pdf)
69. He FJ, MacGregor GA. How far should salt intake be reduced? Hypertension 2003; 42:1093–9.
70. Perry IJ, Beevers DG. Salt intake and stroke: a possible direct effect. J Hum Hypertens 1992; 6:23–5.
71. Kupari M, Koskinen P, Virolainen J. Correlates of left ventricular mass in a population sample aged 36 to 37 years. Focus on lifestyle and salt intake. Circulation 1994; 89:1041–50.
72. Schmieder RE, Messerli FH. Hypertension and the heart. J Hum Hypertens 2000; 14:597–604.
73. Nagata C, Takatsuka N, Shimizu N, Shimizu H. Sodium intake and risk of death from stroke in Japanese men and women. Stroke 2004; 35:1543–7.
74. Tuomilehto J, Jousilahti P, Rastenyte D, et al. Urinary sodium excretion and cardiovascular mortality in Finland: a prospective study. Lancet 2001; 357:848–51.
75. Alderman MH, Madhavan S, Cohen H, Sealey JE, Laragh JH. Low urinary sodium is associated with greater risk of myocardial infarction among treated hypertensive men. Hypertension 1995; 25:1144–52.
76. MacGregor G. Low urinary sodium and myocardial infarction. Hypertension 1996; 27:156.
77. Alderman MH, Cohen H, Madhavan S. Dietary sodium intake and mortality: the National Health and Nutrition Examination Survey (NHANES I). Lancet 1998; 351:781–5.
78. de Wardener HE. Salt reduction and cardiovascular risk: the anatomy of a myth. J Hum Hypertens 1999; 13:1–4.
79. de Wardener H, MacGregor GA. Sodium intake and mortality. Lancet 1998; 351:1508.
80. Engelman K. Sodium intake and mortality. Lancet 1998; 351:1508–9.
81. Karppanen H, Mervaala E. Sodium intake and mortality. Lancet 1998; 351:1509.
82. He J, Ogden LG, Vupputuri S, Bazzano LA, Loria C, Whelton PK. Dietary sodium intake and subsequent risk of cardiovascular disease in overweight adults. JAMA 1999; 282:2027–34.
83. Cianciaruso B, Bellizzi V, Minutolo R, et al. Salt intake and renal outcome in patients with progressive renal disease. Miner Electrolyte Metab 1998; 24:296–301.
84. Heeg JE, de Jong PE, van der Hem GK, de Zeeuw D. Efficacy and variability of the anti-proteinuric effect of ACE inhibition by lisinopril. Kidney Int 1989; 36:272–9.
85. Swift PA, Markandu ND, Sagnella GA, He FJ, MacGregor GA. Modest salt reduction reduces blood pressure and urine protein excretion in black hypertensives. A randomised control trial. Hypertension 2005; 46:308–12.
86. Joossens JV, Hill MJ, Elliott P, et al. Dietary salt, nitrate and stomach cancer mortality in 24 countries. European Cancer Prevention (ECP) and the INTERSALT Cooperative Research Group. Int J Epidemiol 1996; 25:494–504.

87. Tsugane S, Sasazuki S, Kobayashi M, Sasaki S. Salt and salted food intake and subsequent risk of gastric cancer among middle-aged Japanese men and women. Br J Cancer 2004; 90:128–34.
88. Devine A, Criddle RA, Dick IM, Kerr DA, Prince RL. A longitudinal study of the effect of sodium and calcium intakes on regional bone density in postmenopausal women. Am J Clin Nutr 1995; 62:740–5.
89. MacGregor GA, de Wardener HE. Idiopathic edema. In: Schrier RW, Gottschalk CW, eds. Diseases of the Kidney. Boston, MA: Little Brown and Company, 1997:2343–52.
90. Tobian L, Hanlon S. High sodium chloride diets injure arteries and raise mortality without changing blood pressure. Hypertension 1990; 15:900–3.
91. Xie JX, Sasaki S, Joossens JV, Kesteloot H. The relationship between urinary cations obtained from the INTERSALT study and cerebrovascular mortality. J Hum Hypertens 1992; 6:17–21.
92. Levy D, Garrison RJ, Savage DD, Kannel WB, Castelli WP. Prognostic implications of echocardiographically determined left ventricular mass in the Framingham Heart Study. N Engl J Med 1990; 322:1561–6.
93. Laufer E, Jennings GL, Korner PI, Dewar E. Prevalence of cardiac structural and functional abnormalities in untreated primary hypertension. Hypertension 1989; 13:151–62.
94. Schmieder RE, Messerli FH, Garavaglia GE, Nunez BD. Dietary salt intake. A determinant of cardiac involvement in essential hypertension. Circulation 1988; 78:951–6.
95. Du Cailar G, Ribstein J, Daures JP, Mimran A. Sodium and left ventricular mass in untreated hypertensive and normotensive subjects. Am J Physiol 1992; 263:H177–81.
96. Ferrara LA, de Simone G, Pasanisi F, Mancini M. Left ventricular mass reduction during salt depletion in arterial hypertension. Hypertension 1984; 6:755–9.
97. Liebson PR, Grandits GA, Dianzumba S, et al. Comparison of five antihypertensive monotherapies and placebo for change in left ventricular mass in patients receiving nutritional-hygienic therapy in the Treatment of Mild Hypertension Study (TOMHS). Circulation 1995; 91:698–706.
98. Jula AM, Karanko HM. Effects on left ventricular hypertrophy of long-term nonpharmacological treatment with sodium restriction in mild-to-moderate essential hypertension. Circulation 1994; 89:1023–31.
99. Blacher J, Asmar R, Djane S, London GM, Safar ME. Aortic pulse wave velocity as a marker of cardiovascular risk in hypertensive patients. Hypertension 1999; 33:1111–7.
100. Gasowski J, Fagard RH, Staessen JA, et al. Pulsatile blood pressure component as predictor of mortality in hypertension: a meta-analysis of clinical trial control groups. J Hypertens 2002; 20:145–51.
101. Safar ME, Thuilliez C, Richard V, Benetos A. Pressure-independent contribution of sodium to large artery structure and function in hypertension. Cardiovasc Res 2000; 46:269–76.
102. Simon G, Illyes G. Structural vascular changes in hypertension: role of angiotensin II, dietary sodium supplementation, and sympathetic stimulation, alone and in combination in rats. Hypertension 2001; 37:255–60.
103. Avolio AP, Deng FQ, Li WQ, et al. Effects of aging on arterial distensibility in populations with high and low prevalence of hypertension: comparison between urban and rural communities in China. Circulation 1985; 71:202–10.
104. Avolio AP, Clyde KM, Beard TC, Cooke HM, Ho KK, O'Rourke MF. Improved arterial distensibility in normotensive subjects on a low salt diet. Arteriosclerosis 1986; 6:166–9.
105. He FJ, Markandu ND, Macgregor GA. Modest salt reduction lowers blood pressure in isolated systolic hypertension and combined hypertension. Hypertension 2005; 46(1):66–70.
106. Gates PE, Tanaka H, Hiatt WR, Seals DR. Dietary sodium restriction rapidly improves large elastic artery compliance in older adults with systolic hypertension. Hypertension 2004; 44:35–41.
107. Grimm RH, Jr., Svendsen KH, Kasiske B, Keane WF, Wahi MM. Proteinuria is a risk factor for mortality over 10 years of follow-up. MRFIT Research Group. Multiple Risk Factor Intervention Trial. Kidney Int Suppl 1997; 63:S10–4.

108. Gerstein HC, Mann JF, Yi Q, et al. Albuminuria and risk of cardiovascular events, death, and heart failure in diabetic and nondiabetic individuals. JAMA 2001; 286:421–6.
109. Hillege HL, Fidler V, Diercks GF, et al. Urinary albumin excretion predicts cardiovascular and noncardiovascular mortality in general population. Circulation 2002; 106:1777–82.
110. du Cailar G, Ribstein J, Mimran A. Dietary sodium and target organ damage in essential hypertension. Am J Hypertens 2002; 15:222–9.
111. Verhave JC, Hillege HL, Burgerhof JG, et al. Sodium intake affects urinary albumin excretion especially in overweight subjects. J Intern Med 2004; 256:324–30.
112. Beevers DG, Lip GY, Blann AD. Salt intake and Helicobacter pylori infection. J Hypertens 2004; 22:1475–7.
113. Wong BC, Lam SK, Wong WM, et al. Helicobacter pylori eradication to prevent gastric cancer in a high-risk region of China: a randomized controlled trial. JAMA 2004; 291:187–94.
114. Forman D, Newell DG, Fullerton F, et al. Association between infection with Helicobacter pylori and risk of gastric cancer: evidence from a prospective investigation. BMJ 1991; 302:1302–5.
115. Matkovic V, Ilich JZ, Andon MB, et al. Urinary calcium, sodium, and bone mass of young females. Am J Clin Nutr 1995; 62:417–25.
116. Cappuccio FP, Markandu ND, Carney C, Sagnella GA, MacGregor GA. Double-blind randomised trial of modest salt restriction in older people. Lancet 1997; 350:850–4.
117. Cappuccio FP, Kalaitzidis R, Duneclift S, Eastwood JB. Unravelling the links between calcium excretion, salt intake, hypertension, kidney stones and bone metabolism. J Nephrol 2000; 13:169–77.
118. Lin PH, Ginty F, Appel LJ, et al. The DASH diet and sodium reduction improve markers of bone turnover and calcium metabolism in adults. J Nutr 2003; 133:3130–6.
119. Burney P. A diet rich in sodium may potentiate asthma. Epidemiologic evidence for a new hypothesis. Chest 1987; 91143S–8S.
120. Carey OJ, Locke C, Cookson JB. Effect of alterations of dietary sodium on the severity of asthma in men. Thorax 1993; 48:714–8.
121. Mickleborough TD, Lindley MR, Ray S. Dietary salt, airway inflammation, and diffusion capacity in exercise-induced asthma. Med Sci Sports Exerc 2005; 37:904–14.
122. Girgis S, Neal B, Prescott J, et al. A one-quarter reduction in the salt content of bread can be made without detection. Eur J Clin Nutr 2003; 57:616–20.
123. He FJ, Markandu ND, Sagnella GA, MacGregor GA. Effect of salt intake on renal excretion of water in humans. Hypertension 2001; 38:317–20.

13

Influence of Sodium on Pulse Pressure and Systolic Hypertension in the Elderly

Michel E. Safar
Department of Medicine, Paris Descartes University and AP-HP Hôtel-Dieu Hospital, Paris, France

Athanase Benetos
Geriatric Center, Brabois Hospital, University of Nancy II, Nancy, France

For many years, the incidence of systolic hypertension has been increasing in the elderly. The reasons for this evolution are quite simple (1). First, prolongation of life is responsible for an increased number of older individuals with increased systolic blood pressure (SBP). Second, the goal of treatment in middle-aged subjects with systolic–diastolic hypertension was based in the past on reduction of diastolic blood pressure (DBP). Because it is much easier to control DBP (<90 mmHg) than SBP (<140 mmHg) (2) by drug treatment, and because, with age, DBP tends spontaneously to decrease and SBP to increase, this evolution contributes per se to enhance the incidence of systolic hypertension (3). All these findings are quite important to consider for two reasons. First, the pathophysiological mechanisms of systolic hypertension involve, in addition to altered vascular resistance, which is the classical hallmark of hypertension, consistent changes in arterial stiffness and wave reflections, which refer to conduit arteries (mainly the aorta and its principal branches) (1,4). Second, from the different varieties of hypertension in humans, the most sensitive to sodium is hypertension in the elderly (5–7).

The purpose of this review is: (*i*) to provide evidence that in subjects with systolic hypertension, large arteries are not passive conduits and respond actively to Na diet, independently of blood pressure (BP) changes and (*ii*) to show that several modulating factors related to sodium consistently influence the extracellular matrix of the arterial wall, thereby determining the level of arterial stiffness, SBP, and pulse pressure (PP) in each individual with systolic hypertension.

EPIDEMIOLOGICAL DATA

The role of sodium (Na) in hypertensive subjects results from two main clinical observations. Firstly, based on numerous reports (5–7), a positive correlation has been widely observed between urinary Na excretion, an estimate of Na consumption, of various communities around the world, and the upward slope of SBP of their inhabitants with aging. The group of Avolio was one of the first to assess the role of salt diet in the age-related increase in SBP and in arterial stiffness (8,9). These studies have shown that urban and rural Chinese communities exhibit markedly different increases in arterial pressure and pulse wave velocity with age and that the same value of aortic stiffness in a rural community occurred 30 years of age later compared with that of an urban community. This difference in increase in pulse wave velocity with age was similar to the prevalence of hypertension in the two communities. Interestingly, the main difference between the two communities was the consumption of dietary salt which was the double in the urban Chinese population when compared with the rural population.

It has also been reported that, dietary Na restriction lowers systolic pressure and PP, and pulse wave velocity especially in old subjects with isolated or predominantly systolic hypertension, but has only a modest effect on DBP (10–12). Decreased arterial compliance has also been found in the carotid, brachial, and femoral arteries of salt-sensitive subjects with borderline hypertension (13).

Taking into account the role of arterial stiffness on the level of SBP and PP in old subjects, and therefore on cardiovascular risk, it seems likely to relate the effects of Na on the structure and function of, not only small, but also large arteries, and therefore on arterial stiffness.

In animal studies, our group (14,15) has shown that high sodium intake was a significant predictor of mortality in spontaneously hypertensive rats (SHR). Interestingly, mortality was considerably enhanced when sodium intake was given very early during the SHR development (15). The effects of high-salt diet on mortality were considerably attenuated and even tended to disappear when high-sodium diet was associated with blockade of the renin–angiotensin system. Moreover, in rat groups including SHR and Wistar Kyoto (WKY) strains, carotid stiffness increased linearly as function of wall stress when sodium intake was chronically and progressively increased (Fig. 1) (14). Normotensive and hypertensive animals were exactly on the same curve. According to the Laplace law, this finding implies a change in large artery structure and therefore the development of carotid hypertrophy.

SODIUM AND ARTERIAL STRUCTURE AND FUNCTION

Hypertrophy of large vessels, a characteristic feature in the most usual models of animal and human hypertension (1), is due both to an increase in smooth muscle mass and extracellular matrix, primarily involving collagen fibers. Most findings have been obtained from genetic models of hypertension in rats (16–24).

Tobian (16) was the first to show that in stroke-prone SHR, increased sodium intake was associated with more pronounced structural alterations of cerebral and renal arteries, more important than when a low-sodium diet is consumed. Under such conditions, the increased wall thickness was associated with substantially increased collagen content and abnormal collagen cross-linking (16,17). These arterial alterations were reversed by lowering sodium intake, without any change in intra-arterial BP, but in parallel with a lower incidence of strokes (16,18).

In stroke-resistant SHR, the temporal relationship between BP elevation and the appearance of arterial alterations during salt loading was investigated starting at five

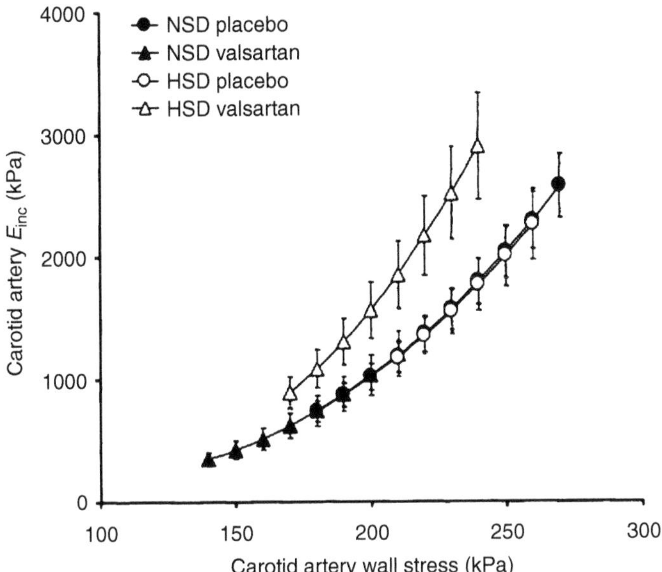

Figure 1 Carotid artery in spontaneously hypertensive rats. Mean incremental elastic modulus (E_{inc}) wall stress curves in placebo- and valsartan-treated rats receiving NSD or HSD. Note that blockade of AT_1 receptors by valsartan shifted the curve upward in the presence of HSD. *Abbreviations*: HSD, high-sodium diet; NSD, normal sodium diet. *Source*: From Ref. 14.

weeks of age (19). Neither BP (assessed by intra-arterial measurements) nor vascular morphology of WKY rats was affected by 1% NaCl in drinking water. In SHR, BP was not affected by a high-sodium diet but rather, between 10 and 20 weeks of age, an increase in arterial media thickness was observed in association with a further accumulation of extracellular matrix and fibronectin (Fn) (19,20). After administration of various diuretic agents to stroke-prone and stroke-resistant SHR (and also sodium-resistant Dahl rats), a reduction of mean arterial pressure (MAP) independent of arterial stiffness was observed (21–24).

In all the experimental models considered in this review, an important prerequisite is the total absence of change in intra-arterial systemic BP along the investigation. Conversely, Partovian and colleagues (20) showed that, when a high-sodium diet was consumed in the long term, intra-arterial BP increased in WKY rats, whereas no structural changes in the aorta were observed. In contrast, in SHR, substantial structural aortic changes developed, without any alteration in BP during the study. Thus a simple comparison of these two strains minimizes the exclusive influence of BP on the changes in arterial structure.

Finally, it is important to remember that, with a high-sodium diet, not only BP may be affected, but also other mechanical factors, such as blood flow. Through changes in shear stress and endothelial function, the sodium diet may be associated with pressure-independent effects on the vascular wall, as previously observed for arterioles (25–27). Interestingly, dietary salt, without altering BP, enhances the production of active transforming growth factor β1 and nitric oxide (NO) synthesis (through increased expression of NO synthase-3) by aortic endothelial cells (28). Similar conclusions can be drawn from experiments performed in the aortas of rats fed a high-salt diet, in which endothelium-dependent relaxation is impaired via reduced NO concentrations and increased production of superoxide (29).

In recent years, the pressure-independent effect of sodium or diuretic compounds, or a combination of both, on the arterial wall, has been confirmed on the basis of molecular biology (30). Stroke-prone (SP)-SHR receiving a high-sodium diet without diuretic treatment were characterized by increased expression of non-muscle myosin in the aorta, and both EIIIA Fn and non-muscle myosin in the coronary arteries. The diuretic agents, chlorothiazide and indapamide, were both without effect on BP, but prevented changes in smooth muscle cell (SMC) contractile phenotype. At the same time, ischemic tissular lesions of cerebral vessels were significantly attenuated and cerebrovascular accidents were consistently reduced.

SODIUM AND CHRONIC BLOCKADE OF THE RENIN–ANGIOTENSIN SYSTEM: EFFECT ON THE ARTERIAL WALL

Salt and water depletion constantly induces powerful vasoactive mechanisms involving mainly the renin–angiotensin–aldosterone and the bradykinin systems (7). Changes in the renin–angiotensin system are traditionally described as acting acutely on arterioles with resulting vasoconstriction. However, in vivo studies showed that such mechanisms involve not only arteriolar but also large artery structure and function, particularly when chronic studies are performed (31,32). The most useful tools are constituted by blockade of the AT_1 receptors of angiotensin II (Ang II) and of bradykinin receptors.

Regarding the long-term effects of Ang II in SHR, AT_1 blockade by valsartan lowers MAP, prevents aortic collagen accumulation, and decreases carotid stiffness in parallel with diminished wall stress. However, the result is observed only in the presence of a low-sodium diet (32). High-sodium diet plus valsartan reduces MAP, but carotid stiffness and aortic collagen accumulation remain elevated, independently of any change in wall stress (Fig. 1). On the other hand, when non-antihypertensive doses of the diuretic indapamide is given to SHR in association with the angiotensin-converting enzyme (ACE) inhibitor perindopril, only the combination of the two agents is able to consistently prevent carotid collagen accumulation and, at the same time, to reduce isobaric carotid stiffness (33,34).

Regarding bradykinin, changes in aortic wall thickness and collagen accumulation have been studied over the long term in SHR and WKY rats in the presence or absence of the specific inhibitor of B_2 receptors, HOE 140 (20). When the effects of chronic high-sodium diet were compared with those of a normal sodium diet, both of them in the absence of HOE 140, carotid and aortic wall thickness and collagen accumulation were significantly increased in SHR, but not in WKY rats. In addition, intra-arterial BP was not significantly changed in SHR. When a high-sodium diet was combined with HOE 140, carotid wall thickness and extracellular matrix increased further, thereby suggesting that endogenous bradykinin might selectively act on arterial structure.

In the recent years, studies in rodents have shown that the stiffness of aortic wall material may be modified in vivo, not only independently of mechanical forces as systemic MAP and wall stress, but also without major modification in the content of collagen and elastin fibers, which represent the principal material modulating vascular elasticity (1). These findings were observed in old people under high-sodium diet, particularly in subjects with diabetes mellitus and/or systolic hypertension (1). Attachment molecules between vascular smooth muscle (VSM) cells, or between VSM cells and extracellular matrix, or between collagen fibers, contribute per se to stiffen the material of the vascular wall (1,35,36).

Collagen cross-links are stabilizers of collagen fibrils, preventing slippage of adjacent molecules under applied tensile stress (37). Particularly with aging, hypertension and diabetes mellitus, they contribute to increase arterial stiffness through formation of end-glycation products (38). In old subjects with systolic hypertension, drug involving collagen cross-link breakers reduce significantly arterial stiffness and PP without any change of MAP (39). These compounds provided the first in vivo evidence that reduction of arterial stiffness can be obtained independently of MAP and without modification in collagen density and content. More recently, other attachment molecules have been described as modifying the stiffness of wall material through (40–47): proteoglycans, Fn, integrins, and even development vascular calcifications, as recently published.

Glycosaminoglycans exhibit viscoelastic properties, which make them candidates as flow-sensing molecules (40). They bind not only sodium and water but also are characterized by calcium cross-linking of the helical chains (40). Removal of 65% of chondroitin–dermatan sulfate-containing glycosaminoglycans from mesenteric resistance arteries increases their stiffness (41). In carotid arteries in SHR, chronic high-Na diet associates reduction of arterial hyaluron and increase of aortic stiffness whereas opposite changes are observed under administration of the diuretic compound indapamide (42). Finally, all these experiments suggest an association between reduction of cell attachments and reduction of arterial stiffness through changes in Na diet and hyaluron.

Because integrins transmit inside-out and outside-in signals capable of modulating changes in vascular responses, Bezie and colleagues suggested that adhesion molecules such as Fn and its $\alpha 1$ $\beta 1$ integrin receptor may contribute, independently of systemic MAP, to modulate arterial wall stiffness (35). Fn matrix polymerization increases tensile strength of model tissue (43). In young and old SHR, studies of aortic Fn measurement have suggested that an increased number of attachment sites between SMCs and extracellular matrix may be responsible for increased arterial rigidity (35). In knockout mice lacking the $\alpha 1$ integrin, studies of changes in carotid stiffness under angiotensin II have shown that a loss of cell–matrix attachments between the $\alpha 1$ integrin receptor and its ligand Fn is associated with a reduction of arterial stiffness at any given value of MAP or wall stress (44). Other arguments in favor of cause-to-effect relationships between integrins, Fn and arterial stiffness result from studies in SHR under different levels of Na diet (14). On a normal sodium diet, angiotensin-converting enzyme inhibition (ACEI) reduces MAP, aortic Fn and $\alpha 1$ $\beta 1$ integrin, together with an increase in isobaric arterial distensibility. Under ACEI plus high-Na diet, MAP is significantly reduced, but increased arterial stiffness and enhanced aortic Fn remain unmodified during the experiment. Similar results are observed under spironolactone (23,45) or chronic administration of aldosterone in association with high-sodium diet. However, under such conditions the findings are reversed by the selective aldosterone antagonist eplerenone (46). Interestingly, aldosterone in the presence of high-sodium diet involves structural and inflammatory changes of the kidney which may be also reversed by eplerenone (47).

In conclusion, all these studies show that local changes in the attachments between cells or between cell and matrix modulate the stiffness of each artery studied individually. This process may not only induce a supplementary increase of vessel wall rigidity, but also is capable, through this procedure, to cause a mismatch in vascular impedance and influence the topography and the diffusion of the various sites of waves reflections (1,2). Taken together such alterations may initiate an increase in PP (2) and, in turn, contribute independently to end-organ damage.

APPLICATIONS TO CLINICAL SITUATIONS IN OLD SUBJECTS WITH HYPERTENSION

In recent years, double-blind studies involving individuals with hypertension have emphasized the importance of the interactions between sodium and the renin–angiotensin system on large artery structure and function. These findings are consistent with the observation that, in hypertensive individuals, moderate salt restriction lowers BP while causing a decrease in arterial stiffness and a dilation of the muscular brachial artery, but not of the musculoelastic carotid artery (9,48).

Pharmacological studies have shown that by comparison with the calcium entry blocker felodipine (49) and the ACE inhibitor perindopril (50), the diuretic hydrochlorothiazide was shown to cause, in hypertensive subjects, minor changes of arterial diameter and stiffness for the same BP reduction. In contrast, when hydrochlorothiazide was combined with the ACE inhibitor captopril (51), the diameter of muscular arteries increased significantly, together with a reduction in arterial stiffness and a delay in carotid wave reflections. In a double-blind study comparing in subjects with essential hypertension the β-blocking agent atenolol and the low-dose combination of the ACE inhibitor perindopril and the diuretic compound indapamide (52), it was shown that, for the same reduction in DBP, SBP was lowered significantly more using a low-dose combination of perindopril/indapamide. This difference was not observed when atenolol was compared with an ACE inhibitor alone, i.e., without any combination with a diuretic compound (53). The observed selective SBP reduction was associated with diminished arterial stiffness and mostly with a delay in wave reflections (54). Because the results became significant only after one year drug treatment, it seems likely that the mechanism of reduction of arterial stiffness was due to the reversibility of structural arteriolar changes, thereby modifying the reflection coefficients and causing in turn a delay of wave reflections, together with reduction of SBP and PP (55).

ACKNOWLEDGMENTS

This study was performed with the help of the Medical School of Paris Descartes University, the Medical School of the University of Nancy and the Inserm. We thank Mrs Maryse Deboute for her helpful assistance.

REFERENCES

1. Safar ME, Levy BI, Struijker-Boudier H. Current perspectives on arterial stiffness and pulse pressure in hypertension and cardiovascular disease. Circulation 2003; 107:2864–9.
2. Black HR. The paradigm has shifted to systolic blood pressure. Hypertension 1999; 34:386–7.
3. Mourad JJ, Blacher J, Blin P, Warzocha U. On behalf of the investigators of the PHASTE study. Conventional antihypertensive drug therapy does not prevent the increase of pulse pressure with age. Hypertension 2001; 38:958–62.
4. Nichols WW, O'Rourke MF, eds. McDonald's Blood Flow in Arteries: Theoretical, Experimental and Clinical Principles. 4th ed. London/Sydney/Auckland: E Arnold Publishing, 1998:54–401.
5. Simpson FO. Blood pressure and sodium intake. In: Laragh JH, Brenner BM, eds. Hypertension: Pathophysiology, Diagnosis and Management. 2nd ed. New York: Ravan Press, 1995:273–81.

6. Intersalt Cooperative Research Group. Intersalt: an international study of electrolyte excretion and blood pressure. Results of 24-hour urinary sodium excretion. BMJ 1988; 297:319–28.
7. Meneton P, Jeunemaitre X, de Wardener HE. Links between dietary salt intake, renal salt handling, blood pressure, and cardiovascular diseases. Physiol Rev 2005; 85:679–715.
8. Avolio AP, Chen SG, Wang RP, Zhang CL, Li MF, O'Rourke MF. Effects of aging on changing arterial compliance and left ventricular load in a northern Chinese urban community. Circulation 1983; 68:50–8.
9. Avolio AP, Deng FQ, Li WQ, et al. Effects of aging on arterial distensibility in populations with high and low prevalence of hypertension: comparison between urban and rural communities in China. Circulation 1985; 71:202–10.
10. Avolio AP, Clyde KM, Beard TC, Cooke HM, O'Rourke MF. Improved arterial distensibility in normotensive subjects on a low salt diet. Arteriosclerosis 1986; 6:166–9.
11. Niarchos AP, Weinstein DL, Laragh JH. Comparison of the effects of diuretic therapy and low sodium intake in isolated systolic hypertension. Am J Med 1984; 77:1061–8.
12. Sacks FM, Stetkey LP, Vollmer WM, et al. Effects on blood pressure of reduced dietary sodium and the dietary approaches to stop hypertension (DASH) diet. N Engl J Med 2001; 344:3–10.
13. Draajier P, Kool MJ, Maessen JM, et al. Vascular distensibility and compliance in salt-sensitive and salt-resistant borderline hypertension. J Hypertens 1993; 11:1199–207.
14. Labat C, Lacolley P, Lajemi M, et al. Effects of valsartan on mechanical properties of the carotid artery in spontaneously hypertensive rats under high-salt diet. Hypertension 2001; 38:439–43.
15. Mercier N, Labat C, Louis H, et al. Sodium, arterial stiffness and cardiovascular mortality in hypertensive rats. Am J Hypertens 2007; 20(3):319–25.
16. Tobian L. Salt and hypertension: lessons from animal models that relate to human hypertension. Hypertension 1991; 17(Suppl. I):I-52--58.
17. Mizutani K, Ikeda K, Kawai Y, et al. Biomechanical properties and chemical composition of the aorta in genetic hypertensive rats. J Hypertens 1999; 17:481–7.
18. Levy BI, Poitevin P, Duriez M, et al. Sodium, survival and the mechanical properties of the carotid artery in stroke-prone hypertensive rats. J Hypertens 1997; 15:251–8.
19. Limas C, Westrum B, Limas CJ, et al. Effect of salt on the vascular lesions of spontaneously hypertensive rats. Hypertension 1980; 2:477–89.
20. Partovian C, Benetos A, Pommies JP, et al. Effects of a chronic high-salt diet on large artery structure: role of endogenous bradykinin. Am J Physiol 1998; 274:H1423–8.
21. Benetos A, Bouaziz H, Albaladejo P, et al. Carotid artery mechanical properties of Dahl salt-sensitive rats. Hypertension 1995; 25:272–7.
22. Levy BI, Curmi P, Poitevin P, et al. Modifications of arterial properties of normotensive and hypertensive rats without arterial pressure changes. J Cardiovasc Pharmacol 1989; 14:253–9.
23. Benetos A, Lacolley P, Safar ME. Prevention of aortic fibrosis by spironolactone in spontaneously hypertensive rats (SHRs). Arterioscler Thromb Vasc Biol 1997; 17:1152–6.
24. Levy BI, Poitevin P, Safar ME. Effects of indapamide on the mechanical properties of the arterial wall in deoxycorticosterone acetate-salt hypertensive rats. Am J Cardiol 1990; 65:28H–32.
25. Matrougui K, Loufrani L, Levy BI, et al. High NaCl intake decreases both flow-induced dilation and pressure-induced myogenic tone in resistance arteries from normotensive rats: involvement of cyclooxygenase-2. Pharmacol Toxicol 2001; 89:183–7.
26. Matrougui K, Schiavi P, Guez D, et al. High sodium intake decreases pressure-induced (myogenic) tone and flow-induced dilation in resistance arteries from hypertensive rats. Hypertension 1998; 32:176–9.
27. Matrougui K, Levy BI, Schiavi P, et al. Indapamide improves flow-induced dilation in hypertensive rats with a high salt intake. J Hypertens 1998; 16:1485–90.
28. Sanders PW. Salt intake, endothelial cell signaling, and progression of kidney disease. Hypertension 2004; 43:142–6.
29. Zhu J, Mori T, Huang T, et al. Effect of high-salt diet on NO release and superoxide production in rat aorta. Am J Physiol 2004; 286:H575–83.

30. Contard F, Sabri A, Glukhova M, et al. Arterial smooth muscle cell phenotype in stroke-prone spontaneously hypertensive rats. Hypertension 1993; 22:665–76.
31. Albaladejo P, Bouaziz H, Duriez M, et al. Angiotensin converting enzyme inhibition prevents the increase in aortic collagen in rats. Hypertension 1994; 23:74–82.
32. Benetos A, Levy BI, Lacolley P, et al. Role of angiotensin II and bradykinin on aortic collagen following converting-enzyme inhibition in spontaneously hypertensive rats. Arterioscler Thromb Vasc Biol 1997; 17:3196–201.
33. Richard V, Joannides R, Henry JP, et al. Fixed-dose combination of perindopril with indapamide in spontaneously hypertensive rats: haemodynamic, biological and structural effects. J Hypertens 1996; 14:1447–54.
34. Joannides R, Richard V, Henry JP, et al. In vivo evidence that chronic antihypertensive treatment increases isobaric carotid compliance and decreases wall thickness in hypertensive rats. Fundam Clin Pharmacol 1993; 7:364 (Abstract).
35. Bezie Y, Lamaziere J-MD, Laurent S, et al. Fibronectine expression and aortic wall elastic modulus in spontaneously hypertensive rats. Arterioscler Thromb Vasc Biol 1998; 18:1027–34.
36. Davies PF. Flow-mediated endothelial mechanotransduction. Physiol Rev 1995; 75:519–60.
37. Huijberts MS, Wolffenbuttel BH, Struijker-Boudier HA, et al. Aminoguanidine treatment increases elasticity and decreases fluid filtration of large arteries from diabetic rats. J Clin Invest 1993; 92:1407–11.
38. Corman B, Duriez M, Poitevin P, et al. Aminoguanidine prevents age-related arterial stiffening and cardiac hypertrophy. Proc Natl Acad Sci USA 1998; 95:1301–6.
39. Kass DA, Shapiro EP, Kawaguchi M, et al. Improved arterial compliance by a novel advanced glycation end-product crosslink breaker. Circulation 2001; 104:1464–70.
40. Bevan JA. Flow regulation of vascular tone. Its sensitivity to changes in sodium and calcium. Hypertension 1993; 22:273–81.
41. Gandley RE, Mclaughlin MK, Koob TJ, Little SA, Mcguffee LJ. Contribution of chondroitin-dermatan sulfate-containing proteoglycans to the function of rat mesenteric arteries. Am J Physiol 1997; 273:H952–60.
42. Et-Taouil K, Schiavi P, Levy BI, Plante GE. Sodium intake, large artery stiffness and proteoglycans in the SHR. Hypertension 2001; 38:1172–6.
43. Gildner CD, Lerner AL, Hocking DC. Fibronectin matrix polymerization increases tensile strength of model tissue. Am J Physiol Heart Circ Physiol 2004; 287:H46–53.
44. Louis H, Li Z, Labat C, et al. Defects in vascular smooth muscle hypertrophic response to angiotensin II in integrin [alpha]1 knockout mice. Hypertension 2004; 43:1349 (Abstract).
45. Lacolley P, Safar ME, Lucet B, et al. Prevention of aortic and cardiac fibrosis by spironolatone in old normotensive rats. J Am Coll Cardiol 2001; 37:662–7.
46. Lacolley P, Labat C, Pujol A. Increased carotid wall elastic modulus and fibronectin in aldosterone–salt treated rats—effects of eplerenone. Circulation 2002; 106:2848–53.
47. Blasi ER, Rocha R, Rudolph AE, Blomme EA, Polly ML, McMahon EG. Aldosterone/salt induces renal inflammation and fibrosis in hypertensive rats. Kidney Int 2003; 63:1791–800.
48. Benetos A, Yang-Yan X, Cuches JL, et al. Arterial effects of salt restriction in hypertensive patients. A 2-month, randomised double-blind, crossover study. J Hypertens 1992; 10:335–60.
49. Gates PE, Tanaka H, Hiatt WR, et al. Dietary sodium restriction rapidly improves large elastic artery compliance in older adults with systolic hypertension. Hypertension 2004; 44:35–41.
50. Asmar R, Benetos A, Chaouche-Teyara K, et al. Comparison of effects of felodipine versus hydrochlorothiazide on arterial diameter and pulse-wave velocity in essential hypertension. Am J Cardiol 1993; 72:794–8.
51. Kool MJ, Lusterman FA, Breed JG, et al. The influence of perindopril and the diuretic combination amiloride + hydrochlorothiazide on the vessel wall properties of large arteries in hypertensive patients. J Hypertens 1995; 13:839–48.
52. Benetos A, Lafleche A, Asmar R, et al. Arterial stiffness, hydrochlorothiazide and converting enzyme inhibition in essential hypertension. J Human Hypertens 1996; 10:77–82.

53. Asmar RG, London GM, O'Rourke ME, et al. Improvement in blood pressure, arterial stiffness and wave reflections with a very-low-dose perindopril/indapamide combination in hypertensive patients: a comparison with atenolol. Hypertension 2001; 38:922–6.
54. Chen CH, Ting CT, Lin SJ, et al. Different effects of fosinopril and atenolol on wave reflections in hypertensive patients. Hypertension 1995; 25:1034–41.
55. London GM, Asmar RG, O'Rourke MF, Safar ME. Mechanism(s) of selective systolic blood pressure reduction after a low-dose combination of perindopril/indapamide in hypertensive subjects: comparison with atenolol. J Am Coll Cardiol 2004; 43:92–9.

14

Salt and Blood Pressure: The Concept of Salt Sensitivity

Murielle Bochud
Institute of Social and Preventive Medicine, University Hospital, University of Lausanne, Lausanne, Switzerland

Michel Burnier
Division of Nephrology and Hypertension Consultation, University Hospital, University of Lausanne, Lausanne, Switzerland

INTRODUCTION

As early as the beginning of the 20th century, Ambard and Beaujard recognized the role of dietary salt restriction in lowering blood pressure in humans (1). In the 1920s, Allen clearly demonstrated the effectiveness of salt restriction in the treatment of hypertension and suggested that salt restriction at the population level would reduce cardiovascular morbidity and mortality (2). In the 1940s, Kempner found that a rice–fruit diet very low in salt was able to lower blood pressure in severely hypertensive patients (3). In the 1960s, Dahl was the first to report a positive association between the dietary salt intake and the prevalence of hypertension across populations (4). In the 1970s, Froment et al. conducted an ecological study (from published data) that analyzed urinary sodium excretion and blood pressure across 28 populations: blood pressure and the age-related blood pressure increases were positively associated with urinary sodium excretion, a proxy for dietary salt intake (5). In the 1980s, the INTERSALT study, a large standardized observational epidemiological study, investigated the relationship between blood pressure and 24-hour urinary sodium excretion in 10,079 participants from 52 populations around the world (6). For the comparison across populations, a 100 mmol difference in salt intake was associated with a 5-7/2-4 mmHg difference in systolic/diastolic blood pressure (7,8). A significant positive association between urinary sodium excretion and blood pressure was also found within populations (except for four isolated populations with very low sodium excretion), for both men and women, and the strength of this association increased with age (9). An overview of data collected for 47,000 non-African subjects from 24 communities confirmed the positive association between blood pressure and urinary sodium excretion across and within populations, and its strengthening with age (10,11).

In the 1980s and 1990s, numerous controlled studies of sodium restriction were conducted in humans to demonstrate the impact of salt intake on blood pressure (12–17). Table 1 summarizes the results of some observational studies and meta-analysis of studies performed on this topic. More recently, in a Cochrane meta-analysis of 28 randomized controlled trials of at least four-week duration, which included 2954 subjects and was last updated in December 2004, He and MacGregor found that a median 78 mmol urinary Na reduction in hypertensive subjects led to a decrease in mean blood pressure of 5.0 mmHg (95% CI: 4.2–5.8) and a median 74 mmol Na reduction in normotensive subjects led to a 2.7 mmHg (95% CI: 2.3–3.2) decrease (18). A significant dose–response effect was found, i.e., trials in which the subjects achieved the greatest reduction in urinary sodium excretion reported the largest blood pressure decrease (18). In another Cochrane meta-analysis of 57 randomized controlled trials that was last updated in March 2004 and included trials of shorter duration, Jurgens and Graudal found only a reduction of 1.27 mmHg (95% CI: 1.76−0.77) and 0.54 mmHg (95% CI: 0.94−0.14), respectively, in systolic and diastolic blood pressure (19). However, unlike the meta-analysis by He and MacGregor, no dose–response effect was observed. A major difference in both meta-analyses is that He and MacGregor restricted their analysis to trials with a sodium reduction of at least 40 mmol and lasting for at least four weeks, while Jurgens and Graudal did not. As a consequence both meta-analyses are answering different questions: the former (18) looks at the "long-term" effect of modest sodium restriction on blood pressure while the latter (19) looks at a mixture of long-term effects of modest sodium reductions and short-term effects of large sodium reductions.

Thus, today, most physicians and researchers would agree on the principle that dietary sodium can influence blood pressure in humans. However, there is no general agreement on whether a decrease in sodium intake should be recommended to all

Table 1 Blood Pressure Reduction (mmHg) per 100 mmol/24 hr[a] Decrease in Urinary Sodium Excretion: A Summary of Large Studies and Meta-Analysis

Study	Study design	*N*	Systolic BP (mmHg)	Diastolic BP (mmHg)
INTERSALT 1988 (7,8)	Observational studies	10,079	5–7	2–4
Law (1991) (11)	Observational studies	47,000	15–19 year: 5	2
			20–29 year: 5	3
			30–39 year: 6	3
			40–49 year: 7	4
			50–59 year: 9	5
			60–69 year: 10	4
Midgley (1996) (13)	Meta-analysis of RCTs	3505	HT: 3.7	HT: 0.9
			NT: 1.0	NT: 0.1
Cutler (1997) (14)	Overview of RCTs	2635	HT: 5.8	HT: 2.5
			NT: 2.3	NT: 1.4
Hooper (2002) (16)	Meta-analysis of RCTs (follow-up >6 month)	3514	7.0	3.4
He (2004) (18)	Meta-analysis of RCTs (follow-up >4 week)	2954	HT: 6–7	HT: 3–4
			NT: 3–4	NT: 1–2

[a] Reduction was extrapolated from available published data assuming linearity.
Abbreviations: HT, hypertensive subjects; NT, normotensive subjects; RCT, randomized controlled trial.

populations. One of the main reasons why this recommendation is not universally accepted lies in the fact that not every individual would respond to a salt restriction.

THE CONCEPT OF SALT SENSITIVITY

Salt sensitivity is a concept that applies to the individual. Despite evidence for a positive association between dietary salt intake and average blood pressure at the population level, the interindividual blood pressure response to dietary sodium intake is definitively heterogeneous. To reflect the interindividual differences, Kawasaki et al., and later on Weinberger et al., have developed the concept of salt sensitivity and salt resistance of blood pressure (20,21). Although it has been clearly shown that the blood pressure response to sodium is a continuously and normally distributed phenotype, and not a bimodal response, both in normotensive and hypertensive individuals, many investigators dichotomize individuals as salt sensitive versus salt-resistant using an arbitrary cutoff (20–22). Others use a trichotomy or tertiles (22–24). The concept of salt sensitivity of blood pressure is confronted to two major issues: the first is the protocol used to assess it, which is by no means standardized, and the second is the reproducibility of the test being used.

How Should One Assess Salt Sensitivity?

Two broad categories of salt-sensitivity protocols have been used: (*i*) the acute blood pressure response to a rapid sodium and volume load or depletion using either an intravenous saline administration or a low-salt diet combined with the administration of a diuretic (21,25) and (*ii*) the blood pressure response to more sustained, but still rather short-term (usually one week), changes in dietary sodium intake using low- and high-salt diets (20). We will refer to the first approach as the "rapid test" and to the second as the "dietary test." While the rapid test is more convenient, the dietary test is more physiological and is considered by some investigators to represent the gold standard. The reason is that the dietary test is performed under steady-state conditions and therefore suffers from less protocol-induced artifacts and is more closely related to the reality (23,24). Various cutoffs have been used to define salt sensitivity, such as an absolute blood pressure difference or a relative 10% difference between the salt-depletion and -repletion phases (20–33). Studies have differed in the way blood pressure was measured (office vs. ambulatory, manual vs. automatic, number of measurements, supine vs. sitting), in the duration of the low- and high-salt diet (from five to seven days), and in the amount of salt in the low- (from 9 to 50 mmol/24 hr) versus high-salt diets (from 170 to 300 mmol/24 hr) (20–36). Usually, compliance with diet is measured using 24-hour urinary sodium excretion. Kato et al. proposed a modified version of the rapid test intended for population-based studies: while participants remain under their usual diet and in their normal environment, a week of salt loading (with sodium supplement of 140 mmol/day) is followed by a week of salt depletion (with diuretic treatment, i.e., hydrochlorothiazide 25 mg/day) (37). Koomans et al. proposed to quantify sensitivity to salt using a sodium-sensitivity index, i.e., the ratio of the difference in mean arterial pressure (mmHg) over the difference in urinary sodium excretion (mmol/24 hr) (38). Some investigators justify the use of such an index by showing that the relationship between urinary sodium excretion and mean arterial pressure is approximately linear across a wide range of salt intakes (1–18 g salt/day) in humans (39,40). Assuming linearity, the sodium-sensitivity index represents the inverse of the slope of the pressure–natriuresis curve (39). Kimura suggested to use a cutoff of 0.05 mmHg/(mmol/24 hr) to identify salt-sensitive subjects, which corresponds to a 10 mmHg blood pressure decrease for a 200 mmol/24 hr decrease in urinary sodium excretion (39).

Although many teams have developed carefully standardized protocols, the lack of standardization across teams greatly limits comparison across studies. Currently available methods are ill-suited for large-scale population-based studies. As a consequence, the vast majority of studies having analyzed salt sensitivity in humans were small-sized. With a few exceptions, most studies could not simultaneously account for all known potential confounding factors, such as age, sex, ethnicity, and other dietary components (e.g., potassium intake). For small sample sizes, a randomization does not ensure that known and unknown confounding factors will be evenly distributed across study groups. Another limitation, due to constraints of human experimental research, is the fact that most currently used protocols are based on the blood pressure response to short-term exposure (usually one week) to diets with extreme salt contents (usually a 10-fold difference). It is not known to what extent the results of these studies apply to the physiological responses to long-term more subtle variations in salt intake in humans, such as those occurring in real life. Thus, the results obtained by Mattes et al. suggest that currently used salt-sensitivity protocols do not reliably reflect blood pressure changes to longer-term dietary salt restriction (41).

While some claim that salt-sensitivity protocols aim at identifying susceptible individuals who may benefit from sodium restriction, we believe that this is neither appropriate nor necessary. In our opinion, currently available salt-sensitivity protocols should rather be viewed as research tools that help further our understanding of physiological and pathophysiological mechanisms. In particular, as noted by Sharma, salt sensitivity is a potentially interesting intermediate phenotype to study the genetic determinants of hypertension (42).

Is Salt Sensitivity a Reproducible Phenotype?

Reproducibility results varied quite substantially across studies. Apart from the fact that this variability may, in part, reflect true variability in intra-individual blood pressure response to sodium, these discrepancies may be due to differences in (*i*) the way study subjects were selected, (*ii*) protocols, and (*iii*) compliance with the dietary changes. In general, studies using more extreme low salt intakes (20 mmol/24 hr) showed a better reproducibility than those using less extreme salt restrictions, which are less difficult to apply (40–60 mmol/24 hr). Reproducibility may also be affected by factors known to influence salt sensitivity itself, such as age and hypertension status. Apart from Mattes et al. (41) who did not find any association between age, sex, ethnicity, body weight and reproducibility of the blood pressure response to a rapid test, the influence of these factors has been barely investigated so far.

Sharma et al. repeated twice the dietary test (20 vs. 220 mmol Na/24 hr) in 10 salt-sensitive and 10 salt-resistant subjects, defined using an absolute 3 mmHg cutoff, and found a kappa statistic of 0.87 after excluding five subjects with poor compliance (i.e., only 1 of 15 compliant subjects were classified differently in the two tests), which reflects a very good agreement (43). However, the blood pressure response to salt between the two tests was not significantly correlated. Weinberger et al. repeated the rapid test in 28 subjects twice within 12 months; a significantly positive correlation was found between the blood pressure response to sodium in the first and second tests; however, 10 of 28 subjects were not consistently classified as salt sensitive, indeterminate and salt resistant, in the two tests (44). Later on, the same authors compared the rapid with the dietary test (<15 vs. >200 mmol Na/24 hr) in 40 hypertensive and normotensive subjects.

The protocols were separated by at least two weeks and given in the same order. A significant positive correlation was found between the blood pressure responses to both protocols ($r=0.40$, $p<0.01$) (34). Galletti et al. compared a modified rapid test with a dietary test (50 vs. 200 mmol Na/24 hr) in 18 non-obese hypertensive patients, 9 of whom were in the lowest and 9 in the highest salt-sensitivity tertiles after the rapid test. They observed that patients in the highest salt-sensitivity tertile significantly lowered their blood pressure under a low-salt diet, whereas those in the lowest tertile did not. Moreover, the blood pressure response to sodium was positively correlated with changes in urinary sodium excretion in the group from the highest salt-sensitivity tertile only (23). Although the authors only analyzed the average group responses and not the individual responses to both tests, they concluded that their data provide evidence for a "reasonably good agreement" between the two tests. Using the data provided in the paper, we calculated a kappa statistic of 0.50 for the two tests, which represents an intermediate to good agreement. Overlack et al. repeated their salt-sensitivity protocol in 31 non-obese white normotensive subjects after three months; the change in mean arterial pressure in response to low- and high-salt diets was highly correlated ($r=0.71$, $p<0.001$) (25); only 3 of 31 participants were classified into a different group in the second study, which suggests a good reproducibility. Draaijer et al. obtained a perfect agreement in salt sensitivity (using a cutoff of 8 mmHg) when a dietary protocol (20 vs. 220 mmol Na/24 hr) was repeated twice in 10 men with borderline hypertension (29).

In contrast to these data, several investigators considered salt-sensitivity tests to have a rather low reproducibility. Sharma et al. compared the rapid with a dietary test (20 vs. 220 mmol Na/24 hr) in 22 healthy male volunteers. A significantly positive correlation was found between the diastolic and mean, but not systolic, blood pressure responses in the two protocols (27). However, the authors considered that the rapid test has a limited ability to reproduce the response to a dietary protocol. A low reproducibility of the classification into salt sensitive and salt resistant was also reported with protocols using both 24-hour ambulatory and clinic blood pressure and a dietary test (40 vs. 170 mmol Na/24 hr) in 14 hypertensive patients (36). The best kappa statistic for the classification into salt sensitive versus salt resistant was obtained for a 10% change in the mean ambulatory blood pressure and was only 0.24. Although ambulatory blood pressure reduces blood pressure variability (45), reproducibility of the salt-induced blood pressure response was similar for ambulatory and clinic blood pressure when assessed using Bland–Altman plots (36). Gerdts et al. repeated a dietary test (50 vs. 250 mmol Na/24 hr) in 30 hypertensive patients using ambulatory versus clinic blood pressure after six months (35). Salt-sensitivity status was only reproducible in 60% when using 24-hour ambulatory blood pressure ($\kappa=0.05$), and in 53% when using clinic blood pressure ($\kappa<0.01$) (35). The salt-induced change in 24-hour blood pressure in the first test (expressed in mmHg/mmol Na) was not significantly correlated with the one in the second test. In addition, there was no significant correlation between the ambulatory and clinic blood pressure responses to salt in the first or second test. These results suggest that ambulatory monitoring does not substantially improve the classification of salt sensitivity over clinic blood pressure and that these two methods identify different subsets of subjects as being salt sensitive. Hence both Gertds et al. and Zoccali et al. observed a similar low reproducibility for ambulatory and clinic blood pressure responses to salt (35,36). Strazullo et al. compared a modified rapid test with a dietary test (50 mmol vs. 150 mmol Na/24 hr) in 94 hypertensive patients; there was a low, but weakly significant, correlation between the response to both tests ($r=0.21$, $p=0.05$), whereas the correlation of the responses to two rapid tests was 0.60 in 19 subjects ($p<0.01$) (22). Only 47% of the subjects were classified into the same salt-sensitivity tertile in the rapid and dietary tests. In this study, the authors found a positive association between the 24-hour urinary sodium excretion on the days preceding the test and the blood pressure response to sodium, which underscores the importance of standardizing salt intake before the procedure. Mattes et al. found a low reproducibility of a dietary test (40 vs. 370 mmol Na/24 hr), with consistent classification (using a 5 mmHg cutoff) in only 30 of 45 participants (41). Using the response to a four-month moderate dietary salt restriction (100 mmol/day) as the gold standard, the sensitivity and specificity of this dietary test were 73% and 60%, respectively; the blood pressure response to sodium during the salt-sensitivity protocol and the four-month low-salt period were not significantly correlated.

Finally, the dietary approaches to stop hypertension (DASH)-sodium trial was the only study reporting the intra-individual blood pressure variability under constant sodium intake (Fig. 1). This intra-individual variability was high and, interestingly, had a similarly wide distribution (i.e., same standard deviation) than that of the blood pressure response to sodium; hence sodium reduction shifted the whole distribution without changing its dispersion (46). Individual data for 188 participants on the control diet were analyzed; each participant was assigned, in random order, to a low (50 mmol/24 hr), medium (100 mmol/24 hr) and high (150 mmol/24 hr) sodium diet, each with a four-week duration. Subjects could be classified as salt sensitive or salt resistant by assessing the changes in blood pressure when going from the low to medium or from the medium to high-salt diet or from the two extremes. Although statistically significant, the rank correlations between the blood pressure responses to the repeated dietary tests were low ($r=0.27, p=0.03$) (Fig. 1). When using a dichotomy, the classification of salt-sensitive and salt-resistant participants showed a poor agreement. This study however had two important limitations: (*i*) the two tests compared differed in the number of blood pressure measurements (two vs. five pairs), in the duration of the diet (two vs. four weeks) and in the absolute levels of dietary sodium intake and (*ii*) although two different tests were compared, bias was not assessed. At last, the changes in sodium intake were relatively modest.

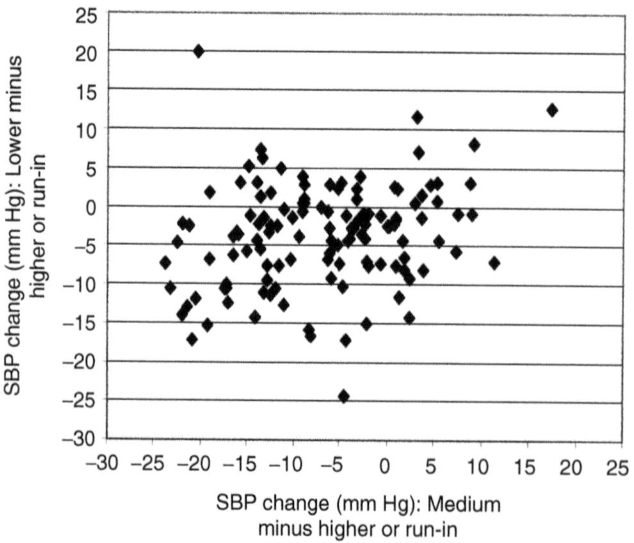

Figure 1 Consistency of systolic blood pressure changes between any greater and smaller sodium level in 129 participants assigned to a low, a medium, and a high sodium intake sequence in the dietary approaches to stop hypertension (DASH) study. *Abbreviation*: SBP, systolic blood pressure. *Source*: From Ref. 46.

Taken together, these data suggest that the reproducibility of salt-sensitivity tests is far from being firmly demonstrated. Nevertheless, one can consider currently available dietary tests to be fairly reproducible, at most, in humans. However, one has also to recognize that there is currently no consensus on what represents a "good reproducibility" for salt sensitivity and several studies having assessed the reproducibility of salt sensitivity in humans suffered from methodological shortcomings. The reproducibility between two different methods can only be good if each of the two methods is itself highly reproducible; hence before comparing the two tests, the authors should provide data on the reproducibility of each test and this was generally not performed. Blood pressure measured in the office is generally not considered as a very reproducible parameter for many reasons and ambulatory blood pressure monitoring has been shown to be more reproducible. Therefore, one would favor protocols using ambulatory blood pressure measurements.

What are the Clinical Characteristics Associated with Salt Sensitivity?

Salt sensitivity of blood pressure has been investigated in several patient populations. Even though there has never been any population-based study on salt sensitivity, several clinical characteristics have been repeatedly associated with the salt-sensitive pattern. These characteristics are summarized in Table 2.

Hypertension

Despite differences in how salt sensitivity was defined using the above-mentioned protocols, several studies reported that about 50% of hypertensive subjects are salt sensitive (20,21). The prevalence among normotensive appears slightly lower with estimates ranging from 18% to 50% (21,47). When analyzed as a continuous variable, the blood pressure response to sodium and/or volume depletion is positively correlated with blood pressure levels (21,25,48,49). This is consistent with the results of randomized controlled trials of sodium restriction which found greater blood pressure reduction in hypertensive than in normotensive subjects.

Age

Numerous studies found that salt sensitivity increases with age (25,50,51), especially among hypertensive subjects (23,44,51), and that the age-related blood pressure increase

Table 2 Characteristics Associated with Salt Sensitivity in Humans

Characteristics	Direction of the effect	Strength of the evidence[a]
Hypertension	↑	+++
Age	↑	+++
Renin–angiotensin–aldosterone system	Blunted in salt sensitivity	++
Insulin resistance	↑	++
Family history of hypertension	↑	+
Female sex	?	(+)
African descent	↑	(+)
Obesity	↑	(+)

[a] Strength of the evidence summarizes both the amount of data available and the consistency of the results across studies. +++, conclusive evidence; ++, strong evidence; +, some evidence, no inconsistency; (+) some evidence, with inconsistency.

is more pronounced in salt-sensitive than in salt-resistant subjects. It is generally widely accepted that older age is associated with increased blood pressure sensitivity to sodium, an effect that may be due to the progressive decline in renal function occurring with age. In the DASH-sodium trial, older individuals showed a larger blood pressure reduction from high-sodium (150 mmol/24 hr) to low-sodium (50 mmol/24 hr) diet than younger individuals among normotensive but not among hypertensive participants (48).

Sex

A few studies found that women tend to be more salt sensitive than men (25,48), whereas others found no sex difference (21,52). The effect of sex has however not been systematically investigated, despite the fact that sex hormones have been shown to influence salt sensitivity. Pechère-Bertschi et al. have investigated the pressure–natriuresis relationship, another approach to salt sensitivity, in women during the various phases of the normal menstrual cycle and after the menopause (53,54). Their data show that normotensive women are rather salt resistant until the menopause. At the menopause, the pressure–natriuresis curve is shifted to the right and flatter, suggesting that more women become salt sensitive, an effect which could be due to aging or changes in sexual hormone profile. More data are needed to understand sex differences in salt sensitivity. For now, separate analyses by sex should always be planned and conducted as one cannot assume that men and women are similar with respect to salt sensitivity of blood pressure.

Family History of Hypertension

The results of several studies suggest that subjects with a positive family history of hypertension are more salt sensitive than subjects with a negative history (25,27,43,55,56). This suggests that salt sensitivity of blood pressure has a genetic component as will be discussed later in this review.

Race

The available evidence suggests that individuals of African descent are more salt sensitive than Caucasians (21,30,48,57), but the observed differences were often not striking. Overall, few studies have compared salt sensitivity across ethnic groups.

Obesity

Animal data suggest that obesity is associated with salt sensitivity (58–61). In humans, data are more inconsistent as some (62–66), but not all (21,23,25,48,51), studies suggested that obesity tends to be associated with salt sensitivity. This research area deserves more attention as a high sodium intake has been associated with an increased risk of cardiovascular disease and all-cause mortality in obese individuals (67).

Renin–Angiotensin–Aldosterone System

Clear associations have been reported between components of the renin–angiotensin–aldosterone system (RAAS) and salt sensitivity. Low salt intake is known to stimulate the RAAS and high salt intake to suppress it (56,68). Salt-sensitive individuals have, on average, lower plasma renin activity (PRA) (20,21,23,25,47,51,69) or a lower plasma aldosterone (20,21,25,70) than salt-resistant individuals. This is consistent with the age-related decrease in PRA levels and increase in salt sensitivity (25). Several studies have shown that the blood pressure decrease following low salt intake was significantly and inversely correlated with the rise in PRA, i.e., individuals with large decreases in blood pressure have small PRA increases (21,34,57,71,72). Some authors (57,72) also found a similar negative correlation for plasma aldosterone. In conclusion, current evidence points toward an association between salt sensitivity and a blunted RAAS.

Insulin Resistance

Data suggest a link between insulin resistance and salt sensitivity in humans as well as in animals. Several studies actually showed a positive association between insulin resistance and salt sensitivity (69,73–82), i.e., salt-sensitive subjects are more insulin resistant. This association appears to be true in both low- and high-salt diets (76) and to also exist in young normotensive individuals (80). However, a few studies either failed to reproduce this observation (70,83,84) or found an inverse association (85). A link between insulin resistance and salt sensitivity has also been found in several rat models of hypertension (86–88) and high-salt diet increases insulin resistance in some rat strains (87–89).

DOES SALT SENSITIVITY AFFECT MORBIDITY AND MORTALITY?

Salt sensitivity has been associated with overall mortality in normotensive subjects (90), with left ventricular hypertrophy (64), hypertensive retinopathy (64), urinary albumin excretion (64,91), insulin resistance (69,73–82), a blunted nocturnal blood pressure decrease (i.e., nondipping) (28,78,92–95) and cardiovascular mortality (33) in hypertensive subjects. In a retrospective cohort study, salt-sensitive subjects had more fatal and nonfatal cardiovascular endpoints than non-salt–sensitive subjects after a mean follow-up of 7.3 years (2.0 vs. 4.3 per 100 person-years, $p<0.01$) (33). After an average follow-up of 26 years, salt-resistant normotensive subjects had a significantly better survival than salt-sensitive normotensive, salt-resistant and salt-sensitive hypertensive subjects ($p<0.0001$) (Fig. 2) (90). Overall, there is substantial evidence to suggest that salt sensitivity is associated with an adverse prognosis. Although these results are very important, few data are available on the long-term prognosis of salt sensitivity in humans. No prospective large-scale population-based study has been conducted so far, so that the generalizability of these results is limited. As a consequence the population-attributable risk of salt sensitivity is unknown. Apart from the reproducibility issues raised before,

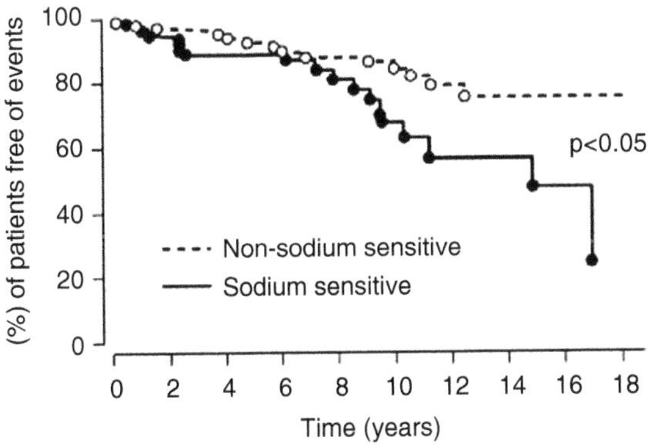

Figure 2 Long-term incidence of cardiovascular complications in subjects according to their salt-sensitivity status. *Source*: From Ref. 33.

an inherent difficulty in determining the true prognosis of salt sensitivity is its strong association with age (20) and kidney function. Dissociating age effect from cohort effect (i.e., the effect of being born on a particular period of time) is no simple task but may be of relevance if the role of prenatal maternal factors (i.e., factors occurring *in utero*) strongly determines the number and function of nephrons.

WHAT IS THE PATHOGENESIS OF SALT SENSITIVITY?

Although it is now widely recognized that an alteration in sodium handling by the kidney plays a crucial role in the pathogenesis of hypertension, less consensus exists with respect to the precise mechanisms that lead to essential hypertension in general and to salt-sensitive hypertension in particular.

Several pathogenic mechanisms have been proposed to explain the heterogeneity of the blood pressure response to salt. Guyton developed the pressure–natriuresis concept using experiments in dogs (96,97). By describing the relationship between systemic blood pressure and sodium balance, Guyton has demonstrated the key role of water and sodium excretion by the kidneys in the long-term regulation of blood pressure (98). Later on, Kimura and Brenner (99) described the different pressure–natriuresis curves in sodium-sensitive and sodium-resistant forms of secondary hypertension. They also proposed that one can differentiate sodium-sensitive from sodium-resistant forms of hypertension by the renal mechanisms involved: (*i*) an increased preglomerular resistance would lead to a rightward shift of the pressure–natriuresis curve and to a non-sodium–sensitive form of hypertension characterized by normal or low glomerular pressure and (*ii*) a reduced ultrafiltration coefficient or an enhanced renal tubular sodium reabsorption would lead to a downward shift (i.e., a depressed slope) of the pressure–natriuresis curve and to sodium-sensitive forms of hypertension characterized by an elevated glomerular pressure (99). Several indirect pieces of evidence suggest that salt sensitivity is indeed associated with an increased glomerular capillary pressure in humans and in animals (100–102) and may thereby lead to renal complications with time (Fig. 3).

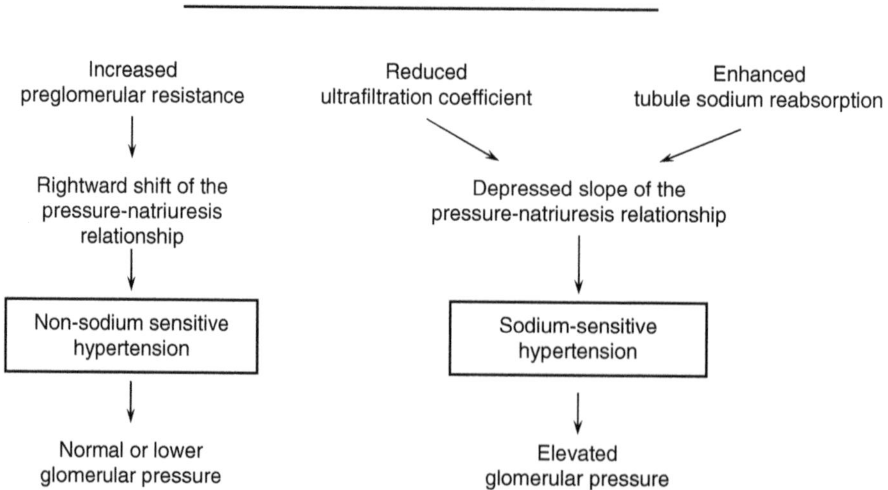

Figure 3 Schematic of the link between the salt sensitivity and the renal risk associated with hyperfiltration.

We have hypothesized that salt sensitivity is associated with an impaired renal handling of sodium by the proximal tubules and demonstrated an increased proximal reabsorption of sodium in patients with salt-sensitive hypertension (Fig. 4) (103,104).

Johnson and colleagues (105,106) have recently formulated the hypothesis that, over time, hypertension may shift from an initially salt-resistant to a subsequent salt-sensitive type once sufficient subtle renal injury has accumulated. Furthermore, Johnson and colleagues have proposed a unifying pathway for the pathogenesis of hypertension (and salt-sensitive hypertension), which combines many of the previously formulated hypotheses (107,108). Salt sensitivity likely results from an imbalance between vasoconstrictors (RAAS and the sympathetic nervous system) and vasodilators (nitric oxide, the kallikrein–kinin system), in parallel with substances and mechanisms leading to progressive glomerular and/or tubular injuries.

GENETIC DETERMINANTS OF SALT SENSITIVITY

The search for genetic determinants of salt sensitivity is motivated by (*i*) the observation that salt sensitivity aggregates in families (109,110) and (*ii*) the fact that almost all monogenetic forms of hypertension are salt sensitive (111). Despite the large number of

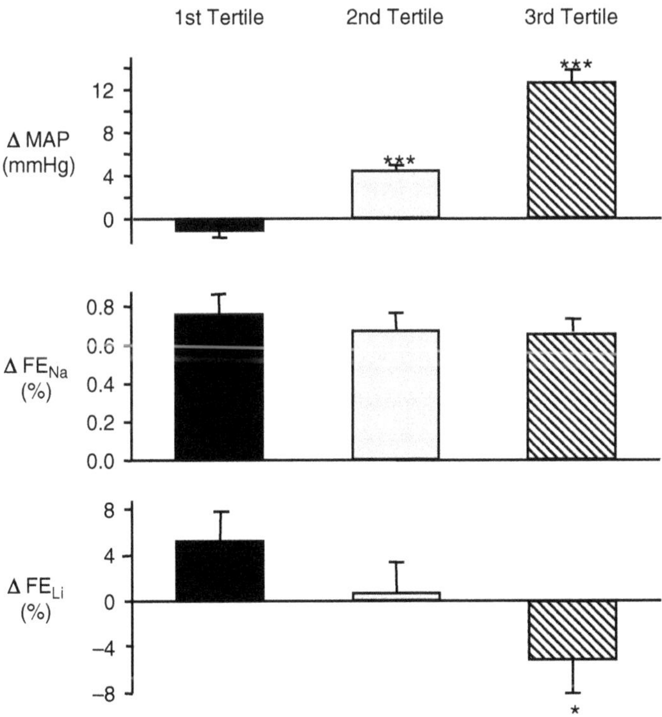

Figure 4 Changes in blood pressure and proximal sodium reabsorption (FE_{Li}) in hypertensive patients distributed in tertiles according to their blood pressure response to a change in sodium intake from a low- to a high-Na diet. Note that patients of the third tertile who are the most salt sensitive exhibit a fall in FE_{Li} suggesting a paradoxical increase in proximal sodium reabsorption when on a high sodium intake. *Abbreviations*: MAP, mean arterial pressure; FE_{Li}, fractional excretion of lithium; FE_{Na}, fractional excretion of sodium. *Source*: From Ref. 103.

candidate genes for blood pressure or hypertension directly or indirectly associated with sodium handling in humans (112), this review will concentrate on the few genes for which an association with salt sensitivity in a broad sense (i.e., either directly using a salt-sensitivity protocol, in a long-term low-salt reduction trial, or indirectly by evaluating the blood pressure response to a diuretic) has been analyzed in humans. Genes potentially involved with salt sensitivity in humans are summarized in Table 3.

Adducin Genes

Adducin is a cytoskeleton protein localized at spectrin–actin junctions (113), where it plays an important role in assembly and regulation of actin filaments and spectrin–actin network. It has been postulated that alterations in cytoskeleton proteins, adducin in particular, influence cell volume and ion transport (114,115). Animal experiments are consistent with the hypotheses that adducin mutant alleles (and interactions between the various subunits) play a role in animal models of hypertension via faster ion transport across cell membrane and via central action in the brain (114,116–121). In humans, the Gly460Trp polymorphism of the α-adducin gene has been repeatedly, but not totally consistently, associated with blood pressure and hypertension, in particular low-renin hypertension. Several studies have analyzed the association of the adducin genes polymorphisms with salt sensitivity in humans. Cusi et al. (122) found a significant association between the Trp allele of the Gly460Trp polymorphism of the α-adducin gene and salt sensitivity, assessed using either an acute protocol or using the blood pressure response to a diuretic treatment in 88 hypertensive subjects (Fig. 5). Manunta et al. (123) observed a less steep pressure–natriuresis curve, hence a higher salt sensitivity, in 28 carriers of the Trp alleles than in 80 Gly/Gly homozygotes, following acute salt-depletion and salt-repletion protocols. The blood pressure response to a diuretic treatment was greater in 55 Trp carrier than in 88 Trp noncarrier hypertensive subjects (124). Moreover, carriers of the Trp allele showed a greater systolic blood pressure response to dietary sodium changes than noncarriers (125) and the Trp allele was associated with a greater

Table 3 Candidate Genes Associated with "Non-Monogenic" Salt Sensitivity in Humans

Gene	Gene symbol	Putative salt-sensitive allele	Strength of the evidence[a]
α-Adducin	ADD1	460Trp	+++
Angiotensinogen	AGT	235T-6A	++
Cytochrome P450 A3 family number 5	CYP3A5	CYP3A5*1	+
G protein β3 subunit	GNB3	825T	(+)
Aldosterone synthase	CYP11B2	-344T(?), intron 2 conversion	(+)
Angiotensin-converting enzyme	ACE	D from I/D	(+)
11β-Hydroxysteroid dehydrogenase type 2	11βHSD2	534G	(+)

[a] Strength of the evidence summarizes both the amount of available data and the consistency of results across studies. +++, conclusive evidence; ++, strong evidence; +, some evidence, no inconsistency; (+) some evidence, but with some inconsistency.

Abbreviations: ACE, angiotensin-converting enzyme; AGT, angiotensinogen; GNB3, G protein β3 subunit; I/D, insertion/deletion.

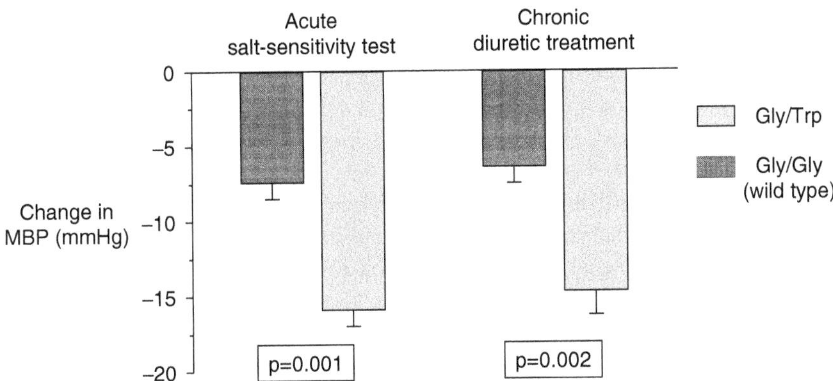

Figure 5 Salt sensitivity in hypertensive patients according to their α-adducin genotype. *Abbreviation*: MBP, mean blood pressure. *Source*: From Ref. 123.

blood pressure response to an acute saline load in 145 hypertensive patients (125). In addition, the Trp allele interacts with the D allele of the insertion/deletion (I/D) polymorphism of the angiotensin-converting enzyme (ACE) gene in blood pressure response to salt loading. These latter results were subsequently confirmed by Sciarrone et al. (126) in 87 never-treated hypertensive subjects. However, Castejon et al. (127) found no association between the Trp allele and salt sensitivity in 90 normotensive Hispanic subjects from Venezuela, but the sodium-dependent modulation of NO production was enhanced in carriers of the Trp allele. Similarly, Ciechanowick (128) did not find any association of the Trp allele with salt sensitivity of blood pressure and PRA in 68 young hypertensive Polish subjects. Of note, the two negative studies (127,128) were conducted in young individuals. Taken together these data suggest that the Gly460Trp polymorphism of the α-adducin gene currently represents one of the best documented and least controversial genetic determinant of salt sensitivity in humans.

Angiotensinogen Gene

Conversion of angiotensinogen (AGT), which is produced in the liver, by renin to form angiotensin I is the first step of the renin–angiotensin system, a key system in blood pressure regulation and renal sodium handling. An early study found a positive correlation between AGT and blood pressure (129). Thereafter, Nakajima et al. (130) identified 44 single nucleotide polymorphisms and 6 of the 21 identified haplotypes explained most variations at the AGT gene in Caucasian and Japanese subjects. However, the most studied polymorphism is M235T. Several studies have described the association between AGT genotypes and/or haplotypes and plasma AGT levels (131,132) and the association of the 235T allele with plasma AGT levels has been confirmed in a recent meta-analysis (133) including nine studies. Animal data have demonstrated that genetic variants which influence plasma AGT levels significantly affect blood pressure (134,135). The AGT gene has been linked and associated with blood pressure in humans (136), but the results have been inconsistent so far (133). Several studies have analyzed the association between the AGT gene and the salt sensitivity in humans. Schorr et al. (137) reported no association between the AGT M235T polymorphism and the blood pressure response to salt in 187 young hypertensive men following a one-week low-salt (20 mmol/day) and one-week high-salt (220 mmol/day) diet protocol. Similarly Giner et al. (138) found no significant association between the AGT M235T polymorphism and the blood pressure response to high salt intake in 50 hypertensive patients following a one-week low-salt (60 mmol/day) and one-week high-salt (260 mmol/day) diet protocol. Poch et al. (139) found no association between the blood pressure response to salt in 71 hypertensive subjects following a one-week low-salt (50 mmol/day) and one-week high-salt (260 mmol/day) diet protocol. Johnson et al. (140) reported that the TT genotype of the M235T polymorphism is associated with a greater salt sensitivity in 46 older hypertensive patients (>60 years old) exposed to increasing dietary salt intakes (4 two-week periods with 50, 100, 200 and 300 mmol/day separated by a two-week low-salt periods). A significantly greater blood pressure decrease to a six-month placebo-controlled low-sodium diet was also reported in 86 hypertensive men and women (aged 55–75 years) carrying the 235T allele than in those carrying the MM genotype (125). In that study, participants in the low-salt diet achieved a 51 mmol/24 hr lower urinary sodium excretion than those in the placebo group. Finally, Hunt et al. (141) found that subjects carrying the AA genotype of the G-6A AGT polymorphism had a greater blood pressure reduction at three years than carriers of the G allele in the 378 participants (aged between 30 and 54 years) in the sodium reduction group of the Trials of Hypertension Prevention II (TOHP II) trial. However those carrying the AA genotype achieved a slightly greater reduction in urinary Na excretion than G carriers. Note that the AA genotype corresponds to the TT genotype of the M235T polymorphism as both polymorphisms are in nearly complete linkage disequilibrium (i.e., nearly completely correlated). Although the results may appear inconsistent at first, studies including older individuals (or having a large sample size) were consistently positive. The 235T allele (or the -6A allele) AGT polymorphism appears to be a marker of salt sensitivity in humans, in particular in older individuals.

CYP3A5 Gene

Enzymes of the human CYP3A family are involved in the metabolism of endogenous substrates, such as steroids, and in the metabolism of many drugs. The genes of the CYP3A family (3A4, 3A43, 3A5, and 3A7) cluster on chromosome 7q21-7q22.1 and show organ-specific patterns of expression. Only the *CYP3A5* gene is expressed in the human kidney (142,143). Several *CYP3A5* alleles have been described, which show different levels of expression and are associated with different amounts of CYP3A5 enzyme. Only carriers of the *CYP3A5*1* express large amounts of CYP3A5 messenger RNA and protein (144). The CYP3A5 enzyme catalyzes the conversion of cortisol to its 6β-hydroxy metabolite in the liver (145) and also accounts for most of the 6β-hydroxylase activity in mammals, including humans (146). A possible link between the *CYP3A5* gene and the blood pressure regulation could be mediated by enhanced renal tubular sodium reabsorption through increased levels of 6β-hydrocortisol. Renal CYP3A5 enzymatic activity has been shown to correlate with systolic blood pressure in the rat (147) and selective inhibitors of the CYP3A5 enzyme decreasing the level of 6β-hydrocortisol have also been shown to lower blood pressure in rats (148). In this species, Warrington et al. (149) observed a significant increase with age of the enzymatic activity of one CYP3A isoform in the kidney, while CYP3A activity decreased with age in the liver. The *CYP3A5* gene has been associated with blood pressure and hypertension (150–153) and with renal sodium handling (152) in humans. A few studies have analyzed the association between the *CYP3A5* gene and the salt sensitivity in humans. Thompson et al. (154) found that the *CYP3A5*3* allele showed an unusual geographical distribution with extreme variation across 52 human populations and significant correlation with distance from the equator. The findings of this ecological study are consistent with the hypothesis formulated by

Kuehl et al. (144) suggesting that the *CYP3A5*1* allele may confer a selective advantage in areas of water shortage by favoring sodium retention. Ho et al. (151) have reported that the *CYP3A5*1* allele is associated with salt sensitive hypertension in blacks but not in whites. In subjects of African descent, Bochud et al. (152) did not assess salt sensitivity using an experimental protocol, but they found nighttime urinary sodium excretion to be a significant determinant of nighttime ambulatory blood pressure in carriers of the *CYP3A5*1* allele, while no such association was observed in noncarriers. This result indirectly suggests that *CYP3A5*1* carriers are more sensitive to salt than noncarriers. Although few studies have been conducted on this gene so far, these results point toward an association of the *CYP3A5* gene with salt sensitivity in individuals of African descent.

G Protein β3 Subunit Gene

Guanine nucleotide regulatory proteins (G proteins) participate in intracellular signaling by relaying signals from more than 1000 receptors to many different intracellular effectors, including enzymes and ion channels (155). The G protein is a trimer composed of an α subunit loosely bound to a dimer made up of tightly associated β and γ subunits. Siffert et al. (156) identified a functional polymorphism (C825T) in the G protein β3 subunit (GNB3) gene that appears to result in significantly enhanced activation of G proteins. The C825T polymorphism has been associated with blood pressure in humans but the exact molecular mechanism responsible for this association is currently unknown (155). An increased sodium hydrogen exchanger (NHE) activity might be the link between the hypertension and the C825T polymorphism (157). This potential link can be explained by two alternative hypotheses (157): (*i*) the enhanced NHE activity in the kidney could results in an increased Na reabsorption and volume expansion, (*ii*) by preventing cells from acidosis during proliferation processes, the enhanced NHE activity might be involved in vascular remodeling of resistance vessels. The three studies (158–160) that have analyzed the association of the C825T polymorphism with salt sensitivity in humans found no significant association. However, Turner et al. (161) reported that the TT genotype of the GNB3 C825T polymorphism is associated with a greater blood pressure response to a four-week thiazide diuretic therapy in 197 black and 190 white hypertensive subjects. Currently available data do not provide a conclusive picture and the association of the GNB3 gene with salt sensitivity in humans remains unclear.

CYP11B2 Gene

The aldosterone synthase gene (*CYP11B2*), located on chromosome 8q22, encodes for the enzyme responsible for the final step of aldosterone synthesis, namely the conversion of deoxycortisone into aldosterone. The *CYP11B2* gene is located near to the *CYP11B1* gene, responsible for the synthesis of cortisol from 11-deoxycortisol. Both genes have a very similar nucleotide sequence. While *CYP11B1* is expressed in the zona fasciculata of the adrenal gland and regulated by adrenocorticotropic hormone (ACTH), *CYP11B2* is expressed in the zona glomerulosa and regulated mainly by angiotensin II and plasma potassium . Mutations in the *CYP11B2* gene are responsible for a rare Mendelian disease, aldosterone synthase deficiency, characterized by salt wasting, hypotension, elevated renin, low aldosterone and elevated deoxycorticosterone. Unequal crossovers between the *CYP11B1* and *CYP11B2* genes are responsible for another rare Mendelian disorder, glucocorticoid remediable aldosteronism, in which aldosterone secretion becomes controlled by ACTH leading to elevated aldosterone and hypertension (162–164). White and Slutker identified a mutation in the 5′-flanking region of the *CYP11B2* gene, the C-344T polymorphism, located in the binding site for a transcription factor (165). The precise functional role of this polymorphism however still remains to be determined (166). The *C-344T* polymorphism is in linkage disequilibrium with (i.e., associated with the same chromosomal strand) a gene conversion in intron 2, in which intron 2 of *CYP11B2* is replaced by that of *CYP11B1*. Although numerous studies in humans have reported an association of the *CYP11B2 C-344T* polymorphism and blood pressure, results were inconsistent with respect to which of the C or T allele is associated with elevated blood pressure. A few studies found the T allele to be associated with high plasma aldosterone levels (167,168) or higher urinary aldosterone secretion (168).

Some studies have analyzed the association of the *CYP11B2 C-344T* polymorphisms with salt sensitivity in humans. In the study by Brand et al. (169), no association between the *CYP11B2 C-344T* polymorphism and the blood pressure response to salt (using one-week high- vs. low-sodium diets with, respectively, 220 and 20 mmol/day) was observed in 163 healthy young normotensive Caucasian men. Furthermore, no association between PRA and plasma aldosterone responses to dietary salt and the *CYP11B2 C-344T* polymorphism was found (169). Later on, Poch et al. (139) also found no association between the C-344T polymorphism, or the gene conversion in intron 2, and blood pressure response to salt (using one-week high- vs. low-sodium diets with, respectively, 260 and 50 mmol/day) in 71 hypertensive patients with a mean age of 47 years. These results contrast with the results of Pamies-Andreu et al. (159) who demonstrated an association between the CYP11B2 intron 2 conversion, but not the C-344T polymorphism, and salt sensitivity measured using a rapid protocol in 102 hypertensive patients.

11βHSD2 Gene

The *11βHSD2* gene encodes for the enzyme that catalyzes the conversion of cortisol into cortisone in the kidney, colon, placenta and salivary glands. Because cortisone has a low affinity for the mineralocorticoid receptor, the presence of *11βHSD2* results in a selective activation of this receptor by aldosterone. A decreased 11βHSD2 activity leads to a cortisol accumulation that stimulates the mineralocorticoid receptor leading to hypertension, hypokalemia and a suppression of the RAAS. Mutations in the *11βHSD2* gene that decrease the 11βHSD2 enzymatic activity induce an increased cortisol-to-cortisone ratio which may lead to severe forms of hypertension. A rare recessive monogenic form of hypertension, called apparent mineralocorticoid excess (AME), has been shown to result from mutations in the *11βHSD2* gene (170,171). To date, more than 20 different mutations, most of which are located in exons 3, 4, or 5, have been identified (172). Hypertension associated with AME is salt sensitive (172). The 11βHSD2 genotype is closely associated with the biochemical phenotype (in vitro cortisol and corticosterone activity) (173) and clinical parameters such as age of hypertension onset or birth weight (174). The presence of a continuum between severe forms of AME due to mutations that fully suppress the 11βHSD2 enzymatic activity and milder forms due to mutations which only slightly affect the 11βHSD2 enzymatic activity suggest that this gene may play an etiological role in primary hypertension as well (172,175). However so far, few studies have been conducted and the role of the *11βHSD2* gene in the etiology of human essential hypertension remains unclear.

The association between the *11βHSD2* gene and salt sensitivity in humans has also been investigated. Poch et al. (139) found a significant association between the salt sensitivity and the *11βHSD2 G534A* polymorphism in 71 hypertensive patients, 35 of whom were classified as being salt sensitive on the basis of their 24-hour ambulatory blood pressure response to a low-salt (50 mmol/24 hr) and a high-salt (260 mmol/24 hr) diet. The CA repeat polymorphism of the *11βHSD2* gene was associated with salt sensitivity as assessed using an acute protocol in 198 mildly hypertensive subjects (176). Moreover, salt-sensitive subjects had a higher cortisol-to-cortisone ratio (a marker of renal 11βHSD2 enzymatic activity) than salt-resistant subjects. In another group of hypertensive patients, salt-sensitive subjects had a lower urinary cortisol metabolite ratio [(tetrahydrocortisol $+5\alpha$-tetrahydrocortisol)/tetrahydrocortisone] than salt-resistant subjects (177). In contrast, Melander et al. (178) and Kertens et al. (179) found no association between salt sensitivity and 11βHSD2 enzymatic activity in normotensive subjects.

ACE Gene

The ACE catalyzes the formation of the decapeptide angiotensin I to the octapeptide angiotensin II, a potent vasoconstrictor that influences sodium and water reabsorption in the kidney. ACE is part of the renin–angiotensin system that regulates blood pressure, and ACE inhibitors represent a major class of antihypertensive drugs. An I/D of a 287-bp Alu repeat in intron 16 of the ACE gene has been associated with serum ACE levels in humans (180). However, many other polymorphisms have been described in the ACE gene. Rieder et al. (181) sequenced the ACE gene in 11 individuals and identified 78 mutations that lead to 13 distinct haplotypes. Interestingly, 17 of the identified mutations were in complete linkage disequilibrium with (i.e., totally associated with) the I/D polymorphism. Although the ACE gene has been one of the most extensively studied hypertension candidate gene in humans, there are about as many negative as positive studies. Most, but not all, positive studies found the D allele to be associated with higher blood pressure levels or with hypertension. Poch et al. (139) reported a significant association between the I allele of the ACE gene I/D polymorphism and the salt sensitivity in 71 hypertensive patients, 35 of whom were classified as being salt sensitive on the basis of their 24-hour ambulatory blood pressure response to a low-salt (50 mmol/24 hr) and a high-salt (260 mmol/24 hr) diet. Similar results were obtained by Hiraga et al. (182) who showed the I allele to be associated with salt sensitivity in a protocol using one-week low-salt (50 mmol/day) and one-week high-salt (340 mmol/day) diets, in 66 hypertensive Japanese patients. Giner et al. (138) found a significant association between the ACE I/D polymorphism and blood pressure response to high salt intake in 50 hypertensive patients. Unlike previous studies, Dengel et al. (183) found a significant association between the D allele of the I/D polymorphism and salt sensitivity in 35 older hypertensive patients following a one-week low-salt (20 mmol/day) diet and one-week high-salt (200 mmol/day) diet protocol. Pamies-Andreu et al. (159) found no evidence for an association between the I/D ACE gene polymorphism and salt sensitivity, assessed using a rapid protocol in 102 hypertensive subjects. Kojima et al. (184) found no association between the I/D polymorphism and the salt sensitivity in 104 hypertensive patients, although there was an association with the PRA response to salt restriction. Johnson et al. (140) found no evidence for an association between the ACE I/D polymorphism with the blood pressure response to increasing amounts of dietary salt intakes (4 two-week periods with 50, 100, 200, and 300 mmol/day interspaced with two-week low-salt periods) in 46 older hypertensive patients. Again, it is difficult, given the inconsistent results, to conclude whether the ACE gene plays a significant role in salt sensitivity in humans.

Taken together, given the known complexity of blood pressure control, there is no reason to believe that the genetic determinants of salt sensitivity do not display a high degree of complexity as well. The majority of studies discussed above had a small sample size (considering a genetic determinant for a complex trait). Therefore, negative studies may have been underpowered to detect a small effect. In addition, most studies have analyzed a single genetic polymorphism per gene, which cannot be expected to fully capture the gene variability. Many investigators failed to properly account for potential confounding factors such as sex, age, body mass index and antihypertensive treatment. And finally, studies conducted so far have not accounted for gene–gene or gene–environment interactions. As a consequence, much remains to be done in order to properly quantify the role of currently identified candidate genes for salt sensitivity in humans.

CONCLUSION

Most clinicians and researchers would agree on the principle that dietary sodium can influence blood pressure in human populations. Salt sensitivity refers to the individual blood pressure response to various dietary salt intakes or to specific maneuvers aiming at modifying the salt load of the organism. There are definitively large interindividual differences in blood pressure response to salt-sensitivity tests. However, the reproducibility of salt-sensitivity tests is far from being firmly demonstrated and one can consider currently available dietary tests to be fairly reproducible, at most, in humans. Despite these limitations, salt sensitivity has been associated with substantial cardiovascular morbidity and mortality. This concept therefore deserves more attention in order to develop a salt-sensitivity test with good reproducibility that would be simple enough to be used in large samples and would allow conducting adequately powered studies. Although it is now widely recognized that an alteration in sodium handling by the kidney plays a crucial role in the pathogenesis of hypertension, no consensus currently exists with respect to the precise genetic and nongenetic mechanisms that lead to salt-sensitive hypertension.

REFERENCES

1. Ambard L, Beaujard E. Causes de l'hypertension artérielle. Arch Gen Med 1904; 1:520–33.
2. Allen FM. Arterial hypertension. J Am Med Assoc 1920; 74:652.
3. Kempner W. Treatment of hypertensive vascular disease with rice diet. Am J Med 1948; 4:545–77.
4. Dahl LK. Possible role of salt intake in the development of essential hypertension. In: Cottier P, Bock DK, eds. Essential Hypertension—An International Symposium. Berlin: Springer, 1960:53.
5. Froment A, Milon H, Gravier C. Relationship of sodium intake and essential hypertension. Contribution to geographical epidemiology. Rev Epidémiol Santé Publique 1979; 27:437–54.
6. The INTERSALT Co-operative Research Group. INTERSALT Study: an international co-operative study on the relation of blood pressure to electrolyte excretion in populations. I. Design and methods. J Hypertens 1986; 4:781–7.
7. Elliott P, Stamler J, Nichols R, et al. Intersalt revisited: further analyses of 24 hour sodium excretion and blood pressure within and across populations. Br Med J 1996; 312:1249–53.
8. The INTERSALT Co-operative Research Group. Intersalt: an international study of electrolyte excretion and blood pressure. Results for 24 hour urinary sodium and potassium excretion. Br Med J 1988; 297:319–28.
9. Stamler J, Rose G, Elliott P, et al. Findings of the International Cooperative INTERSALT Study. Hypertension 1991; 17:I9–15.
10. Frost CD, Law MR, Wald NJ. By how much does dietary salt reduction lower blood pressure? II. Analysis of observational data within populations Br Med J 1991; 302:815–8.
11. Law MR, Frost CD, Wald NJ. By how much does dietary salt reduction lower blood pressure? I. Analysis of observational data among populations Br Med J 1991; 302:811–5.
12. Law MR, Frost CD, Wald NJ. By how much does dietary salt reduction lower blood pressure? III. Analysis of data from trials of salt reduction Br Med J 1991; 302:819–24.

13. Midgley JP, Matthew AG, Greenwood CM, Logan AG. Effect of reduced dietary sodium on blood pressure: a meta-analysis of randomized controlled trials. JAMA 1996; 275:1590–7.
14. Cutler JA, Follmann D, Allender PS. Randomized trials of sodium reduction: an overview. Am J Clin Nutr 1997; 65:643S–51.
15. Whelton PK, Appel LJ, Espeland MA. Sodium reduction and weight loss in the treatment of hypertension of older persons: a randomized controlled trial of nonpharmacologic interventions in the elderly (TONE). JAMA 1998; 279:839–46.
16. Hooper L, Bartlett C, Smith G, Ebrahim S. Systematic review of long term effects of advice to reduce dietary salt in adults. Br Med J 2002; 325:628.
17. Sacks FM, Svetkey LP, Vollmer WM, et al. Effects on blood pressure of reduced dietary sodium and the dietary approaches to stop hypertension (DASH) diet. N Engl J Med 2001; 344:3–10.
18. He FJ, MacGregor GA. Effect of longer-term modest salt reduction on blood pressure. Cochrane Database Syst Rev 2004; 3:CD004937.
19. Jurgens G, Graudal NA. Effects of low sodium diet versus high sodium diet on blood pressure, renin, aldosterone, catecholamines, cholesterols, and triglyceride. Cochrane Database Syst Rev 2004; 1:CD004022.
20. Kawasaki T, Delea CS, Bartter FC, Smith H. The effect of high-sodium and low-sodium intakes on blood pressure and other related variables in human subjects with idiopathic hypertension. Am J Med 1978; 64:193–8.
21. Weinberger MH, Miller JZ, Luft FC, Grim CE, Fineberg NS. Definitions and characteristics of sodium sensitivity and blood pressure resistance. Hypertension 1986; 8:II127–34.
22. Strazzullo P, Galletti F, Fulgheri P, et al. Prediction and consistency of blood pressure salt-sensitivity as assessed by a rapid volume expansion and contraction protocol. Salt-Sensitivity Study Group of the Italian Society of Hypertension. J Nephrol 2000; 13:46–53.
23. Galletti F, Ferrara I, Stinga F, Iacone R, Noviello F, Strazzullo P. Evaluation of a rapid protocol for the assessment of salt sensitivity against the blood pressure response to dietary sodium chloride restriction. Am J Hypertens 1997; 10:462–6.
24. Burnier M, Monod ML, Chiolero A, Maillard M, Nussberger J, Brunner HR. Renal sodium handling in acute and chronic salt loading/depletion protocols: the confounding influence of acute water loading. J Hypertens 2000; 18:1657–64.
25. Overlack A, Ruppert M, Kolloch R, et al. Divergent hemodynamic and hormonal responses to varying salt intake in normotensive subjects. Hypertension 1993; 22:331–8.
26. Grim CE, Luft FC, Fineberg NS, Weinberger MH. Responses to volume expansion and contraction in categorized hypertensive and normotensive man. Hypertension 1979; 1:476.
27. Sharma AM, Schorr U, Cetto C, Distler A. Dietary v intravenous salt loading for the assessment of salt sensitivity in normotensive men. Am J Hypertens 1994; 7:1070.
28. Wilson DK, Sica DA, Miller SB. Ambulatory blood pressure nondipping status in salt-sensitive and salt-resistant black adolescents. Am J Hypertens 1999; 12:159–65.
29. Draaijer P, de Leeuw P, Maessen J, van Hooff J, Leunissen K. Salt-sensitivity testing in patients with borderline hypertension: reproducibility and potential mechanisms. J Hum Hypertens 1995; 9:263–9.
30. Wright JT, Jr., Rahman M, Scarpa A, et al. Determinants of salt sensitivity in black and white normotensive and hypertensive women. Hypertension 2003; 42:1087–92.
31. Luft FC, Weinberger MH, Grim CE, Fineberg NS. Effects of volume expansion and contraction on potassium homeostasis in normal and hypertensive humans. J Am Coll Nutr 1986; 5:357–69.
32. Campese VM, Romoff MS, Levitan D, Saglikes Y, Friedler RM, Massry SG. Abnormal relationship between sodium intake and sympathetic nervous system activity in salt-sensitive patients with essential hypertension. Kidney Int 1982; 21:371–8.
33. Morimoto A, Uzu T, Fujii T, et al. Sodium sensitivity and cardiovascular events in patients with essential hypertension. Lancet 1997; 350:1734–7.
34. Weinberger MH, Stegner JE, Fineberg NS. A comparison of two tests for the assessment of blood pressure responses to sodium. Am J Hypertens 1993; 6:179–84.

35. Gerdts E, Lund-Johansen P, Omvik P. Reproducibility of salt sensitivity testing using a dietary approach in essential hypertension. J Hum Hypertens 1999; 13:375–84.
36. Zoccali C, Mallamaci F, Cuzzola F, Leonardis D. Reproducibility of the response to short-term low salt intake in essential hypertension. J Hypertens 1996; 14:1455–9.
37. Kato N, Kanda T, Sagara M, et al. Proposition of a feasible protocol to evaluate salt sensitivity in a population-based setting. Hypertens Res 2002; 25:801–9.
38. Koomans HA, Roos JC, Boer P, Geyskes GG, Dorhout Mees EJ. Salt sensitivity of blood pressure in chronic renal failure. Evidence for renal control of body fluid distribution in man. Hypertension 1982; 4:190–7.
39. Kimura G, Brenner BM. Implications of the linear pressure–natriuresis relationship and importance of sodium sensitivity in hypertension. J Hypertens 1997; 15:1055–61.
40. Saito F, Kimura G. Antihypertensive mechanism of diuretics based on pressure–natriuresis relationship. Hypertension 1996; 27:914–8.
41. Mattes RD, Falkner B. Salt-sensitivity classification in normotensive adults. Clin Sci (Lond) 1999; 96:449–59.
42. Sharma AM. Salt sensitivity as a phenotype for genetic studies of human hypertension. Nephrol Dial Transplant 1996; 11:927–9.
43. Sharma AM, Schattenfroh S, Kribben A, Distler A. Reliability of salt-sensitivity testing in normotensive subjects. Klin Wochenschr 1989; 67:632–4.
44. Weinberger MH, Fineberg NS. Sodium and volume sensitivity of blood pressure. Age and pressure change over time. Hypertension 1991; 18:67.
45. Zoccali C, Mallamaci F, Leonardis D. Assessment of the salt-arterial pressure relationship in mild hypertensive subjects by 24-hour ambulatory monitoring. Clin Sci (Lond) 1994; 87:635–9.
46. Obarzanek E, Proschan MA, Vollmer WM, et al. Individual blood pressure responses to changes in salt intake: results from the DASH-sodium trial. Hypertension 2003; 42:459–67.
47. Weinberger MH. Salt sensitivity of blood pressure in humans. Hypertension 1996; 27:481–90.
48. Vollmer WM, Sacks FM, Ard J, et al. Effects of diet and sodium intake on blood pressure: subgroup analysis of the DASH-sodium trial. Ann Intern Med 2001; 135:1019–28.
49. Koolen MI, van Brummelen P. Sodium sensitivity in essential hypertension: role of the renin–angiotensin–aldosterone system and predictive value of an intravenous frusemide test. J Hypertens 1984; 2:55–9.
50. Gudmundsson O. Sodium and blood pressure. Studies in young and middle-aged men with a positive family history of hypertension. Acta Med Scand Suppl 1984; 688:1–65.
51. Overlack A, Ruppert M, Kolloch R, Kraft K, Stumpe KO. Age is a major determinant of the divergent blood pressure responses to varying salt intake in essential hypertension. Am J Hypertens 1995; 8:829–36.
52. Ishibashi K, Oshima T, Matsuura H, et al. Effects of age and sex on sodium chloride sensitivity: association with plasma renin activity. Clin Nephrol 1994; 42:376–80.
53. Pechère-Bertschi A, Maillard M, Stalder H, Brunner HR, Burnier M. Blood pressure and renal haemodynamic response to salt during the normal menstrual cycle. Clin Sci (Lond) 2000; 98:697–702.
54. Pechere-Bertschi A, Burnier M. Female sex hormones, salt, and blood pressure regulation. Am J Hypertens 2004; 17:994–1001.
55. Kojima S, Murakami K, Kimura G, et al. A gender difference in the association between salt sensitivity and family history of hypertension. Am J Hypertens 1992; 5:1–7.
56. Sanchez R, Nolly H, Giannone C, Baglivo HP, Ramirez AJ. Reduced activity of the kallikrein–kinin system predominates over renin–angiotensin system overactivity in all conditions of sodium balance in essential hypertensives and family-related hypertension. J Hypertens 2003; 21:411–7.
57. He FJ, Markandu ND, Sagnella GA, McGregor GA. Importance of the renin system in determining blood pressure fall with salt restriction in black and white hypertensives. Hypertension 1998; 32:820–4.

58. Fujiwara K, Hayashi K, Matsuda H, et al. Altered pressure–natriuresis in obese zucker rats. Hypertension 1999; 33:1470–5.
59. Suzuki H, Ikenaga H, Hayashida T, et al. Sodium balance and hypertension in obese and fatty rats. Kidney Int Suppl 1996; 55:S150–3.
60. Radin MJ, Holycross BJ, Hoepf TM, McCune SA. Increased salt sensitivity secondary to leptin resistance in SHHF rats is mediated by endothelin. Mol Cell Biochem 2003; 242:57–63.
61. Rocchini AP, Moorehead C, DeRemer S, Bondie D. Pathogenesis of weight related changes in presssure in the dog. Hypertension 1989; 13:922–8.
62. Rocchini AP, Key J, Bondie D, et al. The effect of weight loss on the sensitivity of blood pressure to sodium in obese adolescents. N Engl J Med 1989; 321:580–5.
63. Nesovic M, Stojanovic M, Nesovic MM, Ciric J, Zarkovic M. Microalbuminuria is associated with salt sensitivity in hypertensive patients. J Hum Hypertens 1996; 10:573–6.
64. Bihorac A, Tezcan H, Ozener C, Oktay A, Akoglu E. Association between salt sensitivity and target organ damage in essential hypertension. Am J Hypertens 2000; 13:864–72.
65. Barbeau P, Litaker MS, Harshfield GA. Impaired pressure natriuresis in obese youths. Obes Res 2003; 11:745–51.
66. Rocchini AP. Obesity hypertension, salt sensitivity and insulin resistance. Nutr Metab Cardiovasc Dis 2000; 10:287.
67. He J, Ogden LG, Vupputuri S, Bazzano LA, Loria C, Whelton PK. Dietary sodium intake and subsequent risk of cardiovascular disease in overweight adults. JAMA 1999; 282:2027–34.
68. He FJ, MacGregor GA. Salt, blood pressure and the renin–angiotensin system. J Renin Angiotensin Aldosterone Syst 2003; 4:11–6.
69. Galletti F, Strazzullo P, Ferrara I, et al. NaCl sensitivity of essential hypertensive patients is related to insulin resistance. J Hypertens 1997; 15:1485–91.
70. Melander O, Groop L, Hulthen UL. Effect of salt on insulin sensitivity differs according to gender and degree of salt sensitivity. Hypertension 2000; 35:827–31.
71. He FJ, Markandu ND, MacGregor GA. Importance of the renin system for determining blood pressure fall with acute salt restriction in hypertensive and normotensive whites. Hypertension 2001; 38:321–5.
72. Parfrey PS, Markandu ND, Roulston JE, Jones BE, Jones JC, MacGregor GA. Relation between arterial pressure, dietary sodium intake, and renin system in essential hypertension. Br Med J 1981; 283:94–7.
73. ter Maaten JC, Voordouw JJ, Bakker SJ, Donker AJ, Gans RO. Salt sensitivity correlates positively with insulin sensitivity in healthy volunteers. Eur J Clin Invest 1999; 29:189–95.
74. Zavaroni I, Coruzzi P, Bonini L, et al. Association between salt sensitivity and insulin concentrations in patients with hypertension. Am J Hypertens 1995; 8:855–8.
75. Bigazzi R, Bianchi G, Baldari D, Campese VM. Clustering of cardiovascular risk factors in salt-sensitive patients with essential hypertension: role of insulin. Am J Hypertens 1996; 9:24–32.
76. Fuenmayor N, Moreira E, Cubeddu LX. Salt sensitivity is associated with insulin resistance in essential hypertension. Am J Hypertens 1998; 11:397–402.
77. Ferri C, Bellini C, Desideri G, et al. Clustering of endothelial markers of vascular damage in human salt-sensitive hypertension: influence of dietary sodium load and depletion. Hypertension 1998; 32:862–8.
78. Suzuki M, Kimura Y, Tsushima M, Harano Y. Association of insuline resistance with salt senstivity and nocturnal fall of blood pressure. Hypertension 2000; 35:864–8.
79. Rocchini AP. The relationship of sodium sensitivity to insulin resistance. Am J Med Sci 1994; 307(Suppl. 1):S75–80.
80. Sharma AM, Ruland K, Spies KP, Distler A. Salt sensitivity in young normotensive subjects is associated with a hyperinsulinemic response to oral glucose. J Hypertens 1991; 9:329–35.
81. Giner V, Coca A, de la Sierra A. Increased insulin resistance in salt sensitive essential hypertension. J Hum Hypertens 2001; 15:481–5.
82. Kuroda S, Uzu T, Fujii T, et al. Role of insulin resistance in the genesis of sodium sensitivity in essential hypertension. J Hum Hypertens 1999; 13:257–62.

83. Cubeddu LX, Hoffmann IS, Jimenez E, et al. Insulin and blood pressure responses to changes in salt intake. J Hum Hypertens 2000; 14(Suppl. 1):S32–5.
84. Raji A, Williams GH, Jeunemaitre X, et al. Insulin resistance in hypertensives: effect of salt sensitivity, renin status and sodium intake. J Hypertens 2001; 19:99–105.
85. Dengel DR, Hogikyan RV, Brown MD, Glickman SG, Supiano MA. Insulin sensitivity is associated with blood pressure response to sodium in older hypertensives. Am J Physiol Endocrinol Metab 1998; 274:E403–9.
86. Sechi LA. Mechanisms of insulin resistance in rat models of hypertension and their relationships with salt sensitivity. J Hypertens 1999; 17:1229–37.
87. Ogihara T, Asano T, Ando K, et al. High-salt diet enhances insulin signaling and induces insulin resistance in dahl salt-sensitive rats. Hypertension 2002; 40:83–9.
88. Hayashida T, Ohno Y, Otsuka K, et al. Salt-loading elevates blood pressure and aggravates insulin resistance in Wistar fatty rats: a possible role for enhanced Na^+-H^+ exchanger activity. J Hypertens 2001; 19:1643–50.
89. Ogihara T, Asano T, Ando K, et al. Insulin resistance with enhanced insulin signaling in high-salt diet-fed rats. Diabetes 2001; 50:573–83.
90. Weinberger MH, Fineberg NS, Fineberg SE, Weinberger M. Salt sensitivity, pulse pressure, and death in normal and hypertensive humans. Hypertension 2001; 37:429–32.
91. Bigazzi R, Bianchi G, Baldari D, Sgherri G, Baldari G, Campese VM. Microalbuminuria in salt-sensitive patients. A marker for renal and cardiovascular risk factors. Hypertension 1994; 23:195–9.
92. Higashi Y, Oshima T, Ozono R, et al. Nocturnal decline in blood pressure is attenuated by NaCl loading in salt-sensitive patients with essential hypertension: noninvasive 24-hour ambulatory blood pressure monitoring. Hypertension 1997; 30:163–7.
93. Uzu T, Kazembe FS, Ishikawa K, Nakamura S, Inenaga T, Kimura G. High sodium sensitivity implicates nocturnal hypertension in essential hypertension. Hypertension 1996; 28:139–42.
94. Uzu T, Ishikawa K, Fujii T, Nakamura S, Inenaga T, Kimura G. Sodium restriction shifts circadian rhythm of blood pressure from nondipper to dipper in essential hypertension. Circulation 1997; 96:1859–62.
95. Uzu T, Kimura G. Diuretics shift circadian rhythm of blood pressure from nondipper to dipper in essential hypertension. Circulation 1999; 100:1635–8.
96. Guyton AC. Renal function curve: a key to understanding the pathogenesis of hypertension. Hypertension 1987; 10:1–6.
97. Guyton AC. Dominant role of the kidneys and accessory role of whole-body autoregulation in the pathogenesis of hypertension. Am J Hypertens 1989; 2:575–85.
98. Guyton AC, Coleman TG, Cowley AWJ, Sheel KW, Manning RDJ, Norman RAJ. Arterial pressure regulation. Overriding dominance of the kidneys in long-term regulation and in hypertension. Am J Med 1972; 52:584–94.
99. Kimura G, Brenner BM. A method for distinghishing salt-sensitive from non-salt-sensitive forms of human and experimental hypertension. Curr Opin Nephrol Hypertens 1993; 2:341–9.
100. Kimura G, Brenner BM. Indirect assessment of glomerular capillary pressure from pressure–natriuresis relationship: comparison with direct measurements reported in rats. Hypertens Res 1997; 20:143–8.
101. Dahl LK. Salt and hypertension. Am J Clin Nutr 1972; 25:231–44.
102. Dahl LK, Heine M, Tassinari L. Role of genetic factors in susceptibility to experimental hypertension due to chronic excess salt ingestion. Nature 1962; 194:480.
103. Chiolero A, Maillard M, Nussberger J, Brunner HR, Burnier M. Proximal sodium reabsorption: an independent determinant of blood pressure response to salt. Hypertension 2000; 36:631–7.
104. Manunta P, Burnier M, D'Amico M, et al. Adducin polymorphism affects renal proximal tubule reabsorption in hypertension. Hypertension 1999; 33:694–7.
105. Johnson RJ, Schreiner GF. Hypothesis: the role of acquired tubulointerstitial disease in the pathogenesis of salt-dependent hypertension. Kidney Int 1997; 52:1169–79.

106. Johnson RJ, Rodriguez-Iturbe B, Nakagawa T, Kang DH, Feig DI, Herrera-Acosta J. Subtle renal injury is likely a common mechanism for salt-sensitive essential hypertension. Hypertension 2005; 45:326–30.
107. Johnson RJ, Herrera-Acosta J, Schreiner GF, Rodriguez-Iturbe B. Subtle acquired renal injury as a mechanism of salt-sensitive hypertension. N Engl J Med 2002; 346:913–23.
108. Johnson RJ, Rodriguez-Iturbe B, Kang DH, Feig DI, Herrera-Acosta J. A unifying pathway for essential hypertension. Am J Hypertens 2005; 18:431–40.
109. Svetkey LP, McKeown SP, Wilson AF. Heritability of salt sensitivity in black Americans. Hypertension 1996; 28:854–8.
110. Miller JZ, Weinberger MH, Christian JC, Daugherty SA. Familial resemblance in the blood pressure response to sodium restriction. Am J Epidemiol 1987; 126:822–30.
111. Lifton RP. Molecular genetics of human blood pressure variation. Science 1996; 272:676–80 (Review; 33 refs).
112. Meneton P, Jeunemaitre X, de Wardener HE, MacGregor GA. Links between dietary salt intake, renal salt handling, blood pressure, and cardiovascular diseases. Physiol Rev 2005; 85:679–715.
113. Matsuoka Y, Li X, Bennett V. Adducin: structure, function and regulation. Cell Mol Life Sci 2000; 57:884–95.
114. Bianchi G, Tripodi G, Casari G, et al. Two point mutations within the adducin genes are involved in blood pressure variation. Proc Natl Acad Sci USA 1994; 91:3999–4003.
115. Bianchi G, Tripodi G. Genetics of hypertension: the adducin paradigm. Ann NY Acad Sci 2003; 986:660.
116. Salardi S, Saccardo B, Borsani G, et al. Erythrocyte adducin differential properties in the normotensive and hypertensive rats of the Milan strain. Characterization of spleen adducin m-RNA. Am J Hypertens 1989; 2:229–37.
117. Ferrari P, Torielli L, Cirillo M, Salardi S, Bianchi G. Sodium transport kinetics in erythrocytes and inside-out vesicles from Milan rats. J Hypertens 1991; 9:703–11.
118. Ferrari P, Torielli L, Salardi S, Rizzo A, Bianchi G. $Na^+/K^+/Cl^-$ cotransport in resealed ghosts from erythrocytes of the Milan hypertensive rats. Biochim Biophys Acta 1992; 1111:111–9.
119. Marro ML, Scremin OU, Jordan MC, et al. Hypertension in β-adducin-deficient mice. Hypertension 2000; 36:449–53.
120. Muro AF, Marro ML, Gajovic S, Porro F, Luzzatto L, Baralle FE. Mild spherocytic hereditary elliptocytosis and altered levels of alpha- and gamma-adducins in beta-adducin-deficient mice. Blood 2000; 95:3978–85.
121. Yang H, Francis SC, Sellers K, et al. Hypertension-linked decrease in the expression of brain γ-adducin. Circ Res 2002; 91:633–9.
122. Cusi D, Barlassina C, Azzani T, et al. Polymorphisms of alpha-adducin and salt sensitivity in patients with essential hypertension. Lancet 1997; 349:1353–7.
123. Manunta P, Cusi D, Barlassina C, et al. Alpha-adducin polymorphisms and renal sodium handling in essential hypertensive patients. Kidney Int 1998; 53:1471–8.
124. Glorioso N, Filigheddu F, Cusi D, et al. α-Adducin 460Trp allele is associated with erythrocyte Na transport rate in North Sardinian primary hypertensives. Hypertension 2002; 39:357–62.
125. Barlassina C, Schork NJ, Manunta P, et al. Synergistic effect of alpha-adducin and ACE genes causes blood pressure changes with body sodium and volume expansion. Kidney Int 2000; 57:1083–90.
126. Sciarrone MT, Stella P, Barlassina C, et al. ACE and α-adducin polymorphism as markers of individual response to diuretic therapy. Hypertension 2003; 41:398–403.
127. Castejon AM, Alfieri AB, Hoffmann IS, Rathinavelu A, Cubeddu LX. Alpha-adducin polymorphism, salt sensitivity, nitric oxide excretion, and cardiovascular risk factors in normotensive Hispanics. Am J Hypertens 2003; 16:1018–24.
128. Ciechanowicz A, Widecka K, Drozd R, Adler G, Cyrylowski L, Czekalski S. Lack of association between Gly460Trp polymorphism of alpha-adducin gene and salt sensitivity of blood pressure in Polish hypertensives. Kidney Blood Press Res 2001; 24:201.

129. Walker WG, Whelton PK, Saito H, Russell RP, Hermann J. Relation between blood pressure and renin, renin substrate, angiotensin II, aldosterone and urinary sodium and potassium in 574 ambulatory subjects. Hypertension 1979; 1:287–91.
130. Nakajima T, Jorde LB, Ishigami T, et al. Nucleotide diversity and haplotype structure of the human angiotensinogen gene in two populations. Am J Hum Genet 2002; 70:108–23.
131. Renner W, Nauck M, Winkelmann BR, et al. Association of angiotensinogen haplotypes with angiotensinogen levels but not with blood pressure or coronary artery disease: the Ludwigshafen Risk and Cardiovascular Health Study. J Mol Med 2005; 83:235–9.
132. Sethi AA, Nordestgaard BG, Agerholm-Larsen B, Frandsen E, Jensen G, Tybjarg-Hansen A. Angiotensinogen polymorphisms and elevated blood pressure in the general population: the Copenhagen City Heart Study. Hypertension 2001; 37:875–81.
133. Sethi AA, Nordestgaard BG, Tybjaerg-Hansen A. Angiotensinogen gene polymorphism, plasma angiotensinogen, and risk of hypertension and ischemic heart disease: a meta-analysis. Arterioscler Thromb Vasc Biol 2003; 23:1269–75.
134. Kim HS, Krege JH, Kluckman KD, et al. Genetic control of blood pressure and the angiotensinogen locus. Proc Natl Acad Sci USA 1995; 92:2735–9.
135. Smithies O, Kim HS. Targeted gene duplication and disruption for analyzing quantitative genetic traits in mice. Proc Natl Acad Sci USA 1994; 91:3612–5.
136. Jeunemaitre X, Soubrier F, Kotelevtsev YV, et al. Molecular basis of human hypertension: role of angiotensinogen. Cell 1992; 71:169–80.
137. Schorr U, Blaschke K, Beige J, Distler A, Sharma AM. Angiotensinogen M235T variant and salt sensitivity in young normotensive Caucasians. J Hypertens 1999; 17:475–9.
138. Giner V, Poch E, Bragulat E, et al. Renin–angiotensin system genetic polymorphism and salt sensitivity in essential hypertension. Hypertension 2000; 35:512–7.
139. Poch E, Gonzalez D, Giner V, Bragulat E, Coca A, de la Sierra A. Molecular basis of salt sensitivity in human hypertension: evaluation of renin–angiotensin–aldosterone system gene polymorphisms. Hypertension 2001; 38:1204–9.
140. Johnson AG, Nguyen TV, Davis D. Blood pressure is linked to salt intake and modulated by the angiotensinogen gene in normotensive and hypertensive elderly subjects. J Hypertens 2001; 19:1053–60.
141. Hunt SC, Cook NRC, Oberman A, et al. Angiotensinogen genotype, sodium reduction, weight loss, and prevention of hypertension. Trials of hypertension prevention, phase II. Hypertension 1998; 32:393–401.
142. Haehner BD, Gorski JC, Vandenbranden M, et al. Bimodal distribution of renal cytochrome P450 3A activity in humans. Mol Pharmacol 1996; 50:52–9.
143. Koch I, Weil R, Wolbold R, et al. Interindividual variability and tissue-specificity in the expression of cytochrome P450 3A mRNA. Drug Metab Dispos 2002; 30:1108–14.
144. Kuehl P, Zhang J, Lin Y, Lamba J, Assem M, Schuetz J, Watkins PB, Daly A, Wrighton SA, Hall SD, et al. Sequence diversity in CYP3A promoters and characterization of the genetic basis of polymorphic CYP3A5 expression. Nat Genet 2001; 27:383–91.
145. Wrighton SA, Brian WR, Sari MA, et al. Studies on the expression and metabolic capabilities of human liver cytochrome P450IIIA5 (HLp3). Mol Pharmacol 1990; 38:207–13.
146. Schuetz EG, Schuetz JD, Grogan WM, et al. Expression of cytochrome P450 3A in amphibian, rat, and human kidney. Arch Biochem Biophys 1992; 294:206–14.
147. Ghosh SS, Basu AK, Ghosh S, et al. Renal and hepatic family 3A cytochromes P450 (CYP3A) in spontaneously hypertensive rats. Biochem Pharmacol 1995; 50:49–54.
148. Watlington CO, Kramer LB, Schuetz EG, et al. Corticosterone 6 beta-hydroxylation correlates with blood pressure in spontaneously hypertensive rats. Am J Physiol 1992; 262:F927–31.
149. Warrington JS, Greenblatt DJ, von Moltke LL. Age-related differences in CYP3A expression and activity in the rat liver, intestine, and kidney. J Pharmacol Exp Ther 2004; 309:720–9.
150. Givens RC, Lin YS, Dowling AL, et al. *CYP3A5* genotype predicts renal CYP3A activity and blood pressure in healthy adults. J Appl Physiol 2003; 95:1297–300.

151. Ho H, Pinto A, Hall SD, et al. Association between the *CYP3A5* genotype and blood pressure. Hypertension 2005; 45:1–5.
152. Bochud M, Eap CB, Elston RC, et al. Association of *CYP3A5* genotypes with blood pressure and renal function in African families. J Hypertens 2006; 24:923–9.
153. Fromm MF, Schmidt BM, Pahl A, Jacobi J, Schmieder RE. *CYP3A5* genotype is associated with elevated blood pressure. Pharmacogenet Genomics 2005; 15:737–41.
154. Thompson EE, Kuttab-Boulos H, Witonsky D, Yang L, Roe BA, Di Rienzo A. CYP3A variation and the evolution of salt-sensitivity variants. Am J Hum Genet 2004; 75:1059–69.
155. Farfel Z, Bourne HR, Iiri T. The expanding spectrum of G protein diseases. N Engl J Med 1999; 340:1012.
156. Siffert W, Rosskopf D, Siffert G, et al. Association of a human G-protein beta-3 subunit variant with hypertension. Nat Genet 1998; 18:45–8.
157. Siffert W. G protein β-3 subunit 825T allele, hypertension, obesity, and diabetic nephropathy. Nephrol Dial Transplant 2000; 15:1298–306.
158. Schorr U, Blaschke K, Beige J, Distler A, Sharma A. G-protein β3 subunit 825T allele and response to dietary salt in normotensive men. J Hypertens 2000; 18:855–9.
159. Pamies-Andreu E, Ramirez-Lorca R, Stiefel Garcia-Junco P, et al. Renin–angiotensin–aldosterone system and G-protein beta-3 subunit gene polymorphisms in salt-sensitive essential hypertension. J Hum Hypertens 2003; 17:187–91.
160. Gonzalez-Nunez D, Giner V, Bragulat E, Coca A, de la Sierra A, Poch E. Absence of an association between the C825T polymorphism of the G-protein beta 3 subunit and salt-sensitivity in essential arterial hypertension. Nefrologia 2001; 21:355–61.
161. Turner ST, Schwartz GL, Chapman AB, Boerwinkle E. C825T polymorphism of the G protein β_3-subunit and antihypertensive response to a thiazide diuretic. Hypertension 2001; 37:739–43.
162. Lifton RP, Dluhy RG, Powers M, et al. Hereditary hypertension caused by chimaeric gene duplications and ectopic expression of aldosterone synthase. Nat Genet 1992; 2:66–74.
163. Lifton RP, Dluhy RG, Powers M, et al. A chimaeric 11β-hydroxylase/aldosterone synthase gene causes glucocorticoid-remediable aldosteronism and human hypertension. Nature 1992; 355:262–5.
164. Pascoe L, Curnow KM, Slutsker L, et al. Glucocorticoid-suppressible hyperaldosteronism results from hybrid genes created by unequal crossovers between CYP11B1 and CYP11B2. Proc Natl Acad Sci USA 1992; 89:8327–31.
165. White PC, Slutsker L. Haplotype analysis of CYP11B2. Endocr Res 1995; 21:437–42.
166. White PC, Rainey WE. Polymorphisms in CYP11B genes and 11-hydroxylase activity. J Clin Endocrinol Metab 2005; 90:1252–5.
167. Barbato A, Russo P, Siani A, et al. Aldosterone synthase gene (CYP11B2) C-344T polymorphism, plasma aldosterone, renin activity and blood pressure in a multi-ethnic population. J Hypertens 2004; 22:1895–901.
168. Davies E, Holloway CD, Ingram MC, et al. Aldosterone excretion rate and blood pressure in essential hypertension are related to polymorphic differences in the aldosterone synthase gene CYP11B2. Hypertension 1999; 33:703–7.
169. Brand E, Schorr U, Ringel J, Beige J, Distler A, Sharma AM. Aldosterone synthase gene (CYP11B2) C-344T polymorphism in caucasians from the Berlin salt-sensitivity trial (BeSST). J Hypertens 1999; 17:1563.
170. Mune T, Rogerson FM, Nikkila H, Agarwal AK, White PC. Human hypertension caused by mutations in the kidney isozyme of 11 beta-hydroxysteroid dehydrogenase. Nat Genet 1995; 10:394–9.
171. Stewart PM, Krozowski ZS, Gupta A, et al. Hypertension in the syndrome of apparent mineralocorticoid excess due to mutation of the 11 beta-hydroxysteroid dehydrogenase type 2 gene. Lancet 1996; 347:88–91.
172. Ferrari P, Lovati E, Frey FJ. The role of the 11beta-hydroxysteroid dehydrogenase type 2 in human hypertension. J Hypertens 2000; 18:241–8.

173. Mune T, White PC. Apparent mineralocorticoid excess: genotype is correlated with biochemical phenotype. Hypertension 1996; 27:1193–9.
174. Nunez BS, Rogerson FM, Mune T, et al. Mutants of 11{beta}-hydroxysteroid dehydrogenase (11-HSD2) with partial activity: improved correlations between genotype and biochemical phenotype in apparent mineralocorticoid excess. Hypertension 1999; 34:638–42.
175. Persu A. 11beta-Hydroxysteroid deshydrogenase: a multi-faceted enzyme. J Hypertens 2005; 23:29–31.
176. Agarwal AK, Giacchetti G, Lavery G, et al. CA-repeat polymorphism in intron 1 of HSD11B2: effects on gene expression and salt sensitivity. Hypertension 2000; 36:187–94.
177. Ferrari P, Sansonnens A, Dick B, Frey FJ. In vivo 11β-HSD-2 activity: variability, salt-sensitivity, and effect of licorice. Hypertension 2001; 38:1330–6.
178. Melander O, Frandsen E, Groop L, Hulthen UL. No evidence of a relation between 11beta-hydroxysteroid dehydrogenase type 2 activity and salt sensitivity. Am J Hypertens 2003; 16:729–33.
179. Kerstens MN, Navis G, Dullaart RP. Salt sensitivity and 11beta-hydroxysteroid dehydrogenase type 2 activity. Am J Hypertens 2004; 17:283–4.
180. Tiret L, Rigat B, Visvikis S, et al. Evidence from combined segregation and linkage analysis, that a variant of the angiotensin I-converting enzyme(ACE) gene controls plasma ACE levels. Am J Hum Genet 1992; 51:197–210.
181. Rieder MJ, Taylor SL, Clark AG, Nickerson DA. Sequence variation in the human angiotensin converting enzyme. Nat Genet 1999; 22:59–62.
182. Hiraga H, Oshima T, Watanabe M, et al. Angiotensin i-converting enzyme gene polymorphism and salt sensitivity in essential hypertension. Hypertension 1996; 27:569–72.
183. Dengel DR, Brown MD, Ferrell RE, Supiano MA. Role of angiotensin converting enzyme genotype in sodium sensitivity in older hypertensives. Am J Hypertens 2001; 14:1178–84.
184. Kojima S, Inenaga T, Matsuoka H, et al. The association between salt sensitivity of blood pressure and some polymorphic factors. J Hypertens 1994; 12:797–801.

15
Renal Sodium Handling in Women

David Z. I. Cherney and Judith A. Miller
Division of Nephrology, Toronto General Hospital, University of Toronto, Toronto, Ontario, Canada

INTRODUCTION

Renal sodium handling is complex and involves an afferent sensory limb, which determines effective circulating volume, and an efferent limb that acts to maintain sodium homeostasis. The afferent mechanisms include neural pathways, arterial volume sensors, renal volume sensors, central nervous system sensors, and hepatic volume sensors. The efferent limb also involves mechanisms that include glomerular and tubular factors, as well as humoral and renal neural components. This chapter focuses on gender differences in the afferent and efferent limbs that have been studied in both animal and human models (Table 1). An understanding of these mechanisms is particularly important as they may contribute to differences in blood pressure (BP) regulation between men and women (1).

AFFERENT MECHANISMS

Neural Mechanisms

The autonomic nervous system is an important consideration in sodium handling because of its influence on efferent systems involved in sodium balance such as the renin–angiotensin system (RAS) and neural pathways. One of the mechanisms leading to hypertension in salt-sensitive Dahl rats may involve alterations in afferent neural signaling. Both male and female rats of this species appear to exhibit an impairment in baroreflex-mediated inhibition of sympathetic nerve activity in response to hypertensive stimuli (2), as well as sympathetically-mediated increases in total peripheral resistance (3). Female rats may be more resistant to these pressor mechanisms, suggesting the presence of a significant afferent neuromodulatory role of estrogen (4), which may blunt potentially hypertensive stimuli. It has been suggested that female rats in the follicular (low estrogen) phase of the menstrual cycle exhibit an increased baroreceptor gain and greater increase in renal nerve activity compared to males, while during the luteal phase baroreceptor gain and maximal increases in nerve activity are blunted (5). This supports the hypothesis that estrogen may exert a protective antihypertensive effect through modulation of baroreceptor afferent signals. Similar findings have been demonstrated in the

Table 1 Mechanisms Responsible for Gender-Based Differences in Renal Sodium Handling

Afferent mechanisms
Neural pathways
Arterial volume receptors
Efferent mechanisms
Sex differences in the pressure natriuresis phenomenon
Sex-steroid effects
Estrogen effects on humoral mediators
Progesterone effects on natriuresis
Testosterone effects on humoral mediators
Humoral mediators
Renin–angiotensin system function differences
Nitric oxide-mediated renal hemodynamic effects
Prostaglandin-mediated renal hemodynamic effects
Endothelin-1-mediated renal hemodynamic effects
Autonomic nervous system effects

normotensive rat model, wherein female rats exhibit an enhanced protective baroreceptor response to the pressor effect of angiotensin II (Ang II) infusion (6). Estrogen may act in the central nervous system by antagonizing Ang II activity in the subfornical and circumventricular organs as well as the area postrema (7,8). This would result in a decreased signal to reabsorb sodium in response to RAS activation. Similar protective baroreceptor effects have been found in postmenopausal women after initiation of hormone replacement therapy (9). These findings may enable females to maintain greater control over effective circulating volume and BP in response to volume expansion or vasopressor stimuli.

Arterial Volume Sensors

Cardiopulmonary baroreceptor mechanisms may also mediate important gender-based differences in renal sodium handling. Increases in effective circulating volume activate cardiopulmonary stretch receptors which inhibit sympathetic activity and result in a reduction in renal sodium reabsorption (5). Although male and female rats have been found to exhibit equivalent right atrial stretch receptor activation and decreases in sympathetic activity in response to effective circulating volume expansion, female rats demonstrate an increase in renal sodium excretion in response to an equivalent stimulus (Fig. 1), suggesting a gender-based difference in renal responsiveness to neurogenic regulatory mechanisms (5). It is unknown, however, whether these afferent mechanisms have clinical implications in humans.

EFFERENT MECHANISMS

Physiologic Principles of Sodium Excretion: Glomerular Hemodynamic Function

Urinary sodium excretion is determined by the rate of tubular reabsorption over a wide range of fluctuations in effective circulating volume. This was demonstrated in a series

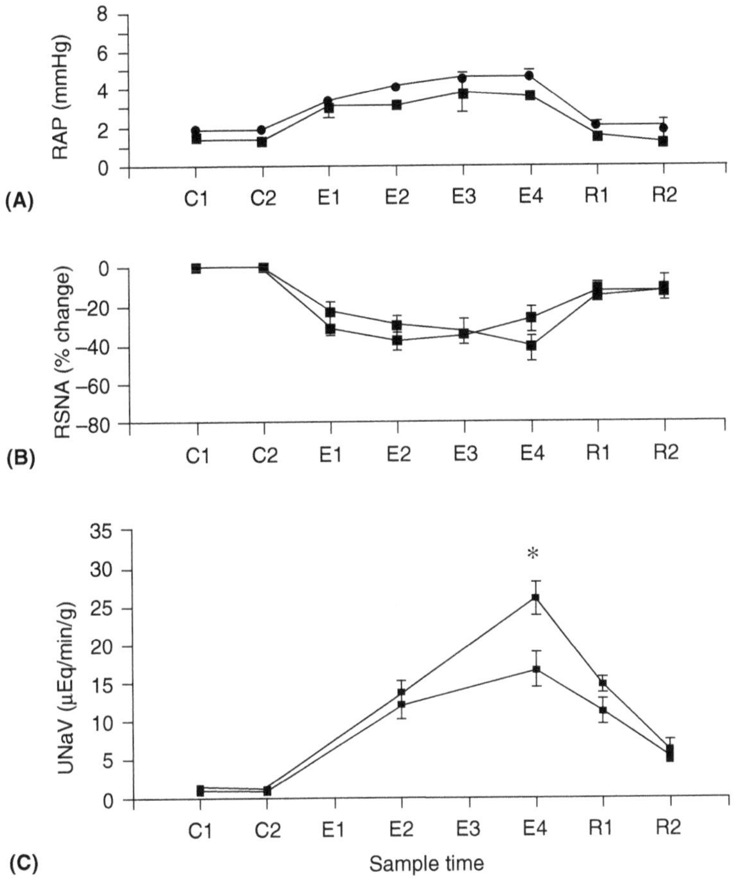

Figure 1 Effects of 5% volume expansion with isotonic saline infusion (1 mL/min) on (**A**) RAP, (**B**) RSNA and (**C**) UNaV in male [filled squares; $n=7$ (**A**,**B**), 9 (**C**)] and female [filled circles; $n=13$ (**A**–**C**)] rats. Measurements were made 30 and 15 minutes prior to volume expansion (C1, C2), during volume expansion (E1, E2, E3, E4) and 15 and 30 minutes after volume expansion (R1, R2). $*p < 0.05$ between males and females. *Abbreviations*: RAP, right atrial pressure; RSNA, renal sympathetic nerve activity; UNaV, urinary sodium excretion. *Source*: From Ref. 5.

of classic physiologic studies (10–12) and is largely independent of glomerular filtration rate (GFR). Sodium handling at the level of the glomerulus is mediated through changes in filtration fraction (FF), which is the ratio of GFR to effective renal plasma flow. This in turn impacts on proximal tubular sodium reabsorptive capacity. As FF increases, hydrostatic pressure in the peritubular capillaries decreases due to preferential efferent vasoconstriction, favoring sodium reabsorption. As the FF increases, the plasma oncotic pressure in the efferent arteriole, which is connected in series to the peritubular capillary bed, rises, which again favors sodium reabsorption.

Physiologic Principles of Sodium Excretion: The Pressure–Natriuresis

The prominent role of the pressure–natriuresis phenomenon in the maintenance of arterial BP homeostasis has been recognized for more than 30 years (13). The model put forward by Guyton et al. as well as others (14) hypothesizes that increases in renal perfusion pressure lead to increases in pressure and flow in the vasa recta. This both raises renal interstitial pressure, which in turn decreases sodium reabsorption in both superficial and deep nephrons, and leads to the washout of the renal medulla solute gradient, with the resultant reduction in sodium reabsorption in the deep nephrons. These changes result in a return of effective circulating volume to normal. Conversely, a shift of the pressure natriuresis curve to the right, which results in a relative state of salt insensitivity, can lead to increases in arterial BP (15). Continuing interest in renal sodium handling and the mechanisms that are responsible for it, such as pressure–natriuresis, has been stimulated by many exciting studies examining gender differences, including animal and human basic science studies, and human epidemiologic studies. Large population-based studies have shown quite consistent positive correlations between alterations in sodium excretion and hypertension in men; this relationship is less certain in premenopausal women, and in younger populations in general (16–18).

The Effect of Sex Hormones and the RAS on Renal Sodium Handling

Extensive animal data has emerged that supports the central role of sex hormones in mediating gender-based BP and sodium handling differences. Reckelhoff et al. have demonstrated that male spontaneously hypertensive rats (SHR) exhibit a blunted pressure–natriuresis response compared to female SHR. Furthermore, castration of the male SHR results in a normalization of the pressure–natriuresis curve (Fig. 2A) (18) and reductions in BP (Fig. 2B), while administration of androgens to the female SHR results in a pressure–natriuresis curve that is similar to that of the males (18). This implicates a prominent role for androgens in mediating gender-based sodium handling differences.

Animal and human renal transplantation studies have also led to interesting insights into gender-based differences in renal sodium handling and hypertension. In rat models, although renal transplantation from a SHR donor to a non-hypertensive rat strain can produce hypertension (19), transplantation of SHR male kidneys to a female rat does not result in a significant rise in BP, and female kidneys do not protect males from hypertension, suggesting a non-renal systemic mediator in the male, possibly androgens (20). Since androgen receptors have been localized to the proximal tubular segment of the nephron, it seems highly likely that androgens can exert a modulatory effect on renal sodium handling (21).

Human transplantation studies, on the other hand, have not been able to address this question as clearly: elegant renal transplantation studies in African American patients in the 1970s examined four men and two women with end-stage renal disease due to clearly documented essential hypertension with no evidence of other primary renal disease after pathologic examination of their native kidneys (22), who underwent renal transplantation. These patients received renal grafts from normotensive individuals and remained free of hypertension after a mean of 4.5 years after the procedure. The gender of the donor was not reported in four of the six cases. These recipients also demonstrated normal renal responses to salt loading and deprivation after transplantation (22). As opposed to the above animal data, these findings suggest an intrarenal cause for hypertension in this group of patients. Further studies in this area would be difficult due to the significant hypertensive effect of modern immunosuppressive drugs such as calcineurin inhibitors.

The RAS is one of the central mechanisms involved in controlling BP, sodium and fluid volume homeostasis (15). An appreciation of gender differences in RAS function is critical to the understanding of gender differences in renal sodium handling. RAS functional differences have been widely suspected to play a central role in the mediation of

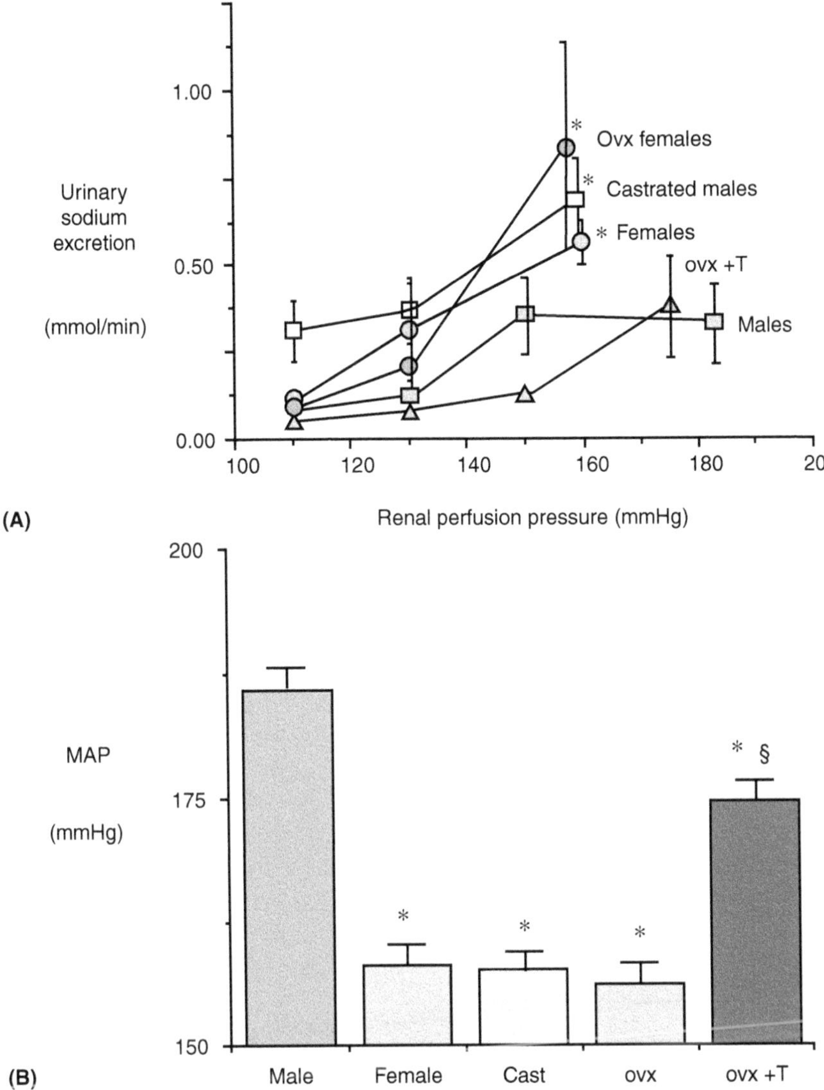

Figure 2 (**A**) Acute pressure–natriuresis relationship comparison in male, female, castrated male, untreated ovariectomized (ovx) female, and ovariectomized female SHR treated chronically for five to six weeks with testosterone (ovx+T). Acute pressure–natriuresis studies were conducted in anesthetized SHR, aged 17 to 19 weeks. Renal perfusion pressure was reduced by tightening a snare around the aorta above the renal arteries in a stepwise fashion. $*p<0.05$ compared with males. (**B**) Mean arterial blood pressure (MAP) measured in anesthetized SHR. MAP measured in anesthetized SHR, aged 17 to 19 weeks, during the established phase of hypertension. Some males and females were castrated (cast) or ovariectomized (ovx) at seven weeks of age. Some ovariectomized females were given testosterone (T) by implantation of silicone elastomer pellets for the last five to six weeks before blood pressure was measured. $*p<0.01$ compared with males and/or testosterone-treated ovariectomized females; $\S p<0.01$ compared with females, castrated males, or ovariectomized females. *Abbreviations*: MAP, mean arterial blood pressure; SHR, spontaneously hypertensive rats. *Source*: From Ref. 18.

gender-based BP disparities, since longitudinal studies in normotensive humans have found increased serum markers of RAS activity, such as plasma renin activity (PRA), in men compared to women (23,24). These differences persist, although to a lesser degree, after the menopause (25). This has been one of the major mechanisms that are thought to be responsible for higher rates of hypertension in men compared to women in most populations (26). An upregulation of RAS activity and the ensuing increase in circulating Ang II increases FF via efferent constriction (27), resulting in a fall in peritubular capillary hydrostatic forces and a simultaneous rise in peritubular plasma oncotic forces, favoring sodium reabsorption, effective circulating volume expansion and hypertension, with a blunting of the pressure–natriuresis curve. Ang II also favors sodium reabsorption by stimulating the basolateral Na^+/HCO_3^- symporter and luminal Na^+/H^+ exchanger, enhancing proximal sodium reabsorption (28). Ang II likely exerts similar sodium-reabsorbing effects in the distal nephron, possibly by increasing the activity of the amiloride-sensitive epithelial sodium channel (29). RAS activation also enhances tubuloglomerular feedback (TGF) sensitivity via an Ang II-mediated reduction in sodium delivery to the macula densa (30). Afferent vasodilatation ensues, thereby maintaining GFR (15,30).

Androgens may mediate some of their pressor effects in rats through neurohormonal mediators (Fig. 3). This has been shown in the following experimental models: (*i*) SHR male rats exhibit higher PRA levels than female rats (32); (*ii*) treatment of female rats with testosterone results in PRA increases (33,34); (*iii*) castration of male rats results in decreases in PRA (33,34), and prevents the development of hypertension (18). At the functional level, increased testosterone levels have been shown to be associated with significant and linear increases in PRA and arterial BP (35). Androgens may mediate this effect by increasing renal angiotensinogen mRNA (33,36), which has in turn been

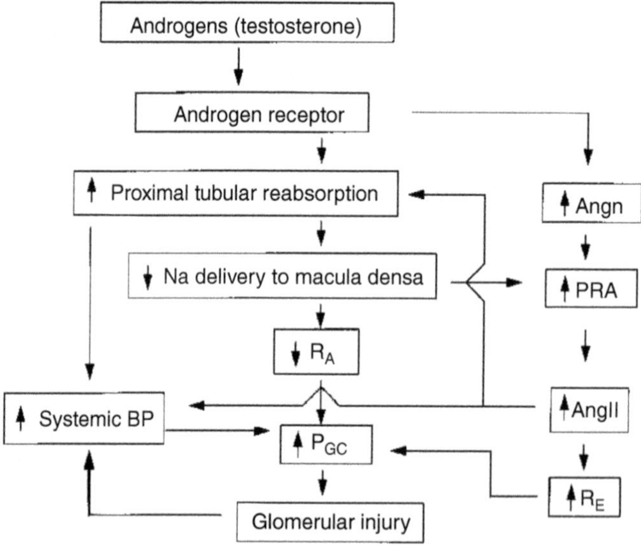

Figure 3 Schematic diagram for the mechanisms by which androgens may increase proximal sodium reabsorption in the kidney and promote renal injury, thereby causing hypertension. *Abbreviations*: Angn, angiotensinogen; Ang II, angiotensin II; P_{GC}, glomerular capillary pressure; PRA, plasma renin activity; R_A, afferent arteriolar resistance; R_E, efferent arteriolar resistance. *Source*: From Ref. 31.

associated with increases in BP (37). An additional hypothesis that could explain the hypertensive effect of androgens is the direct stimulatory role of androgens on proximal tubular sodium reabsorption (38), which could lead to a reduction in distal sodium delivery and a resultant upregulation of renin secretion from the macula densa causing an increase in PRA.

The direct stimulatory effect of androgens on proximal tubular sodium reabsorption has been supported by several additional observations: (*i*) androgen receptors have been localized to nuclear fractions of a renal carcinoma cell line that is functionally similar to proximal tubule cells (38); (*ii*) androgen receptors have been localized to rat proximal tubule cells (21); (*iii*) androgen receptor antagonism with flutamide decreases BP in SHR (39). From a functional perspective, further supportive evidence for the central role of the RAS in mediating androgen-based gender differences in the SHR rat model comes from treatment studies whereby RAS blockade with angiotensin converting enzyme inhibition leads to a greater BP reduction in male SHR and androgenized female SHR than female, castrated male or ovariectomized female rats (40). RAS activity may also be increased by androgen-mediated angiotensin type 1 (AT_1) receptor upregulation, resulting in greater Ang II sensitivity (41) and a resultant blunting of the pressure–natriuresis response. Androgens therefore mediate important direct, as well as indirect sodium-handling effects in animal models.

Physiologic studies in human subjects have also revealed extensive differences in RAS function that may explain gender-based differences in renal sodium handling. In a mechanistic study involving 10 men and 8 women given a sodium load with intravenous hypertonic saline, men exhibited a significant increase in plasma volume (42), and an associated hypertensive effect compared to women in both the luteal and follicular phases of the menstrual cycle. Men also experienced a significantly blunted rise in urinary sodium excretion compared to women. In this short-term study, PRA levels were significantly higher in women who were studied in the luteal phase of the menstrual cycle compared to men and those women in the follicular phase of the menstrual cycle, despite the maintenance of normal BP. Humoral increases in circulating RAS components without a corresponding increase in RAS-mediated physiologic effects during states of high estrogen have been observed elsewhere (43), but the mechanism involved in this RAS-modulating impact of estrogen is poorly understood. Vokes et al. made a similar observation in a group of 15 healthy, young women (44). These investigators administered hypertonic saline during different phases of the menstrual cycle and found the expected expansion of the plasma volume, but failed to demonstrate a rise in BP (44). Humoral RAS activity was not, however, measured in this study. An interesting non-RAS dependent theory that has been put forward to explain this difference in response to saline loading is a differential response in vascular reactivity (45). Male rats exhibit enhanced vascular smooth muscle contraction in response to salt loading compared to female Sprague–Dawley rats, possibly due to an increase in intracellular calcium entry, a process which has also been observed in human lymphocytes (46).

Other human studies have also shown differences in RAS function based on gender. Ang II infusion in normotensive, premenopausal women and age-matched men leads to a rise in BP and a fall in effective renal plasma flow, but only men maintain GFR, resulting in a rise in FF, and possibly intraglomerular pressure. Women, on the other hand, experience a fall in GFR with a greater decrease in effective renal plasma flow, resulting in a blunted rise in FF (Fig. 4). In addition, the Ang II-mediated change in effective renal plasma flow was blunted in high estrogen states (47). In spite of the functional RAS differences that were seen in this study, which would theoretically favor an increase in sodium reabsorption in men, no differences in urinary sodium excretion were observed in response to Ang II. In another study, mean arterial pressure and the humoral RAS response to simulated orthostasis was examined in women during the luteal and the follicular phases of the menstrual cycle (43). Despite augmented circulating RAS components in the luteal phase (Fig. 5), the BP response was discordant, in that women were unable to maintain arterial pressure in response to simulated orthostasis (Fig. 6), whereas in the follicular low estrogen phase, no hypotensive episodes occurred. Therefore, women exhibit a blunted pressor response to Ang II in high estrogen states. Human physiologic studies during the high estrogen state of pregnancy have shown similar findings, with a blunted pressor response to Ang II infusion in pregnant, non-hypertensive women, compared to normal non-gravid women (48,49). Similar findings suggesting renal and peripheral vasodilatation in association with RAS humoral activation were demonstrated in a study examining 16 women during the follicular and luteal phases of the menstrual cycle (50). This highlights the discordance between humoral RAS markers and RAS function in the presence of estrogen. All of these findings suggest a downregulatory tissue response to high Ang II levels during states of high estrogen (43). These studies were not designed to

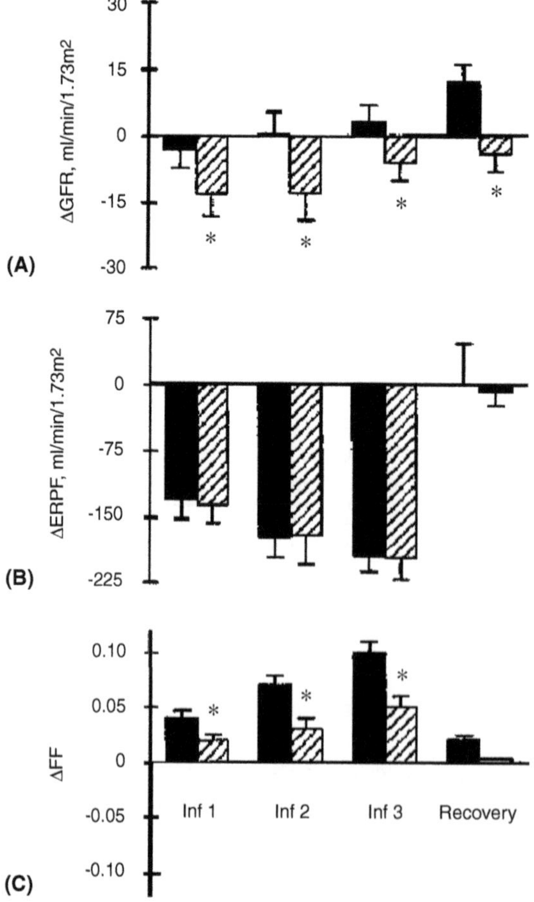

Figure 4 Change in the (**A**) ΔGFR, (**B**) ΔERPF and (**C**) ΔFF in response to angiotensin II infusion at 0.5 ng/kg/min (Inf 1), 1.5 ng/kg/min (Inf 2), 2.5 ng/kg/min (Inf 3), and at recovery in men (■) and women (▧).*$p < 0.05$ versus response in men. *Abbreviations*: ERPF, effective renal plasma flow; FF, filtration fraction; GFR, glomerular filtration rate. *Source*: From Ref. 47.

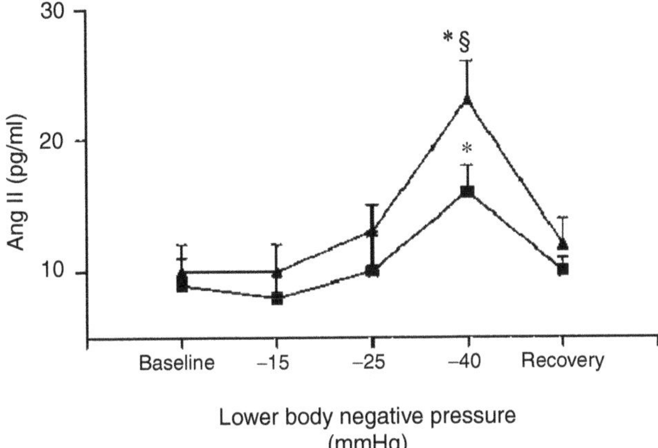

Figure 5 Response of angiotensin II to incremental lower body negative pressure during the follicular phase (■) and the luteal phase (▲) of the normal menstrual cycle. *p <0.05 versus baseline; §p <0.05 versus response during the follicular phase. *Source*: From Ref. 43.

assess possible differences in sodium excretion, but this gender-mediated blunted tissue RAS effect may help to explain the blunted pressure–natriuresis response and relative protection from hypertension seen in women.

RAS activity and renal function in response to salt loading during different parts of the menstrual cycle have been used as physiologic probes of gender differences in the pressure–natriuresis relationship. Burnier et al. demonstrated a salt insensitive, steep pressure–natriuresis response (51) in both the follicular and luteal phases of the menstrual cycle. Compared to the follicular phase, however, the luteal phase was associated with a

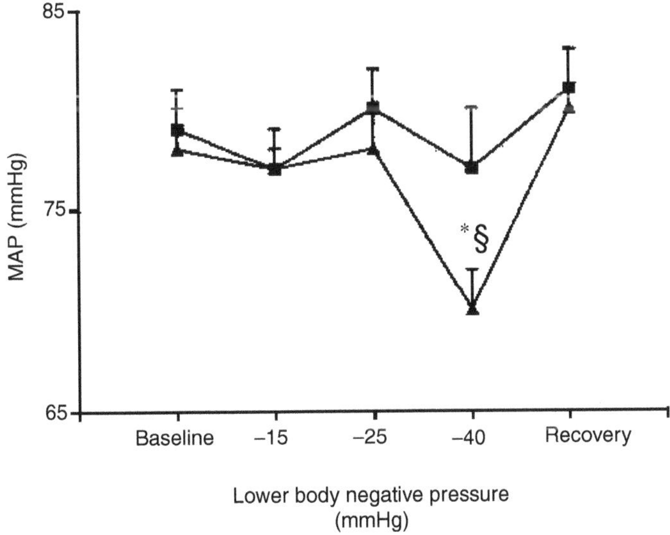

Figure 6 Response of MAP to incremental LBNP during the follicular phase (■) and the luteal phase (▲) of the normal menstrual cycle. *p <0.05 versus baseline; §p <0.05 versus response during the follicular phase. *Abbreviations*: MAP, mean arterial pressure; LBNP, lower body negative pressure. *Source*: From Ref. 43.

blunted suppression of the humoral RAS, even in response to salt-loading maneuvers. Salt loading during the luteal phase was also associated with an increase in the effective renal plasma flow with no change in GFR, resulting in a reduction in FF. The presumed rise in peritubular capillary hydrostatic pressure and fall in plasma oncotic pressure that could be seen under such circumstances could theoretically cause a heightened sensitivity of the pressure–natriuresis curve, although this was not observed in this short-term study. The response to salt loading in normal men is characterized, on the other hand, by increases in effective renal plasma flow and GFR (52). The mechanisms whereby female gender mediates these differences are unknown, but one may speculate that RAS function may be inhibited at a tissue level, or that other counter-RAS mechanisms may be upregulated, such as the nitric oxide (NO) and prostaglandin systems.

In addition to androgens, the direct influence of female sex hormones on renal sodium handling and BP regulation has also been extensively studied. Female Dahl salt-sensitive rats that are fed a high-sodium diet become less hypertensive than male rats. Ovariectomy results in an accelerated form of hypertension (53–55) with a blunted pressure–natriuresis response (53), suggesting either a protective hemodynamic effect of estrogen, or a relative increase in the ratio of deleterious androgen effect compared to the protective effect of female sex hormones. The subsequent finding that dietary phytoestrogens can blunt the hypertensive effect of a high-sodium diet in SHR female rats (Fig. 7) suggests that it is the estrogen effect, rather than merely a relative increase in the ratio of androgens to estrogens, that is responsible for maintaining the pressure–natriuresis response (56).

Studies in humans have also led to important insights into the effect of female sex hormones on renal sodium handling. These studies have supported the concept of a direct action of estrogen on renal sodium handling. Pechère-Bertschi et al. examined a group of 35 premenopausal females during the follicular and luteal phases of the menstrual cycle to study renal segmental sodium handling before and after salt loading (57). They found the same renal vasodilatory response and fall in FF in response to salt loading that they had previously observed in another group of normal women (51), as well as a blunted suppression of PRA. During the follicular phase, both proximal (determined by fractional

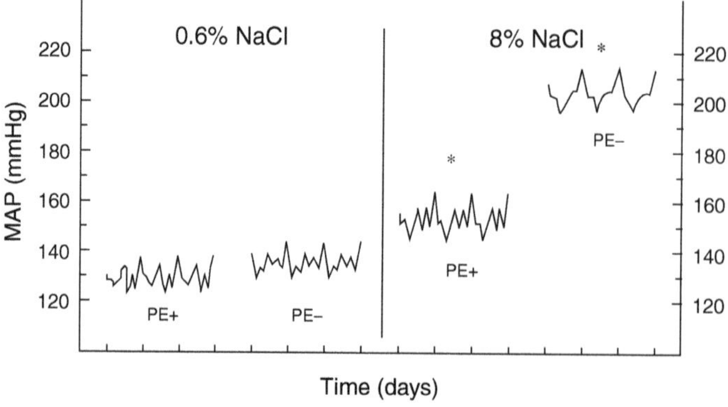

Figure 7 Twenty-four-hour circadian rhythm (PHARMFIT analysis) of arterial pressure in ovariectomized spontaneously hypertensive rats fed either a basal or high-NaCl diet with (PE+) or without (PE−) dietary phytoestrogens. The high-NaCl diet elevated arterial pressure in the PE− group, and removal of dietary phytoestrogens exacerbated the arterial pressure response to NaCl. Elimination of phytoestrogens did not significantly affect arterial pressure in rats fed the basal NaCl diet. *$p < 0.05$ for midline-estimating statistic of rhythm compared with that of all other groups. *Abbreviation*: MAP, mean arterial pressure. *Source*: From Ref. 56.

lithium excretion techniques) and distal (measured by determining the fractional distal reabsorption of sodium) sodium reabsorption was reduced on the high-sodium diet (Fig. 8). A similar pattern was seen in their male subjects. In contrast, during the luteal phase, although proximal tubular sodium reabsorption did not change in response to a high-sodium diet, the fractional distal reabsorption of sodium decreased markedly, suggesting a more prominent role for the distal tubule in sodium handling during the luteal phase (57). A similar pattern to that observed in women in the follicular phase of the menstrual cycle has been demonstrated in men on a high-salt diet (52). These results

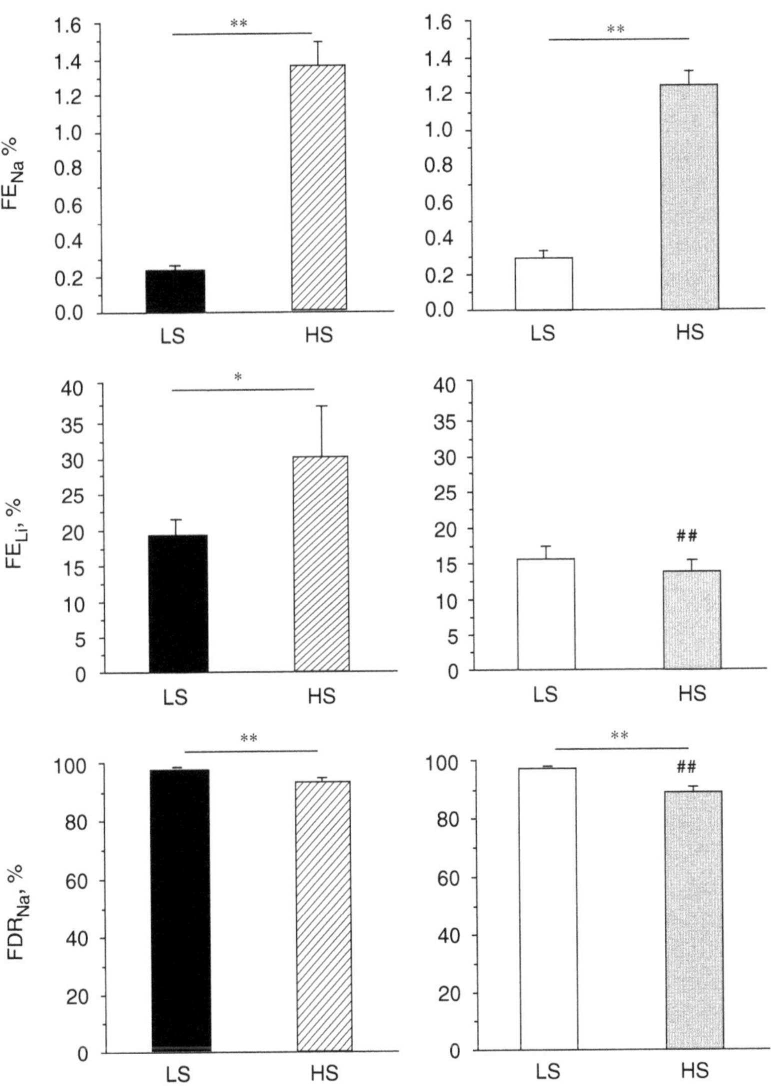

Figure 8 Salt-induced variations in daytime FE$_{Na}$ and FE$_{Li}$ and FDR$_{Na}$ in normotensive women studied during the follicular and the luteal phases of the menstrual cycle. *Abbreviations*: FDR$_{Na}$, fractional distal reabsorption of sodium; FE$_{Na}$, fractional excretions of sodium; FE$_{Li}$, fractional excretions of endogenous lithium; HS, high-salt diet at 250 mmol/day Na; LS, low-salt diet defined as 40 mmol/day Na. $^{**}p < 0.01$ high versus low-salt diet; $^{\#\#}p < 0.01$ high-salt luteal versus high-salt follicular. *Source*: From Ref. 57.

suggest that the physiology underlying relative sodium insensitivity in women may depend on the phase of the menstrual cycle. These results may also help to explain the lack of sodium retention that has been noted in women studied during different phases of the menstrual cycle (58) in spite of relative humoral RAS activation.

Several mechanisms have been postulated to explain the dominant role of distal sodium loss during the luteal phase. First, progesterone, which increases during the luteal phase of the menstrual cycle, has been recognized as possessing anti-mineralocorticoid and therefore natriuretic properties (59). These physiologic effects act to maintain sodium balance, and are thought to be particularly prominent in low aldosterone, high progesterone states, the prototype being salt loading during the luteal phase of the menstrual cycle (57). The blunted decline in PRA that has been observed in these studies may therefore reflect secondary activation of the RAS in response to distal sodium loss and effective circulating volume contraction. The importance of this mechanism is supported by the observation that synthetic progestins that are mineralocorticoid receptor inert fail to cause humoral RAS activation (60). Progestins may also have a minor natriuretic effect at the proximal tubular level in women (61), although this mechanism is not well understood. A second mechanism that has been proposed to explain differences in proximal and distal sodium handling involves changes in TGF. This theory postulates that the renal vasodilatation during the luteal phase is the first step leading to differential sodium handling in the proximal and distal tubules (57). The vasodilatory response could lead to TGF activation and inappropriate proximal sodium reabsorption, which could in turn be compensated for by an increase in distal excretion (57) due to the resulting RAS suppression, similar to sodium handling during pregnancy (50).

Oral Contraceptive Pill Use, Sodium Handling and the RAS

Further insights into gender-mediated differences in renal sodium handling can be gleaned by examining functional changes during states of high estrogen such as use of the oral contraceptive pill (OCP). OCPs are thought to mediate some of their renal and vascular effects through increased angiotensinogen production by the liver (62) after first-pass delivery via the portal circulation, possibly through estrogen receptor-mediated stimulation of angiotensinogen gene transcription (63). The first pass effect likely explains the lack of a rise in plasma angiotensinogen with transdermal estradiol administration (63,64), which bypasses the liver.

OCPs may also induce more subtle increases in BP, which still remain in the normal range (65). These changes may have important public health implications, since small increments in BP in the order of several millimeters of mercury can raise the population incidence of cardiovascular disease (66). Hollenberg et al. demonstrated a reduction in renal blood flow with OCP use, which was felt to be mediated by estrogen-induced RAS activation (67), leading to chronically elevated levels of Ang II, which could cause hypertension in susceptible women through vasoconstriction and sodium retention. Mcareavey et al. demonstrated higher Ang II levels in a group of women who developed hypertension while using the OCP compared to a control group with essential hypertension. This was associated with a higher total body salt content, suggesting that the hypertension was on the basis of a blunted suppression of Ang II in the face of volume expansion and possibly Ang II-mediated sodium retention (68). Kang et al. found similar effects of the OCP in a group of normotensive women, with significant increases in BP, renal vascular resistance and FF as well as humoral markers of RAS activity. The functional effects of the OCP on renal and peripheral vasculature were partially abolished with Ang II blockade (69). This study did not examine the impact of OCPs on renal sodium handling. OCP users also exhibit an augmented renal and peripheral pressor (Fig. 9) response to graded Ang II infusion, in conjunction with skin fibroblast AT_1 receptor upregulation (70). This suggests that non-RAS pathways, such as NO, may protect OCP users from developing hypertension. In contrast to the Mcareavey study, a study involving 27 young women on the OCP for more than six months failed to demonstrate a sodium-reabsorption-mediated hypertensive effect (71). In this study, the pressure–natriuresis relationship did not differ between OCP-users and nonusers during the follicular and luteal phases of the menstrual cycle. In addition, in a study by Ribstein et al., the renal and neurohormonal effects of OCP withdrawal were examined in normal and hypertensive OCP users. Although FF and PRA fell significantly after OCP withdrawal, the rise in 24-hour sodium excretion did not reach statistical significance (72). In summary, therefore, available data suggests that the hypertensive effect of the OCP may be on the basis of hemodynamic alterations rather than major fluctuations in sodium balance.

The Role of NO, Prostaglandins and Endothelin-1

As mentioned above, women appear to have a differential response to salt-loading at the renal hemodynamic level depending on the phase of the menstrual cycle, with a renal vasodilatory response and a fall in FF in the luteal phase, but not the follicular phase (51,57). The NO and prostaglandin systems might play an important role in mediating these differences. Increased estrogen levels that are characteristic of the luteal phase of the menstrual cycle have been shown to augment NO (73,74) and local vasodilatory prostaglandin activity (75,76). These mediators have in turn been associated with physiologic antagonism of Ang II-mediated vasoconstriction (77,78). Blockade of efferent constriction during the luteal phase leads to efferent vasodilatation, a fall in FF and a resultant decrease in sodium reabsorption compared to the follicular phase. Although Ang II is traditionally thought to have predominant efferent constricting effects, it has also been shown in the rat model to have a significant impact on afferent vasoconstriction. NO may

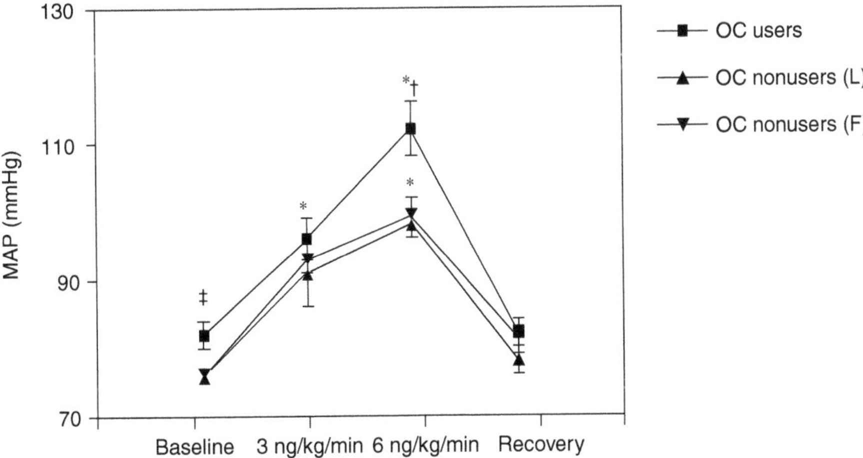

Figure 9 MAP at baseline and in response to 3 and 6 ng/kg/min angiotensin II in OC users (■) and OC nonusers during the luteal (L) phase (▲) and during the follicular (F) phase (▼) of the menstrual cycle. $*p < 0.05$ versus baseline; $^{\dagger}p < 0.05$ versus response of OC nonusers; $^{\ddagger}p < 0.05$ versus baseline value of OC nonusers. *Abbreviations*: MAP, mean arterial pressure; OC, oral contraceptive. *Source*: From Ref. 70.

play an antagonistic role, opposing afferent but not efferent vasoconstriction thereby providing a possible physiologic explanation for differential responses of the renal microcirculation to increases in estrogen levels (79). Under certain circumstances, NO upregulation and subsequent vasodilatation may therefore cause afferent more than efferent vasodilatation, resulting in an increase in GFR and sodium excretion (80), providing a possible mechanism for differences in pressure–natriuresis responses between men and women. NO-induced renal arteriolar vasodilatation may result in increased sodium sensitivity by facilitating more efficient transmission of arteriolar hydrostatic pressure to the renal interstitium, preventing sodium reabsorption (81). This would result in a more efficient pressure–natriuresis response in women. In spite of the ability of L-arginine, the precursor of NO, to abrogate the development of hypertension in salt-sensitive rats, however, it is unknown if there is a differential effect of gender in these models, and whether or not these effects are important in humans (82–85).

Human studies have provided indirect evidence for NO and prostaglandin action as important mediators of glomerular hemodynamic alterations during the menstrual cycle. In the previously mentioned study by Chapman et al., women were studied during the mid-follicular and mid-luteal phases of the menstrual cycle. The renal and peripheral vasodilatation that was observed during the luteal phase, in spite of humoral RAS upregulation, was associated with increases in urinary cyclic adenosine monophosphate, suggestive of prostacyclin activation, as well as urinary cyclic guanosine monophosphate and NO metabolites, suggesting NO activation, although the NO indicators did not reach statistical significance (50). Chapman et al. documented estrogen-mediated increases in vasodilatory prostaglandins through the induction of prostacyclin synthase (86) and cyclooxygenase (87). Estrogen-mediated vasodilatation in humans may also be mediated through inhibition of vasoconstrictors such as endothelin-1 when estrogens are administered in pharmacologic doses, such as the doses given in the case of male-to-female transgender patients (88).

Similarly, studies in SHR and desoxycorticosterone acetate -salt-sensitive hypertensive rats have shown protective antihypertensive and pro-endothelial function effects of estrogen, which are related to an anti-endothelin mechanism (89–92). This suggests that endothelin might play a significant role in salt-sensitive hypertension. The impact of these observations on sodium balance is still unknown, but could theoretically lead to protective antihypertensive effects, both via vasodilatation and sensitization of the pressure–natriuresis curve.

Efferent Effects of the Autonomic Nervous System

The autonomic nervous system may play an important role in gender-mediated differences in renal sodium handling. Induction of central nervous system pharmacologic blockade in SHR can abolish the protective anti-hypertensive effect of estrogen (56), suggesting a modulatory role for estrogens on the balance of sympathetic (93) and parasympathetic (94,95) influences on BP. In the rat model, sympathetic nervous system overactivity may also contribute to Ang II-mediated hypertension. Further, male rats exhibit a greater hypotensive response to sympathetic nervous system blockade during Ang II infusion compared to female rats (6).

Pre-hypertensive Dahl S rats fed a low-sodium diet exhibit an abnormal buffering response to hypertensive stimuli (96). In addition, abnormalities in vascular regulation have been observed under conditions of high-sodium intake in this strain of animals in that they display an elevated total peripheral resistance thought to be secondary to sympathetic overactivation (97). Although this is likely an important element of the hypertension seen in this strain of animals, the etiology of the sympathetic overactivation is unknown. The hypertensive effects of sympathetic activation may be blunted in some female rat models of sodium-sensitive hypertension through the modulating effect of estrogen on pre-junctional peripheral nervous system mechanisms (98). Estrogen possibly exerts antihypertensive effects on the peripheral nervous system, particularly in postmenopausal women. Transdermal estrogen can induce arterial relaxation through the alteration of parasympathetic/sympathetic balance, possibly at the muscarinic receptor level, with a resultant antihypertensive effect (99). Sympathetic activation, due to loss of estrogen, may therefore be in part responsible for postmenopausal hypertension. Another source of sympathetic activation after the menopause is weight gain, which has in turn been associated with increased RAS activity and sodium reabsorption (100).

Sodium Regulation in Postmenopausal Models

Correlations between renal hemodynamic function and salt-sensitivity have further suggested mechanisms that may be responsible for the increased risk of hypertension after the menopause. This is of major importance from a population health perspective since data from the National Health and Nutrition Examination Survey have shown that the prevalence of hypertension in Hispanic and non-Hispanic women increases after the age of 60 to rates that are similar to men, and in non-Hispanic white women, rates of hypertension increase to levels that are higher than men by the age of 70 (101). Similarly, the WHO Cardiovascular Diseases and Alimentary Comparison Study demonstrated a positive correlation between 24-hour urine sodium excretion and BP in postmenopausal women, but not in premenopausal women (102); a prospective study in Finland showed that 24-hour urine sodium excretion correlates positively with BP in men, but not in women (103). Human physiologic studies have also demonstrated a blunted pressure–natriuresis response in postmenopausal women compared to menstruating females and those on the OCP (Fig. 10) (104). Potential mechanisms underlying these differences have derived from both animal and human studies.

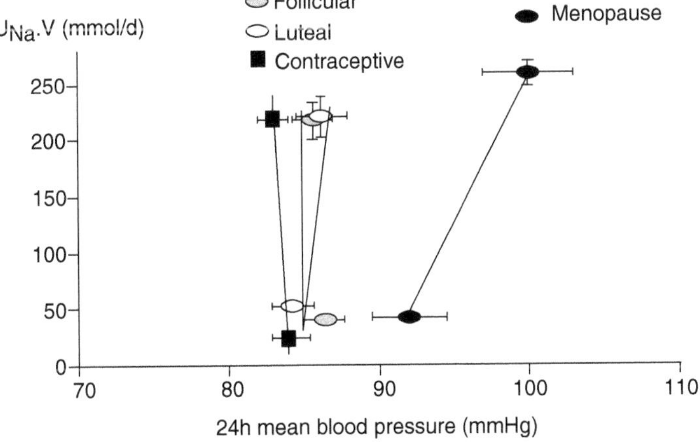

Figure 10 Pressure–natriuresis relationship in normotensive women during the normal menstrual cycle, during use of oral contraceptives, and after menopause. All women received randomly a diet low in sodium (40 mmol Na/day) and high in sodium (250 mmol Na/day) for one week. Blood pressure was measured over 24 hours using ambulatory blood pressure monitoring. *Source*: From Ref. 103.

The Dahl salt-sensitive rat experiences increases in BP with age, regardless of gender (4). However, after ovariectomy, female rats that are fed a high-salt diet exhibit a more marked hypertensive effect, and can demonstrate concomitant increases in PRA (105) compared to intact female rats. Other animal-derived data that support the role of the RAS in the pathogenesis of postmenopausal hypertension include the observation that PRA increases along with BP by 18 months of age in postmenopausal SHR, and this rise in BP can be blocked with AT_1 blockade (105). RAS activation may cause hypertension directly by blunting the pressure–natriuresis response, or through its action on endothelin, causing vasoconstriction and an increase in sodium reabsorption (106). Similarly, follicle stimulating hormone gene knockout mice exhibit low circulating estrogen levels and are hypertensive compared to wild-type animals (107). It is unknown whether or not these observations are due to differences in sodium handling. These studies are also difficult to translate directly into the human arena because postmenopausal rats can demonstrate renal morphologic changes after ovariectomy such as glomerulosclerosis, which may confound differences in renal sodium handling by independently causing hypertension (105).

Human studies examining the impact of hormone replacement therapy on BP have been conflicting, possibly due to different modalities of hormone delivery (oral vs. transdermal) (105), and different durations of follow-up (short-term vs. long-term) (99,108,109). Mechanistically, from the point of view of sodium handling, paradoxical renal vasoconstriction with a rise in FF has been demonstrated in salt-sensitive African Americans after a salt load (110,111); a similar pattern of salt-induced vasoconstriction with a rise in FF has been observed in normotensive menopausal women (112). One might expect these changes to lead to a further rise in sodium reabsorption and an exacerbation of hypertension. The neurohormonal abnormality underlying this finding is poorly understood, but may involve either a impaired NO-mediated vasodilatation due to loss of estrogen, or loss of RAS suppression after salt loading (104).

Although the translation of the effects of estrogen modulation from the salt-sensitive female rat model into the human is fraught with difficulties, it is known that androgens exert direct effects on BP in the postmenopausal state. SHR exhibit significantly elevated testosterone levels compared to cycling, younger females (113). In women, in some studies (114–116), testosterone levels tended to rise late after the menopause, perhaps accounting for some of the increase in BP that can be seen during this period.

After the menopause, women exhibit a response pattern to saline loading that resembles that of men. Stachenfeld et al. demonstrated a significant hypertensive effect of hypertonic saline loading in a group of postmenopausal women (117). They were then able to abolish this effect with oral estradiol administration, in spite of a concurrent reduction in fractional excretion of sodium. This suggests that the pressure–natriuresis curve is shifted to the right in postmenopausal women, possibly due to loss of the effects of estrogen, which blunt RAS activity and increase vasodilatory mediators such as NO. Similarly, hypertensive postmenopausal women who are given oral hormone replacement therapy exhibit an increase in Ang II, but do not demonstrate a rise in BP (118), again suggesting a RAS-blunting effect of estrogen.

Endothelin may also be important in the pathophysiology of postmenopausal hypertension. In addition to its vasoconstrictor activity, endothelin causes increases in renal sodium reabsorption in canine models of hypertension (106). In SHR, endothelin mRNA is increased in the postmenopausal state compared to premenopausal animals (105), and endothelin blockade reduces BP in these animals to levels that are seen in young females. The rise in endothelin may be due to an age-related loss of estrogen-mediated inhibition on endothelin mRNA synthesis (119). Alternatively, endothelin production may be increased in response to the stimulatory influence of Ang II (120). Furthermore, as mentioned previously, testosterone levels can increase after the menopause (113,114,116). Postmenopausal increases in testosterone have also been shown to lead to endothelin activation (87), and may result in enhanced sodium reabsorption and hypertension after the menopause.

CONCLUSIONS AND FUTURE DIRECTIONS

This review emphasizes that most women are protected from hypertension compared to men for reasons that involve both the afferent and efferent limbs of effective circulating volume homeostasis regulation. Both androgens and estrogens are critical in the initiation and maintenance of these differences. Men and women exhibit significant differences in neurohormonal systems that control sodium balance, including the RAS, NO, prostaglandin, and endothelin systems. These differences probably play an important role in the premenopausal protection against hypertension in women, and the subsequent development of postmenopausal hypertension in susceptible individuals. In addition, abnormal sodium handling may play a role in the hypertension that develops in a small minority of women on the OCP, although hemodynamic alterations are likely more important.

The elucidation of these mechanisms could lead to a better understanding and prevention of hypertension. Furthermore, these mechanisms may underlie the gender differences in rates of progression of renal and cardiovascular disease. Lastly, although it is beyond the scope of this chapter, direct and indirect hormonal influences on renal sodium handling and vasoactive mediators may play an important role in the complex pathophysiology that underlies pregnancy-related hypertensive disorders, and will undoubtedly continue to be an area of intense investigation in the future.

REFERENCES

1. August P, Oparil S. Hypertension in women. J Clin Endocrinol Metab 1999; 4:1862–6.
2. Miyajima E, Bunag R. Impaired sympathetic baroreflexes in prehypertensive Dahl hypertension-sensitive rats. Clin Exp Theory Pract 1986; A8:1049–61.
3. Takeshita A, Mark AL, Brody MJ. Prevention of salt-induced hypertension in the Dahl strain by 6-hydroxydopamine. Am J Physiol 1979; 236:H48–52.
4. Hinojosa-Laborde C, Lange DL, Haywood JR. Role of female sex hormones in the development and reversal of Dahl hypertension. Hypertension 2000; 35:484–9.
5. Hinojosa-Laborde C, Chapa I, Lange D, Haywood JR. Gender differences in sympathetic nervous system regulation. Clin Exp Pharmacol Physiol 1999; 26:122–6.
6. Xue B, Pamidimukkala J, Hay M. Sex differences in the development of angiotensin II-induced hypertension in conscious mice. Am J Physiol Heart Circ Physiol 2005; 288:H2177–84.
7. Kisley LR, Sakai RR, Flanagan-Cato LM, Fluharty SJ. Estrogen increases angiotensin II-induced c-Fos expression in the vasopressinergic neurons of the paraventricular nucleus in the female rat. Neuroendocrinology 2000; 72:306–17.
8. Pamidimukkala J, Hay M. 17 beta-Estradiol inhibits angiotensin II activation of area postrema neurons. Am J Physiol Heart Circ Physiol 2003; 285:H1515–20.
9. Hunt BE, Taylor JA, Hamner JW, Gagnon M, Lipsitz LA. Estrogen replacement therapy improves baroreflex regulation of vascular sympathetic outflow in postmenopausal women. Circulation 2001; 103:2909–14.

10. Pamnani MB, Buggy J, Huot SJ, Haddy FJ. Studies on the role of a humoral sodium-transport inhibitor and the anteroventral third ventricle (AV3V) in experimental low-renin hypertension. Clin Sci (Lond) 1981; 61(Suppl. 7):57s–60.
11. Pamnani M, Huot S, Buggy J, Clough D, Haddy F. Demonstration of a humoral inhibitor of the Na^{+}–K^{+} pump in some models of experimental hypertension. Hypertension 1981; 3:II-96–101.
12. Kramer HJ. Natriuretic hormone—a circulating inhibitor of sodium- and potassium-activated adenosine triphosphatase. Its potential role in body fluid and blood pressure regulation. Klin Wochenschr 1981; 59:1225–30.
13. Guyton A, Coleman T, Cowley AJ, Scheel K, Manning R, Norman R. Arterial pressure regulation: overriding dominance of the kidneys in long-tern reulation and in hypertension. Am J Med 1972; 52:584–94.
14. Miller J, Tobe S, Skorecki K. Control of extracellular fluid volume and the pathophysiology of edema formation. In: Brenner B, ed. Brenner and Rector's the Kidney. Vol. 1. Philadelphia, PA: WB Saunders, 1996:817–72.
15. Hall J, Guyton A, Brands M. Control of sodium excretion and arterial pressure by intrarenal mechanisms and the renin–angiotensin system. In: Laragh J, Brenner B, eds. Hypertension: Pathophysiology, Diagnosis, and Management. New York: Raven Press, 1995:1451–75.
16. Staessen J, Bulpitt CJ, Fagard R, et al. Evidence for a curvilinear relation between blood pressure and urinary sodium in men. J Hum Hypertens 1990; 4:19–24.
17. Elliott P, Dyer A, Stamler R. The INTERSALT study: results for 24 hour sodium and potassium, by age and sex. INTERSALT Co-operative Research Group. J Hum Hypertens 1989; 3:323–30.
18. Reckelhoff JF, Zhang H, Granger JP. Testosterone exacerbates hypertension and reduces pressure–natriuresis in male spontaneously hypertensive rats. Hypertension 1998; 31:435–9.
19. Hall J, Mizelle H, Hildebrandt D, Brands M. Abnormal pressure–natriuresis: a cause or a consequence of hypertension. Hypertension 1990; 15:547–59.
20. Harrap SB, Wang BZ, MacLellan DG. Renal transplantation between male and female spontaneously hypertensive rats. Hypertension 1992; 19:431–4.
21. Hennington B, Henegar S, Sinning A, Granger J, Reckehoff J. Localization of androgen receptors in the kidney of male rats. Hypertension 1997; 30:510 (Abstract).
22. Curtis JJ, Luke RG, Dustan HP, et al. Remission of essential hypertension after renal transplantation 1983. J Am Soc Nephrol 2000; 11:2404–12.
23. James GD, Sealey JE, Muller F, Alderman M, Madhavan S, Laragh JH. Renin relationship to sex, race and age in a normotensive population. J Hypertens Suppl 1986; 4:S387–9.
24. Kaplan NM, Kem DC, Holland OB, Kramer NJ, Higgins J, Gomez-Sanchez C. The intravenous furosemide test: a simple way to evaluate renin responsiveness. Ann Intern Med 1976; 84:639–45.
25. Schunkert H, Danser AH, Hense HW, Derkx FH, Kurzinger S, Riegger GA. Effects of estrogen replacement therapy on the renin–angiotensin system in postmenopausal women. Circulation 1997; 95:39–45.
26. Liu PY, Death AK, Handelsman DJ. Androgens and cardiovascular disease. Endocr Rev 2003; 24:313–40.
27. Navat L, Inscho E, Majid S. Paracrine regulation of the renal microcirculation. Physiol Rev 1996; 76:425–536.
28. Geibel J, Giebisch G, Boron WF. Angiotensin II stimulates both Na(+)–H^{+} exchange and Na^{+}/HCO_3^{-} cotransport in the rabbit proximal tubule. Proc Natl Acad Sci USA 1990; 87:7917–20.
29. Wang T, Giebisch G. Effects of angiotensin II on electrolyte transport in the early and late distal tubule in rat kidney. Am J Physiol 1996; 271:F143–9.
30. Braam B, Mitchell KD, Koomans HA, Navar LG. Relevance of the tubuloglomerular feedback mechanism in pathophysiology. J Am Soc Nephrol 1993; 4:1257–74.
31. Reckelhoff JF, Granger JP. Role of androgens in mediating hypertension and renal injury. Clin Exp Pharmacol Physiol 1999; 26:127–31.

32. Reckelhoff J, Fortepiani L, Zhang H, Srivastsava K, Smith M. Gender differences in the response of SHR to acute and chronic superoxide mismutase mimietic TEMPOL. Am J Hypertens 2000; 13:277A (Abstract).
33. Ellison KE, Ingelfinger JR, Pivor M, Dzau VJ. Androgen regulation of rat renal angiotensinogen messenger RNA expression. J Clin Invest 1989; 83:1941–5.
34. Katz F, Roper E. Testosterone effect on renin system in rats. Proc Soc Exp Biol Med 1977; 19:330–3.
35. Reckelhoff JF. Gender differences in the regulation of blood pressure. Hypertension 2001; 37:1199–208.
36. Chen YF, Naftilan AJ, Oparil S. Androgen-dependent angiotensinogen and renin messenger RNA expression in hypertensive rats. Hypertension 1992; 19:456–63.
37. Smithies O. Theodore Cooper Memorial Lecture. A mouse view of hypertension. Hypertension 1997; 30:1318–24.
38. Stefani S, Aguiari GL, Bozza A, et al. Androgen responsiveness and androgen receptor gene expression in human kidney cells in continuous culture. Biochem Mol Biol Int 1994; 32:597–604.
39. Reckelhoff JF, Hennington BS, Moore AG, Blanchard EJ, Cameron J. Gender differences in the renal nitric oxide (NO) system: dissociation between expression of endothelial NO synthase and renal hemodynamic response to NO synthase inhibition. Am J Hypertens 1998; 11:97–104.
40. Reckelhoff JF, Zhang H, Srivastava K, Granger JP. Gender differences in hypertension in spontaneously hypertensive rats: role of androgens and androgen receptor. Hypertension 1999; 34:920–3.
41. Harrison-Bernard LM, Schulman IH, Raij L. Postovariectomy hypertension is linked to increased renal AT1 receptor and salt sensitivity. Hypertension 2003; 42:1157–63.
42. Stachenfeld NS, Splenser AE, Calzone WL, Taylor MP, Keefe DL. Sex differences in osmotic regulation of AVP and renal sodium handling. J Appl Physiol 2001; 91:1893–901.
43. Chidambaram M, Duncan JA, Lai VS, et al. Variation in the renin angiotensin system throughout the normal menstrual cycle. J Am Soc Nephrol 2002; 13:446–52.
44. Vokes TJ, Weiss NM, Schreiber J, Gaskill MB, Robertson GL. Osmoregulation of thirst and vasopressin during normal menstrual cycle. Am J Physiol 1988; 254:R641–7.
45. Barron LA, Green GM, Khalil RA. Gender differences in vascular smooth muscle reactivity to increases in extracellular sodium salt. Hypertension 2002; 39:425–32.
46. Horiguchi M, Kimura M, Skurnick J, Aviv A. Parameters of lymphocyte $Na^+ - Ca_2^+$ regulation and blood pressure: the gender effect. Hypertension 1998; 32:869–74.
47. Miller JA, Anacta LA, Cattran DC. Impact of gender on the renal response to angiotensin II. Kidney Int 1999; 55:278–85.
48. Brown MA, Gallery ED, Ross MR, Esber RP. Sodium excretion in normal and hypertensive pregnancy: a prospective study. Am J Obstet Gynecol 1988; 159:297–307.
49. Brown MA, Broughton Pipkin F, Symonds EM. The effects of intravenous angiotensin II upon blood pressure and sodium and urate excretion in human pregnancy. J Hypertens 1988; 6:457–64.
50. Chapman AB, Zamudio S, Woodmansee W, et al. Systemic and renal hemodynamic changes in the luteal phase of the menstrual cycle mimic early pregnancy. Am J Physiol 1997; 273:F777–82.
51. Pechere-Bertschi A, Maillard M, Stalder H, Brunner H, Burnier M. Blood pressure and renal haemodynamic response to salt during the normal menstrual cycle. Clin Sci 2000; 98:697–702.
52. Burnier M, Monod ML, Chiolero A, Maillard M, Nussberger J, Brunner HR. Renal sodium handling in acute and chronic salt loading/depletion protocols: the confounding influence of acute water loading. J Hypertens 2000; 18:1657–64.
53. Dahl K, Knudson D, Ohanien EV, Muirhead M, Tuthil R. Role of gonads in hypertension-prone rats. J Exp Med 1975; 142:748–59.

54. Masubuchi Y, Kumai T, Uematsu A, Komoriyama K, Hirai M. Gonadectomy-induced reduction of blood pressure in adult spontaneously hypertensive rats. Acta Endocrinol (Copenh) 1982; 101:154–60.
55. Chen YF, Meng QC. Sexual dimorphism of blood pressure in spontaneously hypertensive rats is androgen dependent. Life Sci 1991; 48:85–96.
56. Fang Z, Carlson SH, Chen YF, Oparil S, Wyss JM. Estrogen depletion induces NaCl-sensitive hypertension in female spontaneously hypertensive rats. Am J Physiol Regul Integr Comp Physiol 2001; 281:R1934–9.
57. Pechere-Bertschi A, Maillard M, Stalder H, Brunner HR, Burnier M. Renal segmental tubular response to salt during the normal menstrual cycle. Kidney Int 2002; 61:425–31.
58. Bisson DL, Dunster GD, O'Hare JP, Hampton D, Penney MD. Renal sodium retention does not occur during the luteal phase of the menstrual cycle in normal women. Br J Obstet Gynaecol 1992; 99:247–52.
59. Landrau R, Lugibihl K. Inhibition of the sodium retaining influence of aldosterone by progeserone. Clin Endocrinol 1958; 18:1237–45.
60. Oelkers W, Berger V, Bolik A, et al. Dihydrospirorenone, a new progestogen with antimineralocorticoid activity: effects on ovulation, electrolyte excretion, and the renin-aldosterone system in normal women. J Clin Endocrinol Metab 1991; 73:837–42.
61. Oparil S, Ehrlich EN, Lindheimer MD. Effect of progesterone on renal sodium handling in man: relation to aldosterone excretion and plasma renin activity. Clin Sci Mol Med 1975; 49:139–47.
62. Beckerhoff R, Luetscher J, Beckerhoff I, Nokes G. Effects of oral contraceptives on the renin–angiotensin system and on blood pressure on normal young women. Johns Hopkins Med J 1973; 132:80–7.
63. Gordon MS, Chin WW, Shupnik MA. Regulation of angiotensinogen gene expression by estrogen. J Hypertens 1992; 10:361–6.
64. Oelkers WK. Effects of estrogens and progestogens on the renin-aldosterone system and blood pressure. Steroids 1996; 61:166–71.
65. Staessen J, Bulpitt CJ, Fagard R, Joossens JV, Lijnen P, Amery A. Contraceptive pill use, urinary sodium and blood pressure. A population study in two Belgian towns. Acta Cardiol 1984; 39:55–64.
66. Stamler J, Rose G, Stamler R, Elliott P, Dyer A, Marmot M. INTERSALT study findings. Public health and medical care implications. Hypertension 1989; 14:570–7.
67. Hollenberg NK, Williams GH, Burger B, Chenitz W, Hoosmand I, Adams DF. Renal blood flow and its response to angiotensin II. An interaction between oral contraceptive agents, sodium intake, and the renin–angiotensin system in healthy young women. Circ Res 1976; 38:35–40.
68. McAreavey D, Cumming AM, Boddy K, et al. The renin–angiotensin system and total body sodium and potassium in hypertensive women taking oestrogen–progestagen oral contraceptives. Clin Endocrinol (Oxf) 1983; 18:111–8.
69. Kang AK, Duncan JA, Cattran DC, et al. Effect of oral contraceptives on the renin angiotensin system and renal function. Am J Physiol Regul Integr Comp Physiol 2001; 280:R807–13.
70. Ahmed SB, Kang AK, Burns KD, et al. Effects of oral contraceptive use on the renal and systemic vascular response to angiotensin II infusion. J Am Soc Nephrol 2004; 15:780–6.
71. Pechere-Bertschi A, Maillard M, Stalder H, et al. Renal hemodynamic and tubular responses to salt in women using oral contraceptives. Kidney Int 2003; 64:1374–80.
72. Ribstein J, Halimi JM, du Cailar G, Mimran A. Renal characteristics and effect of angiotensin suppression in oral contraceptive users. Hypertension 1999; 33:90–5.
73. Weiner CP, Lizasoain I, Baylis SA, Knowles RG, Charles IG, Moncada S. Induction of calcium-dependent nitric oxide synthases by sex hormones. Proc Natl Acad Sci USA 1994; 91:5212–6.
74. Rosselli M, Imthurm B, Macas E, Keller PJ, Dubey RK. Circulating nitrite/nitrate levels increase with follicular development: indirect evidence for estradiol mediated NO release. Biochem Biophys Res Commun 1994; 202:1543–52.

75. Terragno NA, Terragno A, McGiff JC. Prostaglandin E—angiotensin II interactions in the gravid uterus. Acta Physiol Lat Am 1974; 24:550–4.
76. Terragno NA, Terragno DA, Pacholczyk D, McGiff JC. Prostaglandins and the regulation of uterine blood flow in pregnancy. Nature 1974; 249:57–8.
77. De Nicola L, Blantz RC, Gabbai FB. Nitric oxide and angiotensin II. Glomerular and tubular interaction in the rat. J Clin Invest 1992; 89:1248–56.
78. Itskovitz HD, Terragno NA, McGiff JC. Effect of a renal prostaglandin on distribution of blood flow in the isolated canine kidney. Circ Res 1974; 34:770–6.
79. Ito S, Arima S, Ren YL, Juncos LA, Carretero OA. Endothelium-derived relaxing factor/nitric oxide modulates angiotensin II action in the isolated microperfused rabbit afferent but not efferent arteriole. J Clin Invest 1993; 91:2012–9.
80. Patel A, Layne S, Watts D, Kirchner K. L-Arginine administration normalizes pressure natriuresis in hypertensive Dahl rats. Hypertension 1993; 22:863–9.
81. Patel AR, Granger JP, Kirchner KA. L-Arginine improves transmission of perfusion pressure to the renal interstitium in Dahl salt-sensitive rats. Am J Physiol 1994; 266:R1730–5.
82. Chen PY, Gladish RD, Sanders PW. Vascular smooth muscle nitric oxide synthase anomalies in Dahl/Rapp salt-sensitive rats. Hypertension 1998; 31:918–24.
83. Chen PY, Sanders PW. L-Arginine abrogates salt-sensitive hypertension in Dahl/Rapp rats. J Clin Invest 1991; 88:1559–67.
84. Chen PY, Sanders PW. Role of nitric oxide synthesis in salt-sensitive hypertension in Dahl/Rapp rats. Hypertension 1993; 22:812–8.
85. Hu L, Manning RD, Jr. Role of nitric oxide in regulation of long-term pressure–natriuresis relationship in Dahl rats. Am J Physiol 1995; 268:H2375–83.
86. Chang W, Nakao J, Orimo H, Murota S. Stimulation of prostaglandin cyclooxygenase and prostacyclin synthase activities by estradiol in rat aortic smooth muscle cells. Biochem Biophys Acta 1980; 620:472–82.
87. Jun S, Chen Z, Pace M, Shaul P. Estrogen upregulatescyclooxygenase-1 gene expression in ovine fetal pulmonary artery endothelium. J Clin Invest 1998; 102:176–83.
88. van Kesteren PJ, Kooistra T, Lansink M, et al. The effects of sex steroids on plasma levels of marker proteins of endothelial cell functioning. Thromb Haemost 1998; 79:1029–33.
89. David FL, Carvalho MH, Cobra AL, et al. Ovarian hormones modulate endothelin-1 vascular reactivity and mRNA expression in DOCA-salt hypertensive rats. Hypertension 2001; 38:692–6.
90. Tostes RC, David FL, Carvalho MH, Nigro D, Scivoletto R, Fortes ZB. Gender differences in vascular reactivity to endothelin-1 in deoxycorticosterone-salt hypertensive rats. J Cardiovasc Pharmacol 2000; 36:S99–101.
91. Dubey RK, Jackson EK, Keller PJ, Imthurn B, Rosselli M. Estradiol metabolites inhibit endothelin synthesis by an estrogen receptor-independent mechanism. Hypertension 2001; 37:640–4.
92. Widder J, Pelzer T, von Poser-Klein C, et al. Improvement of endothelial dysfunction by selective estrogen receptor-alpha stimulation in ovariectomized SHR. Hypertension 2003; 42:991–6.
93. Sturrock ND, Pound N, Peck GM, Soar CM, Jeffcoate WJ. An assessment of blood pressure measurement in a diabetic clinic using random-zero, semi-automated, and 24-hour monitoring. Diabet Med 1997; 14:370–5.
94. Kuo TB, Lin T, Yang CC, Li CL, Chen CF, Chou P. Effect of aging on gender differences in neural control of heart rate. Am J Physiol 1999; 277:H2233–9.
95. Saleh T, Connel B. Centrally mediated effect of 17B-estradiol on parasympathetic tone in male rats. Am J Physiol Regul Integr Comp 1999; 276:R474–81.
96. Miyajima E, Bunag RD. Impaired sympathetic baroreflexes in prehypertensive Dahl hypertension-sensitive rats. Clin Exp Hypertens A 1986; 8:1049–61.
97. Takeshita A, Mark A. Neurogenic contribution to hindquarters vasoconstriction during high sodium intake in Dahl strain of genetically hypertensive rat. Circ Res 1978; 43(Suppl. 1):186–91.

98. Brandin L, Bergstrom G, Manhem K, Gustafsson H. Oestrogen modulates vascular adrenergic reactivity of the spontaneously hypertensive rat. J Hypertens 2003; 21:1695–702.
99. Manhem K, Brandin L, Ghanoum B, Rosengren A, Gustafsson H. Acute effects of transdermal estrogen on hemodynamic and vascular reactivity in elderly postmenopausal healthy women. J Hypertens 2003; 21:387–94.
100. Esler M, Rumantir M, Wiesner G, Kaye D, Hastings J, Lambert G. Sympathetic nervous system and insulin resistance: from obesity to diabetes. Am J Hypertens 2001; 14:304S–9.
101. Burt VL, Whelton P, Roccella EJ, et al. Prevalence of hypertension in the U.S. adult population. Results from the Third National Health and Nutrition Examination Survey, 1988–1991. Hypertension 1995; 25:305–13.
102. Yamori Y, Liu L, Ikeda K, Mizushima S, Nara Y, Simpson FO. Different associations of blood pressure with 24-hour urinary sodium excretion among pre- and post-menopausal women. WHO Cardiovascular Diseases and Alimentary Comparison (WHO-CARDIAC) Study. J Hypertens 2001; 19:535–8.
103. Tuomilehto J, Jousilahti P, Rastenyte D, et al. Urinary sodium excretion and cardiovascular mortality in Finland: a prospective study. Lancet 2001; 357:848–51.
104. Pechere-Bertschi A, Burnier M. Female sex hormones, salt, and blood pressure regulation. Am J Hypertens 2004; 17:994–1001.
105. Reckelhoff JF, Fortepiani LA. Novel mechanisms responsible for postmenopausal hypertension. Hypertension 2004; 43:918–23.
106. Wilkins FC, Jr., Alberola A, Mizelle HL, Opgenorth TJ, Granger JP. Systemic hemodynamics and renal function during long-term pathophysiological increases in circulating endothelin. Am J Physiol 1995; 268:R375–81.
107. Javeshghani D, Touyz RM, Sairam MR, Virdis A, Neves MF, Schiffrin EL. Attenuated responses to angiotensin II in follitropin receptor knockout mice, a model of menopause-associated hypertension. Hypertension 2003; 42:761–7.
108. Cacciatore B, Paakkari I, Hasselblatt R, et al. Randomized comparison between orally and transdermally administered hormone replacement therapy regimens of long-term effects on 24-hour ambulatory blood pressure in postmenopausal women. Am J Obstet Gynecol 2001; 184:904–9.
109. Seely EW, Walsh BW, Gerhard MD, Williams GH. Estradiol with or without progesterone and ambulatory blood pressure in postmenopausal women. Hypertension 1999; 33:1190–4.
110. Schmidlin O, Forman A, Tanaka M, Sebastian A, Morris RC, Jr. NaCl-induced renal vasoconstriction in salt-sensitive African Americans: antipressor and hemodynamic effects of potassium bicarbonate. Hypertension 1999; 33:633–9.
111. Morris RC, Jr., Sebastian A, Forman A, Tanaka M, Schmidlin O. Normotensive salt sensitivity: effects of race and dietary potassium. Hypertension 1999; 33:18–23.
112. Pechere-Bertschi A, Maillard M, Stalder H, Burnier M. Contrasting blood pressure (BP) and renal hemodynamic effects of sodium in pre- and peri-menopausal women. J Am Soc Nephrol 1999; 10:369 (Abstract).
113. Fortepiani LA, Zhang H, Racusen L, Roberts LJ, II, Reckelhoff JF. Characterization of an animal model of postmenopausal hypertension in spontaneously hypertensive rats. Hypertension 2003; 41:640–5.
114. Jiroutek MR, Chen MH, Johnston CC, Longcope C. Changes in reproductive hormones and sex hormone-binding globulin in a group of postmenopausal women measured over 10 years. Menopause 1998; 5:90–4.
115. Baylis C, Reckelhoff JF. Renal hemodynamics in normal and hypertensive pregnancy: lessons from micropuncture. Am J Kidney Dis 1991; 17:98–104.
116. Laughlin GA, Barrett-Connor E, Kritz-Silverstein D, von Muhlen D. Hysterectomy, oophorectomy, and endogenous sex hormone levels in older women: the Rancho Bernardo Study. J Clin Endocrinol Metab 2000; 85:645–51.
117. Stachenfeld NS, DiPietro L, Palter SF, Nadel ER. Estrogen influences osmotic secretion of AVP and body water balance in postmenopausal women. Am J Physiol 1998; 274:R187–95.

118. Umeda M, Ichikawa S, Kanda T, Sumino H, Kobayashi I. Hormone replacement therapy increases plasma level of angiotensin II in postmenopausal hypertensive women. Am J Hypertens 2001; 14:206–11.
119. Earley S, Resta TC. Estradiol attenuates hypoxia-induced pulmonary endothelin-1 gene expression. Am J Physiol Lung Cell Mol Physiol 2002; 283:L86–93.
120. Alexander BT, Cockrell KL, Rinewalt AN, Herrington JN, Granger JP. Enhanced renal expression of preproendothelin mRNA during chronic angiotensin II hypertension. Am J Physiol Regul Integr Comp Physiol 2001; 280:R1388–92.

16
Sodium Balance in Cirrhosis

Andrés Cárdenas and Pere Ginès
Institute of Digestive Diseases and Metabolism, University of Barcelona, Barcelona, Spain

INTRODUCTION

Derangements in fluid and electrolyte balance and renal function commonly occur in the natural history of cirrhosis. Renal abnormalities occur in the setting of a hyperdynamic state characterized by an increased cardiac output, a reduction in total vascular resistance and an activation of neurohormonal vasoactive systems. This circulatory dysfunction, a consequence of intense arterial vasodilation in the splanchnic circulation, is considered a primary feature in the pathogenesis of sodium and water retention in cirrhosis. Sodium retention is the first and main factor involved in the formation of ascites and edema in patients with cirrhosis. The principal event responsible for local splanchnic vasodilation seems to be the overproduction of nitric oxide (NO). Splanchnic vasodilation by decreasing effective arterial blood volume causes homeostatic activation of vasoconstrictor and antinatriuretic factors triggered to compensate for a relative arterial underfilling. The net effect is avid retention of sodium and water as well as renal vasoconstriction in advanced stages. The mechanisms of ascites formation and sodium and water retention in patients with cirrhosis are discussed in this chapter.

FACTORS INVOLVED IN THE DEVELOPMENT OF ASCITES

Portal Hypertension

Portal hypertension is necessary for ascites to occur. Ascites is a consequence of diseases causing sinusoidal portal hypertension, such as cirrhosis, Budd–Chiari syndrome, hepatic veno-occlusive disease, and/or acute alcoholic hepatitis (1). Similar to what occurs with the development of esophageal varices, ascites develops only when the hepatic venous pressure gradient (the gradient between wedged and free hepatic venous pressures) is above 12 mmHg (2). In addition, studies in experimental cirrhosis with rats have demonstrated that these animals will invariably accumulate ascites with advanced liver failure (3,4). In clinical practice cirrhotic patients with ascites subjected to portosystemic shunting by transjugular intrahepatic portosystemic shunting, dramatically decrease ascites with an increase in diuresis and urinary sodium excretion (5).

Lymph Formation

Aside of portal hypertension being the main reason for the development of splanchnic vasodilation, ascites in cirrhosis is the final result of an increased extravasation of fluid from the splanchnic microcirculation. In the initial phases of the disease, this is compensated by an increase in lymph return. Thoracic duct lymph flow, which in normal conditions is lower than 1 L/day, may increase up to more than 20 L/day in cirrhotic patients with portal hypertension (1,6). This is mainly due to marked vasodilation in the splanchnic arterioles secondary to portal hypertension which leads to a large inflow of blood at high pressure into the splanchnic capillaries with a rise in hydrostatic pressure due to both a forward increase in flow and a backward transmission of high portal pressure. Splanchnic arterial vasodilation also has effects on increasing the permeability of capillaries and the net effect is a marked production of lymph from the splanchnic capillaries.

HEMODYNAMIC EVENTS LEADING TO RENAL FUNCTION ABNORMALITIES

Systemic Circulatory Derangements

Cirrhotic patients with ascites show a severe disturbance in their systemic hemodynamics, characterized by a low arterial blood pressure, high cardiac output and a decreased total systemic vascular resistance consequence of an intense splanchnic arterial vasodilation. By contrast, other vascular beds such as the cerebral, upper and lower limbs, and renal circulation are not vasodilated or may be even vasoconstricted (7–9). These circulatory abnormalities increase with the progression of liver disease and become very pronounced in patients with hepatorenal syndrome (HRS) in the late stages of the disease. Contrary to previous belief, recent studies suggest that the development of HRS occurs in the setting of a reduction in cardiac output instead of a markedly elevated cardiac output indicating that the progression of circulatory and renal dysfunction in cirrhosis is not only due to splanchnic vasodilation but also due to a reduction in cardiac output (10). Experimental models of cirrhosis and ascites have shown that the circulatory changes precede sodium and water retention and ascites accumulation, supporting the so-called arterial vasodilation theory of ascites formation and renal dysfunction (4).

Local Circulatory Derangements

An important element in the pathophysiology of portal hypertension is an increase in vascular resistance to portal blood flow arising from the hepatic microcirculation. Experimental data indicate that increased hepatic vascular resistance in cirrhosis is not merely a mechanical consequence of a distorted architecture but there is also an active and dynamic process secondary to contraction of myofibroblasts and activated stellate cells in the intrahepatic circulation (11). Intrahepatic vascular tone is regulated by high levels of endogenous vasoconstrictors (endothelin, leukotrienes, thromboxane A_2, angiotensin II, and others) (12–14) and low levels of intrahepatic NO (15,16). In cirrhosis an increased hepatic vascular resistance is due to an imbalance between vasodilator and vasoconstrictor factors (Fig. 1) (15). Another important factor is that of increased blood flow from

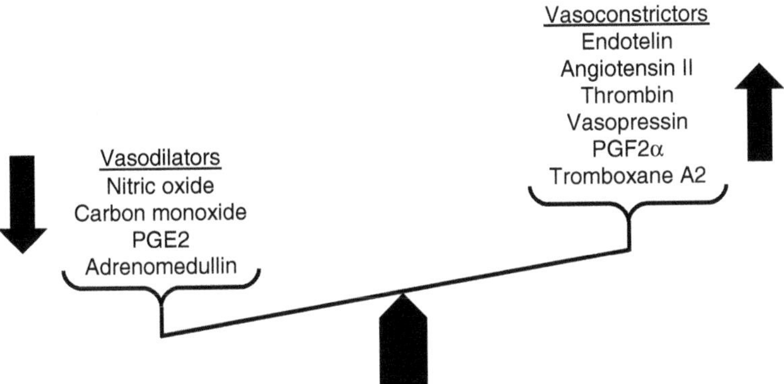

Figure 1 Vasodilators and vasoconstrictors mediating intrahepatic resistance in cirrhosis and portal hypertension. There is a significant decrease in intrahepatic vasodilators (mainly nitric oxide) that along with architectural changes cause portal hypertension. *Abbreviation*: PG, prostaglandin.

the portal venous system due to splanchnic arterial vasodilation. Splanchnic vasodilation mainly caused by a disproportional release of endogenous vasodilators (mainly NO) perpetuates elevated portal pressure (17–19).

Neurohormonal Activation

Several neurohumoral systems with vasoactive properties, namely the renin–angiotensin–aldosterone system (RAAS), sympathetic nervous system (SNS) and arginine vasopressin (AVP), are directly implicated in ascites formation and renal dysfunction in cirrhosis (Table 1). The activity of these vasoconstrictor systems is increased in most cirrhotic patients with ascites, particularly in those with HRS as a homeostatic response to maintain arterial blood pressure within normal limits. However these vasoactive substances may contribute to the progression of liver disease by worsening renal function.

Plasma renin activity, a marker of RAAS activation, is markedly increased in most patients with cirrhosis and ascites; in addition, the plasma levels of angiotensin II and aldosterone, the two main effectors of the RAAS that mediate vasoconstriction and sodium retention, respectively, are also increased in cirrhosis (20,21). RAAS inhibition, either by the administration of angiotensin-converting enzyme inhibitors, angiotensin II antagonists or angiotensin II receptor blockers, is accompanied by a fall in arterial pressure or in some cases a deterioration of renal function (21–23). Activation of the SNS is also present in patients with advanced liver disease as evidenced by increased levels of norepinephrine

Table 1 Neurohormonal Factors Potentially Implicated in Ascites Formation in Cirrhosis

Renin–angiotensin–aldosterone system
Sympathetic nervous system
Arginine vasopressin
Endothelin
Atrial natriuretic peptide
Arachidonic acid metabolites
Adenosine

(NE) and epinephrine (24). Measurements of NE release and spillover in specific vascular beds have shown that the activity of the SNS is increased in many vascular territories, including kidneys, splanchnic organs, heart, and muscle and skin, supporting the concept of a generalized activation of the SNS (24–26). As occurs with RAAS, inhibition of the SNS in human and experimental cirrhosis results in arterial hypotension, suggesting that the SNS is also activated as a homeostatic response to maintain blood pressure in cirrhosis (26–28). Additionally the SNS also contributes to sodium retention (see below). Aside from playing an important role in water retention in cirrhosis (see below), AVP is also a vasoconstrictor that probably contributes to the maintenance of arterial pressure in cirrhosis.

Renal Factors

A significant number of local renal factors participate in the pathogenesis of ascites formation. The presence of arachidonic acid metabolites, adenosine and NO, exert powerful effects on the renal circulation and tubular reabsorption of sodium and water. In cirrhosis one of the arachidonic acid metabolites, the prostaglandins (PGs), normally produced in the kidney via the cyclooxygenase pathway, seem to protect the kidney from the vasoconstrictor effects of the SNS, RAAS, and AVP. The renal PGs namely, PGI2 and PGE2, have vasodilator properties in the kidney and are increased in cirrhosis with ascites (29,30). This increased production of PG contributes to the maintenance of renal hemodynamics.

Adenosine, an endogenous nucleoside produced locally in most cells by the intracellular degradation of adenosine triphosphate, is a potent vasodilator in most vascular beds, except the kidneys, where it causes vasoconstriction (31). Adenosine-1 receptors are present on the afferent arteriole in the kidney and cells of the proximal tubules, whereas adenosine-2 receptors are found in the systemic vasculature (31). Stimulation of adenosine-1 receptors leads to renal vasoconstriction and sodium and water retention, while that of adenosine-2 receptors cause vasodilation (31). The possible role of adenosine in the pathogenesis of renal functional abnormalities in human cirrhosis was evaluated by giving aminophylline (a nonspecific adenosine antagonist) to patients with cirrhosis and ascites (32). This agent caused an increase in renal blood flow (RBF), glomerular filtration rate (GFR), and sodium and water excretion in patients with ascites, while the acute administration of an adenosine-1 receptor antagonist to patients with cirrhosis and ascites induces a marked increase in sodium excretion and urine flow, without changes in renal hemodynamics (33). Conversely, the acute administration of dipyridamole, a drug that acts, at least in part, by increasing the levels of adenosine in the extracellular fluid due to inhibition of the cellular uptake of this substance, is associated with renal vasoconstriction and increased sodium and water retention, particularly in patients with ascites and increased activity of the RAAS (34).

The renal production of NO also participates in the regulation of renal function (35). Under normal circumstances, NO plays a role in the regulation of glomerular microcirculation by modulating the arteriolar tone and the contractility of mesangial cells. Moreover, NO facilitates natriuresis in response to changes in renal perfusion pressure and regulates renin release (35). The inhibition of NO synthesis in rats with cirrhosis and ascites does not result in renal vasoconstriction but induces a marked rise in urinary PG excretion (36). However, the simultaneous inhibition of NO and PGs synthesis results in a marked renal vasoconstriction suggesting that NO interacts with PGs to maintain renal hemodynamics in cirrhosis (37).

FUNCTIONAL RENAL ABNORMALITIES

The functional renal abnormalities that occur in cirrhotic patients are an impaired ability to excrete sodium and solute-free water along with a reduction of RBF and GFR, the latter two being secondary to renal vasoconstriction. Sodium retention is the main factor responsible for ascites and edema formation, whereas impairment in solute-free water excretion is responsible for the development of dilutional hyponatremia. Renal vasoconstriction with disease progression leads to HRS. Typically sodium retention occurs first, whereas dilutional hyponatremia and HRS are late findings (Fig. 2) (1,38,39). In most patients, functional renal abnormalities worsen as liver disease progresses. However, in other patients (particularly abstinent alcoholics) a spontaneous improvement or even normalization of sodium and, less frequently, solute-free water excretion may occur after they stop drinking alcohol.

Sodium Retention

Cirrhosis with ascites is one of the clinical conditions associated with more avid sodium retention. It is the most common abnormality of kidney function in patients with cirrhosis and ascites and plays a fundamental role in the formation of ascites and edema (1,39). As in other sodium-retaining states, the total amount of sodium retained by cirrhotic patients, and the subsequent gain of extracellular fluid, depends on the balance between sodium intake and sodium excretion. If this balance is altered with sodium excretion in urine being lower than that ingested, patients develop ascites and/or edema. By contrast, if the amount of sodium excreted in the urine is greater than that ingested, patients lose extracellular fluid and ascites and/or edema decrease. The important role of sodium

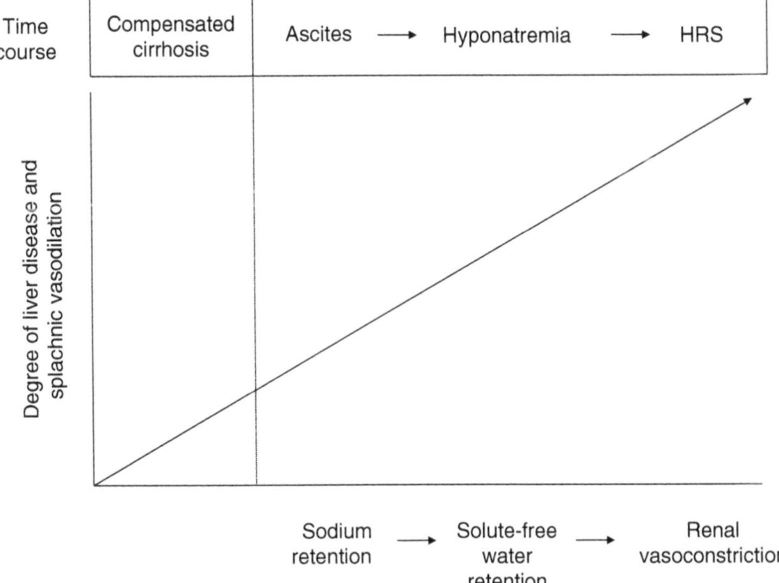

Figure 2 Schematic of the time course of renal functional abnormalities and the relationship to underlying degree of liver disease and splanchnic vasodilation in patients with cirrhosis. *Abbreviation*: HRS, hepatorenal syndrome.

retention in the pathogenesis of ascites formation is further supported by the fact that ascites can disappear by reducing sodium intake and by increasing urinary sodium excretion with the administration of diuretics. Although no studies assessing the chronological relationship between the sodium retention and the formation of ascites have been performed in patients with cirrhosis, studies in experimental animals have provided conclusive evidence indicating that sodium retention precedes ascites formation, further emphasizing the important role of this abnormality of renal function in the pathogenesis of ascites in cirrhosis (4,38).

Sodium is retained along with water iso-osmotically in the kidney (approximately 1 L of water for each 135 mEq of sodium). As a consequence, sodium retention is associated with fluid retention, leading to the expansion of extracellular volume and an increased amount of fluid in the interstitial tissue. The severity of sodium retention varies among patients; some have normal or moderately impaired urine sodium excretion, while many others have severe sodium retention (Fig. 3) (39,41). However, most patients who require hospitalization because of large ascites have marked sodium retention (<10 mEq/day) (41). In those with moderate ascites, the majority excrete ≥ 10 mEq/day spontaneously (without diuretic therapy). The response to diuretics is usually better in patients with moderate sodium retention than in those with marked sodium retention (40).

In cirrhotic patients without ascites or the so-called preascitic stage there is also evidence of subtle sodium retention (Table 2) (42–44). The main findings in these patients relate to increased blood volume (42,45), inability to handle a sodium load (46), and lack of escape to the sodium-retaining effect of mineralocorticoids (42). In preascites most patients have a subtle increase in intravascular fluid volume, which suggests they have experienced episodes of sodium retention (39,44). Additionally a high-sodium diet or intravenous saline may precipitate of ascites and/or edema in preascitic cirrhotic patients (46). Healthy subjects treated with mineralocoticoids for several days experience an early phase characterized by sodium retention that results in increased extracellular fluid volume and plasma expansion, followed by increased sodium excretion with return of extracellular fluid volume and plasma volume to normal values despite the persistent administration of mineralocorticoids (47). This escape phenomenon is aimed at preventing a persistent sodium retention and subsequent development of edema and is due to the suppression of sodium-retaining mechanisms together with activation of natriuretic mechanisms (47). Recently it was reported that the target for this escape mechanism was the thiazide-sensitive NaCl cotransporter (48). When mineralocorticoids are given to cirrhotic patients with preascites, approximately 20% of patients do not show this escape phenomenon and develop marked sodium retention with formation of ascites and edema (42). Another important feature of preascitic cirrhosis is the abnormal natriuretic

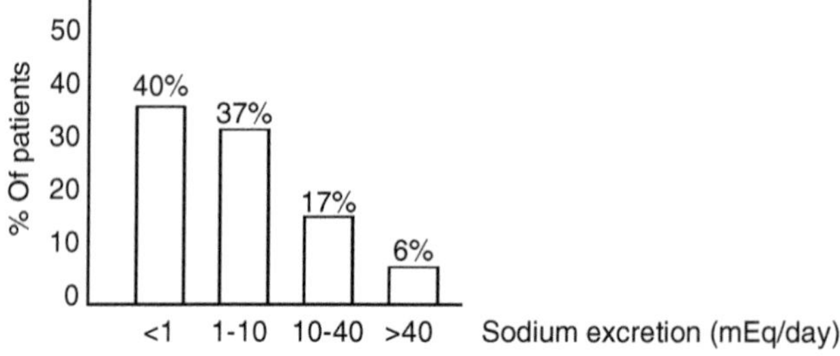

Figure 3 Urinary sodium excretion in a series of patients with cirrhosis hospitalized for treatment of ascites. *Source*: From Ref. 40.

Table 2 Features Indicating the Existence of Impaired Sodium Excretion in the Preascitic Stage of Patients with Cirrhosis

Increased blood volume
Inability to excrete a sodium load
Lack of escape to mineralocorticoids
Reduced sodium excretion in upright position
Increased sodium excretion in recumbence

responses to changes in posture. Cirrhotic patients retain sodium while upright, and show marked natriuresis when lying down when compared with normal subjects (49). A role for antinatriuretic systems such as the RAAS has been implicated in the pathogenesis of sodium retention in preascitic cirrhosis (44,50).

Sites of Sodium Retention

In healthy subjects approximately 95% of filtered sodium is reabsorbed in the renal tubules. Approximately 60% to 70% is absorbed in the proximal tubules, another 30% to 40% gets absorbed in the thick ascending limb and 5% to 10% of sodium is reabsorbed in the collecting ducts (39). Sodium retention in cirrhosis is mainly due to an increased renal tubular reabsorption of sodium because it occurs in the presence of normal or slightly reduced GFR (39). The exact contribution of each segment of the nephron is unknown but both experimental and clinical studies suggest that both proximal and distal tubules are involved (51). Micropuncture studies in rats with cirrhosis and ascites have demonstrated an enhanced reabsorption of sodium in the proximal tubule (39,52). However, the administration of aldosterone antagonists that act mainly on the collecting ducts also prevent the development of a positive sodium balance and the formation of ascites in cirrhotic rats suggesting that the distal ducts are important sites of the increased sodium reabsorption in experimental cirrhosis (4,51). The distal tubules seem to play a key component in sodium reabsorption. A recent study demonstrating protein abundance of renal tubular sodium transporters in rats with carbon tetrachloride (CCL_4)-induced cirrhosis showed an increased expression of the sodium chloride cotransporters of the distal tubule (NCC/TSC) and the epithelial sodium channel of the collecting duct, both of which are regulated by aldosterone, consistent with a major role of hyperaldosteronism in sodium retention in this animal model (53). An increased abundance of the sodium–potassium–two-chloride cotransporter of the thick ascending limb (NKCC/BSC1) and a decreased abundance of the proximal sodium transporters (sodium hydrogen exchanger type 3, and sodium phosphate cotransporter isoform) was also found, consistent with increased sodium reabsorption in the ascending limb of the loop of Henle and reduced reabsorption in the proximal tubule (53).

Investigations in patients with cirrhosis have provided discrepant findings. Results from earlier studies using sodium, water, or phosphate clearances to estimate the tubular handling of sodium suggested that the distal nephron is the main site of sodium retention (39,54). Studies using lithium clearance, which estimates sodium reabsorption in the proximal tubule, suggest that cirrhotic patients with ascites show a marked increase in proximal sodium reabsorption (51,55). Human studies using spironolactone, an aldosterone antagonist, indicate that this agent induces natriuresis in a large proportion of cirrhotic patients with ascites without renal failure, which supports a major role for increased sodium reabsorption in distal sites of the nephron in these patients (56,57). Taken together, these results suggest that in patients with cirrhosis without renal failure, an enhanced reabsorption of sodium in both proximal and distal tubules contributes to sodium retention. Potential mediators of this increased sodium reabsorption include changes in the hydrostatic and colloidosmotic pressures in the peritubular capillaries and increased activity of the SNS and the RAAS. The baroreceptor-mediated activation of these systems arising from a decrease in effective arterial blood volume constitutes a homeostatic response in an attempt maintain arterial pressure within normal limits. Several studies indicate that the activation of RAAS contributes to sodium retention in cirrhosis (21,58,59). In addition, there appears to be an intrarenal activation of RAAS (44). The two final effectors of this system, angiotensin II and aldosterone, induce marked sodium reabsorption by acting in the proximal tubule and the collecting duct, respectively (21). Patients with cirrhosis and ascites have increased urine excretion or plasma levels of aldosterone, which correlate with renal sodium excretion (60). Nonetheless, the strongest evidence for the role of RAAS in sodium derives from the use of medications that antagonize these systems. The administration of aldosterone antagonists successfully promotes diuresis and natriuresis and decreases ascites in cirrhotics (61). In addition, administration of angiotensin II blockers like losartan also induce natriuresis when given at low doses (50,62). The SNS is also commonly activated in advanced cirrhosis and stimulates sodium reabsorption in the proximal tubule, loop of Henle and distal and collecting tubules (24,63). There are elevated levels of NE in plasma and increased rates of NE spillover from different organs in advanced liver disease (24). Additionally, there is an increase in the α-adrenergic receptor tone, which results in an enhanced proximal tubular reabsorption of sodium and an elevation in the β-adrenergic receptor tone, which causes an increase in renin secretion (63).

An unanswered question is why a significant proportion of patients with cirrhosis and ascites present sodium retention despite normal plasma levels of renin, aldosterone and NE levels and increased circulating levels of natriuretic peptides (64). Most of these patients have normal renal plasma flow and GFR. Therefore, sodium retention cannot be explained on the basis of an impaired renal perfusion or a decreased filtered sodium load. It has been suggested that an unknown mechanism (renal or extrarenal), extremely sensitive to changes in effective arterial blood volume would induce sodium retention at the early stages of decompensated cirrhosis. Recently, a role for intrahepatic adenosine causing an increase in portal venous blood flow and triggerring a hepatorenal reflex to regulate sodium and water excretion has been recently proposed as a mechanism that may lead to ascites formation and HRS (65,66). This mechanism by means of increasing sympathetic activity in the kidney probably decreases RBF and GFR (65). In humans, the presence of a hepatorenal reflex has been suggested with observations of reduced RBF following an increase in portal pressure and renal release of endothelin, suggesting that perhaps this vasoconstrictor could play a role in this reflex (66). Further studies in animals and humans are needed in order to elucidate the role of a hepatorenal reflex in ascites formation.

Water Retention

A derangement in the renal capacity to regulate water balance commonly occurs in advanced cirrhosis. The major clinical consequence of this impairment is the appearance of dilutional hyponatremia (sodium serum sodium $\leq$130 mEq/L), which occurs despite avid sodium retention because water is retained in excess of sodium. The estimated prevalence of spontaneous hyponatremia in hospitalized patients with cirrhosis and ascites is near 30% to 35% (67,68). However this figure increases to nearly 70% when water retention is measured as an inability to excrete solute-free water after a water load (Fig. 4) (41). In preascitic cirrhosis patients display similar water-handling mechanisms when

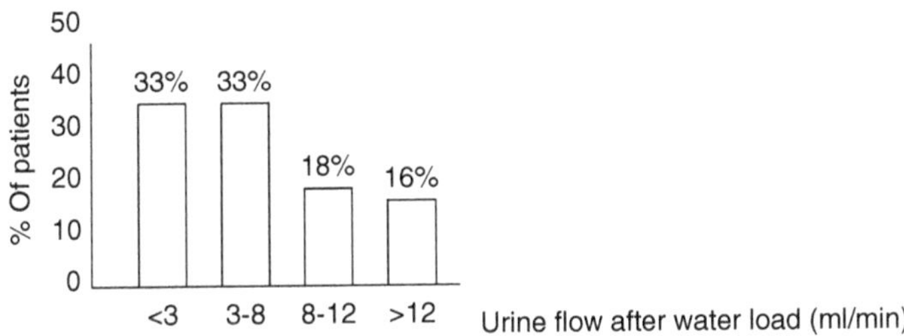

Figure 4 Urine flow after a water load (20 mL/kg body weight of 5% dextrose IV) in a series of patients with cirrhosis and ascites. Normal values for healthy subjects are between 8 and 18 mL/min. *Source*: From Ref. 40.

compared with healthy subjects. Impaired water handling is common in cirrhotics with ascites; as a matter of fact more than two-thirds of hospitalized cirrhotics have an abnormal renal water-handling mechanism as indicated by an impaired ability to generate solute-free water after a water load (Fig. 4) (69). Water retention in cirrhosis usually occurs late in the disease, follows sodium retention and is a poor prognostic indicator (69). The pathogenesis of increased water retention in cirrhosis is complex and involves several factors, including high levels of AVP and reduced delivery of filtrate to the ascending limb of the loop of Henle.

Among these factors, AVP is probably the most important factor in the pathogenesis of water retention in cirrhosis with ascites (70). The high plasma AVP levels seen in cirrhosis are likely to be secondary to a reduced effective intravascular volume. The hemodynamic changes occurring in cirrhosis (low arterial blood pressure, high cardiac output and low total systemic vascular resistance) cause arterial hypotension which unloads the high-pressure baroreceptors and stimulate a nonosmotic release of AVP with the subsequent increase in water reabsorption (70).

The biological effects of AVP are mediated through three types of receptors present in target cells (71). These receptors belong to the superfamily of G protein–coupled receptors and are known as V1a, V1b, and V2. V1a and V1b are associated with the phosphoinositol signaling pathway with intracellular calcium as second messenger. V1a is responsible for vascular smooth muscle cell contraction, platelet aggregation and hepatic glycogenolysis and V1b is expressed in the anterior pituitary where it mediates adrenocorticotropin release (71). The V2 receptors are located on the basolateral (capillary) membrane of the principal cells of the collecting ducts and are responsible for the AVP-induced water reabsorption (72). The effect of AVP on these receptors is mediated by selective water channels, called aquaporins (AQPs). The most important one is AQP2. This water channel has been characterized in human and rat kidneys and is expressed almost exclusively in the principal cells of the collecting ducts (73,74). The binding of AVP to the V2 receptor stimulates adenyl cyclase via the stimulatory G protein and promotes the formation of cyclic AMP (cAMP). This cAMP binds to a regulatory subunit of protein kinase A, which in turn phosphorylates AQP2, which is then translocated from vesicular bodies present in the cytosol to the luminal (apical) plasma membrane of the collecting duct cells, and acts as a water channel thereby increasing water permeability (72–74). The water entering the cell by the luminal plasma membrane leaves the cell through the basolateral membrane and enters the capillaries that are in close contact with tubular cells. AQP 3 and AQP 4 mediate the exiting of water from the cells. In contrast to AQP2, which is translocated from the cytosol to the luminal membrane by the action of AVP, AQP3 and AQP4 are constitutively expressed in the basolateral membrane and their action is not regulated by AVP (73,74). The administration of newly designed V2 receptor antagonists increases free water excretion and improves dilutional hyponatremia in patients with cirrhosis (75).

In most patients, dilutional hyponatremia is asymptomatic, but in some it may be associated with symptoms such as anorexia, headache, poor concentration, lethargy, nausea, vomiting, and occasionally seizures. Presently there is no pharmacological therapy for dilutional hyponatremia and the only therapeutic measure that improves or stops the progressive decrease in serum sodium concentration is water restriction to approximately 1 L/day. The administration of hypertonic saline solutions is not recommended because it invariably leads to further expansion of extracellular fluid volume and accumulation of ascites and edema (75). Preliminary studies show that V2 receptor antagonists of AVP increase solute-free water excretion and increase serum sodium in patients with hyponatremia (76–78). The beneficial effects of V2 receptor antagonists (VPA-985 and tolvaptan) were recently reported in multicenter, randomized, placebo controlled trials in patients with cirrhosis and dilutional hyponatremia (76–78). These compounds when available for use in clinical practice will offer a novel therapeutic approach for the treatment of dilutional hyponatremia in patients with ascites.

Renal Vasoconstriction

Renal vasoconstriction as manifested by the development of HRS is the latest renal functional abnormality in patients with cirrhosis and ascites and its pathogenesis involves several mechanisms, including increased activity of vasoconstrictor factors and probably a reduced activity of renal vasodilator factors. The degree of renal vasoconstriction may range from a modest renal impairment which can be detected only by measuring GFR and renal plasma flow by clearance techniques to a severe renal failure with elevation of blood urea nitrogen and serum creatinine concentration (79,80). The pathogenesis of renal vasoconstriction in cirrhosis is related to changes in systemic hemodynamics. The most accepted theory considers that renal vasoconstriction is the consequence of the extreme underfilling of the arterial circulation present in the latter stages of cirrhosis (80,81). The pathophysiological hallmark of HRS is a vasoconstriction of the renal circulation. Studies of renal perfusion with renal arteriography, ^{133}Xe washout technique, *para*-aminohipuric acid excretion or, more recently, duplex Doppler ultrasonography, have demonstrated the existence of marked vasoconstriction in the kidneys of patients with HRS, with a characteristic reduction in renal cortical perfusion (79,80,82,83).

The mechanism of this vasoconstriction is incompletely understood and possibly multifactorial involving changes in systemic hemodynamics, increased pressure in the portal venous system, activation of vasoconstrictor factors, and suppression of vasodilator factors acting on the renal circulation. Other vascular beds besides the renal circulation are also vasoconstricted in patients with HRS, including the brachial and femoral circulation and the cerebral circulation (7–9). This indicates the existence of a generalized arterial vasoconstriction in nonsplanchnic vascular beds of patients with HRS and suggests that the main vascular bed responsible for arterial vasodilation and reduced total systemic vascular resistance in cirrhosis with HRS is the splanchnic circulation.

The major factors mediating vasoconstriction and vasodilation of the kidney vasculature in cirrhosis are listed in Table 3. Among these the effectors of the RAAS (angiotensin) and SNS (NE) play an important role causing significant renal vasoconstriction, although direct inhibition of these systems carries the risk of inducing hypotension. Other vasoconstrictors such as adenosine and cysteinyl leukotrienes seem to

Table 3 Vasoactive Factors Potentially Involved in Regulation Renal Perfusion and Renal Vasoconstriction in Cirrhosis

Vasodilators
Prostaglandin E2
Nitric oxide
Prostacyclin
Atrial natriuretic peptide
Kallikrein–kinin system
Vasoconstrictors
Angiotensin II
Norepinephrine
Neuropeptide Y
Endothelin-1
Adenosine
Thromboxane A2
Cysteinyl leukotrienes
F2-isoprostanes

play a role in renal vasoconstriction. On the other hand renal vasodilators such as PGs, NO and natriuretic peptides struggle to maintain renal perfusion. As disease progresses the maximal stimulation of vasoconstrictor factors cannot be counterbalanced by either systemic or renal vasodilators and as a consequence, severe vasoconstriction of renal vessels occurs and HRS ensues.

THEORIES OF ASCITES FORMATION

The arterial vasodilation theory was described in an attempt to explain the pathogenesis of ascites and renal dysfunction in cirrhosis (81). It is a rational explanation as to why the hemodynamic changes that occur in cirrhosis are directly related to the development of ascites and renal failure. This theory (Fig. 5) considers that the primary event of renal sodium and water retention in cirrhosis is splanchnic arterial vasodilation secondary to portal hypertension. In the preascitic stage, circulatory homeostasis is maintained by the development of hyperdynamic circulation (high plasma volume, cardiac index, and heart rate). However, as the disease progresses and splanchnic arterial vasodilation increases this compensatory mechanism is insufficient to maintain circulatory homeostasis. Arterial pressure decreases causing stimulation of baroreceptors with a homeostatic increase in the sympathetic nervous activity, renin–angiotensin system activity and circulating levels of AVP. This leads to renal sodium and water retention. Sinusoidal portal hypertension by virtue of causing splanchnic vasodilation produces systemic arterial vascular underfilling and a "forward" increase in the splanchnic capillary pressure and filtration coefficient. In patients with compensated cirrhosis, the degree of portal hypertension and splanchnic arterial vasodilation is moderate. Arterial underfilling is compensated by an increase in plasma volume and cardiac output. In these patients the lymphatic system is able to return the moderate increase in lymph produced to the systemic circulation, thus preventing leakage of fluid into the abdominal cavity. As cirrhosis progresses, portal hypertension and decreased splanchnic vascular resistance turn progressively worse and a critical point is reached in which the consequences of this intense splanchnic arterial vasodilation cannot be compensated for by increasing lymph return, plasma volume, and cardiac

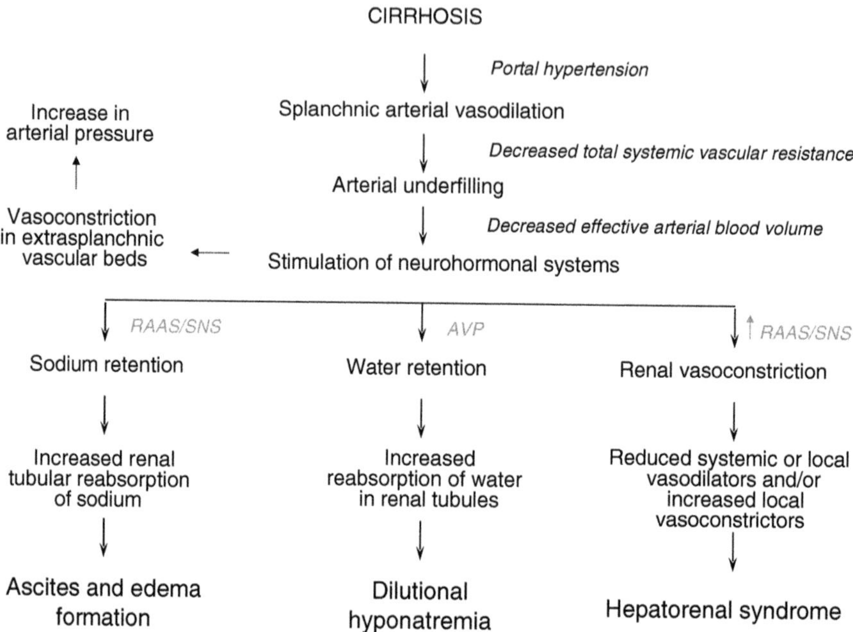

Figure 5 The pathogenesis of ascites formation and renal dysfunction according to the arterial vasodilation theory. The neurohumoral effects of the RAAS, SNS, and AVP on systemic circulation and renal function in cirrhosis with ascites are responsible for sodium and water retention as well as hepatorenal syndrome. The levels of these vasoconstrictors are the highest in patients with hepatorenal syndrome. *Abbreviations*: AVP, arginine vasopressin; RAAS, renin–angiotensin–aldosterone system; SNS, sympathetic nervous system.

output. The maintenance of arterial pressure then requires persistent activation of RAAS, SNS, and AVP, which produce continuous sodium and water retention. The retained fluid is, however, ineffective in refilling the dilated arterial vascular bed because it escapes from the intravascular compartment, due to an imbalance between the excessive lymph production and the ability of the lymphatic system to return it to the systemic circulation. The final consequence of both disorders is persistent renal sodium and water retention with ongoing leakage of fluid into the abdominal cavity and the formation of ascites.

SUMMARY

Ascites is the most common complication of cirrhosis and its existence is associated with profound changes in the splanchnic and systemic circulation as well as renal abnormalities. The development of ascites is related to the existence of severe sinusoidal portal hypertension that causes marked splanchnic arterial vasodilation and a forward increase in the splanchnic production of lymph. Additionally, splanchnic arterial vasodilation decreases effective arterial blood volume and leads to fluid accumulation and renal function abnormalities, which are a consequence of the homeostatic activation of vasoconstrictor and antinatriuretic factors triggered to compensate for a relative arterial underfilling. In addition to changes in splanchnic hemodynamics, cirrhotics with ascites develop a hyperdynamic circulatory state characterized by reduced systemic vascular resistance with low arterial pressure and increased cardiac output. As a consequence of splanchnic vasodilatation, central baroreceptors sense decreased plasma volume triggering RAAS, SNS, and AVP. The net effect is avid retention of sodium and water. The major clinical consequence of impaired solute-free water excretion is dilutional hyponatremia. Renal vasoconstriction develops late in the disease and manifests as HRS with renal failure.

REFERENCES

1. Arroyo V, Ginès P, Planas R, Rodés J. Pathogenesis, diagnosis and treatment of ascites in cirrhosis. In: Bircher J, Benhamou JP, McIntyre N, Rizzetto M, Rodés J, eds. Oxford Textbook of Clinical Hepatology. 2nd ed. Oxford: Oxford University Press, 1999:697–732.
2. Abraldes JG, Tarantino I, Turnes J, Garcia-Pagan JC, Rodes J, Bosch J. Hemodynamic response to pharmacological treatment of portal hypertension and long-term prognosis of cirrhosis. Hepatology 2003; 37:902–8.
3. Jiménez W, Clària J, Arroyo V. Experimental cirrhosis and pathogenesis of ascites formation in chronic liver disease. In: Holstege A, Hahn EG, Scholmerich J, eds. Portal Hypertension. Dordrecht: Kluwer Academic, 1995:15–25.
4. Clària J, Jiménez W. Experimental models of cirrhosis and ascites. In: Ginés P, Arroyo V, Rodes J, Schrier R, eds. Ascites and Renal Dysfunction in Liver Disease. 2nd ed. Oxford: Blackwell Publishing, 2005:215–26.
5. D'Amico G, Luca A, Morabito A, Miraglia R, D'Amico M. Uncovered transjugular intrahepatic portosystemic shunt for refractory ascites: a meta-analysis. Gastroenterology 2005; 129:1282–93.
6. Cárdenas A, Bataller R, Arroyo V. Mechanisms of ascites formation. Clin Liver Dis 2000; 4:447–65.
7. Menon K, Kamath P. Regional and systemic hemodynamic disturbances in cirrhosis. Clin Liver Dis 2001; 5:617–27.
8. Guevara M, Bru C, Ginès P, et al. Increased cerebral vascular resistance in cirrhotic patients with ascites. Hepatology 1998; 28:39–44.
9. Maroto A, Ginès P, Arroyo V, et al. Brachial and femoral artery blood flow in cirrhosis: relationship to kidney dysfunction. Hepatology 1993; 17:788–93.
10. Ruiz del Arbol L, Monescillo A, Arocena C, et al. Circulatory function and hepatorenal syndrome in cirrhosis. Hepatology 2005; 42:439–47.
11. Reynaert H, Thompson MG, Thomas T, Geerts A. Hepatic stellate cells: role in microcirculation and pathophysiology of portal hypertension. Gut 2002; 50:571–81.
12. Titós E, Clària J, Bataller R, et al. Hepatocyte-derived cysteinyl leukotrienes modulate vascular tone in experimental cirrhosis. Gastroenterology 2000; 119:794–805.
13. Graupera M, Garcia-Pagan JC, Abraldes JG, et al. Cyclooxygenase-derived products modulate the increased intrahepatic resistance of cirrhotic rat livers. Hepatology 2003; 37:172–81.
14. Bataller R, Sancho-Bru P, Ginès P, et al. Activated human hepatic stellate cells express the renin–angiotensin system and synthesize angiotensin II. Gastroenterology 2003; 125:117–25.
15. Wiest R, Groszmann R. The paradox of nitric oxide in cirrhosis and portal hypertension: too much, not enough. Hepatology 2002; 35:478–91.
16. Rockey DC, Chung JJ. Reduced nitric oxide production by endothelial cells in cirrhotic rat liver: endothelial dysfunction in portal hypertension. Gastroenterology 1998; 114:344–51.
17. Vorobioff J, Bredfeldt JE, Groszmann RJ. Hyperdynamic circulation in portal-hypertensive rat model: a primary factor for maintenance of chronic portal hypertension. Am J Physiol 1983; 244:G52–7.
18. Wiest R, Groszmann R. Nitric oxide and portal hypertension: its role in the regulation of intrahepatic and splanchnic vascular resistance. Semin Liver Dis 1999; 19:411–26.
19. Moller S, Bendtsen F, Henriksen JH. Vasoactive substances in the circulatory dysfunction of cirrhosis. Scand J Clin Lab Invest 2001; 61:421–9.

20. Asbert M, Jiménez W, Gaya J, et al. Assessment of the renin–angiotensin system in cirrhotic patients. Comparison between plasma renin activity and direct measurement of immunoreactive renin. J Hepatol 1992; 15:179–83.
21. Bernardi M, Domenicali M. The renin–angiotensin system in cirrhosis. In: Ginès P, Arroyo V, Rodes J, Schrier R, eds. Ascites and Renal Dysfunction in Liver Disease. 2nd ed. Oxford: Blackwell Publishing, 2005:43–53.
22. Arroyo V, Bosch J, Mauri M, et al. Effect of angiotensin-II blockade on systemic and hepatic haemodynamics and on the renin–angiotensin–aldosterone system in cirrhosis with ascites. Eur J Clin Invest 1981; 11:221–9.
23. Schneider AW, Kalk JF, Klein CP. Effect of losartan, an angiotensin II receptor antagonist, on portal pressure in cirrhosis. Hepatology 1999; 29:334–9.
24. Dudley F, Esler M. The sympathetic nervous system in cirrhosis. In: Ginès P, Arroyo V, Rodes J, Schrier R, eds. Ascites and Renal Dysfunction in Liver Disease. 2nd ed. Oxford: Blackwell Publishing, 2005:54–72.
25. Henriksen JH, Ring-Larsen H, Christensen NJ. Hepatic intestinal uptake and release of catecholamines in alcoholic cirrhosis. Evidence of enhanced hepatic intestinal sympathetic nervous activity. Gut 1987; 28:1637–42.
26. MacGilchrist AJ, Howes LG, Hawksby C, et al. Plasma noradrenaline in cirrhosis: a study of kinetics and temporal relationship to ascites formation. Eur J Clin Invest 1991; 21:238–43.
27. Esler M, Dudley F, Jennings G, et al. Increased sympathetic nervous activity and the effects of its inhibition with clonidine in alcoholic cirrhosis. Ann Intern Med 1992; 116:446–55.
28. Henriksen JH, Ring-Larsen H, Kanstrup IL, et al. Splanchnic and renal elimination and release of catecholamines in cirrhosis. Evidence of enhanced sympathetic nervous activity in patients with decompensated cirrhosis. Gut 1984; 25:1034–43.
29. Pérez-Ayuso RM, Arroyo V, Camps J, et al. Evidence that renal prostaglandins are involved in renal water metabolism in cirrhosis. Kidney Int 1984; 26:72–80.
30. Laffi G, La Villa G, Pinzani M, et al. Arachidonic acid derivatives and renal function in liver cirrhosis. Semin Nephrol 1997; 17:530–48.
31. Hansen PB, Schnermann J. Vasoconstrictor and vasodilator effects of adenosine in the kidney. Am J Renal Physiol 2003; 285:F590–9.
32. Milani L, Merkel C, Gatta A. Renal effect of aminophylline in hepatic cirrhosis. Eur J Clin Pharmacol 1983; 24:757–60.
33. Stanley AJ, Forrest EH, Dabos K, Bouchier IAD, Hayes PC. Natriuretic effect of an adenosine-1 receptor antagonist in cirrhotic patients with ascites. Gastroenterology 1998; 115:406–11.
34. Llach J, Ginès P, Arroyo V, et al. Effect of dipyridamole on kidney function in cirrhosis. Hepatology 1993; 17:59–64.
35. Blantz RC, Deng A, Lortie M, et al. The complex role of nitric oxide in the regulation of glomerular ultrafiltration. Kidney Int 2002; 61:782–5.
36. Clària J, Jiménez W, Ros J, et al. Pathogenesis of arterial hypotension in cirrhotic rats with ascites: role of endogenous nitric oxide. Hepatology 1992; 15:343–9.
37. Ros J, Clària J, Jiménez W, et al. Role of nitric acid and prostaglandin in the control of renal perfusion in experimental cirrhosis. Hepatology 1995; 22:915–20.
38. Jiménez W, Martínez-Pardo A, Arroyo V, et al. Temporal relationship between hyperaldosteronism, sodium retention and ascites formation in rats with experimental cirrhosis. Hepatology 1985; 5:245–50.
39. Fernandez-Llama P, Ginès P, Schrier RW. Pathogenesis of sodium retention in cirrhosis: the arterial vasodilation hypothesis of ascites formation. In: Ginès P, Arroyo V, Rodes J, Schrier R, eds. Ascites and Renal Dysfunction in Liver Disease. 2nd ed. Oxford: Blackwell Publishing, 2005:201–14.
40. Bernardi M, Laffi G, Salvagnini M, et al. Efficacy and safety of the stepped care medical treatment of ascites in liver cirrhosis: a randomized controlled clinical trial comparing two diets with different sodium content. Liver 1993; 13:156–62.
41. Ginès P, Fernández-Esparrach G, Arroyo V, et al. Pathogenesis of ascites in cirrhosis. Semin Liver Dis 1997; 17:175–89.

42. La Villa G, Salmerón JM, Arroyo V, et al. Mineralocorticoid escape in patients with compensated cirrhosis and portal hypertension. Gastroenterology 1992; 102:2114–9.
43. Wong F, Liu P, Allidina Y, et al. Pattern of sodium handling and its consequences in patients with preascitic cirrhosis. Gastroenterology 1995; 108:1820–7.
44. Bernardi M. Renal sodium retention in preascitic cirrhosis: expanding knowledge, enduring uncertainties. Hepatology 2002; 35:1544–7.
45. Bernardi M, Trevisani F, Santini C, et al. Aldosterone related blood volume expansion in cirrhosis before and after the early phase of ascites formation. Gut 1983; 24:761–6.
46. Caregaro L, Lauro S, Angeli P, et al. Renal water and sodium handling in compensated liver cirrhosis: mechanism of the impaired natriuresis after saline loading. Eur J Clin Invest 1985; 15:360–5.
47. Schrier RW. Peripheral arterial vasodilation in cirrhosis and impaired mineralocorticoid escape. Gastroenterology 1992; 102:2165–8.
48. Wang XY, Masilamani S, Nielsen J, et al. The renal thiazide-sensitive Na–Cl cotransporter as mediator of the aldosterone-escape phenomenon. J Clin Invest 2001; 108:215–22.
49. Bernardi M, Di Marco C, Trevisani F, et al. Renal sodium retention during upright posture in preascitic cirrhosis. Gastroenterology 1993; 105:188–93.
50. Wong F, Liu P, Blendis L. The mechanism of improved sodium homeostasis of low-dose losartan in preascitic cirrhosis. Hepatology 2002; 35:1449–58.
51. Angeli P, Gatta A, Caregaro L, et al. Tubular site of renal sodium retention in ascitic liver cirrhosis evaluated by lithium clearance. Eur J Clin Invest 1990; 20:111–7.
52. López-Novoa JM, Rengel MA, Rodicio JL, et al. A micropuncture study of salt and water retention in chronic experimental cirrhosis. Am J Physiol 1977; 232:F315.
53. Fernández-Llama P, Ageloff S, Fernández-Varo G, et al. Sodium retention in cirrhotic rats is associated with increased renal abundance of sodium transporter proteins. Kidney Int 2005; 67:622.
54. Epstein M, Ramachandran M, DeNunzio AG. Interrelationship of renal sodium and phosphate handling in cirrhosis. Miner Electrolyte Metab 1982; 7:305.
55. Diez J, Simon MA, Anton F, et al. Tubular sodium handling in cirrhotic patients with ascites analysed by the renal lithium clearance method. Eur J Clin Invest 1990; 20:266.
56. Gatta A, Angeli P, Caregaro L, et al. A pathophysiological interpretation of unresponsiveness to spironolactone in a stepped-care approach to the diuretic treatment of ascites in nonazotemic cirrhotic patients. Hepatology 1991; 14:231.
57. Angeli P, Gatta A. Medical treatment of ascites in cirrhosis. In: Ginès P, Arroyo V, Rodes J, Schrier R, eds. Ascites and Renal Dysfunction in Liver Disease. 2nd ed. Oxford: Blackwell Publishing, 2005:227–40.
58. Girgrah N, Liu P, Collier J, et al. Haemodynamic, renal sodium handling, and neurohormonal effects of acute administration of low dose losartan, an angiotensin II receptor antagonist, in preascitic cirrhosis. Gut 2000; 46:114–20.
59. Helmy A, Jalan R, Newby DE, et al. Role of angiotensin II in regulation of basal and sympathetically stimulated vascular tone in early and advanced cirrhosis. Gastroenterology 2000; 118:565–72.
60. Trevisani F, Bernardi M, DePalma R, et al. Circadian variation in renal sodium and potassium handling in cirrhosis. The role of aldosterone, cortisol, sympathoadrenergic tone, and intratubular factors. Gastroenterology 1989; 96:1187–98.
61. Pérez-Ayuso RM, Arroyo V, Planas R, et al. Randomized comparative study of furosemide versus spironolactone in patients with liver cirrhosis and ascites. Relationship between the diuretic response and the activity of the renin–aldosterone system. Gastroenterology 1983; 84:961–8.
62. Yang YY, Lin HC, Lee WC, et al. One-week losartan administration increases sodium excretion in cirrhotic patients with and without ascites. J Gastroenterol 2002; 37:194–9.
63. Esler M, Kaye D. Increased sympathetic nervous system activity and its therapeutic reduction in arterial hypertension, portal hypertension and heart failure. J Auton Nerv Syst 1998; 72:210–9.

64. Salò J, Ginés A, Anibarro L, et al. Effect of upright posture and physical exercise on endogenous neurohormonal systems in cirrhotic patients with sodium retention and normal supine plasma renin, aldosterone and norepinephrine levels. Hepatology 1995; 22:479–87.
65. Ming Z, Smyth DD, Lautt WW. Decreases in portal flow trigger a hepatorenal reflex to inhibit renal sodium and water excretion in rats: role of adenosine. Hepatology 2002; 35:167–75.
66. Jalan R, Forrest EH, Redhead DN, Dillon JF, Hayes PC. Reduction in renal blood flow following acute increase in the portal pressure: evidence for the existence of a hepatorenal reflex in man? Gut 1997; 40:664–70.
67. Arroyo V, Rodés J, Gutiérrez-Lizarraga MA, Revert L. Prognostic value of spontaneous hyponatremia in cirrhosis with ascites. Am J Dig Dis 1976; 21:249–56.
68. Porcel A, Diaz F, Rendon P, et al. Dilutional hyponatremia in patients with cirrhosis and ascites. Arch Intern Med 2002; 162:323–8.
69. Fernández-Esparrach G, Sánchez-Fueyo A, Ginès P, et al. A prognostic model for predicting survival in cirrhosis with ascites. J Hepatol 2001; 34:46–52.
70. Ishikawa S, Schrier RW. Pathogenesis of hyponatremia: the role of arginine vasopressin. In: Ginès P, Arroyo V, Rodes J, Schrier R, eds. Ascites and Renal Dysfunction in Liver Disease. 2nd ed. Oxford: Blackwell Publishing, 2005:305–14.
71. Thibonnier M, Conarty DM, Preston JA, Wilkins PL, Berti-Mattera LN, Mattera R. Molecular pharmacology of human vasopressin receptors. Adv Exp Med Biol 1998; 449:251–76.
72. Verbalis J. Vasopressin V2 receptor antagonists. J Mol Endocrinol 2002; 29:1–9.
73. Kwon TH, Hager H, Nejsum LN, Andersen ML, Frokiaer J, Nielsen S. Physiology and pathophysiology of renal aquaporins. Semin Nephrol 2001; 21:231–8.
74. Nielsen S, Frokiaer J, Marples D, Kwon TH, Agre P, Knepper MA. Aquaporins in the kidney: from molecules to medicine. Physiol Rev 2002; 82:205–44.
75. Cárdenas A, Ginés P. Treatment of hyponatremia in cirrhosis. In: Arroyo V, Navasa M, Foros X, Bataller R, Sanchez-Fueyo A, Rodes J, eds. Update in Treatment of Liver Disease. Barcelona: Ars Medica, 2005:93–102.
76. Wong F, Blei AT, Blendis LM, Thuluvath PJ. A vasopressin receptor antagonist (VPA-985) improves serum sodium concentration in patients with hyponatremia: a multicenter, randomized, placebo-controlled trial. Hepatology 2003; 37:182–91.
77. Gerbes AL, Gulberg V, Ginès P, et al. VPA Study Group. Therapy of hyponatremia in cirrhosis with a vasopressin receptor antagonist: a randomized double-blind multicenter trial. Gastroenterology 2003; 124:933–9.
78. Afdhal N, Cardenas A, Guevara M, et al. For the SALT Study Investigators. Randomized, placebo-controlled trial of tolvaptan, a novel V2-receptor antagonist, in hyponatremia: results of the SALT 2 trial with emphasis on efficacy and safety in cirrhosis. Hepatology 2005; 42:LB19A.
79. Ginès P, Guevara M, Arroyo V, Rodés J. Hepatorenal syndrome. Lancet 2003; 362:1819–27.
80. Guevara M, Ortega R, Ginès P, Rodés J. Pathogenesis of renal vasoconstriction in cirrhosis. In: Ginès P, Arroyo V, Rodés J, Schrier RW, eds. Ascites and Renal Dysfunction in Liver Disease. 2nd ed. Oxford: Blackwell, 2005:329–40.
81. Schrier RW, Arroyo V, Bernardi M, et al. Peripheral arterial vasodilation hypothesis: a proposal for the initiation of renal sodium and water retention in cirrhosis. Hepatology 1988; 8:1151–7.
82. Platt JF, Ellis J, Rubin JM, et al. Renal duplex Doppler ultrasonography: a noninvasive predictor of kidney dysfunction and hepatorenal failure in liver disease. Hepatology 1994; 20:362–9.
83. Maroto A, Ginès A, Saló J, et al. Diagnosis of functional renal failure of cirrhosis by Doppler sonography. Prognostic value of resistive index. Hepatology 1994; 20:839–44.

17
Sodium Balance in Heart Failure

Srinivas Iyengar and William T. Abraham
Division of Cardiovascular Medicine, Ohio State University, Columbus, Ohio, U.S.A.

INTRODUCTION

The incidence of heart failure (HF) has grown to epidemic proportions over the last 20 years, approaching 10 per 1000 in the United States population over the age of 65 years. It is estimated that in the past year, the direct and indirect cost of managing this epidemic in the United States was nearly $30 billion dollars (1). Though this entity has grown, so too has our knowledge of the pathophysiologic mechanisms involved with its progression. Sodium and water balance are integral components in the understanding of how HF propagates itself if left untreated. Renal function and hemodynamics, obviously pivotal to electrolyte and fluid levels in the human body, are active players in the initial compensatory aspect of deteriorating myocardial function. Renal-mediated responses over time can actually contribute to the progression of the overall disease process through their direct interactions with varying hormonal pathways, such as the sympathetic nervous system (SNS), renin-angiotensin-aldosterone system (RAAS), and nonosmotic arginine vasopressin (AVP) release.

ARTERIAL UNDERFILLING

Imagine a pair of dancers, one exceptionally skilled and the other quite clumsy. In order to perform a presentable routine, the skilled dancer will try and compensate for the partner's shortcomings. Though initially this may result in a normal display, without improvement of the untrained partner the continual overcompensation of the skilled individual and resultant decreased effort of the opposite partner will result in a poor overall performance. A situation analogous to this can be found in the pathologic process of HF. The complex interplay between renal and cardiac function in HF can be viewed as a dance of sorts: renal compensatory mechanisms can initially respond to a perceived lack of circulation and temporize a situation until homeostasis can be achieved. Unfortunately in the HF pathway, these compensatory mechanisms, if not mitigated, will result in a continuum of hormonal stimulation and vasoactivity which propagates the disease process. This "vicious cycle" of HF has been well described and currently forms a significant amount of the knowledge base clinicians draw from in order to attempt to treat this entity (2).

Patients with HF often have obvious evidence of fluid retention, yet their kidneys are also in a continuous state of salt and fluid retention. This seemingly paradoxical state can be explained by examining renal function in HF as having both as afferent and efferent limb. Arterial underfilling, as perceived by the renal system as alterations of cardiac output and/or peripheral vascular resistance, has become the central hypothesis for sodium and fluid regulation in HF and is recognized as the most important factor in the afferent limb (Fig. 1) (4–6). According to this hypothesis, a decrease in cardiac output can result in a compensatory phase of sodium and water retention, as the kidneys perceive this reduction of flow as a stimulant to retain essential components for maintaining an effective systemic fluid balance (Fig. 2). Alternatively, peripheral arterial vasodilatation, as seen in states such as high-output cardiac failure, pregnancy, and cirrhosis can also produce the same compensatory mechanisms from the kidneys. This is primarily due to the fact that over 85% of plasma volume is in the low-pressure venous circulation with the remaining volume primarily in the arterial circulation, and expanded blood volume with subsequent vasodilation could still be perceived as arterial underfilling by the kidneys.

Afferent Volume Receptors

As previously mentioned, arterial underfilling forms the basis for the stimulation of afferent volume receptors. High-pressure baroreceptors reside in the aortic arch, carotid sinus, left ventricle, and juxtaglomerular apparatus (JGA), while low-pressure volume receptors are found primarily in the cardiac atria, right ventricle, and pulmonary vessels. Research in mammals has supported the theory that arterial receptors play a larger role in volume control than low-pressure receptors (8–12).

Studies in humans have demonstrated the importance of high-pressure volume receptors in the arterial circulation. Epstein et al. observed that in patients with traumatic arterio-venous fistulae, closure of these fistulae would result in a dramatic increase in sodium excretion independent of renal blood flow (13). The closure of these fistulae was associated with a decreased rate of emptying of the arterial blood into the venous

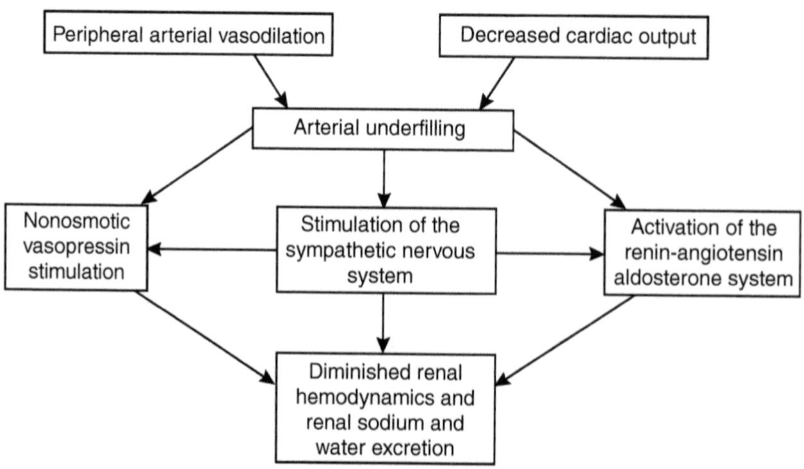

Figure 1 Pathway in which arterial underfilling results in subsequent renal sodium and water retention. *Source*: From Ref. 3.

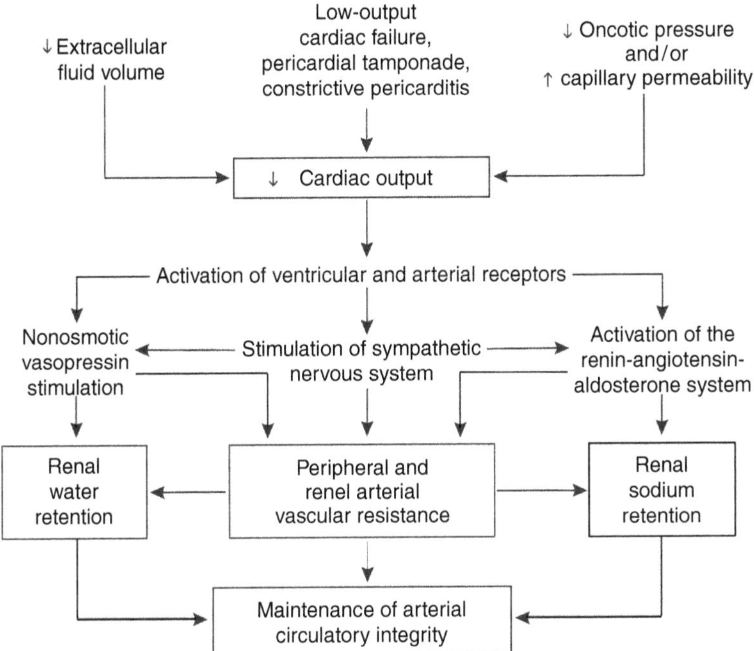

Figure 2 Neurohumoral activation in response to arterial underfilling secondary to a decrease in cardiac output. ↓ = decreased; ↑ = increased. *Source*: From Ref. 7.

circulation, which was shown as closure-induced increases in diastolic arterial pressure and subsequent decreases in cardiac output.

Denervation experiments, either by pharmacologic or surgical means, have also demonstrated that interrupting the sympathetic efferent neural pathways extending from high-pressure receptors can result in a decreased natriuretic response to increased volume (14,15). Hormonal pathways such as the SNS (as activated by alteration of pressure receptors found at the carotid sinus) and the regulation of nonosmotic release of AVP (by sympathetic-mediated stimulation of the supraoptic and paraventricular nuclei in the hypothalamus) are also intimately tied with high-pressure arterial receptors (16–18).

Low-pressure volume receptors also play an important role in volume regulation. Specifically, receptors in the left atria, which have been found to be the sites for the synthesis and release of natriuretic peptides as well as affecting the release of vasopressin in a nonosmotic manner, are also components of the afferent limb (19,20). However, in chronic HF, fluid and sodium retention persists despite increased loading conditions upon the low-pressure receptors. This is thought to occur due to the greater role that arterial high-pressure receptors play in chronic HF and a potentially attenuated response of low-pressure receptors in chronic, as opposed to acute HF states (21–23).

Efferent Mechanisms

Neurohormonal Response

As previously mentioned, alterations in baroreceptors activation by arterial underfilling, whether by a decrease in cardiac output or peripheral vasodilation, can stimulate a number of hormonal pathways that can result in vasoconstriction and sodium and fluid retention

(24,25). This perturbation in receptor sensing results in a decrease of the tonic inhibitory effect of afferent vagal and glossopharyngeal pathways to the central nervous system and results in an increase in sympathetic efferent adrenergic tone with subsequent stimulation of the RAAS and nonosmotic AVP release (Fig. 3). Though initially natriuretic peptide release and vasodilating renal prostaglandins might be serve to offset this process, patients in chronic HF often have a damped response to these counter-regulatory hormonal pathways, the reasons of which are multifactorial, relating most likely to the importance of high-pressure arterial baroreceptors in the role of SNS stimulation as well as concomitant medication use.

Renal Homodynamic

Though it was earlier postulated that glomerular filtration rate (GFR) was decreased in HF, there is evidence to support that GFR can remain stable and even elevate with different forms of HF (26,27). Given that GFR is somewhat difficult to accurately account for in

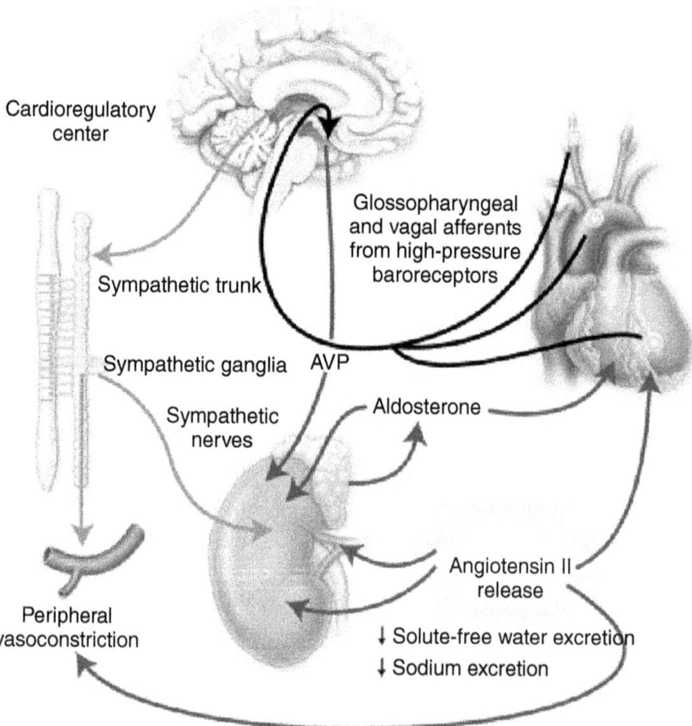

Figure 3 Afferent signals that stimulate specific cardioregulatory areas in the brain are activated by unloading of high-pressure baroreceptors in the left ventricle, carotid sinus, and aortic arch. This results in efferent pathway activation involving the SNS. Renal nerve stimulation by the SNS increases the activity of the renin–angiotensin–aldosterone system as well. Additionally, stimulation of the supraoptic and paraventricular nuclei in the hypothalamus via the SNS results in increased release of nonosmotic arginine vasopressin. Angiotensin II stimulates vasoconstriction, along with the SNS, and also stimulates the release of aldosterone which leads to increased sodium reabsorption. *Abbreviations*: AVP, arginine vasopressin; SNS, sympathetic nervous system. *Source*: From Ref. 2.

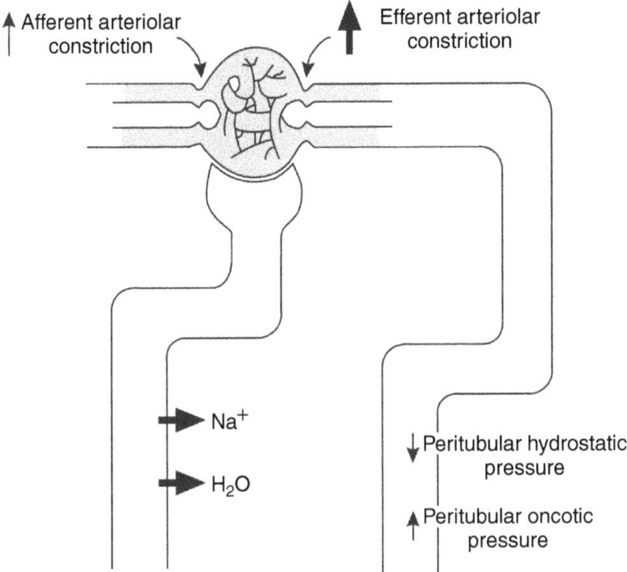

Figure 4 Efferent arteriolar constriction, secondary to increased sympathetic stimulation and exposure to angiotensin II, which increases proximal tubular sodium reabsorption in the presence of arterial underfilling. *Source*: From Ref. 29.

relation to sodium handling, minute changes in GFR might actually represent larger incremental amounts of tubular sodium reabsorption in patients with chronic HF.

Renal blood flow, as opposed to GFR, is affected more profoundly in HF and can be markedly reduced. As a result, filtration fraction is generally increased. This increase results in increased peritubular oncotic pressure in the efferent arterioles of the proximal tubules which then stimulates increased sodium and water reabsorption at this site (28). The mechanisms involved with this response are linked to vasoconstriction of the efferent arterioles of the kidneys, which have been stimulated by increased circulating norepinephrine and angiotensin II (ANG II) (Fig. 4) (30). A decrease in active vasodilating prostaglandins also appears to be factors in relation to renal vasoconstriction in HF (31).

SYMPATHETIC NERVOUS SYSTEM

The SNS has been clearly documented to be highly active in patients with HF (32–35). Not only will stimulation of the SNS result in increased catecholamine circulation, but also subsequent stimulation of nonosmotic AVP release and increased activation of the RAAS. Renal nerve stimulation by the SNS also has a pivotal role in sodium retention in HF states. Animal studies involving stimulation of the renal nerve have demonstrated an increase in sodium reabsorption in renal tubules, as opposed to the countereffect when renal nerves are inhibited (36–38). The mechanism behind this observed increase in sodium retention is thought to be secondary to increased sympathetically mediated efferent arteriolar constriction as well as elevated sodium reabsorption in the proximal convoluted tubule (39).

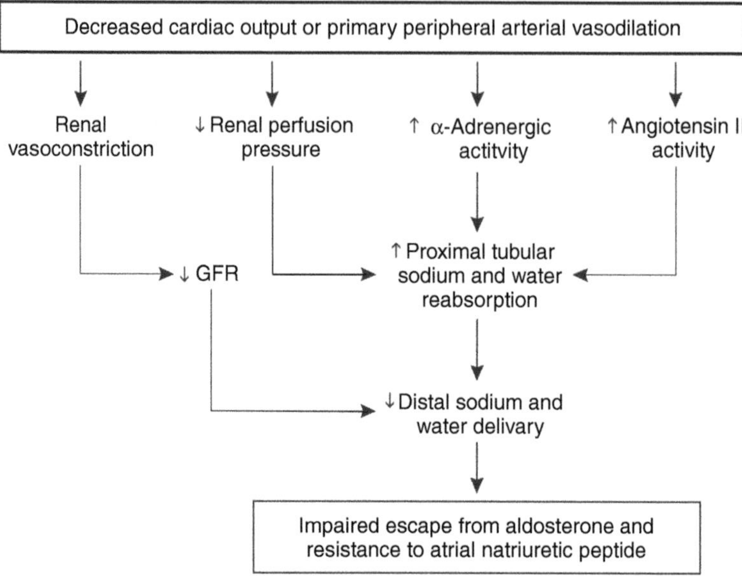

Figure 5 Renal alterations from arterial underfilling results in impaired aldosterone escape and resistance to atrial natriuretic peptide. ↓ = decreased ↑ = increased. *Abbreviation*: GFR, glomerular filtration rate. *Source*: From Ref. 46.

RENIN-ANGIOTENSIN-ALDOSTERONE SYSTEM

The RAAS is also a vital component in the "neurohormonal cascade" of HF. Plasma renin, ANG II, and aldosterone levels are all increased in HF (40–42). As previously mentioned, HF can induce a number of vasoactive responses in the kidneys from SNS stimulation. This includes an increase in renin production from both activation of the renal nerves adjacent to the JGA and increased levels secondary to a decrease in renal blood flow and increase in filtration fraction (43). The increased renin level cleaves angiotensinogen to angiotensin I, which in turn is cleaved by angiotensin-converting enzyme (ACE) to ANG II. ANG II is a potent vasoconstrictor and increases efferent arteriolar resistance and results in increased sodium reabsorption in the proximal tubule (44).

ANG II also increases aldosterone production from the adrenal cortex (45). ANG II-mediated renal vasoconstriction, in addition to proximal tubular reabsorption of sodium, reduces sodium delivery to the distal nephron. This in part serves to impair the ability of patients in HF in escaping the effects of aldosterone (Fig. 5). Hensen and colleagues observed that in patients with HF who were administered the aldosterone antagonist spironolactone (400 mg/day), an increase in urinary sodium, as well as subsequent elevations in plasma renin and norepinephrine, was reported (Fig. 6) (45).

NONOSMOTIC ARGININE VASOPRESSIN SECRETION

As with the previously discussed hormones, plasma AVP is also commonly elevated in patients with HF (47–50). Szatalowicz et al. found that in small cohort of HF patients who were also hyponatremic, plasma AVP could still be identified; given the fact that these patients were in hypo-osmolar states, the authors concluded that the nonosmotic release of

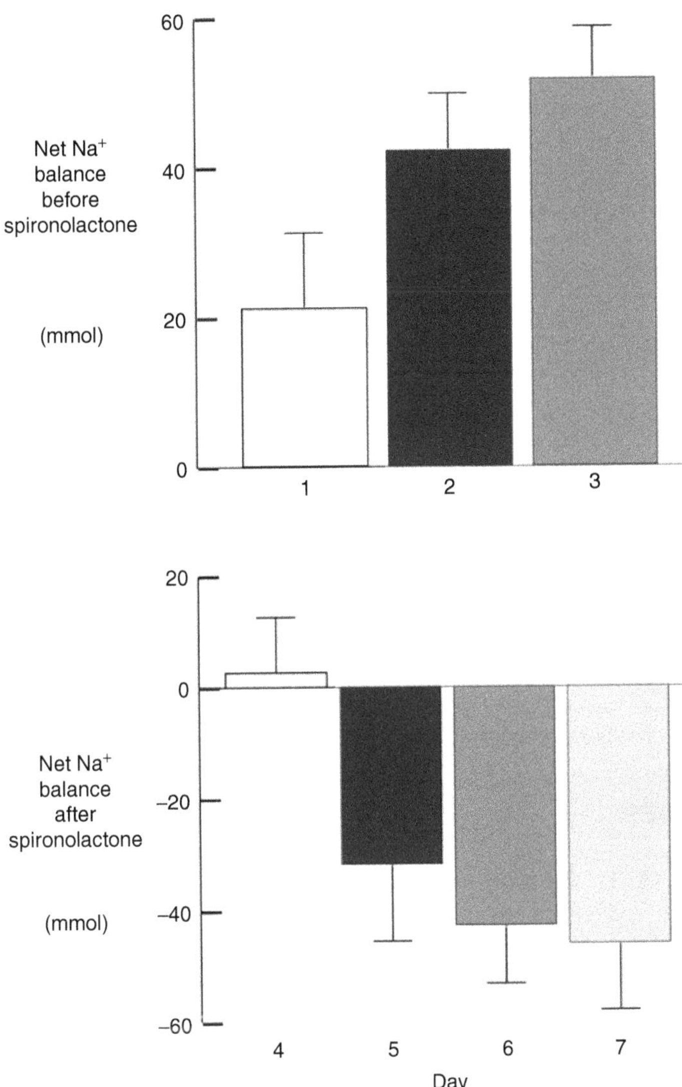

Figure 6 Reversal of sodium retention with the use of an aldosterone antagonist in patients with heart failure. (*Upper panel*) Net positive cumulative sodium balance, by day, for the time period before spironolactone administration. (*Lower panel*) Net negative cumulative sodium balance after the initiation of 400 mg/day of spironolactone. *Source*: Ref. 45.

AVP was due to baroreceptor stimulation secondary to arterial underfilling from HF (47). This initial observation has been verified by additional studies as well (48).

The increased secretion of nonosmotic AVP is also accompanied by an increase in sympathetic tone, which then stimulates the hormonal cascade of the RAAS (51). This increased level of nonosmotic AVP stimulates V_{1a} receptors on vascular smooth muscle beds as a compensatory mechanism to perceived arterial underfilling (52). Vasopressin V_2 receptor stimulation, located on the collecting duct, results in activation of the cyclic AMP pathway that increases aquaporin-2 water channel activity to the apical membrane of the collecting duct. This process results in an overall net increase in fluid reabsorption (Fig. 7) (54,55).

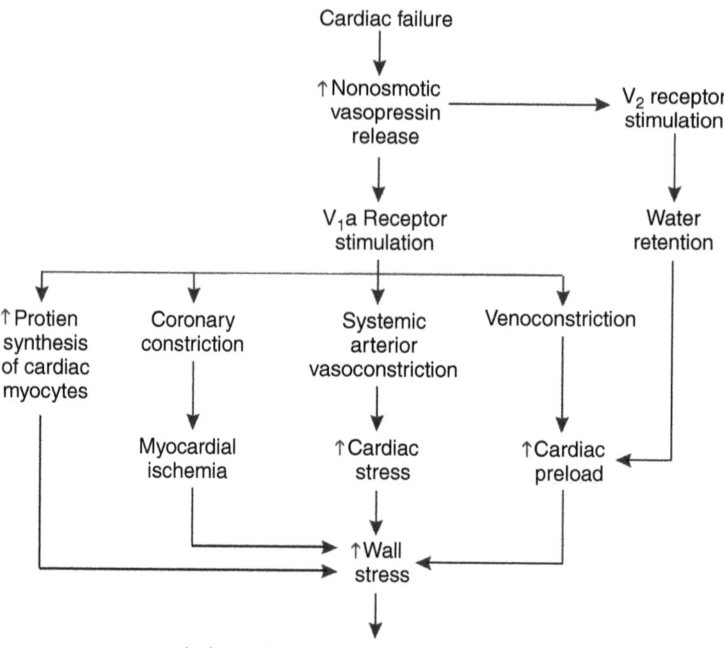

Figure 7 Potential effects of vasopressin on V_1 and V_2 receptors that can further reduce cardiac performance and function by increasing afterload, preload, and wall stress. *Source*: From Ref. 53.

NATRIURETIC PEPTIDES

Atrial natriuretic peptide (ANP) and brain natriuretic peptide (BNP) are hormones that possess both vasodilatory and natriuretic aspects (56). Both hormones are generally elevated in HF states as well and both are secreted from the myocardium in response to increases in end-diastolic pressure (57). This binding triggers activation of the intracellular second messenger cyclic guanosine monophosphate (cGMP), which causes smooth muscle cell relaxation, and dilation of both veins and arteries. In the kidney, this leads to renal arteriolar vasodilatation, enhanced renal perfusion, and increased GFR (58). Atrial natriuretic peptide has been shown not only to vasodilate through peptide receptors, but its beneficial actions also include suppressing the neurohormonal cascade of the RAAS and the SNS (59). Both ANP and BNP have also been demonstrated to inhibit sodium reabsorption in the collecting duct (60).

Though these hormones appear to have effective counter-regulatory functions to the effects of the SNS and RAAS, in chronic HF states, their renal effects are usually blunted. There have been a number of theories postulated on why this may occur: (*i*) downregulation of renal ANP receptors, (*ii*) release of inactive immunoreactive ANP, (*iii*) increased renal neutral endopeptidase activity that can curtail the amount of deliverable ANP to receptor sites, (*iv*) increased aldosterone levels stimulated by increased sodium reabsorption in the distal renal tubule, and (*v*) reduced delivery of sodium to the distal tubule site of ANP action. In HF patients, research has confirmed a positive correlation between plasma ANP and urinary cGMP levels suggesting that decreased distal tubular sodium delivery may be integral in the natriuretic peptide resistance seen in this patient population (61). Additional verification has been demonstrated through animal studies which revealed that after renal denervation, resistance to ANP in HF can be effectively reversed, most likely due to increased distal tubular sodium delivery (62).

PROGNOSTIC SIGNIFICANCE

Sodium levels in HF have prognostic significance as well. Plasma sodium levels have been observed to parallel HF severity (63). This relationship is prognostically significant, as patient survival is adversely affected once the plasma sodium concentration falls below 137 meq/L (64). A similar inverse correlation has been observed between patient survival and the degree of elevation in plasma norepinephrine levels (65). Additionally, plasma sodium concentration below 125 meq/L usually represents patients with end-stage HF.

Hyponatremia can also be a negative predictor of short-term outcomes in patients hospitalized for acute, decompensated HF. Post hoc analysis from the OPTIME-CHF trial, which examined the use of the inotrope milrinone in HF, found that lower admission sodium levels correlated with increased number of days hospitalized for cardiovascular causes and increased mortality within 60 days of discharge (66).

THERAPEUTIC OPTIONS

Numerous trials have demonstrated the efficacy of varying classes of medications (β-blockers, ACE inhibitors, ANG II receptor blockers, aldosterone antagonists) that specifically target the SNS and RAAS and have shown the ability to reduce mortality in the chronic HF population (67–70). The specific treatment of sodium balance in HF, however, has been a more elusive target.

Patients who are in chronic HF and are fluid overloaded or who present in an acutely decompensated state can be treated with a number of therapies including intravenous (IV) diuretics, IV vasodilators, and in cases of cardiogenic shock, IV inotropes and vasopressors. By improving cardiac function with these measures and thus facilitating fluid removal, sodium levels can improve over the course of the admission. Additionally, the use of veno-venous ultrafiltration as an alternate treatment for hypervolemic HF patients is emerging as a viable option for fluid removal with minimal electrolyte derangements (71).

HF patients who are hyponatremic in an outpatient setting are generally advised to pursue fluid restriction as a means of regulating sodium levels. Given the fact that many of these patients are also on chronic oral diuretic therapy, thirst becomes a major limiting factor in this form of therapy. ACE inhibitors, in combination with a loop diuretic, can also improve sodium levels by effectively lowering antidiuretic hormone (ADH), ANG II, and norepinephrine levels and also offsetting the effect of ADH on the collecting tubules (probably through prostaglandin release), thereby decreasing fluid reabsorption at this area (72,73).

Recently, Schrier and colleagues reported the use of tolvaptan, an oral vasopressin (V_2) receptor antagonist, in ambulatory patients with euvolemic or hypervolemic hyponatremia (74). This study was a combined report of two randomized, double-blind, placebo-controlled multicenter trials conducted in a number of sites in both in the United States and abroad (SALT-1 and SALT-2) consisting of 448 patients with hyponatremia (mean plasma sodium 129 meq/L) caused by HF, syndrome of inappropriate antidiuretic hormone, or hepatic cirrhosis. Compared with placebo, the authors found that tolvaptan significantly increased the serum sodium concentration at day 4 (134–135 vs. 130 meq/L) and day 30 (136 vs. 131 meq/L). One week after the discontinuation of the tolvaptan after day 30, hyponatremia was reported to recur.

CONCLUSIONS

Sodium balance in HF constitutes a number of complex mechanisms and hormonal pathways that interact throughout the progression of the disease. Though the underlying theory of arterial underfilling, either by a decrease in cardiac output or peripheral vascular resistance, has formed the foundation of explaining the potential etiology for sodium imbalance in these patients, current treatment options have not completely addressed the exact solution for this problem. The use of vasopressin antagonists as well as ultrafiltration in HF represents exciting novel therapies that have furthered our knowledge of appropriate fluid removal and electrolyte stabilization in this group. Given the fact that hyponatremia is a poor prognostic indicator in patients with HF, only with continual active research in this area can we further elucidate the pathophysiologic mechanisms involved in sodium handling in this patient population.

REFERENCES

1. American Heart Association. Heart and Stroke Statistical Update-2006 Update. Dallas, TX: American Heart Association, 2006.
2. Schrier RW, Abraham WT. Hormones and hemodynamics in heart failure. N Engl J Med 1999; 341:577–85.
3. Cadnapaphornchai MA, Gurevich AK, Weinberger HD. Pathophysiology of sodium and water retention in heart failure. Cardiology 2001; 96:122–31.
4. Schrier RW. Pathogenesis of sodium and water retention in high-output and low-output cardiac failure, nephritic syndrome, cirrhosis, and pregnancy. Part 1. N Engl J Med 1988; 319:1065–72.
5. Schrier RW. Pathogenesis of sodium and water retention in high-output and low-output cardiac failure, nephritic syndrome, cirrhosis, and pregnancy. Part 2. N Engl J Med 1988; 319:1127–34.
6. Schrier RW, Gurevich AK, Cadnapaphornchai MA. Pathogenesis and management of sodium and water retention in cardiac failure and cirrhosis. Semin Nephrol 2001; 21:157–72.
7. Schrier RW. Body fluid volume regulation in health and disease: a unifying hypothesis. Ann Intern Med 1999; 113:155–9.
8. Goetz KL, Bond GC, Bloxham DD. Atrial receptors and renal function. Physiol Rev 1975; 55:157–205.
9. Zucker IH, Earle AM, Gilmore JP. The mechanism of adaptation of left atrial stretch receptors in dogs with chronic congestive heart failure. J Clin Invest 1977; 60:323–31.
10. Schrier RW, Lieberman RA, Ufferman RC. Mechanism of antidiuretic effect of beta adrenergic stimulation. J Clin Invest 1972; 51:97–111.
11. Anderson RJ, Pluss RG, Berns AS, et al. Mechanism of effect of hypoxia on renal water excretion. J Clin Invest 1978; 62:769–77.
12. Schrier RW, Berl T. Mechanism of antidiuretic effect of interruption of parasympathetic pathways. J Clin Invest 1972; 51:2613–20.
13. Epstein FH, Post RS, McDowell M. Effects of an arteriovenous fistula on renal hemodynamics and electrolyte excretion. J Clin Invest 1953; 32:233–41.
14. Gilmore JP, Daggett WM. Response of chronic cardiac denervated dog to acute volume expansion. Am J Physiol 1966; 210:509–12.
15. Pearce JW, Sonnenberg H. Effects of spinal section and renal denervation on the renal response to blood volume expansion. Can J Physiol Pharmacol 1965; 43:211–20.

16. Guyton A, Scanlon CJ, Armstrong GG. Effects of pressoreceptor reflex and Cushing's reflex on urinary output. Fed Proc 1952; 11:61–8.
17. Anderson RJ, Cronin RE, McDonald KM, et al. Mechanism of portal hypertension induces alterations in renal hemodynamics, renal water excretion, and renin secretion. J Clin Invest 1976; 58:964–70.
18. Schrier RW, Berl T, Anderson RJ, et al. Nonosmolar control of renal water excretion. In: Andreoli T, Grantham J, Rector F, eds. Disturbances in Body Fluid Osmolality. Bethesda, MD: American Physiological Society, 1977:149–60.
19. Currie MG, Geller DM, Cole BC, et al. Bioactive cardiac substances: potent vasorelaxant activity in mammalian atria. Science 1983; 221:71–3.
20. Atlas SA, Kleinert HD, Camargo MJ, et al. Purification, sequencing, and synthesis of natriuretic and vasoactive rat atrial peptide. Nature 1984; 309:717–9.
21. Barger AC, Yates FE, Rudolph AM. Renal hemodynamics and sodium excretion in dogs with graded valvular damage, and in congestive failure. Am J Physiol 1961; 200:601–8.
22. Stitzer SO, Malvin RL. Right atrium and renal sodium excretion. Am J Physiol 1975; 228:184–90.
23. Zucker IH, Gorman AJ, Cornish KG, et al. Impaired atrial receptor modulation of renal nerve activity in dogs with chronic volume overload. Cardiovasc Res 1985; 19:411–8.
24. Sklar AH, Schrier RW. Central nervous system mediators of vasopressin release. Physiol Rev 1983; 63:1243–80.
25. Berl T, Henrich WL, Erickson AL, et al. Prostaglandins in the beta-adrenergic and baroreceptor mediated secretion on renin. Am J Physiol 1979; 235:F472–7.
26. Sinclair-Smith B, Kattus AA, Kenest J, et al. The renal mechanism of electrolyte excretion and the metabolic balances of electrolytes and nitrogen in congestive cardiac failure: the effect of exercise, rest, and aminophylline. Bull Johns Hopkins Hosp 1949; 84:369–80.
27. Decaux G, Dumont I, Naeije N, et al. High uric acid and urea clearance in cirrhosis secondary to increased effective vascular volume. Am J Med 1982; 73:328–34.
28. Vander AJ, Malvin RL, Wilde RE, et al. Reexamination of salt and water retention in congestive heart failure. Am J Med 1958; 25:497–502.
29. Schrier RW, Gurevich AK, Abraham WT. Renal sodium excretion, edematous disorders, and diuretic use. In: Schrier RW, ed. Renal and Electrolyte Disorders. Philadelphia, PA: Lippincott Raven, 1997:72–129.
30. Myers BD, Deen WM, Brenner BM. Effects of norepinephrine and angiotensin II on the determinants of glomerular ultrafiltration and proximal tubule fluid reabsorption in the rat. Circ Res 1975; 37:101–10.
31. Henriksen JH, Christensen JJ, Ring-Larsen H. Noradrenaline and adrenaline concentrations in various vascular beds in patients with cirrhosis: relation to hemodynamics. Clin Physiol 1981; 1:293–304.
32. Thomas JA, Marks BA. Plasma norepinephrine in congestive heart failure. Am J Cardiol 1978; 41:233–42.
33. Hasking GJ, Esler MD, Jennings GL, et al. Norepinephrine spillover to plasma in patients with congestive heart failure: evidence of increased overall and cardiorenal sympathetic nervous activity. Circulation 1986; 73:615–21.
34. Levine TB, Francis GS, Goldsmith SR, et al. Activity of the SNS and renin–angiotensin system assessed by plasma hormone levels and their relation to hemodynamic abnormalities in congestive heart failure. Am J Cardiol 1982; 49:1659–66.
35. Abraham WT, Hensen J, Schrier RW. Elevated plasma noradrenaline concentrations in patients with low-output cardiac failure: dependence on increased noradrenaline secretion rates. Clin Sci (Lond) 1990; 79:429–35.
36. Gill JR, Jr., Mason DT, Bartter FC. Adrenergic nervous system in sodium metabolism: effects of guanethidine and sodium-retaining steroids in normal man. J Clin Invest 1964; 43:177–84.
37. DiBona GF, Herman PJ, Sawin LL. Neural control of renal function in edema forming states. Am J Physiol 1988; 254:R1017–24.

38. Bello-Reuss E, Trevino DL, Gottschalk CW. Effect of renal sympathetic nerve stimulation on proximal water and sodium reabsorption. J Clin Invest 1976; 57:1104–7.
39. DiBona GF. Neurogenic regulation of renal tubular sodium reabsorption. Am J Physiol 1977; 233:F73–81.
40. Merril AJ, Morrison JL, Brannon ES. Concentration of renin in renal venous blood in patients with chronic heart failure. Am J Med 1946; 1:468–70.
41. Watkins L, Jr., Burton JA, Haber E, et al. The renin–angiotensin–aldosterone system in congestive heart failure in conscious dogs. J Clin Invest 1976; 57:1606–17.
42. Francis GS, Benedict C, Johnstone DE, et al. Comparison of neuroendocrine activation in patients with left ventricular dysfunction with and without congestive heart failure. A substudy of the Studies of Left Ventricular Dysfunction (SOLVD). Circulation 1990; 82:1724–9.
43. Abraham WT, Schrier RW. Renal salt and water handling in congestive heart failure. In: Hosenpud JD, Greenberg BH, eds. Congestive Heart Failure. Philadelphia, PA: Lippincott Williams and Wilkins, 2000:253–66.
44. Winaver J, Abassi Z, Green J, et al. Control of extracellular fluid volume and the pathophysiology of edema formation. In: Brenner BM, ed. The Kidney. Philadelphia, PA: WB Saunders Company, 2000:795–865.
45. Hensen J, Abraham WT, Durr JA, et al. Aldosterone in congestive heart failure: analysis of determinants and role in sodium retention. Am J Nephrol 1991; 11:441–6.
46. Schrier RW, Better OS. Pathogenesis of ascites formation: mechanism of impaired aldosterone escape in cirrhosis. Eur J Gastroenterol Hepatol 1991; 3:721–9.
47. Szatalowicz VL, Arnold PA, Chaimovitz C, et al. Radioimmunoassay of plasma arginine vasopressin in hyponatremic patients with congestive heart failure. N Engl J Med 1981; 305:263–6.
48. Riegger GA, Niebau G, Kochsiek K. Antidiuretic hormone in congestive heart failure. Am J Med 1982; 72:49–52.
49. Bichet D, Kortasa CK, Mattauer B, et al. Modulation of plasma and platelet vasopressin by cardiac function in patients with severe congestive heart failure. Kidney Int 1986; 29:1188–96.
50. Goldsmith SR, Francis GS, Cowley AW, Jr. Arginine vasopressin and the renal response to water loading in congestive heart failure. Am J Cardiol 1986; 58:295–9.
51. Bichet DG, Van Putten VJ, Schrier RW. Potential role of the increased sympathetic activity in impaired sodium and water excretion in cirrhosis. N Engl J Med 1982; 307:1552–7.
52. Schrier RW, Briner V, Caramelo C. Cellular action and interactions of arginine vasopressin in vascular smooth muscle: mechanism and clinical implications. J Am Soc Nephrol 1993; 4:2–11.
53. Schrier RW. Role of diminished renal function in cardiovascular mortality: marker or pathogenic factor? J Am Coll Cardiol 2006; 47:1–8.
54. Schrier RW, Cadnapaphornchai MA, Ohara M. Water retention and aquaporins in heart failure, liver disease, and pregnancy. J R Soc Med 2001; 94:265–9.
55. Schrier RW, Cadnapaphornchai MA. Renal aquaporin water channels: from molecules to human disease. Prog Biophys Mol Biol 2003; 81:117–31.
56. Mukoyama M, Nakao K, Hosoda K, et al. Brain natriuretic peptide as a novel hormone in humans. Evidence for an exquisite dual natriuretic peptide system, atrial natriuretic peptide and brain natriuretic peptide. J Clin Invest 1991; 87:1402–12.
57. Sato F, Kamoi K, Wakiya Y, et al. Relationship between plasma atrial natriuretic peptide levels and atrial pressure in man. J Clin Endocrinol Metab 1986; 63:823–7.
58. Suga S-I, Nakaao K, Hosoda K, et al. Receptor selectivity of natriuretic peptide family, atrial natriuretic peptide, brain natriuretic peptide and C-type natriuretic peptide. Endocrinology 1992; 130:229–39.
59. Cody RJ, Atlas SA, Laragh JH, et al. Atrial natriuretic factor in normal subjects and heart failure patients. J Clin Invest 1986; 78:1362–74.
60. Dunn BR, Ichikawa I, Pfeffer JM, et al. Renal and systemic hemodynamic effects of synthetic atrial natriuretic peptide in the anesthetized rat. Circ Res 1986; 59:237–46.

61. Abraham WT, Hensen J, Kim JD, et al. Atrial natriuretic peptide and urinary cyclic guanosine monophosphate in patients with congestive heart failure. J Am Soc Nephrol 1992; 2:1697–703.
62. Koepke JP, DiBona GF. Blunted natriuresis to atrial natriuretic peptide in chronic sodium retaining disorders. Am J Physiol 1987; 252:F865–71.
63. Leier CV, Dei Cas L, Metra M. Clinical reliance and management of the major electrolyte abnormalities in congestive heart failure: hyponatremia, hypokalemia, and hypomagnesemia. Am Heart J 1994; 128:564–74.
64. Lee WH, Packer M. Prognostic importance of serum sodium concentration and its modification by converting-enzyme inhibition in patients with severe chronic heart failure. Circulation 1986; 73:257–67.
65. Cohn JN, Levine TB, Olivari MT, et al. Plasma norepinephrine as a guide to prognosis in patients with chronic congestive heart failure. N Engl J Med 1984; 311:819–23.
66. Klein L, O'Connor CM, Leimberger JD, et al. Lower serum sodium is associated with increased short-term mortality in hospitalized patients with worsening heart failure: results from the Outcomes of a Prospective Trial of Intravenous Milrinone for Exacerbations of Chronic Heart Failure (OPTIME-CHF) study. Circulation 2005; 111:2454–60.
67. The CONSENSUS Trial Study Group. Effects of enalapril on mortality in severecongestive heart failure. Results of the Cooperative North Scandinavian Enalapril Survival Study (CONSENSUS). N Engl J Med 1987; 316:1429–35.
68. Packer M, Bristow MR, Cohn JN, et al. The effect of carvedilol on morbidity and mortality in patients with chronic heart failure. N Engl J Med 1996; 334:1349–55.
69. Pitt B, Zannad F, Remme WJ, et al. The effect of spironolactone on morbidity and mortality in patients with severe heart failure. N Engl J Med 1999; 341:709–17.
70. Cohn JN, Tognoni G. A randomized trial of the angiotensin-receptor blocker valsartan in chronic heart failure. N Engl J Med 2001; 345:1667–75.
71. Costanzo MR, Guglin ME, Saltzberg MT, et al. Ultrafiltration versus intravenous diuretics for patients hospitalized for acute decompensated heart failure. J Am Coll Cardiol 2007; 49:675–83.
72. Riegger GA, Kochsiek K. Vasopressin, renin, and norepinephrine levels before and after captopril administration in patients with congestive heart failure due to idiopathic dilated cardiomyopathy. Am J Cardiol 1986; 58:300–3.
73. Rouse D, Dalmeida W, Williamson FC, et al. Captopril inhibits the hydro-osmotic effect of ADH in the cortical collecting tubule. Kidney Int 1987; 32:845–50.
74. Schrier RW, Gross P, Gheorghiade M, et al. Tolvaptan, a selective oral vasopressin V2-receptor antagonist, for hyponatremia. N Engl J Med 2006; 355:2099–112.

18

The Kidney: A Target Organ of Excessive Dietary Salt Intake

Albert Mimran and Jean Ribstein
Department of Medicine, Hospital Lapeyronie, Montpellier, France

INTRODUCTION

In 1904, Leo Ambard, who was credited with the first documentation of a correlation between blood pressure (BP) and salt intake, was in fact searching for the potential antihypertensive effect of protein restriction in patients with presumably "renal" hypertension (1). Forty years later, Walter Kempner, who demonstrated that progressive renal function deterioration may be arrested in patients with malignant hypertension kept on a diet extremely poor in sodium, was convinced that the main characteristic of his rice diet was its low protein content (2). Although it is possible that changes in protein as well as caloric intake are confounding factors in the assessment of the dietary approach of kidney disease, it is difficult to understand why nephrologists have paid so little attention to long-term changes in sodium intake as a factor susceptible to modify the progression of renal damage.

As reviewed elsewhere in this book, salt intake is correlated, albeit weakly, with BP both within and between populations. Nevertheless, in essential hypertension (EH), salt intake may be correlated even more closely with target organ damage—i.e., left ventricular hypertrophy or microalbuminuria—than the BP level itself (3). This suggests that dietary salt may modulate the impact of systemic pressure, the main determinant of organ damage in hypertension. It is a pity, and not easily understandable, that the public health debate on dietary sodium has focused on the effect of salt on the BP in the general population or more narrowly in a subgroup called "salt-sensitive" subjects, i.e., those in whom extreme changes in sodium intake are associated with an increase in BP.

To date, the literature devoted to the influence of long-term changes in sodium intake on renal abnormalities and progression of renal disease, independently of BP, is very poor. Regarding target organs of hypertension, it was found in a small group of patients with left ventricular hypertrophy that a 12-month reduction in sodium intake (by approximately 45%) was associated with a decrease in both systolic BP (by 10%) and left ventricular mass (by 9%) (4).

The consequences of excessive salt intake on cardiovascular and renal parameters have long been ascribed to the occurrence of hypervolemia, and secondary elevation of resistance through "whole-body autoregulation." However, in recent years, the interest in dietary salt has been stimulated by experimental data suggesting that an high salt (HS) intake is needed to "turn on" the deleterious cardiovascular and renal effects of aldosterone, as well as angiotensin and presumably other factors (5–7).

LACK OF DATA ON THE INFLUENCE OF SALT INTAKE ON THE PROGRESSION OF RENAL FAILURE

Most textbooks consider positive sodium balance, and thus indirectly excess dietary salt, as a key factor for the high BP usually associated with chronic kidney disease (CKD). However, no study of acceptable duration has assessed the relationship between dietary salt and renal events, thus precluding any recommendation regarding manipulation of sodium diet as a mean of nephroprotection.

In a retrospective analysis of progression of CKD of both glomerular and tubulointerstitial origin, 57 subjects with baseline creatinine clearance between 10 and 40 mL/min were divided into two groups on the basis of consistent urine sodium excretion rates (considered as the most reliable estimate of sodium intake) of either less than 100 (LS, low salt) or more than 200 mmol/day (HS). The rate of decline in creatinine clearance over a 43-month period was twofold greater in the HS than in the LS group (-0.51 ± 0.09 vs. -0.25 ± 0.07 mL/min per month, $p < 0.05$). Proteinuria increased in the HS group and decreased in the LS group. Of note, the patients' protein intake paralleled their sodium intake, and mean BP as well as its evolution during the observation period did not differ between groups (8). In another small retrospective survey, no correlation was found between urinary sodium excretion and the decline of renal function within the two-year period preceding dialysis treatment (9).

Diuretics are widely used in renal patients in order to treat the volume component of hypertension, and thus control BP. However, the nephroprotective potential of diuretic treatment has not been assessed, and experimental data suggest that it may differ from that of sodium restriction (10). In addition, in a retrospective study of 200 patients followed up for more than six months and maintained on antihypertensive treatment by various agents (except inhibitors of the renin–angiotensin system), diuretics were used as a coprescription in 87%, and as a sole therapy in 14% of the population. The slope of the reciprocal of serum creatinine was steeper in patients on diuretics than those receiving other antihypertensive medication, whereas diastolic BP was similar in both groups (11).

Although no conclusive clinical trial was performed, some studies of small duration suggest that excessive salt intake may induce potentially detrimental effects on renal hemodynamics and function, as reviewed in the following paragraphs.

SHORT-TERM EFFECTS OF SALT INTAKE ON RENAL HEMODYNAMICS AND FUNCTION

In 10 normal and 12 essential hypertensive subjects, an increase in sodium intake from 50 to 180 and 380 mmol/day for four days each resulted in a stepwise increment of glomerular filtration rate (GFR) from 82 to 88 to 93 and from 76 to 80 to 86 mL/min per 1.73 m^2 in normal and EH subjects, respectively. This was associated with expansion of the extracellular fluid volume, but no change in BP (12). Some authors observed a similar salt-induced increase of GFR in patients with mild EH, independent of salt sensitivity and changes in BP (13). In contrast, others reported that GFR only increased in normotensive

(14) and hypertensive (15) salt-sensitive subjects. Interestingly, in the later study, the increase in GFR was not associated with any change in effective renal plasma flow (ERPF), thus resulting in a consistent rise in the filtration fraction (FF) probably suggestive of an increase in intraglomerular pressure; no change in either parameter was observed in salt-resistant patients (15).

In a small group of mostly African-American EH studied on sodium diets of 20 and 200 mmol/day for nine days each, GFR remained unchanged during high sodium intake, whereas ERPF decreased in salt-sensitive and increased in salt-resistant patients. Renal vascular resistance and FF—as well as glomerular pressure calculated by Gomez's equations—rose in salt-sensitive and fell in salt-resistant patients on the HS diet (16).

The larger fall of BP usually associated with acute reduction in salt intake in EH compared with normotensive subjects may be due to a less responsive renin–angiotensin–aldosterone system (17). In a crossover study assessing the effect of three-week periods of low (50 mmol/day) and high (200 mmol/day) sodium intake on renal function, the rise in ERPF associated with the high-sodium diet was blunted in EH patients. In fact, the change in ERPF was inversely correlated, and the change in FF positively correlated with the change in BP, thus suggesting that the sensitivity of BP to excessive salt intake was accompanied by a defect in sodium-induced renal vasodilation in EH (18). Other reported on a subgroup of EH called "non-modulators" in whom the renal vasodilating response to salt loading was abolished—and restored by angiotensin suppression (19).

In diabetic patients, somehow heterogeneous findings were obtained. In response to HS, a parallel increase in GFR (measured as creatinine clearance) and BP during HS intake was observed in normoalbuminuric and albuminuric normotensive type 2 diabetics (20). HS intake was associated with an increase in GFR in the absence of any rise of BP in patients with advanced albuminuria (21). No significant change in GFR occurred in hypertensive type 2 diabetics (22). In patients with glomerulonephritis with or without renal failure, restricting sodium intake from 235 to 35 mmol/day resulted in a decrease in BP, ERPF, and GFR—and an increase in FF (23).

Taken together, these data suggest that in some individuals, HS intake may increase GFR and induce detrimental effects on glomerular hemodynamics, i.e., increased FF and presumably intraglomerular pressure. Underlying mechanisms may include vasoconstriction of the efferent glomerular arterioles due to the inappropriate activation of neuroendocrine systems, or defective vasodilator systems. Several mechanisms may concur to alter the autoregulatory response of the afferent glomerular tone in response to HS intake and increased systemic pressure. It was speculated that in African-Americans prone to develop hypertensive renal injury, habitual consumption of an HS diet may result in tubular hyperperfusion of the macula densa, a rightward and upward resetting of the operating point for the tubuloglomerular feedback, an imbalance between the afferent and efferent vascular tones, a rise in the glomerular capillary hydraulic pressure, and thus hyperfiltration (24).

CLINICAL STUDIES ON THE INFLUENCE OF SALT INTAKE ON URINARY ALBUMIN EXCRETION

In 1992, DuCailar et al. reported on a positive relationship between 24-hour natriuresis and left ventricular mass in a rather small number of normotensive and hypertensive subjects (25). This cross-sectional study was extended in 839 never-treated, healthy subjects with a wide range of BP (3). Sodium intake was higher in men than women, and positively correlated with body mass index (BMI), but not influenced by age. As shown in Table 1,

Table 1 Relationship Between Urinary Sodium Excretion and Target Organ Damage in Hypertension: Results of 450

	Quintiles of natriuresis				
	1	2	3	4	5
UnaV (mmol/24 hr)	36–112	113–150	151–184	185–222	223–470
SAP (mmHg)	158	159	159	160	161
Age (yr)	44	45	47	45	45
MA+ (%)	14.6	26.4	28.9	24.2	41.2
LVH+ (%)	21	20	27	28	36
MA+ LVH+ (%)	10.5	11.1	9.0	19.6	27.7

Abbreviations: LVH, left ventricular hypertrophy defined as $\geq$125 g/m^2; MA, microalbuminuria defined as urinary albumin/creatinine $\geq$1.6 mg/mmol; SAP, systolic arterial pressure.

when men with never-treated EH were analyzed separately, it was found that the prevalence of left ventricular hypertrophy and microalbuminuria was markedly influenced by sodium intake independently of systolic arterial BP which was similar across the five quintiles of sodium intake. Interestingly, the prevalence of patients with combined microalbuminuria and left ventricular hypertrophy was strikingly augmented above a sodium intake higher than 12 g of sodium chloride, NaCl, per day. It would be interesting to study the renal outcome of patients with EH associated with microalbuminuria alone, left ventricular hypertrophy alone, or both, according to sodium intake.

These results were confirmed in a cross-sectional, population-based study of 7850 subjects aged 28 to 75 years (26). In Groningen (26) as well as Montpellier (3), subjects with a higher BMI had higher albuminuria than subjects with a lower BMI at any given level of sodium intake. Such an interaction between salt intake and obesity is consistent with epidemiological observations from the National Health and Nutrition Examination Survey, and the African-American Study of Kidney Disease and Hypertension trial. When the Groningen subjects were studied after a follow-up period of six years, the prevalence of an estimated creatinine clearance lower than 60 mL/min was higher in those with the highest level of albuminuria at baseline (27), thus suggesting that at the population level, albuminuria may be a predictor, among others, of the evolution of renal function.

When 22 essential hypertensive patients were placed on a low- and a high-sodium diet (20 vs. 250 mmol/day), albuminuria was higher at baseline in salt-sensitive than in salt-resistant patients, accentuated by high sodium intake, and correlated with the calculated glomerular capillary pressure (28,29).

In normotensive type 2 diabetics receiving either 80 or 200 mmol sodium/day, the HS diet resulted in a significant increase in albuminuria together with increased GFR (20). In normoalbuminuric type 2 diabetics, switching from a LS to a HS diet did not alter the fractional clearance of the anionic albumin whereas it increased that of the electrically neutral IgG, thus suggesting that the charge selectivity of the glomerular barrier was unaltered (21). In microalbuminuric patients in contrast, the fractional clearances of IgG and albumin rose equally, indicating some neutralization of the pore charge and a shift of the pore size toward a larger diameter. These effects were independent from changes in BP.

In 12 patients with nephrotic range proteinuria (3.2–10.5 g/day), the antiproteinuric effect of the angiotensin-converting enzyme (ACE) inhibitor lisinopril was abolished by increasing salt intake from 50 to 200 mmol/day, and recovered after reinstitution of sodium restriction (30). As shown in Figure 1, administration of hydrochlorothiazide during the HS diet was able to overcome the blunting of the antiproteinuric effect of ACE

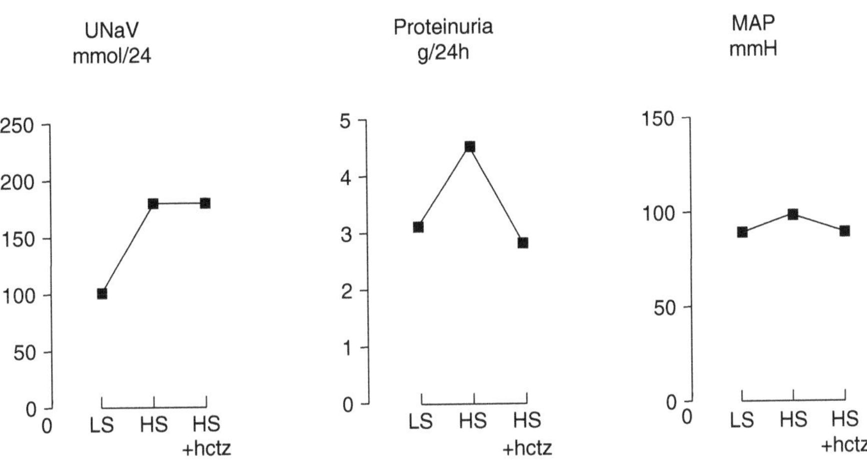

Figure 1 The blunting of the antiproteinuric efficacy of ACEI by high sodium intake (HS) can be restored by hydrochlorothiazide: seven proteinuric patients on chronic ACEI and advised to lower sodium intake to 50 mmol/day (LS), were switched to a high-sodium diet (200 mmol/day), then treated by hydrochlorothiazide 50 mg/day (hctz); median value of creatinine clearance 75 mL/min. *Abbreviations*: ACEI, angiotensin-converting enzyme inhibition; HS, high salt; LS, low salt; MAP, mean arterial pressure. *Source*: Adapted from Ref. 31.

inhibition (31), thus providing a therapeutic alternative for patients poorly compliant to sodium restriction. In type 2 diabetic patients with nephropathy, high sodium intake also impaired the urinary albumin-decreasing effects of diltiazem (32). Thus, a low-sodium diet should be implemented in order to maximize the antiproteinuric effect of most antihypertensive agents, especially the blockers of the renin–angiotensin system.

INAPPROPRIATE SALT STATUS AND THE DELETERIOUS EFFECT OF ALDOSTERONE, CLINICAL AND EXPERIMENTAL

In patients with congestive heart failure, hypertension or diabetic nephropathy, aldosterone breakthrough/escape has been defined as unchanged or increasing level of aldosterone during continued treatment by ACE inhibitors or angiotensin II receptor antagonists. Urinary albumin excretion (33), as well as the rate of decline of GFR (34), was higher in patients with aldosterone escape when compared with those with no escape. It is of interest that in young normotensive and mild hypertensive subjects, urinary aldosterone excretion after an increase in sodium intake by 6 g/day—but not at baseline—was correlated with left ventricular hypertrophy (35). Albuminuria was higher in patients with primary aldosteronism than in EH patients matched for BP levels, and surgical correction was followed by a decrease in GFR, thus suggesting that primary aldosteronism is associated with a relative hyperfiltration (36). In addition, dietary sodium restriction restored a normal nocturnal dipping of BP in patients with primary aldosteronism (37). These observations suggest that aldosterone probably acting in concert with salt status may contribute to the development of target organ damage in various pathological situations.

Far more direct data were obtained in the experimental setting. Almost 25 years ago, it was demonstrated that long-term mineralocorticoid administration resulted in myocardial fibrosis, both interstitial and perivascular, in uninephrectomized rats maintained on high sodium intake (5,6). Neither hypertension nor fibrosis developed when mineralocorticoid treatment was given in animals on a LS diet, even though plasma aldosterone levels were higher in LS when compared with HS diet (5). It later appeared that blood vessels, not cardiac fibroblasts, are the primary target of mineralocorticoids in the presence of salt, and that an excess of salt is needed for activation of inflammatory cells and expression of genes of proinflammatory mediators. These observations were extended to different rat models of hypertension, and the necessity of saline coadministration with angiotensin II as well as aldosterone in order to induce renal lesions was established (7).

THE TOXIC EFFECT OF SALT IN EXPERIMENTAL ANIMALS

In 1958, Meneeley and Ball (38) tested the hypothesis that "excess salt in the diet might manifest itself as a source of degenerative disease, nature unspecified." They observed in rats that, when compared with a control diet containing 0.15% NaCl, a low-sodium diet (0.01% NaCl) was associated with anorexia, diminished growth and survival rate. Progressive increase in sodium content from 0.15% up to 9.8% was associated with a progressive decrease in weight gain and above 7% by "a curious nephrosis-like syndrome" characterized by abrupt onset edema followed by a rapid fall of weight and death. In addition, arterial BP progressively increased, starting at 2.8%, and reaching an increase of 30 mmHg after nine months on the highest level of sodium intake. Moreover, a continuous increase in serum cholesterol was detected. Although serum concentration of urea as well as proteinuria was not measured, heart and kidneys were enlarged and severe arteriolar renal lesions were found. Addition of potassium chloride to the diet was associated with improved survival in rats on the highest sodium. These experiments did not allow to draw conclusions about the BP or non-BP–related renal and cardiac consequences of excessive dietary sodium.

In various studies of extreme changes in sodium intake (to a maximum of 9% NaCl as drinking fluid in rats), no effect on renal function was detected, probably due to the short duration of application of the salt regimen. In contrast, it was recently observed that feeding Sprague–Dawley rats for five months after weaning with an HS (8% NaCl) chow was associated with a consistent (threefold) increase in albuminuria and left ventricular mass, but no significant effect on BP, when compared with rats maintained on 0.8% and 2% NaCl diet. Measurement of renal function using radioactive markers showed a decrease of GFR by 40%, a less marked decrease in ERPF, and consequently a consistent reduction in FF when compared with rats on a normal (0.8% NaCl) or moderately high (2% NaCl) sodium intake. Chronic treatment by spironolactone (100 mg/kg per day) for two weeks prior to termination of studies corrected all abnormalities associated with HS intake (39). The rationale for treatment by spironolactone was the finding that a high-sodium diet given for eight weeks resulted in the expected fall in circulating renin and aldosterone (by 50%) whereas the expression of cardiac angiotensin II type 1 (AT_1) receptor and aldosterone synthesis by cardiac tissue doubled (40).

INFLUENCE OF SODIUM INTAKE ON THE PROGRESSION OF RENAL DISEASE IN EXPERIMENTAL MODELS

Experimental studies have shown that a low-sodium diet may prevent renal alterations in several models of hypertension and renal disease, including chronic infusion of angiotensin II (41), inhibition of nitric oxide synthase (42), antithymocyte serum nephritis (43), and allograft nephropathy (44). In Fisher–Lewis rats, an increase in dietary salt intake to 8% NaCl given from week 3 to 16 after orthotopic transplantation rapidly resulted in a sharp increase in albuminuria together with accentuated histological damage, whereas no such damage occurred in rats maintained on a normal sodium diet (1% NaCl) (44).

The effect of dietary salt restriction to approximately one-fifth of the usual intake (resulting in decreased natriuresis from 0.8 to 0.16 mmol per 100 g of body weight/day and no impairment in body growth) was tested in rats subjected to 5/6 renal ablation, the most widely used model of progressive experimental renal disease. Salt restriction started three days before and continued for eight weeks after surgery prevented the progressive increase in BP and proteinuria, whereas the increase in glomerular pressure was not corrected (45). When salt restriction was started four weeks after injury and continued for four additional weeks, the increase in proteinuria and glomerular volume was not observed (46).

When spontaneously hypertensive rats were uninephrectomized at six weeks of age, a low-sodium diet (0.09% NaCl)—but not hydrochlorothiazide—prevented the progressive increase in proteinuria, compensatory kidney growth and glomerulosclerosis observed four months after nephrectomy, without affecting the level of arterial pressure achieved on standard diet (0.45% NaCl) (10).

These results suggest that the renal protective effect of salt restriction may be independent of changes in systemic arterial as well as intraglomerular pressure, in contrast to observations made with pharmacological blockade of the renin–angiotensin system.

Following streptozotocin injection in rats, GFR and ERPF rapidly (within five to seven days) increased by 30% to 40%, together with the development of renal hypertrophy. Renal hyperfiltration was entirely corrected by five to seven days of sodium-deficient diet (3 mmol/kg chow), but to a lesser extent when rats were studied six weeks after streptozotocin (47,48). Drastic dietary sodium restriction (resulting in a natriuresis of 50 μmol/day) for six days resulted in a consistent and "paradoxical" increase in GFR which was accentuated by concomittant administration of the angiotensin II receptor antagonist losartan in the presence of similar blood glucose levels (49).

Long-term salt restriction (0.05% NaCl for 24 weeks) attenuated the progressive rise in albuminuria of diabetic rats, and prevented the development of renal hypertrophy in the presence of a decreased arterial pressure (48).

It is suggested that chronic substantial reduction in sodium intake may have favorable effects on the progression of nephropathy, probably through correction of renal hyperfiltration associated with the early phase of experimental diabetes.

MECHANISMS

Alteration in the Renin–Angiotensin–Aldosterone System

Although a chronic increase in sodium intake is associated with a marked reduction in the circulating level of renin and angiotensin II, no change in cardiac angiotensin II content has been observed when compared with normal sodium intake (50). In addition to the old findings of a potentiation of angiotensin II-induced vasoconstriction, recent studies have demonstrated that a chronic increase in sodium intake is associated with augmented AT_1 receptor mRNA expression and AT_1 receptor density by approximately 60% in vascular tissue (51,52). In contrast, downregulation of angiotensin II type 2 (AT_2) receptors known to have antihypertrophic properties in resistance arteries was reported in response to high dietary sodium intake (53). As previously discussed, excessive dietary sodium is also associated with increased aldosterone synthase CYP11B2 expression and activity in cardiac tissue despite markedly depressed circulating levels of aldosterone (40). A beneficial role of AT_2 receptor stimulation was also documented in the 5/6 renal ablation model (54). These findings may provide some explanation for the renoprotective effect of dietary sodium restriction via regulation of angiotensin receptors (down-regulation of AT_1 receptors combined with upregulation of AT_2 receptors) in experimental models of renal injury.

In 16-week-old stroke-prone spontaneously hypertensive rats, but nor in Wistar–Kyoto controls, sodium loading (drinking 1% saline for 12 days) resulted in an increase in BP and left ventricular weight. A two- to threefold increase in cardiac ACE activity was observed in both strains (55).

In summary, chronic sodium loading is associated with a substantial decrease in circulating renin as well as renin expression in various tissues, no change in tissue content of angiotensin II, and increased expression of AT_1 receptors and aldosterone synthase.

Overproduction of Transforming Growth Factor-β

Transforming growth factor-β (TGF-β) refers to a family of polypeptides with complex effects on organ development, cell growth and differentiation, expression of extracellular matrix proteins, immune responses, angiogenesis and tissue repair. TGF-β1 is considered the most important of the three mammalian isoforms. The role of TGF-β in the fibrotic response to renal injury was demonstrated using TGF-β antibodies in a model of glomerulonephritis. Renal fibrogenesis was inhibited to a maximum of 45% (i.e., to the same extent when compared with the maximum dose of enalapril). Combined treatment by antibodies and enalapril afforded considerably more protection (56).

When a high (8% NaCl)—rather than a normal (1% NaCl)—sodium diet was given from 8 to 16 weeks of age to normotensive Wistar–Kyoto and spontaneously hypertensive rats, a disproportionate (with respect to the modest rise in BP) widespread fibrosis of heart and kidney developed in both strains. Fibrosis was paralleled by overexpression of TGF-β1 in heart and kidney (57). In normal rats, study of the time course of the effect of high-sodium (8%) versus low-sodium (0.3%) diet showed that kidney production of TGF-β1 mRNA as well as urinary TGF-β1 excretion was markedly enhanced as early as one day after the start of the high-sodium diet, persisted during the two-week duration of experiments, and without any elevation of systemic pressure. Of interest, administration of diuretics in rats maintained on high sodium intake had no effect on the excessive production of TGF-β resulting from salt loading (58). Thus, salt reduction might have a non-angiotensin II effect on intrarenal TGF-β production (59).

A close, positive correlation between urinary sodium and TGF-β excretion was observed in 21 hypertensive and albuminuric patients with type 2 diabetes maintained on a liberal sodium diet. However, short-term sodium restriction (from ~220 to ~85 mmol/day for two weeks) failed to reduce urinary TGF-β excretion (60).

Excessive Oxidative Stress

Free radicals, such as reactive oxygen and nitrogen species, are closely related with regards to generation, interaction, and biological effects. Besides their toxic effects, the production of the latest via an interaction of oxidative stress with nitric oxide or its related products will result in nitric oxide deficiency.

An increased plasma concentration of 8-isoprostanes, a widely used marker of oxidative stress, was observed in rats given an HS intake (10% NaCl to drink for two weeks), and BP was decreased by chronic administration of tempol at a dose shown to reduce superoxide level in kidney and vessels (61). Similarly, an HS diet of one-week duration resulted in increased plasma concentration of 8-isoprostanes and enhanced renal production of superoxide related to increased renal expression and activity of NAD(P)H oxidase (62). An increase in cardiac and aortic production of reactive oxygen species was also observed in rats maintained on a high-sodium diet from weaning to five months of age (39). When seven- to eight-week-old Dahl SS/Rapp rats—a model of salt-sensitive hypertension with renal damage—were placed on either a high-sodium (8%) or a low-sodium (0.3%) diet with or without vitamin E and vitamin C for five weeks, antioxidant treatment decreased arterial pressure, improved renal dysfunction and lessened renal injury (63).

Few clinical studies have been devoted to the effect of sodium intake on superoxide generation. It was recently shown that plasma concentration of isoprostanes was consistently increased after acute sodium loading and reduced after salt depletion, only in subjects with salt-sensitive hypertension (64).

It is of interest that a seven-day HS diet (18 g NaCl/day) increased BP and plasma levels of asymmetrical dimethylarginine while it reduced plasma levels of nitric oxide in salt-sensitive, normotensive Chinese adults. In salt-sensitive but not salt-resistant subjects, potassium supplementation blunted sodium-induced alterations of BP, asymmetrical dimethylarginine and nitric oxide (65).

Insulin Resistance

An HS diet (8% NaCl) given to seven-week-old Sprague–Dawley rats for two weeks almost doubled hepatic glucose production and decreased by two-thirds muscular glucose uptake when compared with controls (66). When Wistar rats were given a low-sodium diet from weaning to adulthood (three months of age), a decrease in insulin sensitivity (also measured by the hyperinsulinemic–euglycemic clamp method) was observed when compared with rats maintained on high dietary sodium. Of interest, improvement in insulin sensitivity was observed after a seven-day period of treatment by captopril, but not by losartan (67). Either late or early steps of insulin signaling were altered in these studies. Conflicting results were also obtained in clinical studies, where insulin sensitivity was deteriorated (68) or unchanged (69) by a short period of high sodium intake. It appears that insulin resistance and salt sensitivity frequently coexist, and it is likely that activation of the sympathetic nervous and renin–angiotensin systems may play a critical role in both syndromes.

Interestingly, several of these putative pathophysiological mechanisms, including inadequate suppression of the renin–angiotensin system, nitric oxide deficiency, and insulin resistance, have been documented even in the earliest stage of renal dysfunction.

Figure 2 summarizes the various mechanisms relating excessive salt intake to target organ damage independently of BP. Some of these mechanisms may result in specific drug therapy. It is presently well accepted that inhibitors of the renin–angiotensin system are protective, as suggested by long-term studies conducted in patients with diabetic nephropathy. The use of aldosterone antagonists is presently under investigation with favorable effects on proteinuria when given on top of renin–angiotensin blockers. Nevertheless, the risk of hyperkalemia makes these drugs difficult to use when renal function is impaired. The role of superoxide radicals, which may result from the effects of angiotensin II or aldosterone, clearly needs to be addressed.

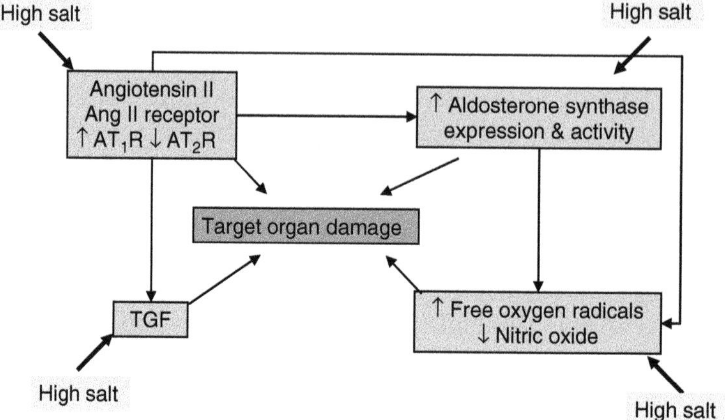

Figure 2 Mechanisms underlying the deleterious cardiorenal effects of excessive dietary sodium. *Abbreviation*: TGF, transforming growth factor.

CONCLUSIONS

A number of experimental data and a handful of clinical results point to a detrimental effect of excessive salt intake on the kidney considered as a target organ of hypertension rather independently of the level of BP itself. Reduction in dietary salt intake affords impressive renal protection in several experimental models of renal disease. In humans, increasing salt intake invariably increases urinary albumin excretion and to a variable extent GFR. The full explanation of the potentiation by excessive salt intake of pathophysiological mechanisms implying angiotensin II and aldosterone is lacking. Whether the possibility that dietary salt is a risk factor for progressive renal damage is restricted to specific genotypes in humans is presently unknown.

This chapter allowed us to review convincing experimental evidence that high-sodium diet may be detrimental to the diseased kidney. The need of clear-cut recommendations in the dietary approach to CKD calls for further pertinent studies in humans, despite the continuous "negationism" of those who do not support salt reduction and the marketing force of the food industry. It is now time to think as rational scientists instead of putting junk science into the debate (70). Renal failure is a well-known state of extracellular volume expansion and at least for this reason, reduction in sodium intake must be proposed as adjunctive antihypertensive therapy in this context. We have produced some evidence for additional effects of excessive dietary salt. At the moment, it is reasonable to measure 24-hour urinary sodium excretion rather than rely on dietary recall in patients with hypertension as well as any degree of renal dysfunction, and to counsel subjects with values in the highest range to cut down their sodium consumption.

REFERENCES

1. Ambard L, Beaujard E. Causes de l'hypertension artérielle. Arch Gen Med 1904; 1:520–33.
2. Kempner W. Treatment of kidney disease and hypertensive vascular disease with rice diet. NC Med J 1944; 5:125–33.
3. Du Cailar G, Ribstein J, Mimran A. Dietary sodium and target organ damage in essential hypertension. Am J Hypertens 2002; 15:222–9.

4. Jula AM, Karanko HM. Effects on left ventricular hypertrophy of long-term nonpharmacological treatment with sodium restriction in mild-to-moderate essential hypertension. Circulation 1994; 89:1023–31.
5. Brilla CG, Weber KT. Mineralocorticoid excess, dietary sodium, and myocardial fibrosis. J Lab Clin Med 1992; 20:893–901.
6. Young M, Fullerton M, Dilley R, et al. Mineralocorticoids, hypertension, and cardiac fibrosis. J Clin Invest 1994; 93:2578–83.
7. Rocha R, Stier CT, Kifor I, et al. Aldosterone: a mediator of myocardial necrosis and renal arteriopathy. Endocrinology 2000; 141:3871–8.
8. Cianciaruso B, Bellizzi V, Minutolo R, et al. Salt intake and renal outcome in patients with progressive renal disease. Miner Electrolyte Metab 1998; 24:296–301.
9. Mazouz H, Kacso I, Ghazali A, et al. Risk factors of renal failure progression two years prior to dialysis. Clin Nephrol 1999; 51:355–66.
10. Benstein JA, Feiner HD, Parker M, et al. Superiority of salt restriction over diuretics in reducing renal hypertrophy and injury in uninephrectomized SHR. Am J Physiol 1990; 258:F1675–81.
11. Brazy PC, Fitzwilliam JF. Progressive renal disease: role of race and antihypertensive medications. Kidney Int 1990; 37:1113–9.
12. Bruun NE, Skott P, Damkjaer Nielsen M, et al. Normal renal tubular response to changes of sodium intake in hypertensive man. J Hypertens 1990; 8:219–27.
13. Mallamaci F, Leonardis D, Bellizzi V, et al. Does high salt intake cause hyperfiltration in patients with essential hypertension? J Hum Hypertens 1996; 10:157–61.
14. Barba G, Cappuccio FP, Russo L, et al. Renal function and blood pressure response to dietary salt restriction in normotensive men. Hypertension 1996; 27:1160–4.
15. Weir MR, Dengel DR, Behrens MT, et al. Salt-induced increases in systolic blood pressure affect renal hemodynamics and proteinuria. Hypertension 1995; 25:1339–44.
16. Campese VM, Parise M, Karubian F, Bigazzi R. Abnormal renal hemodynamics in black salt-sensitive patients with hypertension. Hypertension 1991; 18:805–12.
17. He FJ, Markandu ND, MaGregor GA. Importance of the renin system for determining blood pressure fall with acute salt restriction in hypertensive and normotensive whites. Hypertension 2001; 38:321–5.
18. van Paassen P, de Zeeuw D, Navis G, de Jong PE. Does the renin–angiotensin system determine the renal and systemic hemodynamic response to sodium in patients with essential hypertension? Hypertension 1996; 27:202–8.
19. Shoback DM, Williams GH, Moore TJ, Dluhy RG, Podolsky S, Hollenberg NK. Defect in the sodium-modulated tissue responsiveness to angiotensin II in essential hypertension. J Clin Invest 1983; 72:2115–24.
20. Imanishi M, Yoshioka K, Okumura M, et al. Sodium sensitivity related to albuminuria appearing before hypertension in type 2 diabetic patients. Diabetes Care 2001; 24:111–6.
21. Yoshioka K, Imanishi M, Konishi Y, et al. Glomerular charge and size selectivity assessed by changes in salt intake in type 2 diabetic patients. Diabetes Care 1998; 21:482–6.
22. Campese VM, Wurgaft A, Safa M, et al. Dietary salt intake, blood pressure and the kidney in hypertensive patients with non-insulin dependent diabetes mellitus. J Nephrol 1998; 11:289–95.
23. Cianciaruso B, Bellizzi V, Minutolo R, et al. Renal adaptation to dietary sodium restriction in moderate renal failure resulting from chronic glomerular disease. J Am Soc Nephrol 1996; 7:306–11.
24. Aviv A, Hollenberg NK, Weder AB. Sodium glomerulopathy: tubuloglomerular feedback and renal injury in African Americans. Kidney Int 2004; 65:361–8.
25. Du Cailar G, Ribstein J, Daures JP, Mimran A. Sodium and left ventricular mass in untreated hypertensive and normotensive subjects. Am J Physiol 1992; 263:H177–81.
26. Verhave JC, Hillege HL, Burgerhof JG, et al. Sodium intake affects urinary albumin excretion especially in overweight subjects. J Intern Med 2004; 256:324–30.

27. Verhave JC, Gansevoort RT, Hillege HL, Bakker SJL, de Zeeuw D, de Jong PE. Kidney Int 2004; 66(Suppl. 92):s18–21.
28. Bigazzi R, Bianchi S, Baldari D, et al. Microalbuminuria in salt-sensitive patients. A marker for renal and cardiovascular risk factors. Hypertension 1994; 23:195–9.
29. Weir MR. Salt intake and hypertensive renal injury in African-Americans. A therapeutic perspective. Am J Hypertens 1995; 8:635–44.
30. Heeg JE, de Jong PE, van der Hem GK, et al. Efficacy and variability of the antiproteinuric effect of ACE inhibition by lisinopril. Kidney Int 1989; 36:272–9.
31. Buter H, Hemmelder MH, Navis G, et al. The blunting of the antiproteinuric efficacy of ACE inhibition by high sodium intake can be restored by hydrochlorothiazide. Nephrol Dial Transplant 1998; 13:1682–5.
32. Bakris GL, Weir MR. Salt intake and reductions in arterial pressure and proteinuria. Is there a direct link? Am J Hypertens 1996; 9(12 pt 2):200S–6.
33. Sato A, Saruta T. Aldosterone breakthrough during angiotensin-converting enzyme inhibitor therapy. Am J Hypertens 2003; 16:781–8.
34. Schjoedt KJ, Andersen S, Rossing P, et al. Aldosterone escape during blockade of the renin–angiotensin–aldosterone system in diabetic nephropathy is associated with enhanced decline in glomerular filtration rate. Diabetologia 2004; 47:1936–9.
35. Schlaich MP, Schobel HP, Hilgers K, et al. Impact of aldosterone on left ventricular structure and function in young normotensive and mild hypertensive subjects. Am J Cardiol 2000; 85:1199–206.
36. Ribstein J, du Cailar G, Fesler P, Mimran A. Relative glomerular hyperfiltration in primary aldosteronism. J Am Soc Nephrol 2005; 16:1320–5.
37. Uzu T, Nishimura M, Fujii T, et al. Changes in the circadian rhythm of blood pressure in primary aldosteronism in response to dietary sodium restriction and adrenalectomy. J Hypertens 1998; 16:1745–8.
38. Meneely GR, Ball CO. Experimental epidemiology of chronic sodium chloride toxicity and the protective effect of potassium chloride. Am J Med 1958; 25:713–25.
39. Cordaillat M, Rugale C, Casellas D, et al. Cardiorenal abnormalities associated with high sodium intake: correction by spironolactone in rats. Am J Physiol 2005; 289:R1137–43.
40. Takeda Y, Yoneda T, Demura M, et al. Sodium-induced cardiac aldosterone synthesis causes cardiac hypertrophy. Endocrinology 2000; 141:1901–4.
41. Rugale C, Delbosc S, Cristol JP, et al. Sodium restriction prevents cardiac hypertrophy and oxidative stress in angiotensin II hypertension. Am J Physiol 2003; 284:H1744–50.
42. Fujihara CK, Michellazzo SM, de Nucci G, et al. Sodium excess aggravates hypertension and renal parenchymal injury in rats with chronic NO inhibition. Am J Physiol 1994; 266:F697–705.
43. Suzuki H, Yamamoto T, Ikegaya N, et al. Dietary salt intake modulates progression of anti-thymocyte serum nephritis through alteration of glomerular angiotensin II receptor expression. Am J Physiol 2004; 286:F267–77.
44. Sanders PW, Gibbs CL, Akhi KM, et al. Increased dietary salt accelerates chronic allograft nephropathy in rats. Kidney Int 2001; 59:1149–57.
45. Lax DS, Benstein JA, Tolbert E, et al. Effects of salt restriction on renal growth and glomerular injury in rats with remnant kidneys. Kidney Int 1992; 41:1527–34.
46. Dworkin LD, Benstein JA, Tolbert E, et al. Salt restriction inhibits renal growth and stabilizes injury in rats with established renal disease. J Am Soc Nephrol 1996; 7:437–42.
47. Bank N, Lahorra G, Aynedjian HS, et al. Sodium restriction corrects hyperfiltration of diabetes. Am J Physiol 1988; 254:F668–76.
48. Allen TJ, Waldron MJ, Casley D, et al. Salt restriction reduces hyperfiltration, renal enlargement, and albuminuria in experimental diabetes. Diabetes 1997; 46:19–24.
49. Vallon V, Wead LM, Blantz RC. Renal hemodynamics and plasma and kidney angiotensin II in established diabetes mellitus in rats: effect of sodium and salt restriction. J Am Soc Nephrol 1995; 5:1761–7.

50. Leenen FH, Yuan B. Dietary-sodium-induced cardiac remodeling in spontaneously hypertensive rat versus Wistar–Kyoto rat. J Hypertens 1998; 16:885–92.
51. Nickenig G, Strehlow K, Roeling J, et al. Salt induces vascular AT1 receptor overexpression in vitro and in vivo. Hypertension 1998; 31:1272–7.
52. Wang DH, Du Y, Yao A, et al. Regulation of type 1 angiotensin II receptor and its subtype gene expression in kidney by sodium loading and angiotensin II infusion. J Hypertens 1996; 14:1409–15.
53. Gonzalez M, Lobos L, Castillo F, et al. High-salt diet inhibits expression of angiotensin type 2 receptor in resistance arteries. Hypertension 2005; 45:853–9.
54. Hashimoto N, Maeshima Y, Satoh M, et al. Overexpression of angiotensin type 2 receptor ameliorates glomerular injury in a mouse remnant kidney model. Am J Physiol 2004; 286:F516–25.
55. Kreutz R, Fernandez-Alfonso MS, Liu Y, et al. Induction of cardiac angiotensin I-converting enzyme with dietary NaCl-loading in genetically hypertensive and normotensive rats. J Mol Med 1995; 73:243–8.
56. Yu L, Border WA, Anderson I, et al. Combining TGF-beta inhibition and angiotensin II blockade results in enhanced antifibrotic effect. Kidney Int 2004; 66:1774–84.
57. Yu HC, Burrell LM, Black MJ, et al. Salt induces myocardial and renal fibrosis in normotensive and hypertensive rats. Circulation 1998; 98:2621–8.
58. Ying WZ, Sanders PW. Dietary salt modulates renal production of transforming growth factor-beta in rats. Am J Physiol 1998; 274:F635–41.
59. Sanders PW. Salt intake, endothelial cell signaling, and progression of kidney disease. Hypertension 2004; 43:142–6.
60. Houlihan CA, Akdeniz A, Tsalamandris C, et al. Urinary transforming growth factor-β excretion in patients with hypertension, type 2 diabetes, and elevated albumin excretion rate: effects of angiotensin receptor blockade and sodium restriction. Diabetes Care 2002; 25:1072–7.
61. Williams JM, Pollock JS, Pollock DM. Arterial pressure response to the antioxidant tempol and ETB receptor blockade in rats on a high-salt diet. Hypertension 2004; 44:770–5.
62. Kitiyakara C, Chabrashvili T, Chen Y, et al. Salt intake, oxidative stress, and renal expression of NADPH oxidase and superoxide dismutase. J Am Soc Nephrol 2003; 14:2775–82.
63. Tian N, Thrasher KD, Gundy PD, et al. Antioxidant treatment prevents renal damage and dysfunction and reduces arterial pressure in salt-sensitive hypertension. Hypertension 2005; 45:934–9.
64. Laffer CL, Bolterman RJ, Romero JC, et al. Effect of salt on isoprostanes in salt-sensitive essential hypertension. Hypertension 2006; 47:434–40.
65. Fang Y, Mu JJ, He LC, Wang SC, Liu ZQ. Salt loading on plasma asymmetrical dimethylarginine and the protective role of potassium supplement in normotensive salt-sensitive asians. Hypertension 2006; 48:724–9.
66. Ogihara T, Asano T, Ando K, et al. Insulin resistance with enhanced insulin signaling in high-salt diet-fed rats. Diabetes 2001; 50:573–83.
67. Prada P, Okamoto MM, Furukawa LN, et al. High- or low-salt diet from weaning to adulthood: effect on insulin sensitivity in Wistar rats. Hypertension 2000; 35(1 Pt 2):424–9.
68. Donovan DS, Solomon CG, Seely EW, et al. Effect of sodium intake on insulin sensitivity. Am J Physiol 1993; 264:E730–4.
69. Fliser D, Fode P, Arnold U, et al. The effect of dietary salt on insulin sensitivity. Eur J Clin Invest 1995; 25:39–43.
70. Al-Awqati Q. Evidence-based politics of salt and blood pressure. Kidney Int 2006; 69:1707–8.

19
Sodium Balance in the Metabolic Syndrome and Diabetes

Anne Zanchi
Division of Nephrology, Department of Medicine, Centre Hospitalier Universitaire Vaudois and University of Lausanne, Lausanne, Switzerland

INTRODUCTION

The clustering of high blood pressure (BP), abdominal adiposity, dyslipidemia, impaired glucose tolerance (IGT) or diabetes was originally identified by Reaven and named the metabolic syndrome (1). In 1998, the World Health Organization (WHO) published a definition of the metabolic syndrome, which included insulin resistance as a required component of the syndrome in addition to two of the following three features: abdominal obesity, dyslipidemia, and high BP. The WHO criteria requires special testing of glucose status, which is impractical during routine clinical assessment [impaired fasting glucose (fasting plasma glucose $\geq$6.1 mmol/L or 110 mg/dL)] or IGT (plasma glucose after an oral glucose tolerance test $\geq$11.1 mmol/dL or 200 mg/dL) or hyperinsulinemia (defined as the upper quartile in a non diabetic population). In 2001, guidelines from the adult treatment panel (ATP) III defined the metabolic syndrome as the presence of at least three of the following traits: abdominal obesity (defined as a waist circumference in men >40 inches (102 cm) and in women >35 inches (88 cm); serum triglycerides $\geq$150 mg/dL (1.7 mmol/L); serum high-density lipoprotein cholesterol <40 mg/dL (1 mmol/L) in men and <50 mg/dL (1.3 mmol/L) in women; blood pressure $\geq$130/85 mmHg; and fasting plasma glucose (FPG) $\geq$110 mg/dL (6.1 mmol/L). In order to unify the definitions of the metabolic syndrome worldwide, the International Diabetes Foundation proposed in 2005 the definition to be used as a universally accepted diagnostic tool to identify patients with the metabolic syndrome in the practice setting (Table 1). Central obesity is a prerequisite for the definition and values vary according to different groups. The epidemiological value of this definition is not yet well studied. Most epidemiological studies have used the ATPIII definition.

Insulin resistance is the source of most if not all of the features of the metabolic syndrome (Fig. 1). The metabolic syndrome is a risk factor for the development of cardiovascular disease and diabetes (2). The prevalence differs among countries and is strongly age-dependent (Fig. 2) (3). Because of the emerging cases of childhood obesity worldwide, more and more young people fulfill the diagnostic criteria of the metabolic syndrome (4). In type 2 diabetic subjects, more than 80% have the metabolic syndrome (Fig. 3) (5). Subjects with diabetes and the metabolic syndrome have the highest prevalence of coronary heart disease (5).

Table 1 International Diabetes Foundation Definition of the Metabolic Syndrome

Central obesity defined as waist circumference ≥94 cm for men or ≥80 cm for women (Europids), ≥90 cm for men or ≥80 cm for women (South Asians), ≥90 cm for men or ≥80 cm for women (Chinese), ≥85 cm for men or ≥90 cm for women (Japanese)
Plus any two of the following four factors:
Raised triglyceride level: ≥150 mg/dL (1.7 mmol/L), or specific treatment for this lipid abnormality
Reduced high-density lipoprotein cholesterol: <40 mg/dL (1.03 mmol/L) in males and <50 mg/dL (1.29 mmol/L) in females, or specific treatment for this lipid abnormality
Raised BP: systolic BP≥130 or diastolic BP≥85 mmHg, or treatment of previously diagnosed hypertension
Raised fasting plasma glucose: ≥100 mg/dL (5.6 mmol/L), or previously diagnosed type 2 diabetes

Abbreviation: BP, blood pressure.

Although the clinical identification of the metabolic syndrome involves routinely measured parameters, clinical studies have also identified the clustering of other parameters known to be associated with cardiovascular risk as elevated C-reactive protein and coagulation markers (plasminogen activator inhibitor type 1—and fibrinogen), small low-density lipoprotein (LDL) particles and elevated apolipoprotein B (6).

Therapeutic strategies in the metabolic syndrome and in type 2 diabetes involve non-pharmacological approaches through diet and exercise and pharmacological approaches including lipid lowering, insulin sensitizing and anti-hypertensive drugs. Therapy directed at each individual feature of the metabolic syndrome in type 2 diabetic patients reduces the risk of cardiovascular and microvascular events by 50% as demonstrated in the Steno study (7).

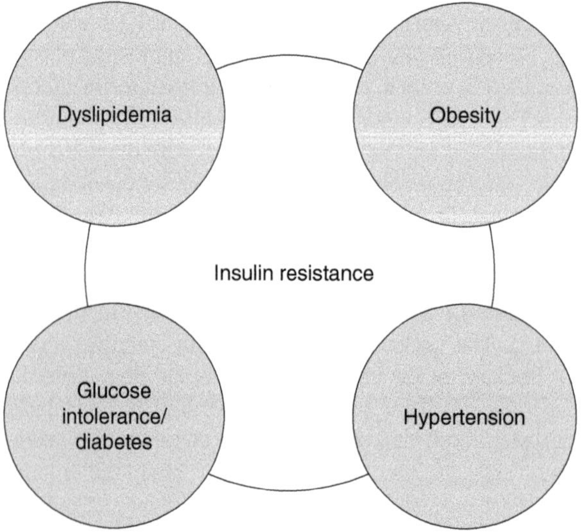

Figure 1 Key features of the metabolic syndrome.

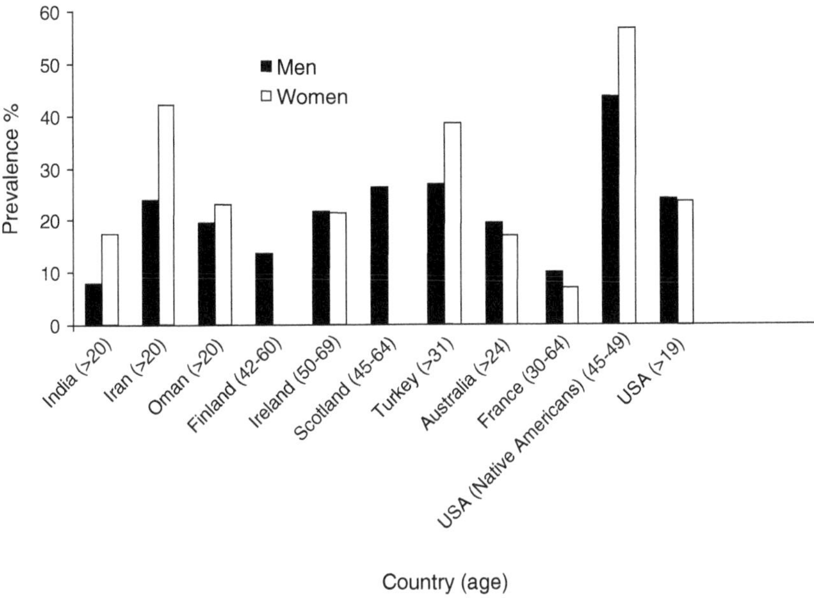

Figure 2 Prevalence of the metabolic syndrome from adult treatment panel III definition. *Source*: From Ref. 3.

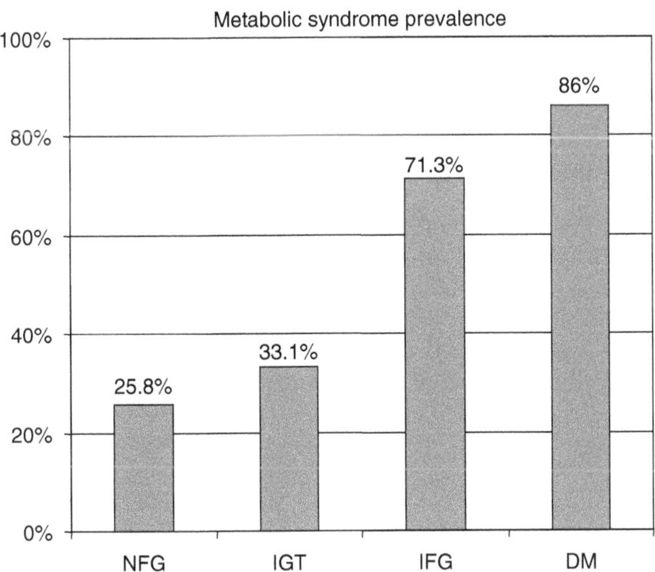

Figure 3 Age-adjusted prevalence of the metabolic syndrome in the U.S. population over 50 years of age categorized by glucose intolerance. *Abbreviations*: DM, diabetes mellitus; IFG, impaired fasting glucose with or without impaired glucose tolerance; IGT, impaired glucose tolerance without impaired fasting glucose; NFG, normal fasting glucose. *Source*: From Ref. 5.

METABOLIC SYNDROME/INSULIN RESISTANCE AND RENAL SODIUM HANDLING

When insulin is given intravenously to healthy volunteers, it reduces sodium excretion and activates the sympathetic nervous system (8–10). Experimental studies show that insulin infusion causes a transient decline in sodium excretion (11), activates renal sodium reabsorption at the proximal tubule (12), the distal tubule (13,14) and loop of Henle (15).

Subjects with insulin resistance have compensatory hyperinsulinemia to counter-balance the decreased sensitivity to insulin. Although the effects of insulin are impaired in the skeletal muscle, the adipose cell and the liver, there does not appear to be an alteration of the renal sodium retaining capacities of insulin nor of the insulin induced activation of the sympathetic nervous system (16,17). Experimental studies show that during a high sodium diet, the kidney is normally able to downregulate the expression of the insulin receptor (18), thus limiting the insulin induced sodium retention in a state of volume expansion. This mechanism is in fact lost in insulin resistant salt-sensitive rats (19). Thus, the anti-natriuretic effects of insulin are preserved during hyperinsulinemia which may contribute to maintaining higher BP levels in insulin resistant subjects.

There is evidence that insulin resistance increases sodium retention through the complex interplay of various other mechanisms as detailed in the table below (Table 2) (20–23). For example, hypertensive subjects have an increased sensitivity to angiotensin II that is tightly correlated to the glucose disposal rate and insulin resistance indexes (24). Studies have shown that with hyperinsulinemia, the angiotensin II induced release of aldosterone is enhanced and may contribute to sodium retention in insulin resistant states (25). Some studies suggest that insulin mediated anti-natriuresis depends on insulin-induced hypokalemia (26) but others do not (27).

Studies are not able to differentiate the contribution of each of these mechanisms of sodium retention in insulin resistant subjects. Indeed, an increase in insulin levels alone is not sufficient to induce hypertension as patients with chronic hyperinsulinemia due to an insulinoma are not always hypertensive (28). Thus, mechanical, genetic and other humoral factors characteristic of the overweight insulin resistant population play a determinant role in sodium retention.

Renal Sodium Handling in the Metabolic Syndrome: Clinical Studies

Increased tubular sodium reabsorption is generally accepted as one of the crucial steps in the genesis of essential hypertension as well as in the pathogenesis of rare monogenic forms of hypertension (29–34). Sodium retention has also been linked to other features of the metabolic syndrome as central obesity (35), glucose intolerance or diabetes (36). Studies performed in subjects with asymptomatic hyperuricemia and features of the metabolic syndrome suggest that the link between the metabolic syndrome and high serum

Table 2 Mechanisms of Sodium Retention During Insulin Resistance

Activation of the sympathetic nervous system
Increased response to angiotensin II and aldosterone release
Direct effects of insulin on renal tubules
Mechanical effects on the kidney related to obesity
Release of adipocytokines
Altered release of natriuretic factors in obesity
Genetic factors

uric acid levels is due to an increase in uric acid reabsorption at the proximal tubule resulting in an increase in serum uric acid levels (37–40). Since serum uric acid levels are closely and independently associated with the reabsorption of sodium at the proximal tubule, these observations indirectly suggest that proximal sodium reabsorption is indeed increased in the metabolic syndrome.

The proximal tubule is responsible for the reabsorption of 60% to 65% of sodium, thus is the main determinant of sodium and fluid balance (41). Several key mechanisms are involved in proximal sodium reabsorption. The apical sodium–proton antiporter allows the entry of luminal sodium by exchange with protons. Intracellular bicarbonates will eventually increase and be removed via basolateral sodium/bicarbonate cotransport. The sodium–potassium ATPase pump located at the basolateral border of the tubular epithelium will create an electrochemical gradient that provides the energy necessary for return of reabsorbed sodium to the extracellular compartment. Activation of the renin–angiotensin system and the sympathetic nervous system plays an important role in the activation of proximal sodium transport. Any abnormalities resulting in increased proximal sodium re-absorption through these mechanisms may result in elevated BP.

Although increased renal sodium reabsorption is well established in the obese-insulin resistant population, studies examining the site of sodium reabsorption (proximal or distal) are rare. As the metabolic syndrome is associated with an activation of the renin–angiotensin system and the sympathetic nervous system, an increase in proximal sodium reabsorption is likely to occur. With the availability of lithium clearance as a marker of proximal sodium reabsorption, some studies have examined the relationship of proximal sodium reabsorption and features of the metabolic syndrome.

Endogenous Lithium Used as a Marker of Proximal Tubular Function

Fractional excretion of endogenous lithium is used as a marker for sodium handling by the proximal segments of the nephron. Lithium is freely filtered at the glomerulus and reabsorbed in the proximal tubule in parallel with sodium and water. Different studies have validated this method in humans and in rats. For example, after acute increases in BP, there are dynamic changes in the baso-lateral sodium–potassium ATPase activity, which parallel the increase in endogenous lithium clearance (42). All these changes are reversible demonstrating the possibility of a rapid adaptation of proximal tubule sodium changes in the distribution of sodium/proton exchanger 3 apical membrane proteins as well as a decreased transport mediated by rapid reversible regulation of sodium pump activity and relocation of apical sodium transporters. Lithium may be reabsorbed beyond the proximal tubule but post proximal reabsorption is probably limited and unimportant in humans (43). In contrast to uric acid, endogenous lithium is not influenced by diet. Therefore, endogenous lithium clearance may be considered to be the best available estimate of proximal tubular sodium handling in humans at basal conditions.

Studies Examining Proximal Sodium Reabsorption and Features of the Metabolic Syndrome

Cappuccio, Strazzullo, and coworkers were the first to perform a cohort study testing the relationship between proximal sodium reabsorption and features of the metabolic syndrome.

Their two first studies have examined in the same population, a white male working population of the Olivetti factory, the relationship between parameters of the metabolic syndrome and proximal sodium reabsorption (32,44). These are the first studies demonstrating an association between the fractional excretion of lithium, serum triglycerides, cholesterol, uric acid, and central adiposity. Both studies used the method of exogenous lithium excretion. The clustering of cardiovascular risk factors was associated with the lowest of fractional excretion of sodium, i.e., those excreting less sodium at the proximal level accumulated more cardiovascular risk factors.

A recent large population study ($n=1190$) examined the relationship between features of the metabolic syndrome and proximal sodium reabsorption (endogenous lithium clearance) in different ethnic groups (45). As expected, insulin resistant indexes were higher in African and South Asian origin subjects than in white subjects. The association of a higher rate of proximal sodium reabsorption with parameters of the metabolic syndrome was again found within white men and women (Table 3). However, these associations were not found within African or South Asian people despite the greater degree of insulin resistance and central adiposity. In this study, there was not a clear stratification of white men and women in their analysis. For this reason, we performed a cohort study in a large group ($n=661$) of healthy white women. The goal was to explore the relationship between variables of the metabolic syndrome and the fractional excretion of lithium taken as an index of proximal sodium handling in healthy women. Our hypothesis was that features of the metabolic syndrome are also associated with an increased proximal tubular sodium reabsorption in women (46). This population-based study confirmed that weight, basal metabolic index, high cholesterol and LDL cholesterol levels were associated with an increase in proximal sodium reabsorption in healthy women. These associations were independent from age, sodium intake, menopausal status and family history of hypertension.

In conclusion, features of the metabolic syndrome are associated with an increase in proximal sodium reabsorption in white subjects. However, this is not the case in other ethnic groups. In white subjects, the metabolic variables accounted for only 4% to 5% of the variance in the fractional excretion of lithium (45) emphasizing the fact that this relationship is weak because it is masked by the complex interplay of genetic, humoral and mechanical factors involved in proximal sodium reabsorption.

Table 3 Fractional Excretion of Lithium versus Metabolic Variables: Age- and Sex-Adjusted Correlation Coefficients by Ethnic Group, Including Subjects on Treatment

Variable	White ($n=426$)	African Origin ($n=397$)	South Asian ($n=367$)
Systolic BP (mmHg)	0.0156	−0.0003	0.0480
Diastolic BP (mmHg)	0.0222	−0.0536	0.0105
BMI (kg/m^2)	−0.1590*	−0.0371	0.0099
Waist (cm)	−0.1479*	−0.0402	0.0016
Hip (cm)	−0.1318*	−0.0254	0.0077
Waist-to-hip ratio	−0.1054*	−0.0316	0.0017
Total cholesterol (mmol/L)	−0.0009	0.0673	−0.0122
High-density lipoprotein cholesterol (mmol/L) δ	0.0987*	−0.0079	−0.0359
Serum triglycerides (mmol/L) δ	−0.1260*	−0.0390	−0.0419
Serum insulin (pmol/L) δ	−0.0873**	−0.0792	0.0020
Serum glucose (mmol/L)	−0.1209*	0.0044	0.0510
Homeostatic model assessment index δ	−0.1097	−0.0730	0.0117

δ Log transformed for analysis. *$p=0.001$; **$p=0.072$. *Abbreviations*: BMI, body mass index; BP, blood pressure. *Source*: From Ref. 45.

Insulin Resistance and Salt-Sensitivity

The definition of salt-sensitivity remains arbitrary with numerous different definitions used in different protocols. Nevertheless, in one study using a reproducible method of salt-sensitivity, 26% of normotensives and 51% of hypertensives were defined as salt sensitive (47).

Normotension

Insulin resistance is correlated to the level of BP (48) and appears to be the main factor contributing to salt-sensitivity in subjects with BP levels within the normal range. In normotensive subjects, salt-sensitivity correlates with insulin resistance as defined by a hyperinsulinemic response to oral glucose (49) or a reduced insulin mediated glucose disposal (50). In the obese normotensive population, plasma insulin levels correlate with salt-induced changes in BP. Conversely, improvement in insulin resistance through weight reduction decreases salt sensitivity (35).

Hypertension

Insulin resistance is correlated to the level of BP (48,51) and the BP response to salt in hypertensive subjects (52–54). When salt-sensitive subjects are stratified according to their renin status, studies show that hypertensive subjects considered to be non-modulators (normal-high renin and unable to modulate efficiently plasma aldosterone levels and paraaminohippurate clearances during angiotensin II infusions) are salt-sensitive and display a clustering of features of the metabolic syndrome (insulin resistance, high LDL cholesterol) as well as an increased erythrocyte Na^+/Li^+ countertransport activity (55,56).

BP $\geq$ 130/85 mmHg is one criteria of the metabolic syndrome. Although insulin resistance is frequent in the hypertensive population, not all hypertensive subjects have the metabolic syndrome. Among 1742 hypertensive patients without cardiovascular disease, the prevalence of the metabolic syndrome was of 34% and doubled the cardiovascular event rate in a prospective study with a mean duration of 4.1 years (57). This was confirmed in a recent study of 354 untreated non diabetic patients with primary hypertension where the presence of the metabolic syndrome (25%) increased markers of end-organ damage (albuminuria, left ventricular hypertrophy, intima-media thickness) (58). Salt-sensitivity is more likely to be present in hypertensive subjects with the metabolic syndrome and defines a group at highest risk for the development of albuminuria and progressive renal disease (59).

All in all, many studies do show a relationship between insulin levels, insulin resistance indexes, features of the metabolic syndrome and BP, increased sodium reabsorption and salt sensitivity. However some studies do not (60,61) particularly in some populations (45), and thus cast some doubt about this relationship.

If insulin resistance were a major contributor to renal sodium reabsorption, all interventions aimed at decreasing insulin resistance as weight loss, exercise, and insulin sensitizers would be expected to reverse the sodium retention linked to insulin resistance.

EFFECTS OF INSULIN SENSITIZERS ON BP CONTROL AND RENAL SODIUM HANDLING

The most natural way of improving insulin sensitivity and salt sensitivity is through weight reduction by diet and/or exercise (35). At present two classes of oral hypoglycemic drugs improve insulin action: biguanides and thiazolidinediones (glitazones). The contribution of each of these pharmacological interventions on BP control and renal sodium handling will be discussed below.

Metformin

Metformin is an insulin sensitizing biguanide used in the treatment of type 2 diabetes since the late 1950s in Europe, which became rapidly the most prescribed oral glucose-lowering drug in Europe. Because of cases of lactic acidosis, biguanides were withdrawn from the U.S. market in the late 1970s and only reintroduced since 1996 (62). The blood glucose lowering properties of metformin are mainly due to the reduced hepatic glucose production and also, to a lesser extent to the increased insulin mediated glucose uptake in muscle and adipose tissue (63). In addition to its blood glucose lowering properties, metformin exerts other effects, which have a favorable impact on cardiovascular morbidity (Table 4) as demonstrated in the U.K. Prospective Diabetes study (64).

In spite of the improvement in insulin sensitivity with metformin, the effects on BP control are sometimes significant (65) but most of times not. For example, in one study (66), metformin improved insulin sensitivity in hypertensive non-obese insulin resistant subjects, increased renal sodium and lithium excretion but had no effect on BP measured over 24 hours. In another study, when metformin was added to intensive insulin treatment in type diabetic subjects, there was no significant effect on BP control (67). Recently, the diabetes prevention program examined prospectively 3234 individuals with IGT. In this study, lifestyle intervention (exercise and low calorie and low fat diet) was able to decrease the cumulative incidence of type 2 diabetes by 58% substantially more than metformin (−31%) after an average follow-up of 2.8 years. The incidence of hypertension was also very efficiently prevented in the lifestyle intervention group. However, unexpectedly, metformin had absolutely no effect on the incidence of hypertension in spite of its effect on the prevention of type 2 diabetes (Fig. 4) (68). Sodium intake was not assessed in this study but was presumably lower in subjects assigned to the lifestyle intervention group. In addition to exercise, subjects assigned to this group followed a low calorie, low fat diet and achieved a much greater weight loss (−5.6 kg) than those assigned to metformin.

PPAR-γ Agonists: Glitazones

The insulin-sensitizing glitazones (or thiazolidinediones) are selective ligands of the nuclear transcription factor peroxisome proliferator-activated receptor (PPAR)-γ and are

Table 4 Direct and Indirect Cardiovascular Protective Effects of Metformin Therapy

Decreases hyperglycemia
Improves diastolic function
Decreases total cholesterol levels
Decreases very low-density lipoprotein cholesterol levels
Decreases low-density lipoprotein cholesterol levels
Increases high-density lipoprotein cholesterol levels
Decreases oxidative stress
Improves vascular relaxation
Decreases plasminogen activator inhibitor-1 levels
Increases tissue plasminogen activator activity
Decreases von Willebrand factor levels
Decreases platelet aggregation and adhesion

Source: From Ref. 63.

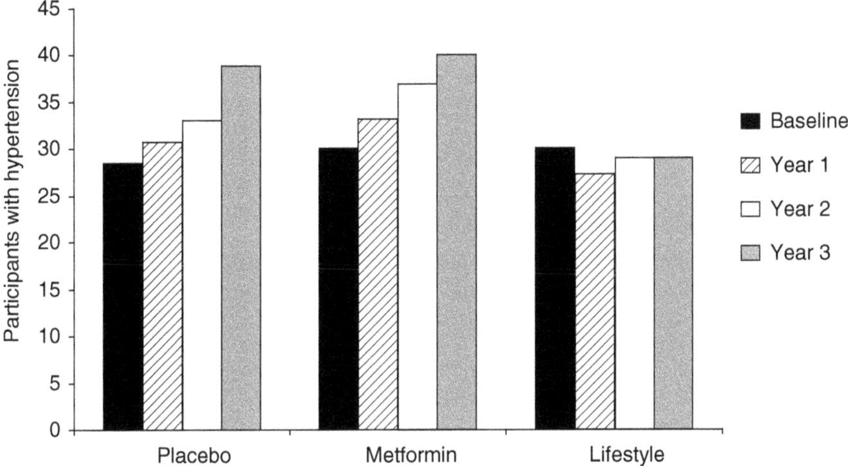

Figure 4 Categorical changes in percent of participants with hypertension over time by treatment assignment. *Source*: From Ref. 68.

currently used as oral hypoglycaemic agents in the treatment of type 2 diabetes (69). Glitazones act predominantly on the adipocyte, influence adipogenesis and increase subcutaneous fat (70,71). They are the most potent insulin sensitizers available for clinical practice. Although exclusively prescribed as hypoglycaemic agents to type 2 diabetic patients, these drugs exert many other effects beyond their glucose lowering properties. They also have anti-inflammatory and antiatherogenic properties (72). They improve endothelial function in insulin resistant subjects (73–75) decrease the intima-media thickness of the carotid artery (76) and have angiotensin II antagonistic properties (77–79).

Glitazones and BP

Glitazones have been shown to decrease BP in the hypertensive (56,80) and diabetic population (81–83). Experimental studies show that pioglitazone is able to dissociate the BP response to accelerated weight gain, hyperphagia and increased salt intake (Table 5) (84). Today, several mechanisms have been proposed to explain the hypotensive properties of glitazones: angiotensin II antagonistic properties (77,85), decreased activity of the sympathetic nervous system due to lower insulin levels (8,10), decreased endothelin-1

Table 5 Average Food and Salt Intake and Final Weight of Obese Zucker Rats in the Various Treatment Groups

	Food intake (g/day)	Salt intake (g/day)	Final weight(g)	MBP (mmHg)	HR (bpm)
Vehicle	28.9±0.3	0.070±0.001	432.0±4.9	116±2*	399±6
Pioglitazone	35.6±0.5‡	0.085±0.001‡	488.1±7.2‡	100±2†	365±5‡
Metformin	27.4±0.5*§	0.066±0.001*§	424.4±4.6§	116±2	385±7

Values are mean±SEM; *$p<0.05$, †$p<0.01$, ‡$p<0.001$ versus vehicle, §$p<0.001$ versus pioglitazone. *Abbreviations*: HR, heart rate; MBP, mean blood pressure.

expression (86,87), improved endothelial function (88) and blockade of calcium uptake by vascular smooth muscle cells (89).

One would expect that by improving insulin sensitivity, sodium retention would consequently decrease. Paradoxically, glitazones promote fluid retention while decreasing efficiently insulin resistance (90).

The Problem of Fluid Retention with Glitazones

The caveat of glitazone therapy is fluid retention and consequently cardiac failure due to fluid overload (90). Type 2 diabetic subjects are at increased risk of heart failure and some case reports have suggested that glitazones may precipitate pulmonary edema (91,92). Still, this remains an area of uncertainty as retrospective cohort studies do not show an increased risk of pulmonary edema, yet of peripheral edema suggesting two independent mechanisms (93). Because the mechanisms of fluid retention are not known, we performed a preliminary study examining the effects of pioglitazone on renal sodium handling in healthy volunteers (non insulin resistant) (94). This was a placebo-controlled, randomized, crossover study. Each volunteer was examined four times with a placebo or pioglitazone and on a high or a low sodium diet. This study integrated renal function studies, ambulatory BP measurements and hormonal studies. It showed that pioglitazone increased plasma renin activity and favored renal proximal sodium reabsorption (Fig. 5).

Based on these findings and experimental studies we hypothesized different mechanisms involved in sodium retention due to glitazones (Fig. 6).

In this study we deliberately chose to investigate normal subjects to study the effects of pioglitazone independently from its effects on glucose tolerance. Similar renal investigations are currently being conducted by our group in diabetic or hypertensive patients to evaluate the impact of glitazones on sodium balance when changes in insulin sensitivity occur simultaneously.

PPAR-γ receptors have been identified in glomeruli, renal vasculature, mesangial cells, and renal tubules (95–100). The activation of these receptors through exogenous ligands (glitazones) has been reported to be protective or deleterious (99). The identification of the precise renal effects of exogenous ligands to PPAR-γ is a complex process as the effects of glitazones may be either direct, through the activation of PPAR response elements of target genes or indirect through for example the attenuation of the effects of endogenous ligands. In other words, glitazones may act as partial PPAR-γ agonists. Some in vitro or ex-vivo studies show that the activation of tubular PPAR-γ receptors by exogenous ligands increases the expression or activity of sodium transporters (101–103). Because the PPAR-γ receptors are predominantly expressed in the collecting duct, two group of investigators hypothesized that sodium retention induced by glitazones occurs predominantly at the collecting duct (104,105). They generated knock out mice lacking the collecting duct PPAR-γ receptor. These mice were resistant to the rapid increase in body weight due to glitazones, mostly due to water as demonstrated by Magnetic Resonance Imaging studies. Furthermore, in vitro studies demonstrated that activation of PPAR-γ in collecting duct cells increased sodium transport through amiloride sensitive channels and increased the transcription of the epithelial Na channel γ. Amiloride prevented the rapid increase in body weight in wild type mice. These results suggest that the rapid increase in body weight induced by glitazones is due to the activation of epitheleal sodium channel and can be prevented by amiloride. The efficiency of amiloride still needs to be demonstrated in clinical studies.

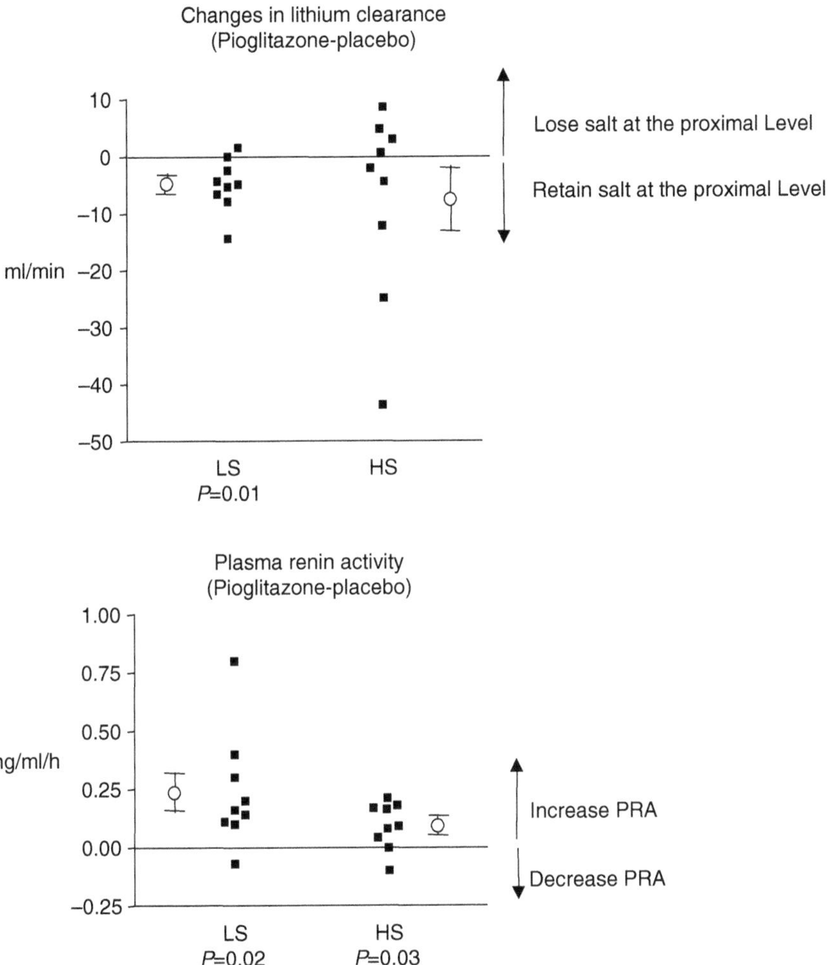

Figure 5 Pioglitazone-induced changes in lithium clearance and PRA from values obtained with placebo on a low-sodium or high-sodium diet. Circles represent mean values with standard error of the mean (SEM). *Abbreviations*: HS, high-sodium; LS, low-sodium; PRA, plasma renin activity.

Effects of PPAR-γ Agonists on the Sodium–Angiotensin II Relationship in Insulin-Resistant Rats

Several studies have demonstrated angiotensin II (Ang II) antagonizing properties of glitazones (77–79,85). Glitazones have been reported to blunt the systemic response to exogenous angiotensin II in rats (85) and also to increase food intake (106). Thus, glitazones may potentially modify the impact of salt on the systemic and renal effects of Ang II. Indeed, sodium is an important physiological modulator of the systemic and renal response to Ang II. On a low sodium intake, the renin–angiotensin system is activated leading to high circulating Ang II levels and a downregulation of Ang II receptors whereas on a high sodium intake, circulating Ang II levels are low and Ang II receptors are up-regulated leading to an increased sensitivity to Ang II (107).

We investigated the effects of pioglitazone on the relation between sodium and the systemic effects of angiotensin II in the insulin resistant obese Zucker rat model (84). Pioglitazone increased food intake, body weight and decreased very significantly

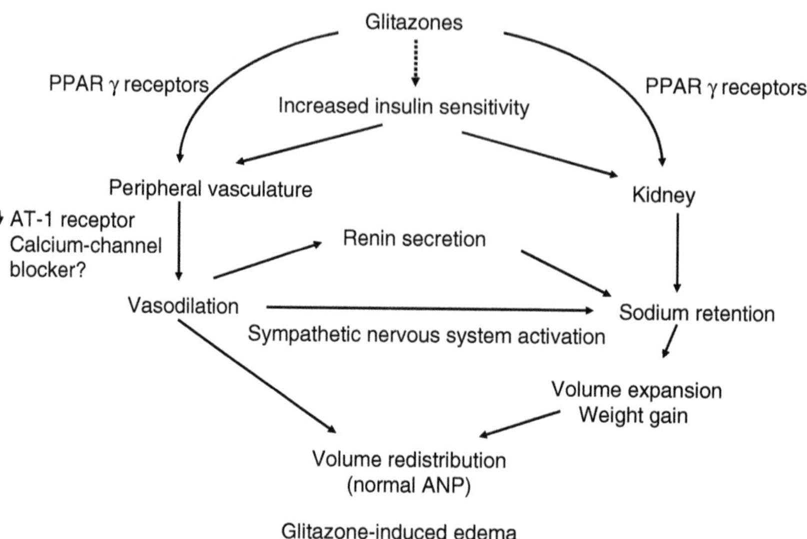

Figure 6 Possible mechanisms involved in glitazone-induced edema. *Abbreviations*: ANP, atrial natriuretic peptide; AT1, angiotensin II type 1; PPAR, peroxisome proliferator-activated receptor.

the insulin levels. Despite a higher food and sodium intake and a net gain in weight, basal BP and its response to exogenous Ang II was significantly reduced in obese rats treated with pioglitazone. These Ang II antagonistic effects were however not found in the lean Zucker rat. As expected, the BP response to exogenous Ang II increased in the obese Zucker rats receiving a high sodium diet. Pioglitazone abolished totally the salt-induced enhanced responsiveness independently from any change in insulin sensitivity (Fig. 7). Moreover, in the obese rat, pioglitazone modified the renal hemodynamic response to

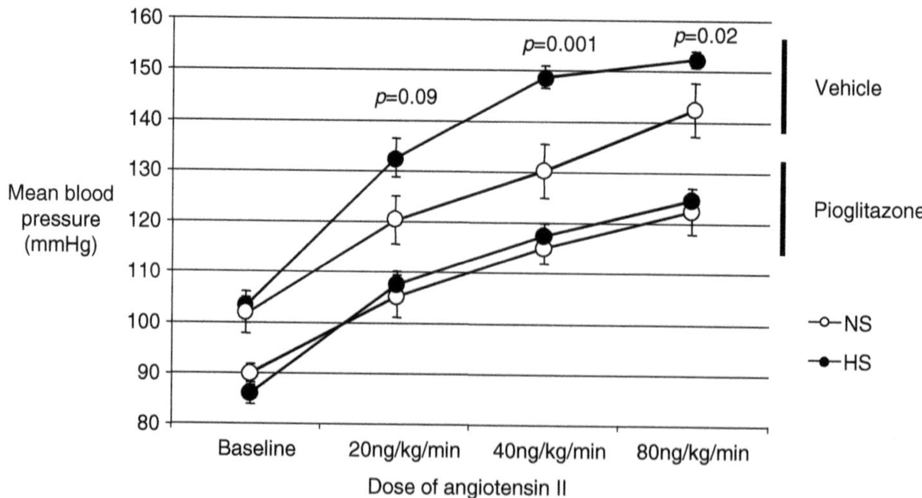

Figure 7 Effects of a high-sodium diet on the angiotensin II induced increase in BP in obese Zucker rats, vehicle or pioglitazone treated. BP levels achieved after 30 minutes of perfusion of angiotensin II. *p* value versus vehicle- NS. *Abbreviations*: BP, blood pressure; HS, high sodium diet; NS, normal sodium diet.

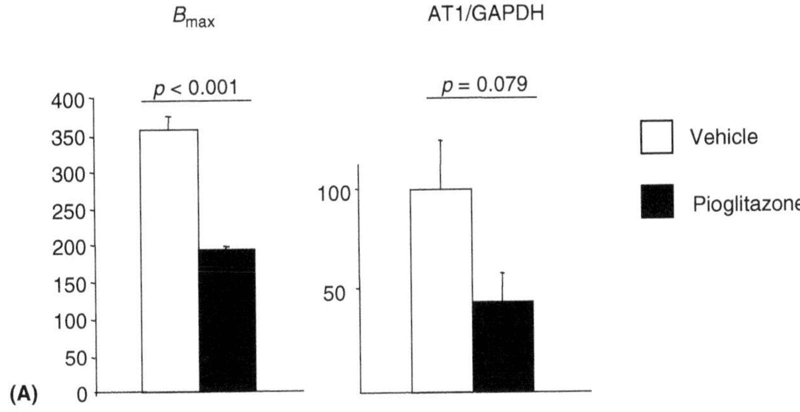

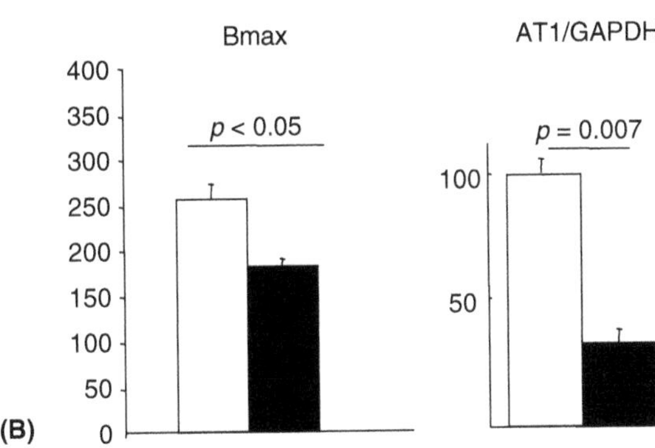

Figure 8 Renal angiotensin type 1 receptor binding studies and mRNA expression. Pioglitazone-dependent changes in number (B_{max}) and mRNA expression of angiotensin II subtype I receptors in kidneys of obese normal sodium diet (**A**) and high sodium diet (**B**) treated Zucker rats. Values are mean ± SEM. *Abbreviation*: AT1, angiotensin II type 1.

changes in salt intake while maintaining a lower filtration fraction at baseline and during Ang II perfusion. These effects were associated with a lower number and expression of the Ang II angiotensin type 1 receptor in the kidney of pioglitazone treated rats (Fig. 8). Taken together, these results confirm the Ang II antagonistic effects of pioglitazone and demonstrate that pioglitazone modifies the physiological relation between sodium and Ang II both at the vascular and renal level in obese insulin resistant rats.

In summary, glitazones have a very complex relationship with sodium in insulin resistant subjects. They definitely can promote sodium retention, but they blunt the increased vascular responsiveness to angiotensin II induced by a high sodium intake. Consequently, in spite of sodium retention and weight gain, BP is lower with glitazones (83).

CONCLUSIONS

Subjects with insulin resistance, accumulating the features of the metabolic syndrome with/or without diabetes are at increased risk of sodium retention. Body weight reduction through diet and exercise will decrease the sodium retention. Moderate sodium restriction may have a favorable impact on the risk of diabetes and cardiovascular morbidity (108,109). Diuretics, beta-blockers, angiotensin-converting enzyme inhibitors and angiotensin II antagonists will decrease the tendency toward sodium retention and are efficient in treating hypertension. Doses of thiazide diuretics and beta-blockers should however be kept relatively low in accord with current recommendations because higher doses can worsen insulin resistance and dyslipidemia (110). Insulin sensitizers do not have parallel effects on sodium balance to those on the improvement of insulin sensitivity. Studies of the effects of metformin on sodium handling are scarce. Metformin effects on BP control are insignificant. Nevertheless, they may decrease macrovascular morbidity particularly in obese type 2 diabetic patients. There are consistent data on the favorable effects of glitazones on BP control and response to angiotensin II in spite of a gain in weight, hyperphagia, increased sodium intake and sodium retention. Further studies are needed to explore the mechanisms on how glitazones are able to dissociate the BP response to salt and weight gain.

Overall, a multifactorial approach is needed in patients with the metabolic syndrome, by decreasing insulin resistance through exercise, weight loss, and the use of insulin sensitizers in case of diabetes. Improvement with insulin sensitizers may have a favorable impact on cardiovascular risk factors though they are not natriuretic. Whether they decrease cardiovascular disease and mortality still needs to be demonstrated in diabetic subjects.

REFERENCES

1. Reaven GM. Banting lecture 1988. Role of insulin resistance in human disease. Diabetes 1988; 37:1595–607.
2. Dandona P, Aljada A, Chaudhuri A, et al. Metabolic syndrome: a comprehensive perspective based on interactions between obesity, diabetes, and inflammation. Circulation 2005; 111:1448–54.
3. Cameron AJ, Shaw JE, Zimmet PZ. The metabolic syndrome: prevalence in worldwide populations. Endocrinol Metab Clin North Am 2004; 33:351–75 (table of contents).
4. Eckel RH, Grundy SM, Zimmet PZ. The metabolic syndrome. Lancet 2005; 365: 1415–28.
5. Alexander CM, Landsman PB, Teutsch SM, Haffner SM. NCEP-defined metabolic syndrome, diabetes, and prevalence of coronary heart disease among NHANES III participants age 50 years and older. Diabetes 2003; 52:1210–4.
6. Grundy SM, Hansen B, Smith SC, Jr., et al. Clinical management of metabolic syndrome: report of the American Heart Association/National Heart, Lung, and Blood Institute/ American Diabetes Association conference on scientific issues related to management. Circulation 2004; 109:551–6.
7. Gaede P, Vedel P, Larsen N, et al. Multifactorial intervention and cardiovascular disease in patients with type 2 diabetes. N Engl J Med 2003; 348:383–93.
8. Anderson EA, Hoffman RP, Balon TW, et al. Hyperinsulinemia produces both sympathetic neural activation and vasodilation in normal humans. J Clin Invest 1991; 87:2246–52.
9. DeFronzo RA, Cooke CR, Andres R, et al. The effect of insulin on renal handling of sodium, potassium, calcium, and phosphate in man. J Clin Invest 1975; 55:845–55.
10. Rowe JW, Young JB, Minaker KL, et al. Effect of insulin and glucose infusions on sympathetic nervous system activity in normal man. Diabetes 1981; 30:219–25.
11. Hall JE, Brands MW, Mizelle HL, et al. Chronic intrarenal hyperinsulinemia does not cause hypertension. Am J Physiol 1991; 260:F663–9.
12. Baum M. Insulin stimulates volume absorption in the rabbit proximal convoluted tubule. J Clin Invest 1987; 79:1104–9.

13. Skott P, Vaag A, Bruun NE, et al. Effect of insulin on renal sodium handling in hyperinsulinaemic type 2 (non-insulin-dependent) diabetic patients with peripheral insulin resistance. Diabetologia 1991; 34:275–81.
14. DeFronzo RA, Goldberg M, Agus ZS. The effects of glucose and insulin on renal electrolyte transport. J Clin Invest 1976; 58:83–90.
15. Kirchner KA. Insulin increases loop segment chloride reabsorption in the euglycemic rat. Am J Physiol 1988; 255:F1206–13.
16. Kuroda S, Uzu T, Fujii T, et al. Role of insulin resistance in the genesis of sodium sensitivity in essential hypertension. J Hum Hypertens 1999; 13:257–62.
17. Egan BM. Insulin resistance and the sympathetic nervous system. Curr Hypertens Rep 2003; 5:247–54.
18. Sechi LA, Griffin CA, Schambelan M. Effect of dietary sodium chloride on insulin receptor number and mRNA levels in rat kidney. Am J Physiol 1994; 266:F31–8.
19. Catena C, Cavarape A, Novello M, et al. Insulin receptors and renal sodium handling in hypertensive fructose-fed rats. Kidney Int 2003; 64:2163–71.
20. Gonzalez-Albarran O, Ruilope LM, Villa E, Garcia Robles R. Salt sensitivity: concept and pathogenesis. Diabetes Res Clin Pract 1998; 39(Suppl.):S15–26.
21. Engeli S, Sharma AM. The renin–angiotensin system and natriuretic peptides in obesity-associated hypertension. J Mol Med 2001; 79:21–9.
22. Hall JE. Mechanisms of abnormal renal sodium handling in obesity hypertension. Am J Hypertens 1997; 10:49S–55.
23. Wolf G. After all those fat years: renal consequences of obesity. Nephrol Dial Transplant 2003; 18:2471–4.
24. Gaboury CL, Simonson DC, Seely EW, et al. Relation of pressor responsiveness to angiotensin II and insulin resistance in hypertension. J Clin Invest 1994; 94:2295–300.
25. Rocchini AP, Moorehead C, DeRemer S, et al. Hyperinsulinemia and the aldosterone and pressor responses to angiotensin II. Hypertension 1990; 15:861–6.
26. Friedberg CE, van Buren M, Bijlsma JA, Koomans HA. Insulin increases sodium reabsorption in diluting segment in humans: evidence for indirect mediation through hypokalemia. Kidney Int 1991; 40:251–6.
27. Quinones-Galvan A, Ferrannini E. Renal effects of insulin in man. J Nephrol 1997; 10:188–91.
28. O'Brien T, Young WF, Jr., Palumbo PJ, et al. Hypertension and dyslipidemia in patients with insulinoma. Mayo Clin Proc 1993; 68:141–6.
29. Doris PA. Renal proximal tubule sodium transport and genetic mechanisms of essential hypertension. J Hypertens 2000; 18:509–19.
30. Burnier M, Biollaz J, Magnin JL, et al. Renal sodium handling in patients with untreated hypertension and white coat hypertension. Hypertension 1994; 23:496–502.
31. Chiolero A, Wurzner G, Burnier M. Renal determinants of the salt sensitivity of blood pressure. Nephrol Dial Transplant 2001; 16:452–8.
32. Cappuccio FP, Strazzullo P, Siani A, Trevisan M. Increased proximal sodium reabsorption is associated with increased cardiovascular risk in men. J Hypertens 1996; 14:909–14.
33. Weder AB. Red-cell lithium–sodium countertransport and renal lithium clearance in hypertension. N Engl J Med 1986; 314:198–201.
34. Manunta P, Burnier M, D'Amico M, et al. Adducin polymorphism affects renal proximal tubule reabsorption in hypertension. Hypertension 1999; 33:694–7.
35. Rocchini AP, Katch V, Kveselis D, et al. Insulin and renal sodium retention in obese adolescents. Hypertension 1989; 14:367–74.
36. Nosadini R, Sambataro M, Thomaseth K, et al. Role of hyperglycemia and insulin resistance in determining sodium retention in non-insulin-dependent diabetes. Kidney Int 1993; 44: 139–46.
37. Rathmann W, Funkhouser E, Dyer AR, Roseman JM. Relations of hyperuricemia with the various components of the insulin resistance syndrome in young black and white adults: the CARDIA study. Coronary Artery Risk Development in Young Adults. Ann Epidemiol 1998; 8:250–61.

38. Facchini F, Chen YD, Hollenbeck CB, Reaven GM. Relationship between resistance to insulin-mediated glucose uptake, urinary uric acid clearance, and plasma uric acid concentration. JAMA 1991; 266:3008–11.
39. Reaven GM. The kidney: an unwilling accomplice in syndrome X. Am J Kidney Dis 1997; 30:928–31.
40. Vuorinen-Markkola H, Yki-Jarvinen H. Hyperuricemia and insulin resistance. J Clin Endocrinol Metab 1994; 78:25–9.
41. Vander AJ. Renal physiology. New York: McGraw-Hill, 1994.
42. Zhang Y, Magyar CE, Norian JM, et al. Reversible effects of acute hypertension on proximal tubule sodium transporters. Am J Physiol 1998; 274:C1090–100.
43. Boer WH, Koomans HA, Dorhout Mees EJ, et al. Lithium clearance during variations in sodium intake in man: effects of sodium restriction and amiloride. Eur J Clin Invest 1988; 18:279–83.
44. Strazzullo P, Barba G, Cappuccio FP, et al. Altered renal sodium handling in men with abdominal adiposity: a link to hypertension. J Hypertens 2001; 19:2157–64.
45. Barbato A, Cappuccio FP, Folkerd EJ, et al. Metabolic syndrome and renal sodium handling in three ethnic groups living in England. Diabetologia 2004; 47:40–6.
46. Zanchi A, Bochud M, Decosterd D, et al. Metabolic determinants of proximal sodium reabsorption in healthy women. Am J Hypertens 2003; 16:263A.
47. Weinberger MH, Fineberg NS. Sodium and volume sensitivity of blood pressure. Age and pressure change over time. Hypertension 1991; 18:67–71.
48. Kanauchi M, Yamano S, Kanauchi K, Saito Y. Homeostasis model assessment of insulin resistance, quantitative insulin sensitivity check index, and oral glucose insulin sensitivity index in nonobese, nondiabetic subjects with high-normal blood pressure. J Clin Endocrinol Metab 2003; 88:3444–6.
49. Sharma AM, Ruland K, Spies KP, Distler A. Salt sensitivity in young normotensive subjects is associated with a hyperinsulinemic response to oral glucose. J Hypertens 1991; 9:329–35.
50. Sharma AM, Schorr U, Distler A. Insulin resistance in young salt-sensitive normotensive subjects. Hypertension 1993; 21:273–9.
51. Ferrannini E, Buzzigoli G, Bonadonna R, et al. Insulin resistance in essential hypertension. N Engl J Med 1987; 317:350–7.
52. Suzuki M, Kimura Y, Tsushima M, Harano Y. Association of insulin resistance with salt sensitivity and nocturnal fall of blood pressure. Hypertension 2000; 35:864–8.
53. Giner V, Coca A, de la Sierra A. Increased insulin resistance in salt sensitive essential hypertension. J Hum Hypertens 2001; 15:481–5.
54. Vedovato M, Lepore G, Coracina A, et al. Effect of sodium intake on blood pressure and albuminuria in Type 2 diabetic patients: the role of insulin resistance. Diabetologia 2004; 47:300–3.
55. Ferri C, Bellini C, Desideri G, et al. Relationship between insulin resistance and non-modulating hypertension: linkage of metabolic abnormalities and cardiovascular risk. Diabetes 1999; 48:1623–30.
56. Raji A, Williams GH, Jeunemaitre X, et al. Insulin resistance in hypertensives: effect of salt sensitivity, renin status and sodium intake. J Hypertens 2001; 19:99–105.
57. Schillaci G, Pirro M, Vaudo G, et al. Prognostic value of the metabolic syndrome in essential hypertension. J Am Coll Cardiol 2004; 43:1817–22.
58. Leoncini G, Ratto E, Viazzi F, et al. Metabolic syndrome is associated with early signs of organ damage in nondiabetic, hypertensive patients. J Intern Med 2005; 257:454–60.
59. Johnson RJ, Segal MS, Srinivas T, et al. Essential hypertension, progressive renal disease, and uric acid: a pathogenetic link? J Am Soc Nephrol 2005; 16:1909–19.
60. Lind L, Lithell H, Gustafsson IB, et al. Metabolic cardiovascular risk factors and sodium sensitivity in hypertensive subjects. Am J Hypertens 1992; 5:502–5.
61. Saad MF, Lillioja S, Nyomba BL, et al. Racial differences in the relation between blood pressure and insulin resistance. N Engl J Med 1991; 324:733–9.
62. Bailey CJ, Turner RC. Metformin. N Engl J Med 1996; 334:574–9.

63. Kirpichnikov D, McFarlane SI, Sowers JR. Metformin: an update. Ann Intern Med 2002; 137:25–33.
64. UK Prospective Diabetes Study (UKPDS) Group. Effect of intensive blood-glucose control with metformin on complications in overweight patients with type 2 diabetes (UKPDS 34). Lancet 1998; 352:854–65.
65. Landin K, Tengborn L, Smith U. Treating insulin resistance in hypertension with metformin reduces both blood pressure and metabolic risk factors. J Intern Med 1991; 229:181–7.
66. Dorella M, Giusto M, Da Tos V, et al. Improvement of insulin sensitivity by metformin treatment does not lower blood pressure of nonobese insulin-resistant hypertensive patients with normal glucose tolerance. J Clin Endocrinol Metab 1996; 81:1568–74.
67. Wulffele MG, Kooy A, Lehert P, et al. Does metformin decrease blood pressure in patients with Type 2 diabetes intensively treated with insulin? Diabet Med 2005; 22:907–13.
68. Ratner R, Goldberg R, Haffner S, et al. Impact of intensive lifestyle and metformin therapy on cardiovascular disease risk factors in the diabetes prevention program. Diabetes Care 2005; 28:888–94.
69. Yki-Jarvinen H. Thiazolidinediones. N Engl J Med 2004; 351:1106–18.
70. Miyazaki Y, Mahankali A, Matsuda M, et al. Effect of pioglitazone on abdominal fat distribution and insulin sensitivity in type 2 diabetic patients. J Clin Endocrinol Metab 2002; 87:2784–91.
71. Smith SR, De Jonge L, Volaufova J, et al. Effect of pioglitazone on body composition and energy expenditure: a randomized controlled trial. Metabolism 2005; 54:24–32.
72. Barbier O, Pineda Torra I, Duguay Y, et al. Pleiotropic actions of peroxisome proliferator-activated receptors in lipid metabolism and atherosclerosis. Arterioscler Thromb Vasc Biol 2002; 22:717–26.
73. Quinones MJ, Hernandez-Pampaloni M, Schelbert H, et al. Coronary vasomotor abnormalities in insulin-resistant individuals. Ann Intern Med 2004; 140:700–8.
74. Caballero AE, Saouaf R, Lim SC, et al. The effects of troglitazone, an insulin-sensitizing agent, on the endothelial function in early and late type 2 diabetes: a placebo-controlled randomized clinical trial. Metabolism 2003; 52:173–80.
75. Watanabe Y, Sunayama S, Shimada K, et al. Troglitazone improves endothelial dysfunction in patients with insulin resistance. J Atheroscler Thromb 2000; 7:159–63.
76. Langenfeld MR, Forst T, Hohberg C, et al. Pioglitazone decreases carotid intima-media thickness independently of glycemic control in patients with type 2 diabetes mellitus: results from a controlled randomized study. Circulation 2005; 111:2525–31.
77. Takeda K, Ichiki T, Tokunou T, et al. Peroxisome proliferator-activated receptor gamma activators downregulate angiotensin II type 1 receptor in vascular smooth muscle cells. Circulation 2000; 102:1834–9.
78. Diep QN, El Mabrouk M, Cohn JS, et al. Structure, endothelial function, cell growth, and inflammation in blood vessels of angiotensin II-infused rats: role of peroxisome proliferator-activated receptor-gamma. Circulation 2002; 105:2296–302.
79. Ryan MJ, Didion SP, Mathur S, et al. PPAR{gamma} agonist rosiglitazone improves vascular function and lowers blood pressure in hypertensive transgenic mice. Hypertension 2004; 43(3):661–6.
80. Fullert S, Schneider F, Haak E, et al. Effects of pioglitazone in nondiabetic patients with arterial hypertension: a double-blind, placebo-controlled study. J Clin Endocrinol Metab 2002; 87:5503–6.
81. Ogihara T, Rakugi H, Ikegami H, et al. Enhancement of insulin sensitivity by troglitazone lowers blood pressure in diabetic hypertensives. Am J Hypertens 1995; 8:316–20.
82. Bennett SM, Agrawal A, Elasha H, et al. Rosiglitazone improves insulin sensitivity, glucose tolerance and ambulatory blood pressure in subjects with impaired glucose tolerance. Diabet Med 2004; 21:415–22.
83. Dormandy JA, Charbonnel B, Eckland DJ, et al. Secondary prevention of macrovascular events in patients with type 2 diabetes in the PROactive Study (PROspective pioglitAzone

Clinical Trial In macroVascular Events): a randomised controlled trial. Lancet 2005; 366:1279–89.

84. Zanchi A, Perregaux C, Maillard M, et al. The PPARgamma agonist pioglitazone modifies the vascular sodium–angiotensin II relationship in insulin-resistant rats. Am J Physiol Endocrinol Metab 2006; 291:E1228–34.
85. Kotchen TA, Zhang HY, Reddy S, Hoffmann RG. Effect of pioglitazone on vascular reactivity in vivo and in vitro. Am J Physiol 1996; 270:R660–6.
86. Satoh H, Tsukamoto K, Hashimoto Y, et al. Thiazolidinediones suppress endothelin-1 secretion from bovine vascular endothelial cells: a new possible role of PPARgamma on vascular endothelial function. Biochem Biophys Res Commun 1999; 254:757–63.
87. Iglarz M, Touyz R, Amiri F, et al. Effect of peroxisome proliferator-activated receptor-α and -γ activators on vascular remodeling in endothelin-dependent hypertension. Arterioscler Thromb Vasc Res 2003; 23:45–51.
88. Fujishima S, Ohya Y, Nakamura Y, et al. Troglitazone, an insulin sensitizer, increases forearm blood flow in humans. Am J Hypertens 1998; 11:1134–7.
89. Buchanan TA, Meehan WP, Jeng YY, et al. Blood pressure lowering by pioglitazone. Evidence for a direct vascular effect. J Clin Invest 1995; 96:354–60.
90. Nesto RW, Bell D, Bonow RO, et al. Thiazolidinedione use, fluid retention, and congestive heart failure: a consensus statement from the American Heart Association and American Diabetes Association. Circulation 2003; 108:2941–8.
91. Kermani A, Garg A. Thiazolidinedione-associated congestive heart failure and pulmonary edema. Mayo Clin Proc 2003; 78:1088–91.
92. Jamieson A, Abousleiman Y. Thiazolidinedione-associated congestive heart failure and pulmonary edema. Mayo Clin Proc 2004; 79:571 (author reply 575–7).
93. Tang WH, Francis GS, Hoogwerf BJ, Young JB. Fluid retention after initiation of thiazolidinedione therapy in diabetic patients with established chronic heart failure. J Am Coll Cardiol 2003; 41:1394–8.
94. Zanchi A, Chiolero A, Maillard M, et al. Effects of the peroxisomal proliferator-activated receptor-gamma agonist pioglitazone on renal and hormonal responses to salt in healthy men. J Clin Endocrinol Metab 2004; 89:1140–5.
95. Guan Y, Zhang Y, Davis L, Breyer MD. Expression of peroxisome proliferator-activated receptors in urinary tract of rabbits and humans. Am J Physiol 1997; 273:F1013–22.
96. Guan Y, Breyer MD. Peroxisome proliferator-activated receptors (PPARs): novel therapeutic targets in renal disease. Kidney Int 2001; 60:14–30.
97. Nicholas SB, Kawano Y, Wakino S, et al. Expression and function of peroxisome proliferator-activated receptor-gamma in mesangial cells. Hypertension 2001; 37:722–7.
98. Yang T, Michele DE, Park J, et al. Expression of peroxisomal proliferator-activated receptors and retinoid X receptors in the kidney. Am J Physiol 1999; 277:F966–73.
99. Chana RS, Lewington AJ, Brunskill NJ. Differential effects of peroxisome proliferator activated receptor-gamma (PPAR gamma) ligands in proximal tubular cells: thiazolidinediones are partial PPAR gamma agonists. Kidney Int 2004; 65:2081–90.
100. Panchapakesan U, Pollock CA, Chen XM. The effect of high glucose and PPAR-gamma agonists on PPAR-gamma expression and function in HK-2 cells. Am J Physiol Renal Physiol 2004; 287:F528–34.
101. Song J, Walsh M, Igwe R, et al. Troglitazone reduces contraction by inhibition of vascular smooth muscle Ca2+ currents and not endothelial nitric oxide production. Diabetes 2002; 46:659–64.
102. Muto S, Miyata Y, Imai M, Asano Y. Troglitazone stimulates basolateral rheogenic Na+/HCO3− cotransport activity in rabbit proximal straight tubules. Exp Nephrol 2001; 9:191–7.
103. Hong G, Lockhart A, Davis B, et al. PPARgamma activation enhances cell surface ENaCalpha via up-regulation of SGK1 in human collecting duct cells. FASEB J 2003; 17:1966–8.
104. Guan Y, Hao C, Cha DR, et al. Thiazolidinediones expand body fluid volume through PPARgamma stimulation of ENaC-mediated renal salt absorption. Nat Med 2005; 11:861–6.

105. Zhang H, Zhang A, Kohan DE, et al. Collecting duct-specific deletion of peroxisome proliferator-activated receptor gamma blocks thiazolidinedione-induced fluid retention. Proc Natl Acad Sci USA 2005; 102:9406–11.
106. Wang Q, Dryden S, Frankish HM, et al. Increased feeding in fatty Zucker rats by the thiazolidinedione BRL 49653 (rosiglitazone) and the possible involvement of leptin and hypothalamic neuropeptide Y. Br J Pharmacol 1997; 122:1405–10.
107. Nickenig G, Strehlow K, Roeling J, et al. Salt induces vascular AT1 receptor overexpression in vitro and in vivo. Hypertension 1998; 31:1272–7.
108. Hu G, Jousilahti P, Peltonen M, et al. Urinary sodium and potassium excretion and the risk of type 2 diabetes: a prospective study in Finland. Diabetologia 2005; 48:1477–83.
109. He J, Ogden LG, Vupputuri S, et al. Dietary sodium intake and subsequent risk of cardiovascular disease in overweight adults. JAMA 1999; 282:2027–34.
110. Chobanian AV, Bakris GL, Black HR, et al. The seventh report of the Joint National Committee on Prevention, Detection, Evaluation, and Treatment of High Blood Pressure: the JNC 7 report. JAMA 2003; 289:2560–72.

20
Drug-induced Alterations of Sodium Balance: The Example of Nonsteroidal Anti-inflammatory Agents

Marc P. Maillard and Michel Burnier
Division of Nephrology and Hypertension Consultation, University Hospital, University of Lausanne, Lausanne, Switzerland

INTRODUCTION

As discussed in previous chapters, several neuro-humoral and renal tubular transport systems are involved in the maintenance of sodium balance. Many of these systems actually represent therapeutic targets for which specific drugs have been developed. It is therefore not surprising that many drugs have a major impact on sodium and water balance. The best example is of course that of diuretics, which act at different sites along the renal tubule to increase urinary sodium excretion, or blockers of the renin–angiotensin–aldosterone system, which promote sodium excretion by interfering with the renal hemodynamic and tubular properties of angiotensin II and aldosterone (1). In these cases, the impact of the drug is clearly understood and is due to an expected and eventually desired interference of the drug with a physiological renal function. With these compounds, the renal effects may even contribute to the overall beneficial effects of the drug class (2,3).

With some other drugs, the impact on urinary sodium and water excretion is considered a side effect that may or may not be due to an interference with renal mechanisms. Thus, pure arterial vasodilators can induce sodium retention and peripheral edema because of the peripheral vasodilation and the secondary, reflex activation of the renin–angiotensin and sympathetic nervous systems. Recently, a similar mechanism has been evoked for the water and sodium retention induced by the peroxisome proliferators-activated receptor (PPAR)-γ agonists, the thiazolidinediones (3), although in this latter case, an interaction between PPAR-γ receptors and the activity of the renal epithelial sodium channel has also been suggested (4,5). As shown in Table 1, numerous drugs can interfere either with water or sodium balance and hence can cause clinical disorders such as hypo- and hypernatremia, diabetes insipidus, sodium retention leading to peripheral edema or congestive heart failure or dehydration due to sodium and water losses.

Table 1 Drugs with the Potential to Interfere with Urinary Sodium and Water Excretion

Drugs associated with hyponatremia	Drugs associated with diabetes insipidus	Drugs with natriuretic properties	Drugs with antinatriuretic properties
Antidiuretic analogs	Lithium	*Proximal tubular diuretics*	NSAIDs and COX2-inhibitors
Deamino-D-arginine vasopressin	Demeclocycline	Mannitol	Glitazones
Oxytocin	Gliburide	Acetazolamide	Calcineurin inhibitors
Drugs enhancing ADH release or action	Amphotericine	*Loop diuretics*	Pure vasodilators
Chlorpropamide	Foscarnet	Furosemide	Fludrocortisone and Mineralocorticoids
Clofibrate	Vasopressin antagonists	Torasemide	
Carbamazepine		Bumetanide	
Vincristine		*Distal tubular diuretics*	
Nicotine		Thiazides	
Narcotics		Chlorthalidone	
Antipsychotique, antidepressant		Metolazone	
Ifosfamide		*Potassium sparing diuretics*	
Cyclophosphamide		Amiloride	
NSAIDs		Spironolactone	
Acetaminophene		Eplerenone	
Unknown mechanisms		*Nondiuretic agents*	
Haloperidol		ACE inhibitors	
Fluphenazine		Angiotensin receptor blockers	
Amitriptyline		Calcium channel blockers	
Serotonin inhibitors		Aminophylline	
Ectasy		Dopamine	
		Phosphodiesterase inhibitor	
		Vasopeptidase inhibitors	

Abbreviations: ACE, angiotensin-converting enzyme; ADH, antidiuretic hormone; NSAIDs, non-steroidal anti-inflammatory drugs.

Discussing the impact of all these drugs on renal sodium and water handling is beyond the scope of this chapter but we would like to focus on non-steroidal anti-inflammatory drugs (NSAIDs), which belong to the most frequently used class of drugs worldwide, either prescribed or over-the-counter. NSAIDs are well recognized as drugs promoting salt and water retention and inducing peripheral edema and eventually acute renal failure.

BIOCHEMISTRY OF RENAL PROSTAGLANDINS

Prostaglandins (PGs) with biological activity in the kidneys are derived from arachidonic acid (Fig. 1), a tetranenoic unsaturated 20-carbon fatty acid. They belong to the dienoic

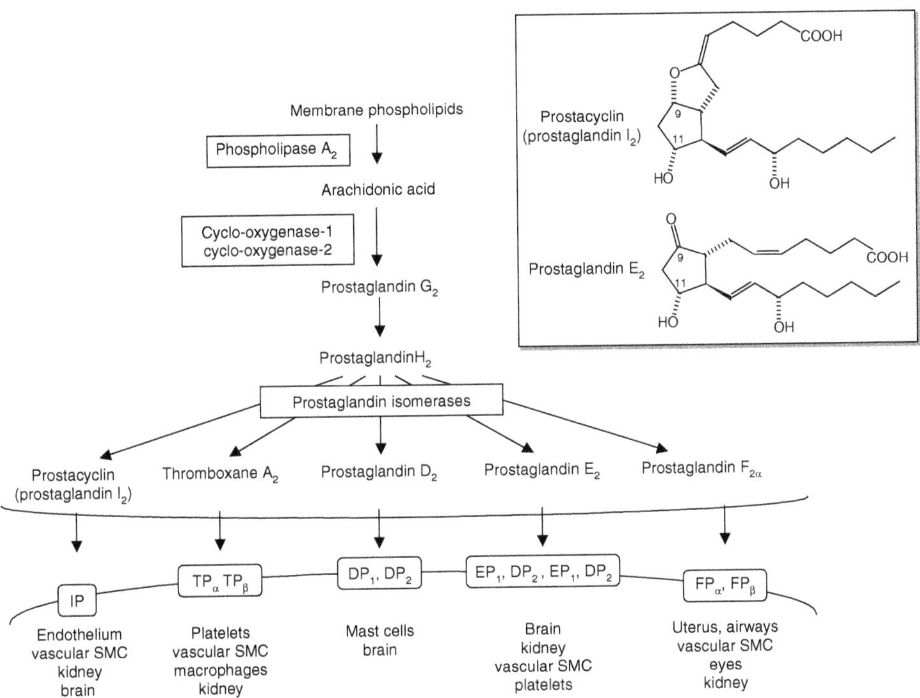

Figure 1 Schematic representation of prostaglandin (PG) synthetic pathways and enzymes that catalyze the specific reactions, together with the respective tissue-specific G-protein transmembrane PG receptors.

series of PGs and are thus designated by the suffix 2 (i.e., PGE_2), while in contrast, those which are derived from trienoic or pentaenoic derivatives of arachidonic acid are designed by the suffixes 1 and 3 respectively (i.e., PGE_1 and PGE_3) and are produced in too low concentrations to act biologically in the kidney (6). Arachidonic acid is released from membrane phospholipids primarily by the action of phospholipase A2, an enzyme which can be activated by a series of factors such as angiotensin II (7), bradykinin (8), vasopressin (9), norepinephrine (10) and ischemia (11) and can be inhibited by glucocorticoids (12) and non-steroidal anti-inflammatory agents (13). Through the action of cyclo-oxygenases (the COX exists as two isoforms: COX-1 and COX-2, which differ mainly in their regulation and expression as will be discussed below), molecular oxygen is then added to arachidonic acid, resulting in the formation of the endoperoxide PGG_2, which, with the liberation of a free superoxide radical is converted to the endoperoxide PGH_2. This unstable endoperoxide intermediate is then metabolized by several PG isomerases expressed in a relatively tissue-specific manner to form PGE_2, $PGF_{2\alpha}$ or PGD_2. PGE_2 can also be converted to $PGF_{2\alpha}$ by 9-ketoreductase, an enzyme that can be stimulated by high salt intake (14) and inhibited by the loop diuretic furosemide. PGH_2 is also metabolized by prostacyclin synthase to form PGI_2 (also known as prostacyclin), and by thromboxane synthase to form thromboxane A_2.

After formation all these PGs are rapidly degraded into inactive products, mainly by the renal 15-hydroxyprostaglandin dehydrogenase, or for those escaping the kidney, by the lung. Therefore, due to their short half-lives, PGs act as autacoids rather than circulating hormones and activate membrane receptors at, or close to, their site of formation. Single receptors have been cloned for prostacyclin (IP), $PGF_{2\alpha}$ (the FPs) and

TXA_2 (the TPs), while four distinct PGE_2 receptors (the EPs 1-4) and two PGD_2 (DP1 and DP2) receptors have been identified (15,16). Stimulation of these G-protein-coupled receptors result in the activation of various intracellular signal transduction systems which can initiate a highly diverse array of signaling events (17) and thus have a variety of physiologic and pathologic functions (Table 2) (16).

Under normal physiologic conditions, PGs are constitutively produced. Besides their effects on renal function which will be discussed below, they play an essential role in cytoprotection of gastric mucosa, platelet aggregation and gestation and parturition. However, it has been demonstrated that in some pathological situations such as inflammation, the tissue expression of the COX-2 enzyme can increase several folds and thereby COX-2-mediated PGs contribute directly to the inflammatory process and the development of pain and fever (18).

The finding of a constitutive COX-1 and inducible COX-2 enzyme has generated the elegant hypothesis according to which the physiological effects of PGs are mediated by the COX-1 enzyme and the pathological effects of PGs result from the induction of COX-2. According to this hypothesis, COX-1 (also named PG endoperoxyde H synthase-1) which is constitutively expressed in the gastric mucus, in platelets and in most tissues, is responsible for the production of homeostatic prostanoids or "physiological" PGs. For example, PGE_2 and PGI_2 are produced by the GI tract to protect epithelial cells against ulceration (19). However, COX-1 is also involved in TXA_2 production in platelets and is associated with prothrombic activity (20). Some other products like prostacyclin ensure the protection of the stressed or inadequately perfused kidney (21). On the other hand, the COX-2 is responsible for the generation of "pathological" PGs as observed in inflammatory processes. It is true that COX-2 is essentially an inducible enzyme, the expression of which is not only increased by inflammatory mediators but also by non-inflammatory stimuli. Both isoforms of COX have been observed in the endothelium but

Table 2 Physiological Activity of Prostaglandins

Eicosanoid	Site of production	Physiological actions
PGE_2	Kidney	Vasodilation
		Maintenance of GFR
	Kidney	Renin release
		Excretion of sodium and water
	Gastrointestinal tract	Mucus production
		Bicarbonate secretion
		Mucosal blood flow
		Epithelial proliferation
		Mucosal resistance to injury
	Mast cells	Inflammation process
PGI_2=prostacyclin	Kidney	Vasodilation
		Maintenance of GFR
		Excretion of sodium and water
		Renin release
$PGF_{2\alpha}$	Kidney	Excretion of sodium and water
TXA_2	Platelets	Prothrombotic activity
	Kidney	Vasoconstriction, contraction of the glomerulus (regulation of GFR)

Abbreviation: GFR, glomerular filtration rate.

COX-2 was only detectable in cells stimulated by inflammatory stimuli (22) or shear stress (23). Unfortunately, this hypothesis appeared to be an oversimplification. Thus, COX-2 has been shown to be constitutively present in several organs including the brain and the kidneys (24) and it has appeared that COX-2 mRNA and protein expression in the mammalian kidney are among the highest observed in any tissues (25).

In fact, both COX-1 and COX-2 are constitutively expressed within the normal adult kidney: COX-1 is present in the glomerulus, the afferent arteriole and in tubular cells and COX-2 has been located in the afferent and efferent arterioles, the podocytes, the macula densa, interstitial cells and in some tubular cells, mainly in the thick ascending limb and the collecting tubules (26,27). As reviewed recently by several authors, intrarenal PGs participate actively in the regulation of renal perfusion and glomerular filtration rate (GFR) (24,28). Of note, PGs appear to play no role in the regulation of renal perfusion in the basal state when their secretion rate is relatively low but PG synthesis is increased (mostly within the glomeruli) by vasoconstrictors such as angiotensin II, norepinephrine, vasopressin (acting via the V1 receptor), and endothelin (29–31). Each of these hormones activates phosphatidylinositol turnover, leading to the formation of diacylglycerol, which contains arachidonic acid at position 2. PGs can then be released from diacylglycerol by the action of phospholipase A2. The ensuing PG-induced vasodilation partially counteracts the neurohumoral vasoconstriction, thereby minimizing the degree of renal ischemia (30).

Besides their activities as important regulators of renal hemodynamics through their effects on afferent arterioles, COX-2-derivatives are also implicated in the maintenance of sodium, potassium, chloride and water homeostasis and in the regulation of renin secretion (24,28,32). Several recent studies by Harris and colleagues have contributed to the understanding of the role COX-2 in the kidney and its implication in the progression of renal diseases (33). Thus, these authors have demonstrated that COX-2 expression is locally increased in high renin states such as salt restriction (33), in the 5/6 nephrectomy model of chronic renal failure (34), during angiotensin-converting-enzyme-inhibition (35,36) or in renovascular hypertension (37). Of note, salt loading also induced COX-2 expression in the medulla of rats, suggesting a role of this isoform in facilitating urinary sodium excretion (38). During water deprivation, COX-2 expression was enhanced to promote medullary interstitial cell survival during the hypertonic stress of dehydration (39,40). Finally, upregulated expression of medullary COX-2, but not COX-1, occurred in an experimental heart failure model in rats, suggesting that this isoform produces PGs that maintain medullary blood flow and natriuresis in the face of decreased renal perfusion from congestive heart failure (CHF) (Table 3) (41).

The PGs (Fig. 1) PGE_2, PGI_2 together with $PGF_{2\alpha}$ and TXA_2 have been shown to be the major biologically active PGs in the kidneys (42). PGE_2 and $PGF_{2\alpha}$ are produced mainly not only by the medullary interstitial cells, but also by the papillary collecting tubules and glomeruli. Arteriolar endothelium appears to be the major site of production of PGI_2, although this compound has also been found in papillary collecting tubules and glomeruli (42). Thromboxane A2 has been shown to be present in glomeruli, but it may actually originate from circulating platelets (43).

As already stated, the early paradigm linking COX-1 to physiological homeostasis and COX-2 to inflammation is too simplistic to fully explain the complex and often interdependent roles of these two isoenzymes in the kidney. The differential expression and localization of the two COX isoforms however suggests that they may have different physiological functions within the kidney. This separation of COX-mediated functions in the kidney is based in part on the physiologic/anatomic distribution of COX-1 compared to COX-2 and in part on the observation that blockade of either or both of these enzymes can have different effects on renal function (Table 4).

Table 3 Upregulated Renal Expression of COX-2 Iso-Enzyme

Stimulus	Renal localization	Consequences
Salt restriction	Renal cortex Macula densa	Vasodilation Renin secretion
Reduced renal mass (5/6 nephrectomy)		Compensatory renal hypertrophy
ACE inhibitors/Angiotensin II receptor antagonists	Renal cortex	Vasodilation
	Macula densa	Renin secretion
Salt loading	Renal medulla Medullary interstitial cells	Natriuresis
Water deprivation	Medullary interstitial cells	Vasodilation, cell survival
Experimental heart failure	Renal medulla	Maintenance of renal blood flow Natriuresis

EFFECTS OF PGS ON RENAL SALT AND WATER EXCRETION

The most important PGs in kidneys are PGE_2 and PGI_2 (prostacyclin). Other arachidonic acid derivatives, such as TXA_2 and other eicosanoids can also affect renal function, but their clinical significance is less well understood (44,45). Thromboxane concentrations are very low in kidneys of normal subjects and inhibition of its synthesis has only little effect on renal function (44). However, this PG is a known cause of renal vasoconstriction and mesangial cells contraction and hence can contribute to the fall in GFR and increase in urinary protein excretion frequently seen in glomerular diseases (44).

Table 4 Major Renal Biological Effects of Prostaglandins and Thromboxane

Agent	Renal localization	Synthesized by	Mode of action	Direct consequences
PGE_2, PGI_2	Intrarenal arterioles	COX-1	Vasodilation	Increased renal perfusion (more pronounced in inner cortical and medullary regions)
PGI_2	Glomeruli	COX-1	Vasodilation	Increase filtration rate
PGE_2, PGI_2	Efferent arterioles	COX-1 and COX-2	Vasodilation	Increase Na excretion through increased post-glomerular perfusion
PGE_2, PGI_2, $PGF_{2\alpha}$	Distal tubules	COX-2	Decreased transport	Increase Na excretion, decrease maximum medullary hypertonicity
PGE_2, (PGI_2, $PGF_{2\alpha}$)	Distal tubules	COX-2	Inhibition of cAMP synthesis	Interference with ADH action
PGE_2, PGI_2	Juxtaglo-merular apparatus	COX-2	cAMP stimulation?	Increase in renin secretion
TXA_2	Intrarenal arterioles	COX-1	Vasocon-striction	Decreased renal perfusion

Abbreviations: ADH, antidiuretic hormone; cAMP, cyclic adenosine monophosphate.

As already mentioned, renal PGs have both vascular and tubular actions, resulting from the activation of their distinct cell surface receptors.

Clinical data available today suggest that the intrarenal function of COX-2 is predominantly associated with the maintenance of sodium and water homeostasis, while COX-1 derivatives, which may also influence sodium and water homeostasis, have a more defined role in the maintenance of glomerular filtration function (46).

PGE_2 is involved in the regulation of sodium reabsorption in the tubule and it acts as a counter-regulatory factor under conditions of increased sodium reabsorption.

PGE_2 is present primarily in the thick ascending limb of the loop of Henle, where it promotes diuresis and natriuresis by inhibiting reabsorption of sodium and water through the inhibition of the Na–K–2Cl cotransporter, a finding confirmed by in vitro studies on isolated renal epithelial cells systems (47), microperfusion of isolated nephron segments (48) and clearance studies in humans (Fig. 2) (47,49). The natriuretic effect of other PGs have also been studied (47), and only PGI_2 was found to act as a diuretic, though in a markedly lesser extent than PGE_2 (50). In fact, PGI_2 is rather kaliuretic since prostacyclin increases potassium secretion, mainly by stimulating secretion of renin and activating the renin–angiotensin system, ultimately resulting in increased secretion of aldosterone (51). In addition, this vasodilatory PG increases renal blood flow and GFR under conditions associated with decreased effective circulating volume, resulting in greater tubular flow and secretion of potassium (51).

Besides their natriuretic activity, PGs have been shown to modulate water transport in several vasopressin-sensitive epithelial cell systems as well as in in vivo models (43,47). PGE_2, for example, modified renal vasopressin V-2 receptors signaling, resulting in a reduced insertion of water channels (aquaporin 2) into luminal membrane and therefore in a decreased water reabsorption.

In summary, renal PGs do not appear to contribute actively to the regulation of sodium and water homeostasis in healthy hydrated individuals. However, under conditions of reduced or compromised renal perfusion, the production of renal PGs serves as an important regulatory mechanism (32). Therefore, medical treatments that interfere with

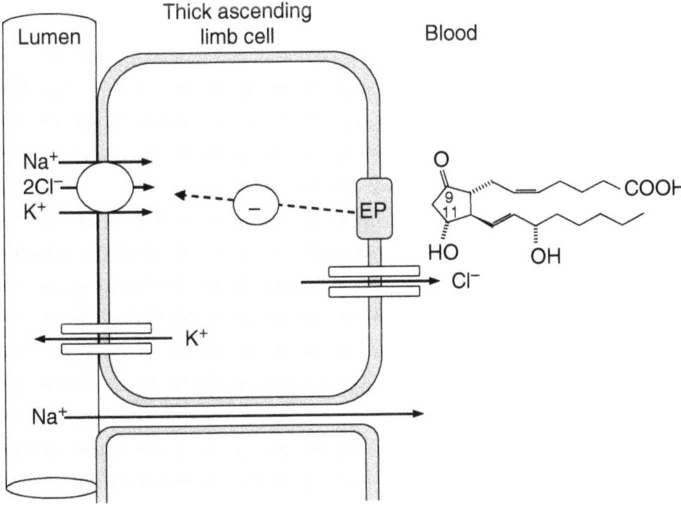

Figure 2 Schematic representation of the impact of prostaglandins on sodium transport in the thick ascending limb of the loop of Henle.

the biosynthesis of PGs will very likely have a major impact on renal function and water and electrolytes balance in high-risk patients, i.e., patients with a preexisting renal dysfunction, a low-effective arterial volume or dehydrated subjects. Among drugs inhibiting the biosynthesis of PGs, NSAIDs and selective COX-2 inhibitors are the most commonly prescribed agents.

EFFECTS OF NSAIDS ON RENAL FUNCTION

NSAIDs represent a class of compounds that are widely used. These drugs have analgesic, antipyretic and anti-inflammatory effects and are mainly used by patients with acute or chronic pain due to osteoarthritis and rheumatoid arthritis (52,53). The clinical use of NSAIDs is often limited by the occurrence of side effects such as gastrointestinal erosions, bleeding, salt retention and occasionally, acute renal failure. The development of these side effects is directly linked to the inhibition of cyclo-oxygenase in the stomach, platelets and kidneys. The discovery of the two isoforms of COXs has led to the development of selective COX-2 inhibitors. These drugs were developed with the intention to provide a treatment of pain and inflammation without inducing the potentially serious gastrointestinal side effects associated with the inhibition of gastric COX-1 derivatives.

NSAIDs in fact represent a heterogeneous class of drugs which includes aspirin (ASA), the traditional non-selective COX-1/COX-2 inhibitors (tNSAIDs) as well as the recently developed selective inhibitors of COX-2, the coxibs. Clinically, traditional non-selective NSAIDs and selective COX-2 appear to be equally effective in the treatment of chronic pain (53). More recently, selective COX-2 inhibitors have also been shown to be as effective as conventional NSAIDs in the treatment of gout and ankylosing spondylitis (54,55). Finally, like aspirin, the COX-2 inhibitor celecoxib is approved for the reduction of number of adenomatous colorectal polyps in familial adenomatous polyposis (56) and may contribute to the prevention of colorectal cancers (57).

Effects of COX-Inhibition on Renin Secretion

The renin–angiotensin system is an important regulator of sodium balance and PGs have been shown to play an important role in the regulation of renin secretion. In fact both COX-1 and COX-2 have been identified and localized in the juxtaglomerular apparatus (58). Harding et al. (59) have demonstrated that the selective inhibition of COX-2 in the mouse abolishes renin secretion stimulated by a low-sodium diet. This finding suggests that COX-2 is responsible for the formation of PGs which participate in the synthesis and release of renin. Renin production, secretion and release is also mediated by the type I nitric oxide (NO) synthase which is also present in the macula densa (58,60,61). Kurtz et al. have shown that there are close relations between COX-2, NO and the renin–angiotensin system (62). These authors have demonstrated that inhibition of the renin–angiotensin system is associated with an overexpression of COX-2 at the macula densa. Thus, COX-2 activity in the macula densa participates in the negative feedback that angiotensin II exerts on renin secretion (62,63). Wang et al. have nicely demonstrated in a rat model of renovascular hypertension that COX-2 activity is enhanced in the cortex of the stenotic kidney which secretes renin and that renin activity can be blunted by the administration of a COX-2 inhibitor. In that case, COX-2 inhibition is associated with a significant decrease in blood pressure (37). Taken together, these observations suggest that PGs play an essential role on the regulation of renin secretion and thereby participate in the regulation of sodium balance.

Effects of NSAIDs on Salt Retention

Renal complications of NSAIDs are not uncommon, and adverse reactions such as acute renal failure, hyperkalemia, hyponatremia and peripheral edema are listed in the package insert of most of these drugs. As described above, renal PGs, and particularly PGE_2, decrease sodium reabsorption in the thick ascending limb of the loop of Henle. It is therefore not surprising that administration of NSAIDs, by decreasing tubular PGE_2 increases sodium reabsorption and hence favor salt retention and the development of peripheral edema in humans. Sodium retention is a well-known complication that has been reported to occur in up to 25% of the NSAIDs-treated patients (64). In rare instances, the weight gain can be very marked with a 70-year-old patient treated with ibuprofen gaining as much as 15 kg over 17 days (65). However, practical knowledge regarding, for example, the magnitude of sodium retention induced by these agents, and the variation in response among individuals, is lacking (66). Because NSAIDs inhibit the physiologic role of renal PGs and because these PGs are predominantly produced in clinical conditions of decreased renal perfusion, NSAIDs produce their renal side effects mainly in high-risk situations, that is, in patients with a low-effective intravascular volume or in patients with preexisting renal disease (21). In these patients, the disease-induced reduction in the capacity to excrete sodium is aggravated by the administration of NSAIDs. Moreover, it is important to note that the sodium retention induced by NSAIDs reduce the therapeutic efficacy of several drugs classes including blockers of the renin–angiotensin system and diuretics. Thus, several studies have shown that the natriuretic efficacy of loop diuretics may decrease by 15% to 20% (64,67).

With this background, several studies have been designed to evaluate whether some NSAIDs might be less deleterious on renal function and in particular, whether the selective COX-2 inhibitors might differ in their effects on the kidney.

Catella-Lawson et al. (68) studied 36 older adults on a normal salt diet. Subjects were randomized under double-blind conditions to receive the specific COX-2 inhibitor rofecoxib (50 mg/day), indomethacin (50 mg 3×/day), or placebo for two weeks. The urinary sodium excretion decreased transiently but significantly during the first 72 hours of the rofecoxib administration and subsequently returned to baseline, while sodium excretion remained slightly but not significant diminished in the indomethacin group. These results suggested that despite differences in effect on COX iso-enzymes, there was no difference in terms of sodium reabsorption in elderly patients consuming a typical salt diet. A similar transient decrease ($p < 0.05$) in urinary sodium excretion was observed by Whelton et al. (69) who compared the effects of an another selective COX-2 inhibitor, celecoxib (200 mg 2×/day for five days, followed by 400 mg 2×/day for 10 days) with naproxen (500 mg 2×/day for 15 days) on renal function in 29 healthy elderly subjects in a single-blind, randomized, crossover study. Sodium excretion values returned to baseline by the end of the study.

As already stated several times, the properties of NSAIDs to retain sodium are most notable in patients who are already sodium avid, such as those with mild heart failure (70) or with liver disease (71). Thus studies in sodium-restricted subjects are more susceptible to clarify the effect of NSAIDs in high-risk patients, including those who are volume-depleted and patients who are taking diuretics. In this context, we performed a randomized, parallel study involving 40 salt-depleted normotensive young volunteers in which we compared the renal effects of celecoxib 200 and 400 mg bid, naproxen 500 mg bid and a placebo (72). As shown in Figure 3, we found also a transient but significant decrease in urinary sodium excretion with celecoxib and naproxen (72), suggesting that COX-2 is a key element for the regulation of sodium balance in salt-restricted conditions. In addition, in this study, we also

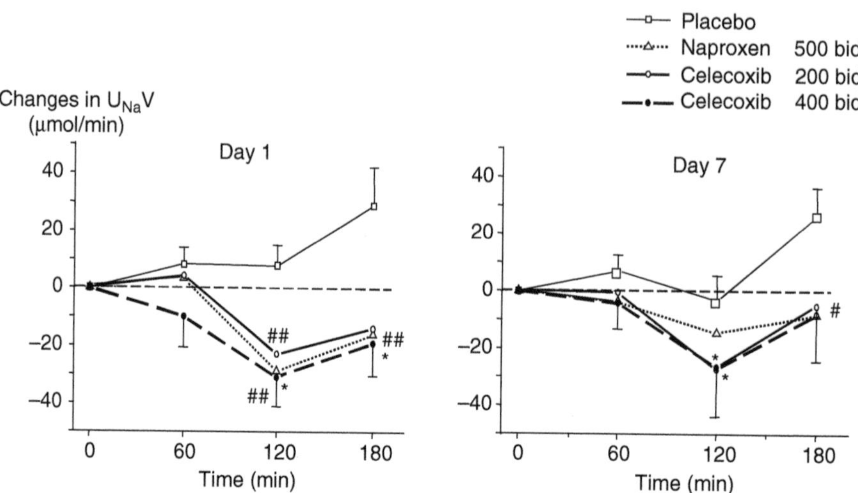

Figure 3 Acute changes in sodium excretion after selective and nonselective cyclo-oxygenase 2 inhibition in salt-depleted subjects. * $p<0.05$ versus baseline. #$p<0.05$ and ##$p<0.01$ versus placebo. *Source*: From Ref. 72.

measured the endogenous lithium clearance as an index of proximal sodium reabsorption and found that both celecoxib and indomethacin decreased lithium clearance indicating that both the COX-2 inhibitor and the traditional NSAID increase sodium reabsorption through an effect on the proximal segments of the nephron (72).

Apart these small phase II studies, large clinical trials have confirmed that coxibs can cause salt and water retention leading to edema and worsening hypertension (26,73,74). Thus, in a post hoc analysis of the renal safety of celecoxib, including data from more than 50 clinical studies involving more than 13,000 subjects (75), the most common side effects were peripheral edema (2.1%) and hypertension (0.8%). The incidence of the side effects reported with celecoxib was similar to that observed with other traditional NSAIDs, and were not time- or dose-related. In the CLASS trial (Celecoxib Long-term Arthritis Safety Study) that compared diclofenac, ibuprofen and celecoxib in patients with osteoarthritis and rheumatoid arthritis, the incidence of peripheral edema was 2% to 0.8% in the celecoxib group and 3.5% in the other NSAIDs groups (p=non-significant) (76).

As mentioned earlier, another aspect to consider in these patients, is that NSAIDs blunt the natriuretic effect of diuretics. Two studies performed in elderly patients have demonstrated that the use of NSAIDs is associated with an increased risk of developing congestive heart failure (70,77). One of them was a large cohort study in more than 10,000 patients, where a doubling of the risk for hospitalization for CHF was observed in patients taking diuretics and NSAIDs versus those ingesting diuretics alone (77). Similarly, in a case-control study, a twofold increase in risk of first hospital admission with CHF has been reported in patients treated with NSAIDs as compared with patients who did not receive these drugs (70).

Effects of NSAIDs on Renal Hemodynamics

Evaluation of COX-2 selective inhibitors on renal function in human subjects has improved our understanding of the role of the COX-2 isoform in the human kidney and provided insight into the effects of these drugs on GFR. Indeed, besides the effect of

NSAIDs on sodium retention, most studies mentioned above have also estimated the GFR before and after treatment.

In the study of Catella-Lawson et al. (68), selective inhibition of COX-2 by rofecoxib did not cause any significant decrease in GFR, compared to indomethacin that caused a decline in GFR. The same results were observed in the older patients studied by Whelton who observed that after the first dose, the trend was for a greater decrease in GFR with naproxen (-5.31 mL/min per 1.73 m^2) compared with celecoxib (-0.86 mL/min per 1.73 m^2). The treatment difference became statistically significant on sixth day (-7.53 vs. -1.11 mL/min per 1.73 m^2 for naproxen and celecoxib, respectively; $p=0.004$) (69). These two studies suggested that selective COX-2 inhibition in healthy elderly subjects might spare renal hemodynamic function because depression of GFR seemed to be mainly due to the non-selective inhibition of COX. Our study in salt-depleted subjects unfortunately contradict these observations. Indeed, in our salt-depleted healthy subjects the highest dose of celecoxib (400 mg twice a day) lowered GFR [(almost equal to) -20 mL/min] and effective plasma flow [(almost equal to) -100 mL/min] significantly, whereas naproxen had no such effect (72). After one week of administration, renal blood flow and GFR were decreased with both celecoxib and naproxen in these subjects (Fig. 4). A second study evaluating the effect of selective COX-2 drugs on GFR was undertaken in a slightly higher risk group. The renal effects of multiple doses of rofecoxib and indomethacin were studied in a group of salt-restricted elderly subjects (78). Sixty patients whose creatinine clearances ranged between 30 and 80 mL/min were randomized into one of four groups that received 12.5 mg of rofecoxib per day, 25 mg of rofecoxib per day, 50 mg of indomethacin three times per day, or placebo for six days. The 12.5- and 25-mg rofecoxib doses significantly decreased GFR by 10.2 and 9.6 mL/min, respectively, whereas indomethacin similarly decreased GFR by 7.8 mL/min. These data suggest that administration of a selective COX-2 inhibitor to salt-depleted subjects or to patients with mild to moderate chronic kidney disease is associated with a high risk of an

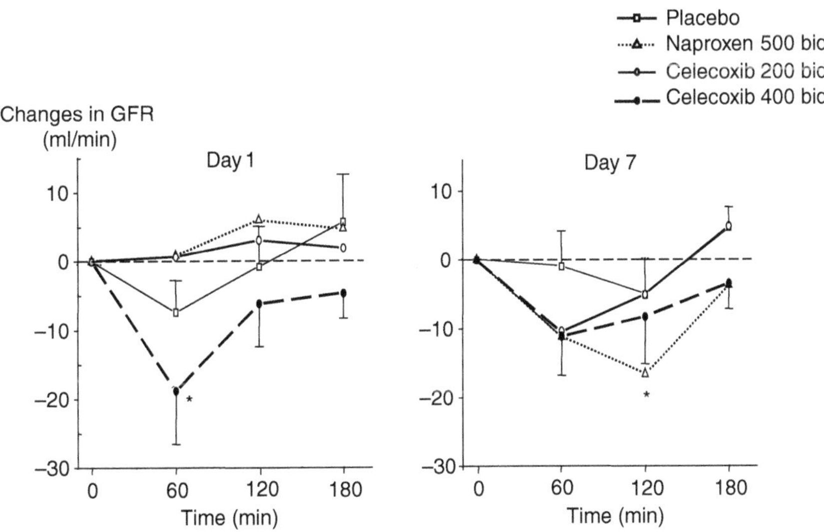

Figure 4 Acute changes in glomerular filtration GFR after selective and nonselective cyclo-oxygenase 2 inhibition in salt-depleted subjects. $*p<0.05$ versus baseline. $\#p<0.05$ and $\#\#p<0.01$ versus placebo. *Source*: From Ref. 72.

aggravation of renal function which is reminiscent of the traditional NSAID renal toxicity.

Decrements of GFR induced by NSAIDs may also occasionally result in acute renal failure. The pathogenesis is attributed to the renal vasoconstriction secondary to inhibition of vasodilatory PGs together with the unopposed effects of vasoconstrictive neurohormonal systems such as the renin–angiotensin and sympathetic nervous systems that lead to renal ischemia (71). Once again, this kind of side effect is observed predominantly in patients with clinical predispositions, such as patients with decompensated cirrhosis and ascites and/or edema or in patients with diseases states implying a low-effective arterial volume (71,79,80).

Effects of NSAIDs on Cardiovascular Events

Although it is not the main purpose of this chapter, it is not possible to discuss the renal effects of NSAIDs without dealing with their effects on cardiovascular safety, and particularly in view of the recent polemic that rose up after the withdrawal from the market of two selective-COX-2 inhibitors, rofecoxib and valdecoxib. Several reviews have been published on this topic (21,81–84). Schematically, as recently mentioned by G.A. FitzGerald in an editorial "the inhibition of PG formation, either by NSAIDs, aspirin or COX-2 inhibitors is remarkably well tolerated by otherwise healthy individual" (85). Hence, the cardiovascular complications of PG inhibition appear to occur mainly among patients at high risk, such as patients with heart failure, hypertension and previous cardiovascular events.

Among the different mechanisms evoked to support the eventual deleterious effects of selective COX-2 and NSAIDs on the occurrence of CV events, the most important pathway is certainly the integrity of the equilibrium between the vasodilator and potent inhibitor of platelet aggregation prostacyclin (PGI_2), produced by the endothelium via the COX-2 enzyme and the COX-1-mediated generation of TXA_2 by platelets as suggested experimentally by Cheng et al. (86). The use of low-dose aspirin for secondary prevention of myocardial infarction and stroke is based essentially on the fact that aspirin suppresses TXA_2 generation for the lifetime of platelets without any sustained effects on other PG synthesis. In contrast, coxibs suppress the COX-2-mediated production of prostacyclin and do not affect TXA_2 synthesis leading to a prothrombotic state. This is probably the main reason underlying the cardiovascular risk of coxibs in high-risk patients (21). In contrast to aspirin which irreversibly inhibits the production of TXA_2, most traditional NSAIDs are competitive and reversible inhibitors of platelet COX-1 with various potencies. Since they produce a shorter and reversible inhibition of thromboxane formation, they are often less potent and may not induce a sustained inhibition of platelet aggregation even though they are administered several times a day. One exception may be naproxen which has a longer half life (20,87). However, data are quite discordant and one cannot conclude that there is clear evidence to support a cardiovascular hazard from the administration of naproxen or non-naproxen NSAIDs (84). Therefore, and as it is the case in patients with preexistent kidney diseases or renal insufficiency, and in the absence of clear cut data, physicians will have to use traditional NSAIDs (or coxibs) in patients with a high cardiovascular risk on the basis of their common sense rather than on evidence-based medicine. For these patients, one should not forget that an inadequate long-term control of cardiovascular risk factors such as a hypertension, dyslipidemia, diabetes, smoking and weight excess is definitively more deleterious in term of cardiovascular mortality than the administration of NSAIDs itself.

CONCLUSION

Drugs can produce almost any kind of clinical side effects including disturbances in renal function and urinary water and electrolyte excretion. The example of NSAIDs and selective COX-2 inhibitors is an excellent demonstration of the multiple impacts that drugs can have on renal hemodynamics, GFR, renin secretion and renal sodium, potassium and water excretion. The case of NSAIDs not only illustrates the multiple possible facets of the drug-kidney interaction; it also reflects the importance of understanding the physiological and pharmacological mechanisms leading to these interactions. Indeed, knowing how drugs interfere with renal function and produce potential side effects is crucial in order to identify patients at risk of developing these complications and hence to prevent or reduce their occurrence.

REFERENCES

1. Burnier M, Brunner HR. Renal effects of angiotensin II receptor blockade and angiotensin-converting enzyme inhibition in healthy subjects. Exp Nephrol 1996; 4(Suppl. 1):41–6.
2. Wuerzner G, Chiolero A, Maillard M, et al. Angiotensin II receptor blockade prevents acute renal sodium retention induced by low levels of orthostatic stress. Kidney Int 2004; 65(1):238–44.
3. Zanchi A, Chiolero A, Maillard M, et al. Effects of the peroxisomal proliferator-activated receptor-gamma agonist pioglitazone on renal and hormonal responses to salt in healthy men. J Clin Endocrinol Metab 2004; 89(3):1140–5.
4. Nofziger C, Chen L, Shane MA, et al. PPARgamma agonists do not directly enhance basal or insulin-stimulated Na(+) transport via the epithelial Na(+) channel. Pflugers Arch 2005; 451(3):445–53.
5. Guan Y, Hao C, Cha DR, et al. Thiazolidinediones expand body fluid volume through PPARgamma stimulation of ENaC-mediated renal salt absorption. Nat Med 2005; 11(8):861–6.
6. Dusting GJ, Moncada S, Vane JR. Prostaglandins, their intermediates and precursors: cardiovascular actions and regulatory roles in normal and abnormal circulatory systems. Prog Cardiovasc Dis 1979; 21(6):405–30.
7. Jacobs LS, Douglas JG. Angiotensin II type 2 receptor subtype mediates phospholipase A2-dependent signaling in rabbit proximal tubular epithelial cells. Hypertension 1996; 28(4):663–8.
8. Siragy HM, Jaffa AA, Margolius HS. Bradykinin B2 receptor modulates renal prostaglandin E2 and nitric oxide. Hypertension 1997; 29(3):757–62.
9. Breyer MD, Jacobson HR, Hebert RL. Cellular mechanisms of prostaglandin E2 and vasopressin interactions in the collecting duct. Kidney Int 1990; 38(4):618–24.
10. Matsumura Y, Ozawa Y, Suzuki H, et al. Synergistic action of angiotensin II on norepinephrine-induced prostaglandin release from rat glomeruli. Am J Physiol 1986; 250(5 Pt 2):F811–6.
11. Slimane MA, Ferlicot S, Conti M, et al. Expression of cyclooxygenase 2 and prostaglandin E synthase after renal ischemia-reperfusion. Transplant Proc 2002; 34(7):2841–2.
12. Vishwanath BS, Frey FJ, Bradbury MJ, et al. Glucocorticoid deficiency increases phospholipase A2 activity in rats. J Clin Invest 1993; 92(4):1974–80.
13. Franson RC, Eisen D, Jesse R, et al. Inhibition of highly purified mammalian phospholipases A2 by non-steroidal anti-inflammatory agents. Modulation by calcium ions. Biochem J 1980; 186(2):633–6.
14. Weber PC, Larsson C, Scherer B. Prostaglandin E2-9-ketoreductase as a mediator of salt intake-related prostaglandin–renin interaction. Nature 1977; 266(5597):64–6.
15. Narumiya S, Sugimoto Y, Ushikubi F. Prostanoid receptors: structures, properties, and functions. Physiol Rev 1999; 79(4):1193–226.
16. Narumiya S, FitzGerald GA. Genetic and pharmacological analysis of prostanoid receptor function. J Clin Invest 2001; 108(1):25–30.

17. Grosser T. The pharmacology of selective inhibition of COX-2. Thromb Haemost 2006; 96(4):393–400.
18. Vane JR, Bakhle YS, Botting RM. Cyclooxygenases 1 and 2. Annu Rev Pharmacol Toxicol 1998; 38:97–120.
19. Wight NJ, Gottesdiener K, Garlick NM, et al. Rofecoxib, a COX-2 inhibitor, does not inhibit human gastric mucosal prostaglandin production. Gastroenterology 2001; 120(4):867–73.
20. Catella-Lawson F, Reilly MP, Kapoor SC, et al. Cyclooxygenase inhibitors and the antiplatelet effects of aspirin. N Engl J Med 2001; 345(25):1809–17.
21. Chioléro A, Maillard MP, Burnier M. Cardiovascular hazard of selective COX-2 inhibitors: myth or reality? Expert Opin Drug Saf 2002; 1(1):45–52.
22. Camacho M, Lopez-Belmonte J, Vila L. Rate of vasoconstrictor prostanoids released by endothelial cells depends on cyclooxygenase-2 expression and prostaglandin I synthase activity. Circ Res 1998; 83(4):353–65.
23. Okahara K, Sun B, Kambayashi J. Upregulation of prostacyclin synthesis-related gene expression by shear stress in vascular endothelial cells. Arterioscler Thromb Vasc Biol 1998; 18(12):1922–6.
24. Komers R, Anderson S, Epstein M. Renal and cardiovascular effects of selective cyclooxygenase-2 inhibitors. Am J kidney Dis 2001; 38(6):1145–57.
25. Breyer MD, Hao C, Qi Z. Cyclooxygenase-2 selective inhibitors and the kidney. Curr Opin Crit Care 2001; 7(6):393–400.
26. Harris RC. Cyclooxygenase-2 inhibition and renal physiology. Am J Cardiol 2002; 89(6 Suppl. 1):10D–7.
27. Komhoff M, Grone HJ, Klein T, et al. Localization of cyclooxygenase-1 and -2 in adult and fetal human kidney: implication for renal function. Am J Physiol 1997; 272(4 Pt 2):F460–8.
28. Harris RC, Breyer MD. Physiological regulation of cyclooxygenase-2 in the kidney. Am J Physiol Renal Physiol 2001; 281(1):F1–11.
29. Scharschmidt LA, Dunn MJ. Prostaglandin synthesis by rat glomerular mesangial cells in culture. Effects of angiotensin II and arginine vasopressin. J Clin Invest 1983; 71(6):1756–64.
30. Oliver JA, Pinto J, Sciacca RR, et al. Increased renal secretion of norepinephrine and prostaglandin E2 during sodium depletion in the dog. J Clin Invest 1980; 66(4):748–56.
31. Chou SY, Dahhan A, Porush JG. Renal actions of endothelin: interaction with prostacyclin. Am J Physiol 1990; 259(4 Pt 2):F645–52.
32. Whelton A. Renal and related cardiovascular effects of conventional and COX-2 specific NSAIDS and non-analgesics. Am J Ther 2000; 7(2):63–74.
33. Harris RC, McKanna JA, Akai Y, et al. Cyclooxygenase-2 is associated with the macula densa of rat kidney and increases with salt restriction. J Clin Invest 1994; 94(6):2504–10.
34. Wang JL, Cheng HF, Zhang MZ, et al. Selective increase of cyclooxygenase-2 expression in a model of renal ablation. Am J Physiol 1998; 275(4 Pt 2):F613–22.
35. Cheng HF, Wang JL, Zhang MZ, et al. Genetic deletion of COX-2 prevents increased renin expression in response to ACE inhibition. Am J Physiol Renal Physiol 2001; 280(3):F449–56.
36. Cheng H-F, Wang CJ, Moeckel GW, et al. Cyclooxygenase-2 inhibitor blocks expression of mediators of renal injury in a model of diabetes and hypertension. Kidney Int 2002; 62(3):929–39.
37. Wang J-L, Cheng H-F, Harris RC. Cyclooxygenase-2 inhibition decreases renin content and lowers blood pressure in a model of renovascular hypertension. Hypertension 1999; 34(1):96–101.
38. Yang T, Singh I, Pham H, et al. Regulation of cyclooxygenase expression in the kidney by dietary salt intake. Am J Physiol 1998; 274(3 Pt 2):F481–9.
39. Yang T, Schnermann JB, Briggs JP. Regulation of cyclooxygenase-2 expression in renal medulla by tonicity in vivo and in vitro. Am J Physiol 1999; 277(1 Pt 2):F1–9.
40. Hao CM, Yull F, Blackwell T, et al. Dehydration activates an NF-kappaB-driven, COX2-dependent survival mechanism in renal medullary interstitial cells. J Clin Invest 2000; 106(8):973–82.

41. Abassi Z, Brodsky S, Gealekman O, et al. Intrarenal expression and distribution of cyclooxygenase isoforms in rats with experimental heart failure. Am J Physiol Renal Physiol 2001; 280(1):F43–53.
42. Garella S, Matarese RA. Renal effects of prostaglandins and clinical adverse effects of nonsteroidal anti-inflammatory agents. Medicine (Baltimore) 1984; 63(3):165–81.
43. Levenson DJ, Simmons CE, Jr., Brenner BM. Arachidonic acid metabolism, prostaglandins and the kidney. Am J Med 1982; 72(2):354–74.
44. Remuzzi G, FitzGerald GA, Patrono C. Thromboxane synthesis and action within the kidney. Kidney Int 1992; 41(6):1483–93.
45. Carroll MA, Cheng MK, Jiang H, et al. Regulation of renal microvascular 20-hydroxyeicosatetraenoic acid (20-HETE) levels. Adv Exp Med Biol 2003; 525:55–8.
46. Whelton A. COX-2-specific inhibitors and the kidney: effect on hypertension and oedema. J Hypertens Suppl 2002; 20(Suppl. 6):S31–5.
47. Raymond KH, Lifschitz MD. Effect of prostaglandins on renal salt and water excretion. Am J Med 1986; 80(1A):22–33.
48. Stokes JB. Effect of prostaglandin E2 on chloride transport across the rabbit thick ascending limb of Henle. Selective inhibitions of the medullary portion. J Clin Invest 1979; 64(2):495–502.
49. Kaojarern S, Chennavasin P, Anderson S, et al. Nephron site of effect of nonsteroidal anti-inflammatory drugs on solute excretion in humans. Am J Physiol 1983; 244(2):F134–9.
50. Villa E, Garcia-Robles R, Haas J, et al. Comparative effect of PGE2 and GI2 on renal function. Hypertension 1997; 30(3 Pt 2):664–6.
51. DeMaria AN. NSAIDs, coxibs and cardio-renal Physiology: a mechanism-based evaluation. Medscape Online 2002. www.medscape.com.
52. American College of Rheumatology. Recommendations for the medical management of osteoarthritis of the hip and knee: 2000 update. American College of Rheumatology Subcommittee on Osteoarthritis Guidelines. Arthritis Rheum 2000; 43(9):1905–15.
53. FitzGerald GA, Patrono C. The coxibs, selective inhibitors of cyclooxygenase-2. N Engl J Med 2001; 345(6):433–42.
54. Rubin BR, Burton R, Navarra S, et al. Efficacy and safety profile of treatment with etoricoxib 120 mg once daily compared with indomethacin 50 mg three times daily in acute gout: a randomized controlled trial. Arthritis Rheum 2004; 50(2):598–606.
55. Gossec L, van der HD, Melian A, et al. The efficacy of cyclooxygenase-2 inhibition by etoricoxib and naproxen on the axial manifestations of ankylosing spondylitis in the presence of peripheral arthritis. Ann Rheum Dis 2005; 64(11):1563–7.
56. Steinbach G, Lynch PM, Phillips RK, et al. The effect of celecoxib, a cyclooxygenase-2 inhibitor, in familial adenomatous polyposis. N Engl J Med 2000; 342(26):1946–52.
57. Asano TK, McLeod RS. Non steroidal anti-inflammatory drugs (NSAID) and aspirin for preventing colorectal adenomas and carcinomas. Cochrane Database Syst Rev 2004; (2):CD004079. www.mrw.interscience.wiley.com.
58. Schnermann JB. Juxtaglomerular cell complex in the regulation of renal salt excretion. Am J Physiol 1998; 274:R263–79.
59. Harding P, Sigmon DH, Alfie ME, et al. Cyclooxygenase-2 mediates increased renal renin content induced by low-sodium diet. Hypertension 1997; 29(1 Pt 2):297–302.
60. Schricker K, Hamann M, Kurtz A. Nitric oxide and prostaglandins are involved in the macula densa control of the renin system. Am J Physiol 1995; 269(6 Pt 2):F825–30.
61. Kurtz A, Wagner C. Role of nitric oxide in the control of renin secretion. Am J Physiol 1998; 275(6 Pt 2):F849–62.
62. Wolf K, Castrop H, Hartner A, et al. Inhibition of the renin–angiotensin system upregulates cyclooxygenase-2 expression in the macula densa. Hypertension 1999; 34(3):503–7.
63. Cheng HF, Wang JL, Zhang MZ, et al. Angiotensin II attenuates renal cortical cyclooxygenase-2 expression. J Clin Invest 1999; 103(7):953–61.
64. Brater DC, Harris RC, Redfern JS, et al. Renal effects of COX-2 selective inhibitors. Am J Nephrol 2001; 21(1):1–15.

65. Schooley RT, Wagley PF, Lietman PS. Edema associated with ibuprofen therapy. JAMA 1977; 237(16):1716–7.
66. Zawada ET, Jr. Renal consequences of nonsteroidal antiinflammatory drugs. Postgrad Med 1982; 71(5):223–30.
67. Whelton A. Nephrotoxicity of nonsteroidal anti-inflammatory drugs (NSAID): physiologic foundations and clinical implications. Am J Med 1999; 106(5B):13S–24.
68. Catella-Lawson F, McAdam B, Morrison BW, et al. Effects of specific inhibition of cyclooxygenase-2 on sodium balance, hemodynamics and vaso-eicosanoids. J Pharmacol Exp Ther 1999; 289(2):735–41.
69. Whelton A, Schulman G, Wallemark C, et al. Effects of celecoxib and naproxen on renal function in the elderly. Arch Intern Med 2000; 160(10):1465–70.
70. Page J, Henry D. Consumption of NSAIDs and the development of congestive heart failure in elderly patients: an underrecognized public health problem. Arch Intern Med 2000; 160(6):777–84.
71. Epstein M. Non-steroidal anti-inflammatory drugs and the continuum of renal dysfunction. J Hypertens Suppl 2002; 20(6):S17–23.
72. Rossat J, Maillard M, Nussberger J, et al. Renal effects of selecive cyclooxygenase-2 inhibition in normotensive salt-depleted subjects. Clin Pharmacol Ther 1999; 66:76–84.
73. Stichtenoth DO, Frolich JC. COX-2 and the kidneys. Curr Pharm Des 2000; 6(17):1737–53.
74. Frishman WH. Effects of nonsteroidal anti-inflammatory drug therapy on blood pressure and peripheral edema. Am J Cardiol 2002; 89(6 Suppl. 1):18D–25.
75. Whelton A, Maurath CJ, Verburg KM, et al. Renal safety and tolerability of celecoxib, a novel cyclooxygenase-2 inhibitor. Am J Ther 2000; 7(3):159–75.
76. Silverstein FE, Faich G, Goldstein JL, et al. Gastrointestinal toxicity with celecoxib vs nonsteroidal anti-inflammatory drugs for osteoarthritis and rheumatoid arthritis: the CLASS study: a randomized controlled trial. Celecoxib Long-term Arthritis Safety Study. JAMA 2000; 284(10):1247–55.
77. Heerdink ER, Leufkens HG, Herings RM, et al. NSAIDs associated with increased risk of congestive heart failure in elderly patients taking diuretics. Arch Intern Med 1998; 158(10):1108–12.
78. Swan SK, Rudy DW, Lasseter KC, et al. Effect of cyclooxygenase-2 inhibition on renal function in elderly persons receiving a low-salt diet. A randomized, controlled trial. Ann Intern Med 2000; 133(1):1–9.
79. Epstein M, Lifschitz MD. Volume status as a determinant of the influence of renal PGE on renal function. Nephron 1980; 25(4):157–9.
80. Epstein M. Renal prostaglandins and the control of renal function in liver disease. Am J Med 1986; 80(1A):46–55.
81. Wong D, Wang M, Cheng Y, et al. Cardiovascular hazard and non-steroidal anti-inflammatory drugs. Curr Opin Pharmacol 2005; 5(2):204–10.
82. Wong M, Chowienczyk P, Kirkham B. Cardiovascular issues of COX-2 inhibitors and NSAIDs. Aust Fam Physician 2005; 34(11):945–8.
83. Konstantinopoulos PA, Lehmann DF. The cardiovascular toxicity of selective and nonselective cyclooxygenase inhibitors: comparisons, contrasts, and aspirin confounding. J Clin Pharmacol 2005; 45(7):742–50.
84. Maillard M, Burnier M. Comparative cardiovascular safety of traditional nonsteroidal anti-inflammatory drugs. Expert Opin Drug Saf 2006; 5(1):83–94.
85. FitzGerald GA. The choreography of cyclooxygenases in the kidney. J Clin Invest 2002; 110(1):33–4.
86. Cheng Y, Austin SC, Rocca B, et al. Role of prostacyclin in the cardiovascular response to thromboxane A2. Science 2002; 296(5567):539–41.
87. Capone ML, Tacconelli S, Sciulli MG, et al. Clinical pharmacology of platelet, monocyte, and vascular cyclooxygenase inhibition by naproxen and low-dose aspirin in healthy subjects. Circulation 2004; 109(12):1468–71.

21

Position of Diuretics in the Management of Hypertension

Bernard Waeber
Division of Clinical Pathophysiology and Hypertension Consultation, Department of Medicine, University Hospital, University of Lausanne, Lausanne, Switzerland

Michel Burnier
Division of Nephrology and Hypertension Consultation, University Hospital, University of Lausanne, Lausanne, Switzerland

INTRODUCTION

Hypertension is a common condition that still represents worldwide a main cause of mortality (1). Major efforts have been directed during the last decades not only to screen and treat patients with high blood pressure, but also to explore the mechanisms involved in the abnormal blood pressure elevation (2–4). It is now apparent that essential hypertension is very heterogeneous and that both genetic and environmental factors may contribute to the pathogenesis of this disease. The position of the sodium ion is in this respect exemplary: there exists in the general population a direct relationship between the amount of dietary sodium and blood pressure levels, and some genetically predisposed persons are more salt-sensitive than others (5,6).

Lowering total body sodium by decreasing salt intake is an effective approach to preventing and treating hypertension (5,6). Negativation of sodium balance can also been achieved pharmacologically using natriuretic agents. Such medications, especially thiazide and thiazide-like diuretics, have become a mainstay in the management of hypertension (7–10). The trend is to use them at low doses, either as monotherapy or in combination with other types of antihypertensive agents. Loop diuretics are reserved principally for patients with impaired renal function or resistant hypertension. Also available are potassium-sparing diuretics, in particular competitive antagonists of aldosterone, which are considered more and more as valuable antihypertensive drugs (11).

This chapter aims to review the experience accumulated with diuretics in the management of patients with high blood pressure. Focus is on the current recommendations regarding the position of these low-cost drugs in the therapeutic strategy of hypertension.

CLASSIFICATION AND MECHANISMS OF ANTIHYPERTENSIVE ACTION OF DIURETICS

A common feature of all diuretics is their natriuretic action, which leads to a decrease in total body sodium (12). The most potent diuretics, known as loop diuretics (main representatives: furosemide, bumetanide, ethacrynic acid, torasemide) decrease sodium reabsorption by interfering with the Na^+–K^+–$2Cl^-$ cotransport system in the thick ascending loop of Henle. These diuretics act at a site where a large fraction of sodium (30%) is normally resorbed. Thiazide (main representatives: hydrochlorothiazide, bendroflumethiazide) and thiazide-like diuretics (main representatives: chlortalidone, metolazone and indapamide) inhibit the Na^+/Cl^- cotransporter located in the early portion of the distal convoluted tubule. Only a small fraction of filtered sodium (7%) is normally reabsorbed at this site of the nephron, which accounts for the limited natriuretic activity of this type of diuretics. In the cortical collecting duct, the sodium ion is transported at the apical level of the tubular cell through the amiloride-sensitive epithelial sodium channel (ENaC). The hormone aldosterone (secreted by the adrenal glomerulosa) reaches the tubular cell cytoplasm where it stimulates a mineralocorticoid receptor, increasing thereby the number of sodium channels and sodium reabsorption. To go out of the cell, the sodium ion is then exchanged against a potassium ion at the basal membrane owing to the enzyme Na^+–K^+-ATPase. The activity of this energy-dependent enzyme is enhanced by aldosterone. The reabsorption of sodium is paralleled with a urinary loss of potassium droved to maintain intracellular electroneutrality. Spironolactone and eplerenone are competitive antagonists of aldosterone and, consequently, have a natriuretic effect while exerting a potassium-retaining action (11). Amiloride and triamterene are, like aldosterone antagonists, potassium-sparing diuretics, but have only a weak natriuretic activity. They act by blocking the apical sodium channel.

The mechanisms responsible for the blood pressure lowering effects of diuretics are complex and still poorly understood (12). At initiation of treatment the diuretic-induced extracellular fluid volume depletion is reflected by a loss of body weight, a blood pressure decrease, a reduction in plasma volume and a diminution in venous return and cardiac output (13). Concomitantly, because of an activation of both the renin–angiotensin and the sympathetic nervous system, total peripheral vascular resistance is increased (14,15). In the longer term, the antihypertensive effect persists despite a return of plasma volume and cardiac output towards pretreatment values.

Notably, the diuretic-mediated blood pressure lowering is almost wholly attributable with time to a reduction of total peripheral vascular resistance (16). Several hypotheses have been proposed to explain this phenomenon. The initial decrease in tissue blood flow consecutive to the contraction of plasma volume might be progressively restored as part of a whole body autoregulation process (17). Also, thiazides and thiazide-like diuretics may have direct vasodilating properties (18), and an increased release of nitric oxide and prostacyclin from the endothelium has been observed using furosemide (19). Finally, the diuretic-induced salt depletion is expected to attenuate the vasocontractile response to pressor stimuli (20), and the possibility exists that diuretics, by reducing total body sodium, promote the extrusion of calcium from vascular smooth muscle cells (via the sodium–calcium exchanger located in the cell membrane), facilitating thereby the relaxation of the vasculature (21).

FACTORS INFLUENCING THE BLOOD-PRESSURE RESPONSE TO DIURETICS

The blood pressure response to an increase in salt intake is highly variable. Actually, only a subset of individuals raises their blood pressure when switched from a low to a high sodium intake. This observation led to the concept of salt sensitivity and salt resistance (5,22,23). Salt sensitive subjects exhibit an incapacity of the kidneys to excrete the whole intake of sodium until renal perfusion pressure (and consequently systemic blood pressure) increases, allowing the elimination of sodium via the so-called pressure–natriuresis mechanism (24). Subtle functional or structural abnormalities in renal sodium handling may exist in salt-sensitive subjects (23). Many studies have shown a relationship between genetic factors and hypertension (5,25) and some variants of genes with a bearing on renal sodium retention have been linked with salt-sensitivity (26).

The prevalence of salt-sensitivity is increased in patients with low-renin levels, a form of hypertension which is commonly encountered in older individuals and black populations (27,28). As expected therefore diuretics tend to be more effective in lowering blood pressure in older than in younger patients, and in black than in white patients. This is exemplified by the results of a double-blind trial in which 1292 men with diastolic blood pressures of 95 to 109 mmHg were assigned to a one-year treatment with either placebo or six monotherapies, including hydrochlorothiazide (HCTZ) ($n=188$). There was an initial two-month titration phase during which the dose of the diuretic could be increased to reach the target diastolic blood pressure of less than 90 mmHg (29). Patients were considered responders if they had achieved the blood pressure goal at the end of the titration phase and exhibited a diastolic blood pressure of less than 95 mmHg at one year. Figure 1 depicts the placebo-corrected response rate. The success rate was greater in older (≥ 60 years) than in younger (<60 years) patients, both in blacks and in whites. HCTZ was more effective, regardless of age, in black than in white patients. Notably, HCTZ appeared particularly effective in reducing pulse pressure compared with other classes of antihypertensive agents (30). In the elderly thiazide diuretics and calcium antagonists are on the average superior to angiotensin converting enzyme (ACE) inhibitors and β-blockers (BB), as indicated by the results of a trial in which elderly patients with isolated systolic hypertension received according to a cross-over design each of the four classes of antihypertensive agents (31).

Numerous trials have demonstrated the effectiveness of diuretics in the management of hypertension (11,32,33). Overall, when considering groups of patients, the blood pressure lowering effect of diuretics is very similar to that of the main classes of antihypertensive agents. The blood pressure response to diuretics may however greatly differ from patient to patient, which is also the case for all medications used to treat hypertension.

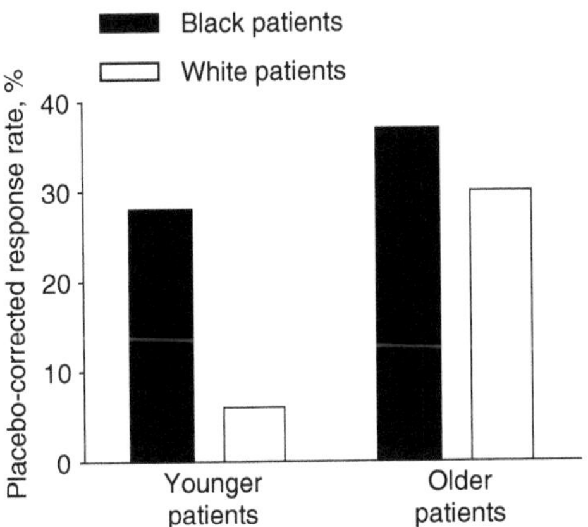

Figure 1 Placebo-corrected response rate, as defined as diastolic blood pressure <90 mmHg at the end of the titration phase and a diastolic blood pressure <95 mmHg at one-year follow-up. Younger patients were aged <60 years and older patients ≥ 60 years. *Source*: From Ref. 29.

The diuretic-induced salt depletion and the ensuing activation of the renin–angiotensin system is a major factor limiting the magnitude of the blood pressure response (15). During recent years pharmacogenetic approaches has been used in an attempt to tailor antihypertensive drug therapy. Some gene polymorphisms seem to contribute to the prediction of the blood pressure lowering effect of thiazide diuretics, but the search for such polymorphisms is not yet clinically useful for taking therapeutic decisions (34).

DIURETICS: A PIVOTAL ROLE IN COMBINATION THERAPY

The rationale for combination therapy is now well documented (35–37). The blood pressure lowering effect of antihypertensive drugs is often blunted because of the activation of feed-back mechanisms. The association of two drugs that mutually interfere with compensatory responses therefore increases the blood pressure control rate. Furthermore, the doses needed when two agents are co-administered are generally lower than those required when the components are used as single agents. This has a major advantage in terms of tolerability as the incidence of adverse effects shows a clear-cut dose-dependent character for some classes of antihypertensive agents.

Diuretics enhance the efficacy of all classes of antihypertensive drugs. This is particularly true for agents that block the renin–angiotensin system (38). The diuretic-induced negativation of sodium balance triggers the release of renin, and concomitant treatment with an ACE inhibitor or an AT_1-receptor blocker allows the neutralization of this reactive hyperreninemia, making it possible to derive maximal benefit from sodium depletion. Blockers of the renin–angiotensin system represent therefore the prototype of antihypertensive drugs which complementary mechanisms of action. Noteworthy, during inhibition of the renin–angiotensin system, diuretic therapy with HCTZ 25 mg/day or moderate sodium restriction (approximately 100 mmol/day) provide equivalent blood pressure reductions (39).

With regard to antihypertensive drugs that do not block the renin–angiotensin axis, they lead to some degree of renal sodium retention whenever they lower blood pressure, so that the co-administration of a diuretic is often required to maintain their long-term efficacy. Calcium antagonists may cause some natriuresis themselves (40), but their effectiveness is also increased by diuretics (41,42).

MORBIDITY–MORTALITY TRIALS

Placebo-Controlled Trials

Most earlier morbidity–mortality trials in the field of hypertension compared thiazide-based strategies and placebo (43). A meta-analysis of these trials showed significant benefits of reducing blood pressure on risks of cardiovascular events (44). Figure 2 illustrates the observations made with low-dose diuretics (generally 12.5–25 mg/day of chlortalidone or HCTZ as initial therapy). The active treatment lowered total mortality by 10% and cardiovascular mortality by 19%. This was associated with a reduction in risk of stroke, coronary heart disease (CHD), and congestive heart failure (CHF) of 29%, 21%, and 49%, respectively.

The importance of high blood pressure as a cardiovascular risk factor raises with aging. Arterial stiffness increases over years, leading to a preferential elevation of systolic blood pressure and a widened pulse pressure manifesting by a high prevalence of isolated systolic hypertension in the elderly (45). With advancing age systolic blood pressure

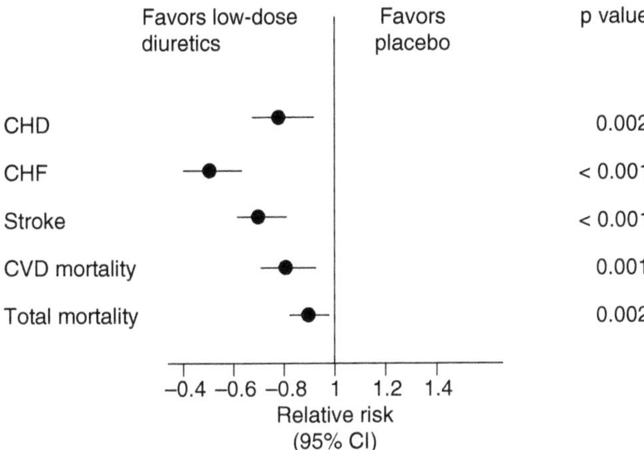

Figure 2 Effects of a therapeutic strategy based on a low-dose thiazide diuretic compared with placebo on the relative risk of cardiovascular complications. *Abbreviations*: CHD, coronary heart disease; CHF, congestive heart failure; CI, confidence interval; CVD, cardiovascular disease. *Source*: From Ref. 44.

becomes a better predictor of cardiovascular events than diastolic blood pressure. Randomized placebo-controlled trials carried-out in elderly patients have shown that thiazide-type diuretics are effective in reducing the incidence of cardiovascular events, at least up to the age of 80, in both systolodiastolic and isolated systolic hypertension (46,47). Significant benefits were observed with regard to stroke, heart failure and myocardial infarction.

The Systolic Hypertension in the Elderly Program (SHEP) trial has to be discussed in more detail since it was performed to assess the effects of a thiazide-based treatment in patients with isolated systolic hypertension, as defined by a systolic blood pressure ranging from 160 to 219 mmHg together with a diastolic blood pressure <90 mmHg (48). A total of 4736 patients aged 60 years or above were randomized for a mean follow-up of 4.5 years to either chlortalidone, 12.5 mg/day, or placebo. There was the possibility to double the dose of chlortalidone, and then to add the BB atenolol, 25 to 50 mg/day, if necessary to reach the target systolic blood pressure (systolic blood pressure <160 mmHg if baseline systolic blood pressure >180 mmHg, or reduction of systolic blood pressure by at least 20 mmHg if baseline systolic blood pressure was between 160 and 179 mmHg). The active treatment significantly reduced the risk of stroke (−37%) and myocardial infarction (−33%), but almost half of the patients were not on chlortalidone monotherapy anymore at the end of the trial.

Comparison with Other Drug Classes

Most event-based trials aimed to evaluate different therapeutic strategies included a thiazide diuretic as first or second step medication (49–51). The majority of these trials took only diastolic blood pressure as a target, accounting for a rather poor control of systolic blood pressure (52). Diuretics and BBs are the principal representative of older therapies, and calcium antagonists, ACE inhibitors and AT_1-receptor blockers those of newer ones. An important question is whether the older, conventional drug regimens provide equivalent protection against cardiovascular events in comparison with the modern classes of antihypertensives. This issue was addressed in a meta-analysis of 15 interventional trials involving 120,574 hypertensive patients (51). No significant advantage of the most modern drugs emerged, in terms of total and cardiovascular mortality, fatal and non-fatal stroke as well as fatal and non-fatal myocardial infarction.

As already pointed out thiazide diuretics used as single agents bring blood pressure under control in only a fraction of hypertensive patients. This is illustrated by the observations made in five recent randomized trials in which the goal was to normalize both systolic and diastolic blood pressure (53–57). To reach these target blood pressures various therapeutic strategies allowing a stepwise intensification of treatment were pre-established. Thiazide diuretics were part of the drug regimens in at least one treatment arm of each of the trials, either as step 1 or step 2 therapy. Table 1 summarizes the comparative impact of the various drug regimens on the incidence of stroke and myocardial infarction. Overall the observations made in these large interventional trials confirmed that combination therapy is required in the majority of patients in order to normalize at the same time systolic and diastolic blood pressure. Trials with predefined systolic and diastolic goal pressures reflect therefore more the results obtained with combination than with single-drug therapies. Some of the therapeutic strategies evaluated in the trials described above were found to protect more effectively than others against cardiovascular complications, which in most cases could be accounted for by differences in the level of blood pressure achieved during antihypertensive therapy. The most consistent findings were a better prevention of stroke by a regimen comprising a calcium antagonist and an ACE inhibitor, or an AT_1-receptor blocker and a thiazide diuretic, compared with a strategy based on BB and a thiazide diuretic (56,57). In one trial, however, fewer strokes were observed in the patients allocated to a thiazide-BB treatment than in patients randomized to an ACE inhibitor–BB therapy (53), but the superiority of the diuretic-based regimen was seen only in black patients, i.e., patients who are generally poor responders to renin–angiotensin and β-adrenoceptor blockade.

Table 1 Presence or Absence of Significant Difference in Blood Pressure and Incidence of Cardiovascular Complications (Stroke and Myocardial Infarction) during Treatment with Various Drug Regimens

Trial	Treatment strategies (1 vs. 2)	Difference in blood pressure	Difference in fatal and non-fatal stroke	Difference in fatal and non-fatal myocardial infarction
ALLHAT	D±BB vs. ACE-I±BB	+	+	−
	CA±BB vs. ACE-I±BB	−	−	−
	D±BB vs. CA±BB	−	−	−
LIFE	AT_1-B±D vs. BB±D	−	+	−
VALUE	AT_1±B±D vs. CA±D	+	−	+
INVEST	CA±ACE-I vs. BB±D	−	−	−
ASCOT	CA±ACE-I vs. BB±D	+	+	+[a]

Drug regimen: First-step drug±Second-step drug. *Abbreviations*: ACE-I, angiotensin converting enzyme inhibitor; AT_1-B, AT_1-receptor blocker; BB, β-blocker; CA, calcium antagonist; D, diuretic; ALLHAT, Antihypertensive and Lipid-Lowering Treatment to prevent Heart Attack Trial; ASCOT, Anglo-Scandinavian Cardiac Outcomes Trial; INVEST, International Verapamil-Trandolapril Study; LIFE, Losartan Intervention for Endpoint Reduction in Hypertension Trial; VALUE, Valsartan Antihypertensive Long-term Use Evaluation Trial. + significant difference in favor of treatment strategy 1; − no significant difference.

[a] Non-fatal myocardial infarction (excluding silent)+fatal coronary heart disease.

EFFECTS OF DIURETICS ON LARGE ARTERIES

Impaired endothelial function is a very early marker of endothelial suffering. It precedes the development of the structural changes observed in the arterial wall (58) and is frequently associated with essential hypertension (59). Angiotensin II is known to increase the endothelial production of superoxide, a reacting oxygen species leading to the generation of peroxynitrite (devoid of vasodilatory activity) from nitric oxide (60). Potentially diuretics might therefore, by stimulating the renin–angiotensin system, fail to improve endothelial function, as it could be expected when blood pressure is lowered. This issue has been addressed in a double-blind trial involving 60 patients with essential hypertension: endothelial function was assessed before and after a six-week treatment with either HCTZ, 25 mg/day, valsartan, 80 mg/day, or placebo (61). Evidence was found in the forearm circulation for an improvement in basal nitric oxide production during AT_1-receptor blockade, but not with the diuretic and placebo. Notably, the magnitude of the blood pressure fall was similar in the two groups of patients having received the active compounds.

Abnormalities in the function and/or morphology of large arteries can be evaluated non-invasively by measuring pulse-wave velocity, which accelerates when the distensibility of the arterial wall decreases, in response for instance to an increased thickness of the arterial wall (62). Despite significant reductions in blood pressure thiazide diuretics, unlike the other main classes of antihypertensive agents, have no clear-cut effect on pulse wave velocity (63).

The intima-media thickness of the carotid artery, as measured by ultrasonography, represents a strong indicator of cardiovascular risk (64). Carotid artery imaging was performed in an ancillary study to the prospective morbidity–mortality International Nifedipine Study Intervention as a Goal in Hypertension Treatment (INSIGHT) in which hypertensive patients were randomized to receive once daily for four years a nifedipine gastrointestinal transport system, 30 mg ($n=115$), or a fixed-dose combination containing HCTZ, 25 mg, and amiloride, 2.5 mg ($n=127$), with the possibility to add other drugs than a calcium antagonist or a diuretic when required to reach a target blood pressure of less than 140/90 mmHg (65). A greater reduction of intima-media thickness was found in the calcium antagonist than in the diuretic-based treatment group. In another randomized double-blind trial (The Plaque Hypertension Lipid-Lowering Italian Study) hypercholesterolemic patients with asymptomatic carotid atherosclerosis were allocated to different treatment groups, including the diuretic HCTZ, 25 mg/day ($n=127$) or the ACE inhibitor fosinopril, 20 mg/day ($n=127$) (66). Nifedipine gastrointestinal therapeutic system (30 mg/day) could be added if needed to control diastolic blood pressure. Clinic and ambulatory blood pressures were not significantly different between the two groups. Carotid intima-media thickness progressed significantly during the mean 2.6-year follow-up in the HCTZ group, but not in the fosinopril group.

In another sub-study of the INVEST trial progression of coronary atherosclerosis was assessed by dual-section spiral computed tomography (67). Coronary calcifications significantly increased during a 3-year observation period in patients who had a reduced renal function at baseline (estimated creatinine clearance <60 mL/min, $n=53$), but not in those with a normal renal function at beginning ($n=53$). The thiazide-based therapy was associated with a faster progression compared to the nifedipine-based regimen (Odds ratio$=1.66$, 95% confidence interval: 1.09–2.51).

Overall these data indicate that, for a given blood pressure reduction, diuretics may not be as effective as other types of antihypertensive agents in improving endothelial function, regressing arterial wall hypertrophy and preventing the development of atherosclerosis. Co-administering a diuretic and a blocker of the renin–angiotensin system may restore the full benefit on the atherosclerotic process that is expected from the blood pressure lowering, but this remains to be verified.

EFFECTS OF DIURETICS ON CARDIAC HYPERTROPHY

Left ventricular hypertrophy has been established as an independent cardiovascular risk factor (68,69) and may lead to overt CHF (70). Relevantly, regression of cardiac hypertrophy during antihypertensive treatment allows a marked reduction in risk of a subsequent morbid event (71). One placebo-controlled trial examined in 844 mild hypertensive patients the specific effects of different monotherapies [thiazide diuretic (chlortalidone), calcium antagonist (amlodipine), BB (acebutolol), ACE inhibitor (enalapril)] on left ventricular mass (72). The patients received nutritional-hygienic therapy in addition to the pharmacological treatments for four years. A significant decrease in left ventricular mass was evidenced by echocardiography in all groups, including in patients randomized to placebo on the background of the nonpharmacological approach. The effects of the various treatments on left ventricular mass were very similar, with a modest advantage in favor of the diuretic. In another trial 1105 men with mild to moderate hypertension were randomly allocated to double-masked treatment with various monotherapies [diuretic (HCTZ), BB (atenolol), ACE inhibitor (captopril), calcium antagonist (diltiazem), α_1-blocker (prazosin), or centrally-acting sympatholytic agent (clonidine)] (73). Within the one-year follow-up echocardiographically determined left ventricular mass was reduced in patients with adequate blood pressure control on HCTZ, captopril, and atenolol, but not in corresponding patients having received the other compounds.

Double-blind, randomized controlled trials that assessed in hypertensive patients the effects of diuretics, BB, calcium antagonists, ACE inhibitors, or AT_1-receptor blockers on echocardiographic left ventricular mass were recently reviewed (74). This meta-analysis is based on 80 trials comprising 146 treatments arms ($n=3767$ patients). Figure 3 shows the percentage change in left ventricular mass obtained with the five drug classes. The calcium antagonists and the blockers of the renin–angiotensin system were more effective than the diuretics and the BB, but the difference achieved a significant levels only with the latter.

EFFECTS OF DIURETICS ON RENAL FUNCTION

There exists a direct relationship between the level of blood pressure and renal disease progression (75) and blood pressure lowering in hypertensive patients represents the most effective way in slowing the glomerular filtration rate decline (76). This is well recognized in recent hypertension guidelines which recommend to lower blood pressure below 130/80 mmHg in patients with chronic renal disease (8,77). An important issue is therefore the comparative efficacy of different drug classes, including diuretics, on the progression of hypertensive kidney disease. In the ALLHAT trial, no significant difference was observed in the incidence of end stage renal disease or 50% or greater decrease in glomerular filtration rate between patients assigned to the chlortalidone-based strategy compared with those randomized to the amlodipine- or the lisinopril-based regimen (78). In the INSIGHT study, creatinine clearance fell significantly ($p<0.05$) more in patients allocated to the nifedipine than to the hydrochlorothiazide/amiloride-treatment, despite similar reductions in blood pressure (79). Renal failure, defined as a serum creatinine

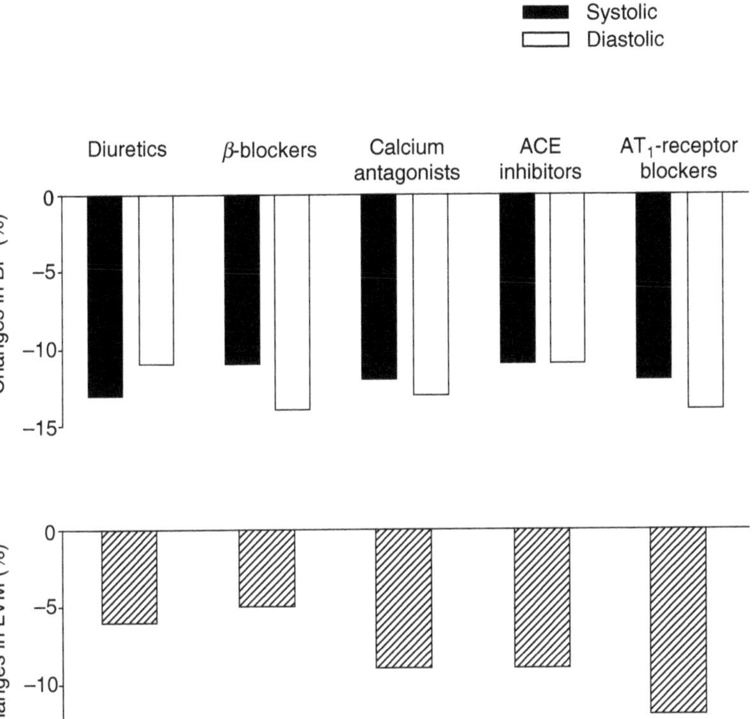

Figure 3 Mean changes in BP and LVM index, expressed as percentage from baseline, obtained with different classes of antihypertensive agents. *Abbreviations*: ACE, angiotensin converting enzyme; AT_1, angiotensin II type 1 receptor; BP, blood pressure; LVM, left ventricular mass. *Source*: From Ref. 74.

level of 260 μmol/L or higher developed in 2% of patients receiving nifedipine and 5% of patients receiving the diuretic combination ($p<0.01$).

Hypertensive patients with type 2 diabetes and microalbuminuria are at markedly increased risk for cardiovascular and renal events (80) and reduction in microalbuminuria using an ACE-inhibitor has a clear-cut protective effect in these patients (81). A double-blind comparison of the diuretic indapamide (slow-release formulation, 1.5 mg/day) and the ACE inhibitor enalapril (10 mg/day) was performed in 570 hypertensive patients with type 2 diabetes and microalbuminuria. The aim was to reach a target blood pressure of 140/90 mmHg, with the possibility of adding amlodipine, atenolol, or both whenever required (in more than half of the patients in both groups). The two drug regimens were equally effective in reducing blood pressure and microalbuminuria. Creatinine clearance decreased over the one-year follow-up by an average of 3.6 mL/min in the indapamide group, compared with 4.0 mL/min in the enalapril group ($p>0.05$).

Growing evidence suggests that blockers of the renin–angiotensin system, by lowering intraglomerular pressure and exerting an anti-inflammatory action, have a kidney protective effect exceeding that expected from the blood pressure lowering per se (82). The diuretic-induced negativation of sodium balance activates the renin–angiotensin system. It is not known however whether diuretics afford a better renal protection when co-administered with an ACE inhibitor or an AT_1-receptor blocker than when given as single agents.

Diuretics assume a key therapeutic position for the control of volume and blood pressure in patients with chronic renal disease (83). Loop diuretics are generally required when glomerular filtration rate decreases below 40 mL/min, and high doses of these agents, up to 500 mg/day furosemide for instance, may be needed in patients with end stage renal disease. Whenever possible it seems today preferable to co-administer a loop diuretic with a thiazide-like diuretic such as metolazone, since this compound still exerts a natriuretic activity when renal function is impaired. This allows the loop diuretic to be used at a lower dose, which is associated with a better tolerability. Aldosterone antagonists should not be used in the presence of impaired renal function, as they increase the risk of severe hyperkalemia (84).

DIURETIC-RELATED SIDE EFFECTS

Metabolic Effects

Hypertension and type 2 diabetes frequently coexist, which amplifies considerably the adverse impact of both conditions on the development of both micro and macrovascular complications (85). The use of some antihypertensive drugs, particularly high-dose diuretics and BB, is associated with an increased risk of new-onset diabetes (86–88). The diabetogenic effect of thiazides may be increased by co-administering a BB, but decreased by combining a blocker of the renin–angiotensin system (87). For example, in the Losartan Intervention For Endpoint reduction in hypertension study hypertensive patients with left ventricular hypertrophy were randomized to a double-blind four-year treatment based on either the AT_1-receptor blocker losartan, 50 mg/day, or the BB atenolol, 50 mg/day, with the possibility to add hydrochlorothiazide, 12.5 mg/day, to reach a blood pressure of ≤ 140 mmHg systolic and ≤ 90 mmHg diastolic (57). The dosage of all drugs could be doubled when needed. Notably, most patients were on ≥ 2 drugs at the end of the study (85.1% in the losartan group and 84.6% in the atenolol group). The incidence of new-onset diabetes during the trial was significantly greater in the atenolol–hydrochlorothiazide group (8.0%) than in the losartan–hydrochlorothiazide group (6.0%). Another prospective double-blind trial randomized newly diagnosed hypertensive patients to a one-year treatment with the AT_1-receptor blocker candesartan (16 mg/day, $n = 196$), or hydrochlorothiazide, 25 mg/day ($n = 196$) (89). It was possible to add, as needed, a calcium antagonist (felodipine extended release, 2.5–5 mg/day) in the candesartan group or a BB (atenolol, 50–100 mg/day) in the hydrochlorothiazide group. The blood pressure reduction was of similar magnitude in the two treatment arms. New-onset diabetes was observed during the follow-up in eight hydrochlorothiazide-treated patients (4.1%) compared with only one in the patients receiving candesartan (0.5%, $p = 0.03$). Table 2 shows the mean changes in plasma glucose and serum insulin concentrations observed during the trial.

Different mechanisms may contribute to the glucose intolerance of thiazide diuretics, including a reduced secretion on insulin by the pancreas and a decreased tissue sensitivity to insulin (90,91), in relation possibly to the diuretic-induced potassium depletion (92,93). The clinical consequences of the increased incidence of type 2 diabetes observed in hypertensive patients on thiazide therapy remain unclear, partly because of the shortness of treatment periods (94). Blood pressure-lowering drug regimens protect against cardiovascular events whether they contain or not a diuretic, regardless of the presence or not of type 2 diabetes (95).

Table 2 Effects of Candesartan- and Hydrochlorothiazide-based Therapy on Plasma Glucose and Serum Insulin Concentrations

	Candesartan ($n=196$)	Hydrochlorothiazide ($n=196$)
Plasma glucose concentration[a], mmol/L		
Baseline	5.17 ± 0.58	5.29 ± 0.98
Change	-0.06 ± 0.46 ($p<0.001$)	0.13 ± 0.69 ($p<0.001$)
Serum insulin concentration[a], mU/L		
Baseline	9.25 ± 7.90	9.65 ± 6.09
Change	-0.30 ± 6.50 ($p=0.003$)	0.35 ± 6.09 ($p=0.003$)

[a] Means ± SD.
Source: From Ref. 89.

Thiazide diuretics have modest adverse effects on lipid metabolism during long-term therapy (86,88,96). This is exemplified by the observations made in the SHEP study (97). This placebo-controlled trial included patients with isolated systolic hypertension, aged 60 years or older. The active treatment consisted of chlortalidone, 12.5 to 25 mg/day as first step, and atenolol 25 to 50 mg/day as second step. Over a three-year follow-up the active treatment, compared with placebo, induced small but significant changes in fasting lipid levels—total cholesterol: +0.09 mmol/L, $p<0.01$; high-density lipoprotein-cholesterol: −0.02 mmol/L, $p<0.01$; triglycerides: +0.9 mmol/L, $p<0.001$.

An association between the level of serum uric acid and cardiovascular risk has been identified in the general population and, more particularly among hypertensive patients, in whom hyperuricemia appears to be linked to an increased risk of renal disease progression (98–100). The development of hyperuricemia and gout is a well-known side effect of diuretic therapy (88). In the SHEP study, uricemia increased by an average of 35 μmol/L (active treatment versus placebo, $p<0.001$). There is some evidence that increased serum uric acid levels still represent an independent cardiovascular risk factor during antihypertensive treatment (101,102). Notably, addition of the AT_1-receptor blocker losartan to hydrochlorothiazide attenuates the diuretic-induced hyperuricemia (103). This is because the mother compound of losartan inhibits an anion-proton exchanger in the proximal tubules of the renal glomeruli, with an ensuing enhanced urate elimination (104).

Effects on Plasma Electrolytes

Therapy with thiazide diuretics represent a common cause of hyponatremia and hypokalemia (86,88,105). The diuretic-induced potassium depletion is of particular concern because it may increase the risk of cardiac arrhythmias and sudden death (106,107). The thiazide-induced decrease in total body potassium occurs in a dose-dependent fashion (108). Low-dose diuretic therapy appears more effective in preventing CHD than high-dose diuretic therapy (109). In the SHEP study, after one year of treatment, 7.2% of the participants allocated to the thiazide-based treatment had a serum potassium <3.5 mmol/L, compared with 1% in the placebo group ($p<0.001$) (110). Relevantly, the patients who had developed hypokalemia did not derive benefit in terms of cardiovascular prevention, as opposed to those who did not have hypokalemia. The thiazide-induced hypokalemia can be prevented by the simultaneous use of a potassium-sparing diuretic (108), and effectively attenuated by the co-administration of a blocker of the renin–angiotensin system (38).

Hyponatremia is another common complication of diuretic therapy, especially in hospitalized patients (111,112). When severe, this disorder is associated with a high level of morbidity and mortality. Hyponatremia usually develops within the first few weeks of therapy, but can occur at any time during thiazide administration (112,113).

The frequency of hypokalemia and hyponatremia amongst patients taking a thiazide diuretic has been evaluated recently by a computerized analysis of the electronic prescribing and laboratory records of 951 patients in a primary care setting. Prescription of a thiazide diuretic led to hypokalemia and/or hyponatremia in 20.6% of patients (105). Figure 4 shows the fraction of patients having such electrolyte disturbances. The frequency of hypokalemia and hyponatremia was markedly greater in older than in younger patients.

Potassium-sparing diuretics may occasionally lead to hyperkalemia (88). The risk exists mainly in patients with impaired renal function, especially when they receive potassium supplements or potassium-containing salt-substitutes, or take a blocker of the renin–angiotensin system, a nonsteroidal anti-inflammatory drug or heparin therapy.

Both thiazide and loop diuretics increase urinary magnesium excretion (88). Hypomagnesemia may lead to neurological manifestations and cardiac arrhythmias. A large fraction of patients with hypokalemia exhibit at the same time hypomagnesemia (114). This should be kept in mind as it may be impossible to correct hypokalemia unless the underlying magnesium deficit is corrected (115).

Other Adverse Effects of Diuretics

Thiazide and thiazide-like diuretics have an adverse impact on male sexual function (decreased libido, erectile dysfunction, trouble in ejaculating), which represents a major cause of withdrawal from antihypertensive therapy (88,116). Impotence, decreased libido and gynecomastia are the main adverse effects of spironolactone in men (88,117). In women spironolactone may cause menstrual irregularities, hirsutism, and deepening of voice. The recently developed aldosterone antagonist eplerenone has the advantage to be devoid of the endocrine adverse effects seen using spironolactone (117).

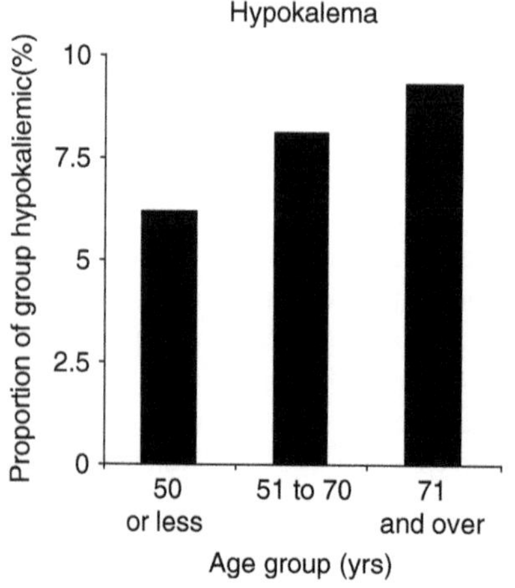

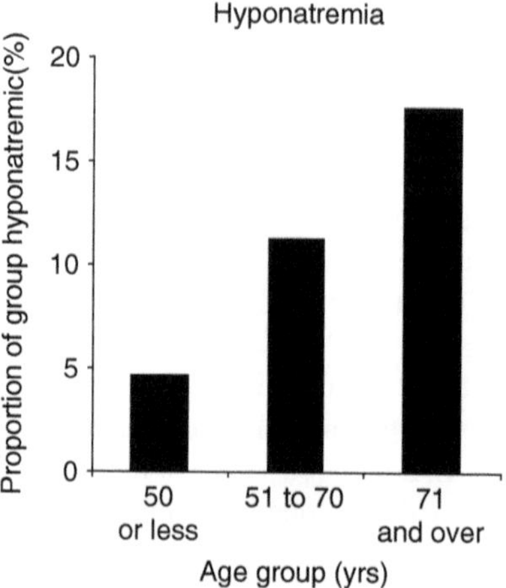

Figure 4 Fraction of patients (according to age) prescribed a thiazide and exhibiting hypokalemia (<3.5 mmol/L, left panel) or hyponatremia (<135 mmol/L, right panel). *Source*: From Ref. 105.

Photosensitivity dermatitis may occur during therapy with a thiazide or a thiazide-like diuretic. Necrotizing vasculitis or pancreatitis, and allergic interstitial nephritis are rare complications. Notably, chronic diuretic therapy might be associated with an increased risk of renal cell carcinoma, but this critical issue remains debated (118).

EFFECTS OF DIURETICS ON BONE

In the kidney thiazides decrease calciuria, resulting in a mild increase in calcemia and a decrease in parathyroid hormone and bone turnover (119). The data accumulated so far indicate that thiazide diuretics increase discretely bone mineral density and reduce the risk of fracture. These agents, given alone or in combination with other drugs, may be therefore particularly useful in osteoporotic and postmenopausal hypertensive women.

PERSISTENCE ON THERAPY

In actual practice unsatisfactory blood pressure control and intolerance to the treatment are by far the major causes of drug discontinuation. A number of studies have looked at the continuation rate of the major classes of antihypertensive drugs in newly diagnosed hypertensive patients. Figure 5 summarizes the persistence rate observed after one year in four studies having surveyed a large number of patients in different countries (120–123). The percentage of patients staying on AT_1-receptor blockers was the greatest and that of the thiazide diuretics the lowest in all studies. The 1-year continuation rate for the AT_1-receptor blockers averaged 42% when considering the four studies together, the corresponding values for the ACE inhibitors, the calcium antagonists, the BB, and the thiazides being 37.9%, 34.6%, 28.2%, and 21.2%, respectively. The fraction of patients still on the same therapy after four years was also the largest for AT_1-receptor blockers and the smallest for diuretics. These observations are meaningful:they show that thiazide diuretics are not necessarily the best drugs to use to initiate antihypertensive therapy, even if at first glance such a low cost approach may appear the most appealing.

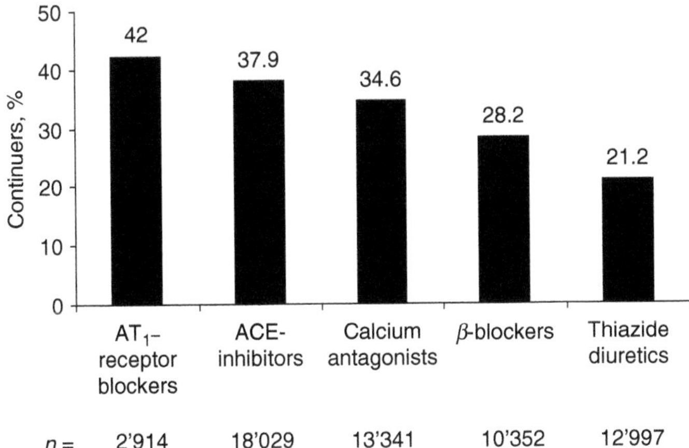

Figure 5 Percentage of patients remaining on initial antihypertensive therapy over one year. *Abbreviations*: ACE, angiotensin converting enzyme; AT_1, angiotensin II type 1 receptor. *Source*: From Refs. 120–123.

POSITION OF DIURETICS IN THE TREATMENT OF HYPERTENSION

Experts in the field of hypertension consider thiazide diuretics as a valuable first-line option to treat patients with high blood pressure (8–10,124,125). They also recognize the necessity to combine drugs in the majority of hypertensive patients in order to normalize blood pressure. The co-administration of a diuretic and a blocker of the renin–angiotensin system appears particularly attractive, as it allows blood pressure normalization in most patients without having detrimental effects on their quality of life. This accounts for the exploding number of fixed-dose preparations combining such agents.

REFERENCES

1. Ezzati M, Lopez AD, Rodgers A, Vander Hoorn S, Murray CJ. Selected major risk factors and global and regional burden of disease. Lancet 2002; 360:1347–1360.
2. Hamet P, Pausova Z, Adarichev V, Adaricheva K, Tremblay J. Hypertension: genes and environment. J Hypertens 1998; 16:397–418.
3. Waeber B. Treatment strategy to control blood pressure optimally in hypertensive patients. Blood Press 2001; 10:62–73.
4. Staessen JA, Wang J, Bianchi G, Birkenhager WH. Essential hypertension. Lancet 2003; 361:1629–1641.
5. Meneton P, Jeunemaitre X, de Wardener HE, MacGregor GA. Links between dietary salt intake, renal salt handling, blood pressure, and cardiovascular diseases. Phys Rev 2005; 85:679–715.
6. Weinberger MH. Sodium and blood pressure 2003. Curr Opin Cardiol 2004; 19:353–356.
7. Kaplan NM. The place of diuretics in preventing cardiovascular events. J Hum Hypertens 2004; 18(Suppl. 2):29–32.
8. European Society of Hypertension–European Society of Cardiology Guidelines Committee. 2003 European Society of Hypertension–European Society of Cardiology guidelines for the management of arterial hypertension. J Hypertens 2003; 21:1011–1053.
9. Chobanian AV, Bakris GL, Black HR, et al. Seventh report of the Joint National Committee on Prevention, Detection, Evaluation, and Treatment of High Blood Pressure. Hypertension 2003; 42:1206–1252.
10. Whitworth JA. 2003 World Health Organization (WHO)/International Society of Hypertension (ISH) statement on management of hypertension. J Hypertens 2003; 21:1983–1992.
11. Pratt-Ubunama MN, Nishizaka MK, Calhoun DA. Aldosterone antagonism: an emerging strategy for effective blood pressure lowering. Curr Hypertens Rep 2005; 7:186–192.
12. Hughes AD. How do thiazide and thiazide-like diuretics lower blood pressure? J Renin Angiotensin Aldosterone Syst 2004; 5:155–160.
13. Tarazi RC, Dustan HP, Frohlich ED. Long-term thiazide therapy in essential hypertension. Evidence for persistent alteration in plasma volume and renin activity. Circulation 1970; 41:709–717.
14. Lake CR, Ziegler MG, Coleman MD, Kopin IJ. Hydrochlorothiazide-induced sympathetic hyperactivity in hypertensive patients. Clin Pharmacol Ther 1979; 26:428–432.
15. Brunner HR, Nussberger J, Waeber B. Responsiveness of renin secretion: a key mechanism in the maintenance of blood pressure. J Hypertens 1986; 4(Suppl.):89–94.
16. Shah S, Khatri I, Freis ED. Mechanism of antihypertensive effect of thiazide diuretics. Am Heart J 1978; 95:611–618.
17. Tobian L. Why do thiazide diuretics lower blood pressure in essential hypertension? Annu Rev Pharmacol 1967; 7:399–408.
18. Pickkers P, Hughes AD, Russel FG, Thien T, Smits P. Thiazide-induced vasodilation in humans is mediated by potassium channel activation. Hypertension 1998; 32:1071–1076.

19. Wiemer G, Fink E, Linz W, Hropot M, Scholkens BE, Wohlfart P. Furosemide enhances the release of endothelial kinins, nitric oxide and prostacyclin. J Pharmacol Exp Ther 1994; 271:1611–1615.
20. Aleksandrow D, Wysznacka W, Gajewski J. Influence of chlorothiazide upon arterial responsiveness to norepinephrine in hypertensive subjects. N Engl J Med 1959; 261:1052–1055.
21. Blaustein MP. Sodium ions, calcium ions, blood pressure regulation, and hypertension: a reassessment and a hypothesis. Am J Physiol 1977; 232:C165–C173.
22. Weinberger MH. Sodium sensitivity of blood pressure. Curr Opin Nephrol Hypertens 1993; 2:935–939.
23. Chiolero A, Wurzner G, Burnier M. Renal determinants of the salt sensitivity of blood pressure. Nephrol Dial Transplant 2001; 16:452–458.
24. Guyton AC. Dominant role of the kidneys and accessory role of whole-body autoregulation in the pathogenesis of hypertension. Am J Hypertens 1989; 2:575–585.
25. Luft FC, Miller JZ, Weinberger MH, Christian JC, Skrabal F. Genetic influences on the response to dietary salt reduction, acute salt loading, or salt depletion in humans. J Cardiovasc Pharmacol 1988; 12(Suppl. 3):49–55.
26. Beeks E, Kessels AG, Kroon AA, van der Klauw MM, de Leeuw PW. Genetic predisposition to salt-sensitivity: a systematic review. J Hypertens 2004; 22:1243–1249.
27. Weinberger MH, Miller JZ, Luft FC, Grim CE, Fineberg NS. Definitions and characteristics of sodium sensitivity and blood pressure resistance. Hypertension 1986; 8:II127–II134.
28. Nesbitt SD. Hypertension in black patients: special issues and considerations. Curr Hypertens Rep 2005; 7:244–248.
29. Materson BJ, Reda DJ, Cushman WC, et al. Single-drug therapy for hypertension in men. A comparison of six antihypertensive agents with placebo. The Department of Veterans Affairs Cooperative Study Group on Antihypertensive Agents. N Engl J Med 1993; 328:914–921.
30. Cushman WC, Materson BJ, Williams DW, Reda DJ. Pulse pressure changes with six classes of antihypertensive agents in a randomized, controlled trial. Hypertension 2001; 38:953–957.
31. Morgan TO, Anderson AI, MacInnis RJ. ACE inhibitors, beta-blockers, calcium blockers, and diuretics for the control of systolic hypertension. Am J Hypertens 2001; 14:241–247.
32. Carter BL, Ernst ME, Cohen JD. Hydrochlorothiazide versus chlorthalidone: evidence supporting their interchangeability. Hypertension 2004; 43:4–9.
33. Robinson DM, Wellington K. Indapamide sustained release: a review of its use in the treatment of hypertension. Drugs 2006; 66:257–271.
34. Turner ST, Chapman AB, Schwartz GL, Boerwinkle E. Effects of endothelial nitric oxide synthase, alpha-adducin, and other candidate gene polymorphisms on blood pressure response to hydrochlorothiazide. Am J Hypertens 2003; 16:834–839.
35. Brunner HR, Menard J, Waeber B, et al. Treating the individual hypertensive patient: considerations on dose, sequential monotherapy and drug combinations. J Hypertens 1990; 8:3–11.
36. Ruzicka M, Leenen FH. Monotherapy versus combination therapy as first line treatment of uncomplicated arterial hypertension. Drugs 2001; 61:943–954.
37. Law MR, Wald NJ, Morris JK, Jordan RE. Value of low dose combination treatment with blood pressure lowering drugs: analysis of 354 randomised trials. BMJ 2003; 326:1427–1431.
38. Waeber B. Combination therapy with ACE inhibitors/angiotensin II receptor antagonists and diuretics in hypertension. Expert Rev Cardiovasc Ther 2003; 1:43–50.
39. Singer DR, Markandu ND, Cappuccio FP, Miller MA, Sagnella GA, MacGregor GA. Reduction of salt intake during converting enzyme inhibitor treatment compared with addition of a thiazide. Hypertension 1995; 25:1042–1044.
40. Pearce CJ, Wallin JD. Calcium antagonists and the kidney. New Horiz 1996; 4:123–128.
41. Luscher TF, Waeber B. Efficacy and safety of various combination therapies based on a calcium antagonist in essential hypertension: results of a placebo-controlled randomized trial. J Cardiovasc Pharmacol 1993; 21:305–309.

42. Burris JF, Weir MR, Oparil S, Weber M, Cady WJ, Stewart WH. An assessment of diltiazem and hydrochlorothiazide in hypertension. Application of factorial trial design to a multicenter clinical trial of combination therapy. JAMA 1990; 263:1507–1512.
43. Fuchs FD. Diuretics: drugs of choice for the initial management of patients with hypertension. Expert Rev Cardiovasc Ther 2003; 1:35–41.
44. Psaty BM, Lumley T, Furberg CD, et al. Health outcomes associated with various antihypertensive therapies used as first-line agents: a network meta-analysis. JAMA 2003; 289:2534–2544.
45. Franklin SS, Gustin W, Wong ND, et al. Hemodynamic patterns of age-related changes in blood pressure. The Framingham Heart Study. Circulation 1997; 96:308–315.
46. Beard K, Bulpitt C, Mascie-Taylor H, O'Malley K, Sever P, Webb S. Management of elderly patients with sustained hypertension. BMJ 1992; 304:412–416.
47. Hanon O, Seux ML, Lenoir H, Rigaud AS, Girerd X, Forette F. Diuretics for cardiovascular prevention in the elderly. J Hum Hypertens 2004; 18(Suppl. 2):15–22.
48. SHEP Cooperative Research Group. Prevention of stroke by antihypertensive drug treatment in older persons with isolated systolic hypertension. Final results of the Systolic Hypertension in the Elderly Program (SHEP). JAMA 1991; 265:3255–3264.
49. Turnbull F. Effects of different blood-pressure-lowering regimens on major cardiovascular events: results of prospectively-designed overviews of randomised trials. Lancet 2003; 362:1527–1535.
50. Williams B. Recent hypertension trials: implications and controversies. J Am Coll Cardiol 2005; 45:813–827.
51. Staessen JA, Wang JG, Thijs L. Cardiovascular prevention and blood pressure reduction: a quantitative overview updated until 1 March 2003. J Hypertens 2003; 21:1055–1076.
52. Mancia G, Grassi G. Systolic and diastolic blood pressure control in antihypertensive drug trials. J Hypertens 2002; 20:1461–1464.
53. ALLHAT Officers and Coordinators for the ALLHAT Collaborative Research Group. Major outcomes in high-risk hypertensive patients randomized to angiotensin-converting enzyme inhibitor or calcium channel blocker vs diuretic. JAMA 2002; 288:2977–2981.
54. Pepine CJ, Handberg EM, Cooper-DeHoff RM, Marks RG, Kowey P, Messerli FH, Mancia G, Cangiano JL, Garcia-Barreto D, Keltai M, et al. A calcium antagonist vs a non-calcium antagonist hypertension treatment strategy for patients with coronary artery disease. The International Verapamil-Trandolapril Study (INVEST): a randomized controlled trial. JAMA 2003; 290:2805–2816.
55. Julius S, Kjeldsen SE, Weber M, et al. Outcomes in hypertensive patients at high cardiovascular risk treated with regimens based on valsartan or amlodipine: the VALUE randomised trial. Lancet 2004; 363:2022–2031.
56. Dahlöf B, Sever PS, Poulter NR, et al. Prevention of cardiovascular events with an antihypertensive regimen of amlodipine adding perindopril as required versus atenolol adding bendroflumethiazide as required, in the Anglo-Scandinavian Cardiac Outcomes Trial-Blood Pressure Lowering Arm (ASCOT-BPLA): a multicentre randomised controlled trial. Lancet 2005; 366:895–906.
57. Dahlöf B, Devereux RB, Kjeldsen SE, et al. Cardiovascular morbidity and mortality in the Losartan Intervention For Endpoint reduction in hypertension study (LIFE): a randomised trial against atenolol. Lancet 2002; 359:995–1003.
58. Davignon J, Ganz P. Role of endothelial dysfunction in atherosclerosis. Circulation 2004; 109:III27–III32.
59. Brunner H, Cockcroft JR, Deanfield J, Donald A, Ferrannini E, Halcox J, Kiowski W, Luscher TF, Mancia G, Natali A, et al. Endothelial function and dysfunction. Part II: Association with cardiovascular risk factors and diseases. A statement by the Working Group on Endothelins and Endothelial Factors of the European Society of Hypertension. J Hypertens 2005; 23:233–246.
60. Waeber B, Feihl F. Oxidative stress: a pivotal link among cardiovascular risk factors? Curr Hypertens Rep 2005; 7:229–230.

61. Klingbeil AU, John S, Schneider MP, Jacobi J, Handrock R, Schmieder RE. Effect of AT_1 receptor blockade on endothelial function in essential hypertension. Am J Hypertens 2003; 16:123–128.
62. Benetos A, Waeber B, Izzo J, et al. Influence of age, risk factors, and cardiovascular and renal disease on arterial stiffness: clinical applications. Am J Hypertens 2002; 15:1101–1108.
63. Mahmud A, Feely J. Antihypertensive drugs and arterial stiffness. Expert Rev Cardiovasc Ther 2003; 1:65–78.
64. Simon A, Gariepy J, Chironi G, Megnien JL, Levenson J. Intima-media thickness: a new tool for diagnosis and treatment of cardiovascular risk. J Hypertens 2002; 20:159–169.
65. Gariepy J, Simon A, Chironi G, Moyse D, Levenson J. Large artery wall thickening and its determinants under antihypertensive treatment: the IMT-INSIGHT study. J Hypertens 2004; 22:137–143.
66. Zanchetti A, Crepaldi G, Bond MG, et al. Different effects of antihypertensive regimens based on fosinopril or hydrochlorothiazide with or without lipid lowering by pravastatin on progression of asymptomatic carotid atherosclerosis: principal results of PHYLLIS–a randomized double-blind trial. Stroke 2004; 35:2807–2812.
67. Bursztyn M, Motro M, Grossman E, Shemesh J. Accelerated coronary artery calcification in mildly reduced renal function of high-risk hypertensives: a 3-year prospective observation. J Hypertens 2003; 21:1953–1959.
68. Levy D, Garrison RJ, Savage DD, Kannel WB, Castelli WP. Prognostic implications of echocardiographically determined left ventricular mass in the Framingham Heart Study. N Engl J Med 1990; 322:1561–1566.
69. Koren MJ, Devereux RB, Casale PN, Savage DD, Laragh JH. Relation of left ventricular mass and geometry to morbidity and mortality in uncomplicated essential hypertension. Ann Intern Med 1991; 114:345–352.
70. Mann DL. Mechanisms and models in heart failure: a combinatorial approach. Circulation 1999; 100:999–1008.
71. Verdecchia P, Angeli F, Borgioni C, et al. Changes in cardiovascular risk by reduction of left ventricular mass in hypertension: a meta-analysis. Am J Hypertens 2003; 16:895–899.
72. Liebson PR, Grandits GA, Dianzumba S, et al. Comparison of five antihypertensive monotherapies and placebo for change in left ventricular mass in patients receiving nutritional-hygienic therapy in the Treatment of Mild Hypertension Study (TOMHS). Circulation 1995; 91:698–706.
73. Gottdiener JS, Reda DJ, Massie BM, Materson BJ, Williams DW, Anderson RJ. Effect of single-drug therapy on reduction of left ventricular mass in mild to moderate hypertension: comparison of six antihypertensive agents. The Department of Veterans Affairs Cooperative Study Group on Antihypertensive Agents. Circulation 1997; 95:2007–2014.
74. Klingbeil AU, Schneider M, Martus P, Messerli FH, Schmieder RE. A meta-analysis of the effects of treatment on left ventricular mass in essential hypertension. Am J Med 2003; 115:41–46.
75. Whelton PK, Perneger TV, He J, Klag MJ. The role of blood pressure as a risk factor for renal disease: a review of the epidemiologic evidence. J Hum Hypertens 1996; 10:683–689.
76. Peterson JC, Adler S, Burkart JM, et al. Blood pressure control, proteinuria, and the progression of renal disease. The Modification of Diet in Renal Disease Study. Ann Intern Med 1995; 123:754–762.
77. Chobanian AV, Bakris GL, Black HR, et al. The Seventh Report of the Joint National Committee on Prevention, Detection, Evaluation, and Treatment of High Blood Pressure: the JNC 7 report. JAMA 2003; 289:2560–2572.
78. Rahman M, Pressel S, Davis BR, Nwachuku C, Wright JT, Jr., Whelton PK, Barzilay J, Batuman V, Eckfeldt JH, Farber M, et al. Renal outcomes in high-risk hypertensive patients treated with an angiotensin-converting enzyme inhibitor or a calcium channel blocker vs a diuretic: a report from the Antihypertensive and Lipid-Lowering Treatment to Prevent Heart Attack Trial (ALLHAT). Arch Intern Med 2005; 165:936–946.

79. de Leeuw PW, Ruilope LM, Palmer CR, et al. Clinical significance of renal function in hypertensive patients at high risk: results from the INSIGHT trial. Arch Intern Med 2004; 164:2459–2464.
80. Mogensen CE. Microalbuminuria predicts clinical proteinuria and early mortality in maturity-onset diabetes. N Engl J Med 1984; 310:356–360.
81. Heart Outcomes Prevention Evaluation Study Investigators. Effects of ramipril on cardiovascular and microvascular outcomes in people with diabetes mellitus: results of the HOPE study and MICRO-HOPE substudy. Lancet 2000; 355:253–259.
82. Remuzzi G, Ruggenenti P, Perico N. Chronic renal diseases: renoprotective benefits of renin–angiotensin system inhibition. Ann Intern Med 2002; 136:604–615.
83. Sica DA, Gehr TW. Diuretic use in stage 5 chronic kidney disease and end-stage renal disease. Curr Opin Nephrol Hypertens 2003; 12:483–490.
84. Mantero F, Lucarelli G. Aldosterone antagonists in hypertension and heart failure. Ann Endocrinol 2000; 61:52–60.
85. Sowers JR, Epstein M. Diabetes mellitus and associated hypertension, vascular disease, and nephropathy. An update. Hypertension 1995; 26:869–879.
86. Perez-Stable E, Caralis PV. Thiazide-induced disturbances in carbohydrate, lipid, and potassium metabolism. Am Heart J 1983; 106:245–251.
87. Mason JM, Dickinson HO, Nicolson DJ, Campbell F, Ford GA, Williams B. The diabetogenic potential of thiazide-type diuretic and beta-blocker combinations in patients with hypertension. J Hypertens 2005; 23:1777–1781.
88. Sica DA. Diuretic-related side effects: development and treatment. J Clin Hypertens 2004; 6:532–540.
89. Lindholm LH, Persson M, Alaupovic P, Carlberg B, Svensson A, Samuelsson O. Metabolic outcome during 1 year in newly detected hypertensives: results of the Antihypertensive Treatment and Lipid Profile in a North of Sweden Efficacy Evaluation (ALPINE study). J Hypertens 2003; 21:1563–1574.
90. Pollare T, Lithell H, Berne C. A comparison of the effects of hydrochlorothiazide and captopril on glucose and lipid metabolism in patients with hypertension. N Engl J Med 1989; 321:868–873.
91. Harper R, Ennis CN, Sheridan B, Atkinson AB, Johnston GD, Bell PM. Effects of low dose versus conventional dose thiazide diuretic on insulin action in essential hypertension. BMJ 1994; 309:226–230.
92. Helderman JH, Elahi D, Andersen DK, et al. Prevention of the glucose intolerance of thiazide diuretics by maintenance of body potassium. Diabetes 1983; 32:106–111.
93. Zillich AJ, Garg J, Basu S, Bakris GL, Carter BL. Thiazide diuretics, potassium, and the development of diabetes: a quantitative review. Hypertension 2006; 48:219–224.
94. Elliott WJ. Differential effects of antihypertensive drugs on new-onset diabetes? Curr Hypertens Rep 2005; 7:249–256.
95. Turnbull F, Neal B, Algert C, et al. Effects of different blood pressure-lowering regimens on major cardiovascular events in individuals with and without diabetes mellitus: results of prospectively designed overviews of randomized trials. Arch Intern Med 2005; 165:1410–1419.
96. Lithell HO. Effect of antihypertensive drugs on insulin, glucose, and lipid metabolism. Diabetes Care 1991; 14:203–209.
97. Savage PJ, Pressel SL, Curb JD, Schron EB, Applegate WB, Black HR, Cohen J, Davis BR, Frost P, Smith W, et al. Influence of long-term, low-dose, diuretic-based, antihypertensive therapy on glucose, lipid, uric acid, and potassium levels in older men and women with isolated systolic hypertension: The Systolic Hypertension in the Elderly Program. SHEP Cooperative Research Group. Arch Intern Med 1998; 158:741–751.
98. Bengtsson C, Lapidus L, Stendahl C, Waldenstrom J. Hyperuricaemia and risk of cardiovascular disease and overall death. A 12-year follow-up of participants in the population study of women in Gothenburg, Sweden. Acta Med Scand 1988; 224:549–555.

99. Messerli FH, Frohlich ED, Dreslinski GR, Suarez DH, Aristimuno GG. Serum uric acid in essential hypertension: an indicator of renal vascular involvement. Ann Intern Med 1980; 93:817–821.
100. Johnson RJ, Segal MS, Srinivas T, et al. Essential hypertension, progressive renal disease, and uric acid: a pathogenetic link? J Am Soc Nephrol 2005; 16:1909–1919.
101. Alderman MH, Cohen H, Madhavan S, Kivlighn S. Serum uric acid and cardiovascular events in successfully treated hypertensive patients. Hypertension 1999; 34:144–150.
102. Hoieggen A, Alderman MH, Kjeldsen SE, Julius S, Devereux RB, De Faire U, Fyhrquist F, Ibsen H, Kristianson K, Lederballe-Pedersen O, et al. The impact of serum uric acid on cardiovascular outcomes in the LIFE study. Kidney Int 2004; 65:1041–1049.
103. Soffer BA, Wright JT, Jr., Pratt JH, Wiens B, Goldberg AI, Sweet CS. Effects of losartan on a background of hydrochlorothiazide in patients with hypertension. Hypertension 1995; 26:112–117.
104. Burnier M, Waeber B, Brunner HR. Clinical pharmacology of the angiotensin II receptor antagonist losartan potassium in healthy subjects. J Hum Hypertens 1995; 13(Suppl. 1):S23–S28.
105. Clayton JA, Rodgers S, Blakey J, Avery A, Hall IP. Thiazide diuretic prescription and electrolyte abnormalities in primary care. Br J Clin Pharmacol 2006; 61:87–95.
106. Cohen JD, Neaton JD, Prineas RJ, Daniels KA. Diuretics, serum potassium and ventricular arrhythmias in the Multiple Risk Factor Intervention Trial. Am J Cardiol 1987; 60:548–554.
107. Grobbee DE, Hoes AW. Non-potassium-sparing diuretics and risk of sudden cardiac death. J Hypertens 1995; 13:1539–1545.
108. Kohvakka A, Salo H, Gordin A, Eisalo A. Antihypertensive and biochemical effects of different doses of hydrochlorothiazide alone or in combination with triamterene. Acta Med Scand 1986; 219:381–386.
109. Psaty BM, Smith NL, Siscovick DS, et al. Health outcomes associated with antihypertensive therapies used as first-line agents. A systematic review and meta-analysis. JAMA 1997; 277:739–745.
110. Franse LV, Pahor M, Di Bari M, Somes GW, Cushman WC, Applegate WB. Hypokalemia associated with diuretic use and cardiovascular events in the Systolic Hypertension in the Elderly Program. Hypertension 2000; 35:1025–1030.
111. Adrogue HJ, Madias NE. Hyponatremia. N Engl J Med 2000; 342:1581–1589.
112. Fichman MP, Vorherr H, Kleeman CR, Telfer N. Diuretic-induced hyponatremia. Ann Intern Med 1971; 75:853–863.
113. Chow KM, Szeto CC, Wong TY, Leung CB, Li PK. Risk factors for thiazide-induced hyponatraemia. QJM 2003; 96:911–917.
114. Whang R, Oei TO, Aikawa JK, et al. Predictors of clinical hypomagnesemia. Hypokalemia, hypophosphatemia, hyponatremia, and hypocalcemia. Arch Intern Med 1984; 144:1794–1796.
115. Dyckner T, Wester PO. Effects of magnesium infusions in diuretic induced hyponatraemia. Lancet 1981; 1:585–586.
116. Bansal S. Sexual dysfunction in hypertensive men. A critical review of the literature. Hypertension 1988; 12:1–10.
117. Magni P, Motta M. Aldosterone receptor antagonists: biology and novel therapeutic applications. Curr Hypertens Rep 2005; 7:206–211.
118. Grossman E, Messerli FH, Goldbourt U. Does diuretic therapy increase the risk of renal cell carcinoma? Am J Cardiol 1999; 83:1090–1093.
119. Pérez-Castrillon JL, Justo I, Sanz-Cantalapiedra A, Pueyo C, Hernandez G, Duenas A. Effect of antihypertensive treatment on the bone mineral density and osteoporotic fracture. Curr Hypertens Rev 2005; 1:61–66.
120. Conlin PR, Gerth WC, Fox J, Roehm JB, Boccuzzi SJ. Four-year persistence patterns among patients initiating therapy with the angiotensin II receptor antagonist losartan versus other artihypertensive drug classes. Clin Ther 2001; 23:1999–2010.

121. Degli Esposti L, Degli Esposti E, Valpiani G, et al. A retrospective, population-based analysis of persistence with antihypertensive drug therapy in primary care practice in Italy. Clin Ther 2002; 24:1347–1357.
122. Mazzaglia G, Mantovani LG, Sturkenboom MC, et al. Patterns of persistence with antihypertensive medications in newly diagnosed hypertensive patients in Italy: a retrospective cohort study in primary care. J Hypertens 2005; 23:2093–2100.
123. Perreault S, Lamarre D, Blais L, et al. Persistence with treatment in newly treated middle-aged patients with essential hypertension. Ann Pharmacother 2005; 39:1401–1408.
124. Lemogoum D, Seedat YK, Mabadeje AF, et al. Recommendations for prevention, diagnosis and management of hypertension and cardiovascular risk factors in sub-Saharan Africa. J Hypertens 2003; 21:1993–2000.
125. Williams B, Poulter NR, Brown MJ, et al. British Hypertension Society guidelines for hypertension management 2004 (BHS-IV): summary. BMJ 2004; 328:634–640.

22

Sodium Status and the Response to Blockade of the Renin-Angiotensin System

Friso L. H. Muntinghe and Gerjan J. Navis
Department of Medicine, University Medical Center Groningen, Groningen, The Netherlands

INTRODUCTION

Blockade of the renin–angiotensin–aldosterone system (RAAS) has proven a highly effective pharmacological tool for intervention in hypertension and renal disease, and for the prevention and treatment of heart failure. The design of the first angiotensin-converting enzyme (ACE) inhibitors was the result of rational drug design, purposefully aiming at blockade of the RAAS by inhibiting the enzyme converting the biologically inactive angiotensin I to the effector hormone angiotensin II (1). At the introduction of the first orally active ACE inhibitor, captopril, it was anticipated that RAAS blockade would be particularly suited for the treatment of high-renin conditions, such as renovascular hypertension. However, within a few years, it was apparent that ACE inhibitors were also effective in conditions that were not characterized by a high level of renin in the circulation. Several explanations have been forwarded for this unexpected efficacy, such as the inhibition of bradykinin breakdown. Moreover, over the years, a large body of evidence has accumulated that points toward an independent pathophysiological role of the tissue RAAS, which is not reflected by circulating parameters of RAAS activity. Accordingly, in target tissues RAAS activity may have a pathophysiological impact that is not reflected in the circulation, and in spite of the absence of signs of RAAS activation in the circulation, target organ damage may well be driven by RAAS activity at tissue level. Interference with the RAAS at tissue level may thus account for the efficacy of RAAS blockade in so-called low-renin conditions, but obviously, this if difficult to prove in humans (2).

Notwithstanding the efficacy of ACE inhibitors in several low-renin conditions, induction of a high-renin status by sodium depletion has consistently been shown to potentiate the response to ACE inhibition. This potentiation can sometimes result in unwanted side effects, such as the so-called first-dose hypotension, but it can also be deliberately used to obtain a better therapeutic effect, by combining the ACE inhibitor with a diuretic and/or dietary sodium restriction. Thus, the interaction between sodium status and RAAS blockade can be used as a tool to improve the outcome of therapy with RAAS blockade. This emphasizes the potential clinical importance of this interaction, as, in spite of the progress afforded by the availability of RAAS blockade in the treatment of renal and cardiovascular end organ damage, in many instances the therapeutic benefit is still insufficient. In renal patients, for instance, the rate of renal function loss can often be retarded, but renal function loss can usually not be stopped or reversed, and also in cardiac populations the prognosis remains grim. Therefore, strategies to improve the outcome of therapy are highly important: these should focus on identification of factors improving therapy response and elucidation of the underlying mechanisms. In this respect it is somewhat surprising that the potentiating effects of low sodium (and/or diuretic), and conversely the adverse effect of excess sodium intake on the response to RAAS blockade, got relatively little emphasis over the years. In fact, excess sodium intake has long since been recognized to exert an adverse effect on the response to ACE inhibition as high sodium intake consistently blunts the efficacy of ACE inhibition, in human conditions as well as experimental renal disease. The modulating effect of sodium status on the response to ACE inhibition has been described in different conditions, and this appears to occur irrespective of the underlying condition that is being treated. Yet, it may be relevant that most conditions where ACE inhibitors are used (hypertension, renal disease, heart failure) are associated with impaired renal sodium handling, so some degree of volume excess may be present in most patients, even when sodium intake is not excessive. Here, we will systematically review the interactions between sodium status and the response to RAAS blockade, both with respect to the available clinical data and the underlying mechanisms, from the perspective of improvement of outcome of therapy.

THE RAAS: EFFECTS OF SODIUM STATUS AND RAAS BLOCKADE

The RAAS plays an important role in homeostasis of blood pressure, renal function, and sodium status. Moreover, it is a key player in the pathophysiology of cardiovascular and renal target organ damage. Renin is synthesized and released from juxtaglomerular cells, its release is the first and possibly rate-limiting step in activation of the RAAS cascade. The main physiological stimuli for renin secretion are low blood pressure and renal hypoperfusion, increased sympathetic activity and a decreased supply of sodium and chloride to the macula densa. Renin initiates a sequence of events starting with the cleavage of the decapeptide angiotensin I from angiotensinogen. Angiotensin I is rapidly converted to the octapeptide angiotensin II by the ACE. Angiotensin II is a potent vasoconstrictor with effects on both the systemic and the renal vascular bed, and moreover promotes renal retention of sodium and water, both by direct effects on the proximal tubulus and by stimulating the release of aldosterone that promotes distal tubular sodium reabsorption.

Thus, under conditions of sodium depletion the RAAS is activated with proportional increases in renin, angiotensin I, angiotensin II and aldosterone. This RAAS activation plays a main role in the homeostasis of blood pressure, renal function and circulation volume, by the combined effects of maintenance of blood pressure, glomerular filtration pressure, and sodium handling. During pharmacological blockade of the RAAS, these homeostatic functions are blunted, which is a main factor underlying the interaction between sodium status and the effects of RAAS blockade. Generally speaking, RAAS blockade blunts the buffering effects of changes in sodium status on blood pressure and glomerular filtration pressure, and thus changes in sodium status are more directly translated in changes in blood pressure and glomerular filtration pressure. Sodium depletion does not appear to modulate circulating ACE activity, but there is evidence suggesting that tissue ACE activity may be increased by high sodium intake (3–5).

The effects of angiotensin II are mediated by binding to specific receptors: angiotensin II type 1 (AT_1) and type 2 (AT_2) receptors. The vascular and renal tubular actions, as well as the negative feedback on renin activity are primarily mediated by the AT_1 receptor. Sodium depletion suppresses, and sodium repletion increases the systemic and renal vascular responsiveness to angiotensin II, presumably by down- and upregulation of the receptor, respectively, whereas this effect appears to be opposite for the adrenal sensitivity to angiotensin (6). Recently, a new homologue of ACE, called ACE2, was identified. ACE2 also cleaves angiotensin I, but at a different site, leading to generation of angiotensin (1-9) instead of angiotensin II. Angiotensin (1-9), which has no vascular activity, can be cleaved to angiotensin (1-7), a vasodilator with antiproliferative properties. In addition, ACE2 promotes the breakdown of angiotensin II to angiotensin (1-7). This has led to a renewed interest in these smaller angiotensin peptides. Because of this cleavage profile, and because cardiac pathology of ACE2-knockout mice is prevented by the additional knockout of ACE, ACE2 has been suggested to act as the natural counterpart of ACE. Its precise functional significance, however, remains to be explored. Whether sodium status affects ACE2 is unknown.

Different classes of drugs are available for intervention in the RAAS that can be classified by the level of interference with the RAAS cascade. ACE inhibitors block the conversion of angiotensin I to angiotensin II, and AT_1 receptor blockers block the receptor for angiotensin II, both leading to a decrease in angiotensin II-mediated effects. These two classes of drugs have been extensively used in cardiovascular and renal disease for many years now, and most experience with RAAS blockade derives from these two classes. Several renin inhibitors are available as well, blocking the effects of renin at angiotensinogen. Their pharmacodynamics support the efficacy of blockade of the RAAS at its initial step, but poor bio-availability hampered the clinical introduction of several renin-inhibiting compounds so far. Experiences in the clinical setting therefore are limited and await further clinical testing of more recently developed compounds. Vasopeptidase inhibitors (VPI) provide a mode of dual blockade of both ACE and endopeptidase, which limits breakdown of atrial natriuretic peptide (ANP) and thus enhances natriuresis. Thus, VPI were assumed to represent an ACE inhibitor with an inherent diuretic effect, which would be particularly effective in conditions of volume overload, where monotherapy ACE inhibition is less effective. Promising results were obtained in experimental animals with volume-overload hypertension (such as the deoxycorticosterone acetate–salt model) and in man. However, idiosyncratic side effects hampered their clinical introduction.

Pharmacological blockade of the RAAS has clear-cut effects on the circulating components of the RAAS, but does not eliminate the effect of sodium status. This has been best documented for ACE inhibition, as shown in Figure 1 providing short-term data on patients with essential hypertension.

ACE inhibition elicits a clear-cut reactive rise in plasma renin activity, and it is readily apparent that the stimulation by low sodium persists during ACE inhibition, albeit at a higher overall level. The stimulating effect of low sodium on plasma aldosterone also persists during ACE inhibition, albeit at a lower overall level than in the untreated condition. Whether these short-term data bear relevance to long-term treatment has not been studied; but it would be of interest to see whether sodium status is relevant to the so-called aldosterone escape phenomenon. Interestingly, during ACE inhibition, sodium status also modulates the level of the reactive rise in angiotensin I, and, accordingly the vasodilator angiotensin (1-7), with higher levels during low sodium (Fig. 2).

Whereas some studies suggest a contribution of changes in angiotensin (1-7) in the effects of ACE inhibition the impact of the sodium-induced effects on angiotensin (1-7) during ACE inhibition on the eventual response to treatment has not been established (9).

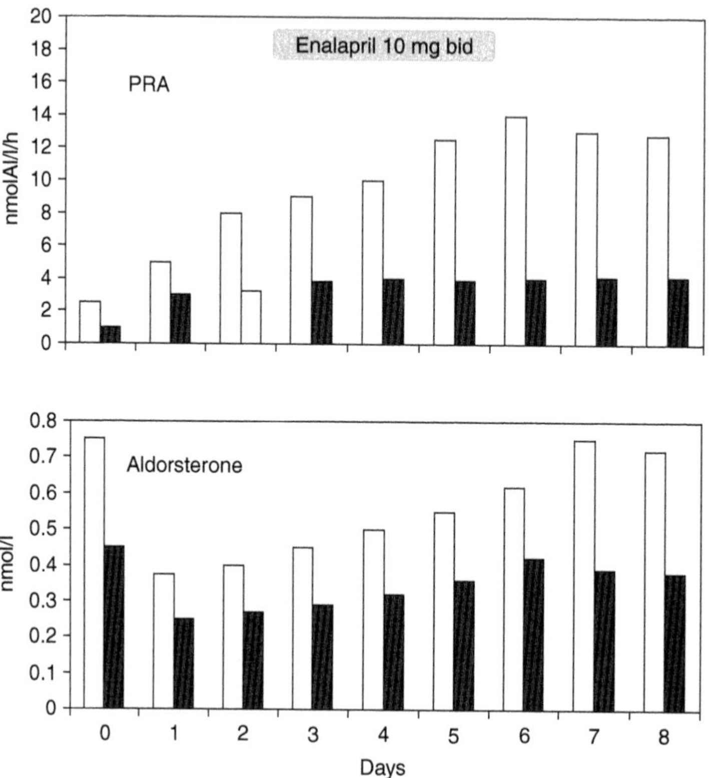

Figure 1 Effects of angiotensin-converting enzyme inhibition on PRA and plasma aldosterone concentration in essential hypertensive subjects, on low (50 mmol Na^+/day) and high sodium intake (200 mmol Na^+/day) respectively, with each subject as his/her own control. *Abbreviation*: PRA, plasma renin activity. *Source*: From Ref. 7.

Taken together, the available data show that the RAAS cascade remains responsive to changes in sodium status despite pharmacological blockade, but a systematical appraisal of these effects for the eventual response to therapy is not available.

EFFECTS OF SODIUM STATUS ON THE THERAPY RESPONSES TO RAAS BLOCKADE

Hypertension

Sodium restriction has long since been recommended in the therapy of hypertension, either as a life style measure that is mainly effective in those with sodium sensitive hypertension, or as an adjunct measure to pharmacological intervention with, for instance, diuretics and beta-blockers. Already early after the introduction of ACE inhibitors it was shown that dietary sodium restriction enhances the effects of ACE inhibition as well. In a group of essential hypertensives in whom sodium restriction as such did not affect blood pressure, the effect of enalapril was slightly but significantly more pronounced during dietary sodium restriction of 50 mmol Na^+/day than during a liberal sodium intake of 200 mmol Na^+/day (Fig. 3) (7,10). This difference in sodium intake corresponded to a change in body weight, reflecting a change in extracellular volume status, of approximately 2 kg.

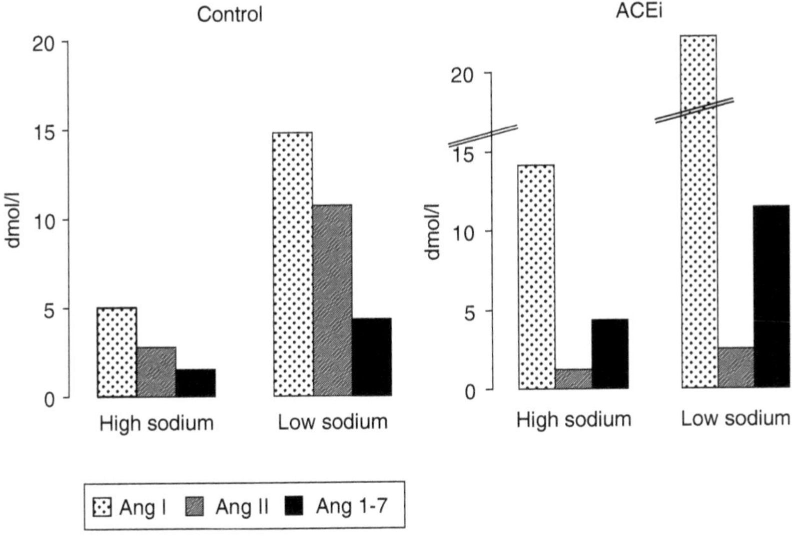

Figure 2 Angiotensins during placebo control and ACEi, on high (200 mmol Na^+/day) and low (50 mmol Na^+/day) sodium intake in 17 healthy male volunteers. During placebo (*left panel*) angiotensin I, angiotensin (1-7) and angiotensin II concentrations were approximately threefold higher on the low-sodium diet. ACE inhibition (*right panel*) elicited a significant rise in angiotensin I on both sodium intakes, and a rise in angiotensin (1-7) that reached significance during low sodium only. It shows that during ACE inhibition sodium intake still affects angiotensin levels. *Abbreviation*: ACE, angiotensin-converting enzyme. *Source*: From Ref. 8.

The potentiation of the blood pressure response was in line with other data in essential hypertension, showing that co-treatment with an ACE inhibitor and sodium restriction resulted in an extra 9% reduction in blood pressure compared to treatment with an ACE inhibitor alone (11). Put the other way round, ACE inhibition induces or enhances sodium sensitivity of blood pressure, thus rendering sodium restriction also effective in subjects in whom blood pressure was not sodium sensitive to start with. The potentiating effect of sodium depletion has also been reported for AT_1 receptor blockade.

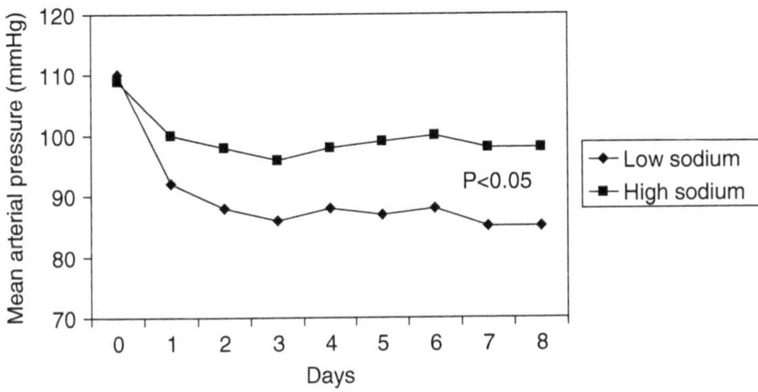

Figure 3 Effects of angiotensin-converting enzyme inhibition on mean arterial pressure in essential hypertensive subjects on low (50 mmol Na^+) and liberal (200 mmol Na^+/day) sodium, respectively, with each subject as his/her own control. Mean value is given. *Source*: From Ref. 7.

After sodium depletion, treatment with the AT_1 receptor blocker losartan caused a greater response in blood pressure in healthy volunteers compared to placebo, whereas this effect was not seen in salt replete persons (12). In type 2 diabetic patients with hypertension and albuminuria the antihypertensive and antiproteinuric effects of losartan were potentiated by a low-sodium diet as well (13). Thus, during low-sodium the antihypertensive effect of both ACE inhibition and AT_1 receptor blockade is potentiated in various clinical conditions. From their mechanism of action, which includes a diuretic effect, VPI were anticipated to be effective in sodium replete conditions as well. Indeed, the blood pressure lowering effect of omapatrilat in normotensive volunteers persisted despite high sodium intake, in contrast to blunting of the effect of fosinopril (14). The effect of RAAS blockade on renal hemodynamics, characterized by renal vasodilation that is particularly apparent for the efferent arteriole, is modified by sodium status as well: in essential hypertensives the vasodilation leading to a rise in effective renal plasma flow and glomerular filtration rate during ACE inhibition was somewhat more pronounced during low-sodium diet, because the ACE inhibitor reversed the renal vasocontriction induced by low-sodium diet (10).

Renal Disease

RAAS blockade is a cornerstone for treatment of hypertension and proteinuria in renal patients, and has been shown to prevent against progressive renal function loss in diabetic and non-diabetic chronic renal disease. In renal patients, sodium restriction also potentiates the blood pressure response to RAAS blockade, as has been shown early on for lisinopril in non-diabetic proteinuric patients. In addition, sodium status is an important determinant of the therapy response to RAAS blockade with respect to renal hemodynamics and proteinuria (10,15). During sodium excess, either due to excess sodium intake or to avid sodium retention due to nephrotic syndrome, the effect of ACE inhibition on blood pressure and proteinuria is considerably and often completely blunted. This blunting is reversible upon correction of sodium status, either by sodium restriction and/or diuretic therapy (Fig. 4) (16).

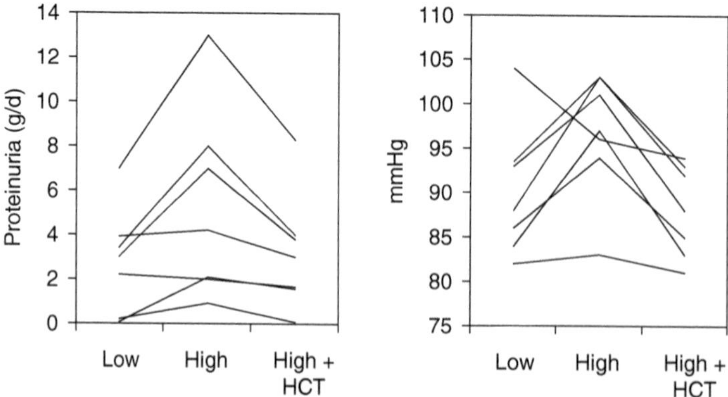

Figure 4 The individual values of proteinuria (g/day, *left panel*) and mean arterial pressure (*right panel*) during low sodium, high sodium and high sodium plus hydrochlorothiazide in seven patients with non-diabetic proteinuria on maintenance therapy angiotensin-converting enzyme inhibitor. *Source*: From Ref. 16.

The drop in blood pressure and proteinuria by low sodium is often accompanied by a slight drop in renal function, presumably due to lower filtration pressure by the concomitant effects of lower blood pressure and efferent vasodilation. It is generally reversible upon volume repletion. As mentioned above in the study of Houlihan besides a better antihypertensive effect, also a better antiproteinuric was seen in type 2 diabetic patients treated with an AT_1 receptor antagonist during low sodium, demonstrating that the early findings on ACE inhibition also apply to AT_1 receptor blockade, and to diabetic subjects (13). In general, in renal patients, the potentiating effects of sodium depletion on proteinuria and blood pressure tend to run more or less in parallel. Interestingly, sodium depletion by diuretic plus sodium restriction also potentiated the effect of the combination of ACE inhibition and AT_1 receptor blockade—a regimen with enhanced potency in itself by the dual RAAS blockade—on proteinuria and blood pressure, as shown recently. An increase in serum creatinine was observed during the sodium depletion regimen (17).

The effect of VPI on proteinuria and the effects of sodium status have been studied in a normotensive, nephrotic rat model. Remarkably, the renoprotective effect of the VPI gemopatrilat was fully blunted by a high-sodium diet. Moreover, lisinopril was more effective than the VPI (18).

Heart Failure

Intervention in the RAAS with an ACE inhibitor is a well established therapy to attenuate the progression of left ventricular (LV) dysfunction and to prevent cardiovascular events and mortality. ACE inhibition even improves cardiac function (19). Whereas, formerly sodium restriction was a cornerstone of the therapy of heart failure, currently sodium restriction meets reluctance due to the neurohumoral activation that it elicits that could be detrimental for cardiac prognosis. Whereas these may be true in the untreated condition, an appraisal of the effects of low sodium during RAAS blockade is not available and currently, in patients with LV dysfunction, sodium depletion is not deliberately being used as a strategy to potentiate the response to ACE inhibition. On the other hand, sodium restriction is routinely advised to patient with LV dysfunction to reduce fluid retention. Recent experimental data in a rat model of LV dysfunction, post-myocardial infarction showed a positive effect of dietary sodium restriction added to ACE inhibitor on LV ACE activity, LV hypertrophy and early mortality (20). These data prompt for further investigation of the role of modulating volume status in subjects with LV dysfunction treated with RAAS blockade.

So, taken together, it appears that a modulating effect of sodium status on response to RAAS blockade occurs irrespective of the underlying clinical condition with both ACE inhibition and AT_1 receptor blockade. Thus, the interaction with sodium status appears to be a characteristic that is linked to RAAS blockade as such, which would be in line with the known physiology of the RAAS. Whether differences in the level of interference with the RAAS are relevant to the sodium-dependency of therapy response has not been investigated. The only between-class comparisons on sodium-dependency of therapy response have been made between ACE inhibition and VPI, where differences presumably are due to effects on ANP degradation, but not to differences in the level of interference with the RAAS.

In general, sodium excess blunts the therapeutic effects of RAAS blockade on blood pressure, renal hemodynamics and proteinuria, and the other way round, sodium depletion by dietary sodium restriction or by diuretic co-treatment enhances it. In almost all studies, the interaction between sodium status and RAAS blockade was investigated

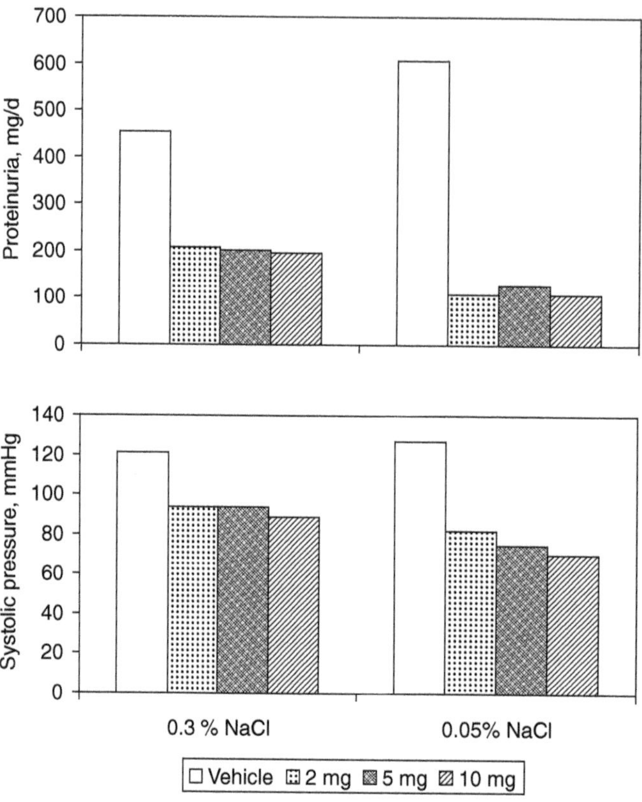

Figure 5 Effects of sodium intake on dose response for proteinuria (*upper panel*) and blood pressure (*lower panel*) in rats with adriamycin-induced proteinuria. Doses lisinopril were 0, 2, 5, and 10 mg/kg body weight/24 hr. Sodium restriction augments the effect of angiotensin-converting enzyme inhibition by shifting the top of the dose response, both for blood pressure and proteinuria: for each dose the responses on low sodium are significantly larger. Mean values are given. *Source*: From Ref. 21.

at fixed doses without considering dose–response, but the scanty data in animal and man seem to indicate that low sodium shifts the top of the dose–response, as suggested by animal data and in man (Fig. 5).

The shift in the top of the dose–response would implicate that sodium depletion can be used to enhance the maximum response and not just to reduce the required dose of the RAAS blocker. Thus, sodium depletion can potentially serve to increase the overall therapeutic benefit, provided that no adverse effects occur. The "dose" of the sodium status has not been addressed in a graded fashion either: the available studies typically compare the sodium-replete condition with a single condition of sodium depletion that is obtained either by low-sodium diet or by diuretic. Studies applying graded volume depletion by stepwise lowering of sodium intake during RAAS blockade are not available, and only a single study published in abstract form reports on the separate versus the combined effects of diuretic and low-sodium diet on the response to AT_1 receptor blockade, in proteinuric patients (22). Considering the potential of volume depletion as a tool for improvement of the response to RAAS blockade, studies pursuing a better, systematic approach taking into account both type and dose of the RAAS blocker, and a graded modulation of sodium status would be important to define the optimal combination of pharmacological RAAS blockade and volume depletion for specific clinical conditions. Nevertheless, in some clinical settings such as the symptomatic treatment of proteinuria or severe heart failure, considerable clinical experience is available on the effect of aggressive volume depletion in patients on RAAS blockade, as in these settings the clinical condition can prompt for such aggressive volume depletion. In those conditions the attempts to enhance the response to RAAS blockade by further dose increase and/or depletion of (excess) volume are often limited by hypotension, renal function impairment, or both (23).

Considering the consistency of the interaction between sodium status and RAAS blockade it might seem logical to conclude that sodium restriction and/or diuretic treatment should be recommended in all patients that use RAAS blockade, at least in those in whom blood pressure or proteinuria have not yet reached target, and in whom no pharmacological side effects occur. However, several issues should be considered before such a general recommendation can be made. First, in man, no studies are available that report on hard end points, such as cardiovascular events, mortality, renal death, and on long-term safety. Studies reporting on effects of sodium status on RAAS blockade so far all address intermediate end points, such as blood pressure, renal hemodynamics and proteinuria. Whereas both blood pressure and proteinuria are considered valid predictors of long-term outcome, it would be important to see whether improved responses of these intermediate parameters indeed result in an improved long-term morbidity and mortality. It would also be important to substantiate this for the different underlying conditions as the clinical impact of sodium restriction or diuretic may not be similar for, for instance, subjects with chronic renal disease and subjects with heart failure. Thus, it should not a priori be assumed that sodium restriction is always harmless. In specific patient populations, such as subjects with diabetes, sodium restriction can elicit an unfavorable renal hemodynamic profile (24), and in heart failure excess neurohumoral activation can occur, with detrimental cardiac effects. This notion is reinforced by animal data on adverse effects of low-sodium diet on the effects of RAAS blockade on target tissues. In nephrotic rats, low sodium added to RAAS blockade resulted in improvement of proteinuria and blood pressure without a correspondingly improved protection against renal structural damage (21). In studies, further exploring this dissociation between the intermediate response parameters and eventual target organ damage we found that low sodium added to RAAS blockade led to renal interstitial fibrotic changes in healthy rats and in rats with cardiac failure as well as nephrotic rats (21,25,26). In the latter, the pro-fibrotic effect of low sodium added to ACE inhibition occurred in spite of a clear-cut antiproteinuric effect. This dissociation is remarkable, and also worrisome, because a good antiproteinuric response is assumed to indicate a beneficial effect on the kidney, and in this case thus masks a concomitant unfavorable effect. For obvious reasons, no comparable data are available in man. Moreover, rat studies suggest that during ACE inhibition volume depletion by low sodium can induce impairment of endothelial function in the renal vascular bed (27). Whereas, it remains unclear whether these findings in rats have bearing for the human clinical condition, they prompt for caution in not simply considering favorable effects on intermediate parameters sufficient proof for the eventual clinical benefit. Empirical evidence is needed to see whether, during ACE inhibition, possible unwanted effects of sodium restriction are neutralized or overcome by the improvement of therapy response with regards to hard end points.

Second, the added effect of volume depletion appears to be considerably different between individual patients, with a pronounced effect in some individuals, and an almost negligible effect in others (16). This prompts for identification of predictors of the effect of sodium depletion on the response to RAAS blockade, and elucidation of its mechanisms, rather than institute sodium depletion for all.

INDIVIDUAL DIFFERENCES IN THE EFFECT OF SODIUM STATUS ON THE RESPONSE TO RAAS BLOCKADE: GENE–ENVIRONMENT INTERACTION

The difference between individuals in their blood pressure response to sodium restriction, the so-called sodium sensitivity of blood pressure, is one of the most extensively studied issues in the field of hypertension. However, individual differences in the sodium sensitivity of therapy response have drawn little attention so far. Yet, from the available data it is readily apparent that the individual differences in the added effect of sodium depletion in the response to RAAS blockade are considerable. This is not only of clinical interest in allocating sodium restriction or diuretic to those most likely to benefit, it could also provide clues as to mechanisms of action of drug response, and thus guide improved intervention strategies.

Individual factors in drug response have gained increasing interest due to the rapid developments in genetics. Indeed, several genetic variations have been identified that are involved in determining responsiveness to pharmacological interventions (28,29). As to the response to RAAS blockade, many studies addressed the impact of ACE (I/D) genotype on the response to ACE inhibition, and other studies addressed the impact of AT_1 receptor genotype on the response to AT_1 receptor blockade. The results, however, tend to be conflicting, indicating that either these genetic variants in the RAAS are not relevant to the response to RAAS blockade, or that therapy response is a complex phenotype, with factors other than genetic variation being involved as well, either or not in gene–environment interaction. Indeed, as to the response to RAAS blockade, sodium status is a well-established environmental factor that modifies therapy response, which should not be overlooked in pharmacogenetic analyses on the response to RAAS blockade. In addition, in experimental renal disease, the severity of structural renal damage at onset of therapy has also been identified as a determinant of the response to RAAS blockade and retrospective data suggest this to be true in man as well (30,31). Obviously, however, this factor is difficult to reliably account for in human pharmacogenetic analyses.

Several large trials addressed the effect of ACE (I/D) genotype on the response to ACE inhibition in renal patients, and hypertensive patients, respectively. Data from the Ramipril Efficacy In Nephropathy trial provide evidence for an interaction between ACE genotype, response to ACE inhibition and gender (32). However, genetic analysis in the Antihypertensive and Lipid-Lowering Treatment to Prevent Heart Attack Trial study showed no relation between the response to antihypertensive treatment and ACE I/D genotype (33). Data from smaller studies suggest that effects of sodium intake may be involved in these discrepancies. In a retrospective, cross-sectional analysis in renal patients a blunted response for blood pressure and proteinuria to ACE inhibition was found in patients with the ACE DD genotype on high sodium intake but not in subjects with ACE ID or II genotype (Fig. 6) (34).

Remarkably, the poor response was not seen in DD subjects that ingested less sodium. This suggests, first, that sodium intake differently affects therapy response in subjects with different ACE genotype with a larger sodium-dependency in DD genotype, and moreover, that high sodium intake can unmask an unfavorable phenotype in DD homozygotes. The latter assumption was substantiated prospectively in healthy volunteers, where angiotensin I elicited significantly larger rises in blood pressure and aldosterone (providing a functional index for angiotensin I conversion or tissue ACE activity) in subjects with the ACE DD genotype compared to ACE ID or II genotype during high sodium intake, whereas the difference between the genotypes was blunted when the same subjects were studied during low sodium (4). Moreover, recent data published in abstract

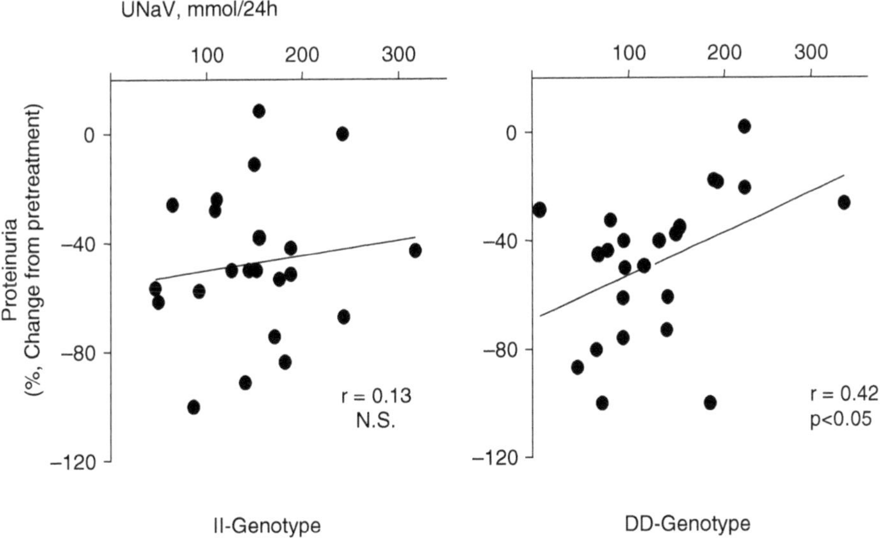

Figure 6 Scatterplot of cross-sectional data showing change in proteinuria from baseline (*Y*-axis, %) and the prevalent urinary sodium excretion (*X*-axis, mmol/24 hr) by ACE (I/D) genotype. In DD genotype (*right panel*), a higher sodium excretion is significantly correlated to a worse antiproteinuric response: in the II genotype (*left panel*) this association was not observed. For ID genotype (not shown) data were in between. Data on blood pressure response corresponded to those of proteinuria. *Source*: From Ref. 34.

form, suggest that the responsiveness to sodium status during RAAS blockade in volunteers was determined by ACE genotype, with therapy resistance of blood pressure to ACE inhibition during high sodium particularly in the DD genotype (35). Thus, for the moment the available evidence is consistent in supporting a gene–environment interaction between sodium status and the genotype–phenotype relationship for ACE genotype, and it appears that this may also apply to therapy response. Obviously, the latter assumption needs confirmation in patient populations. If true, it would implicate that particularly DD subjects would benefit from sodium depletion during RAAS blockade. As to AT_1 receptor blockade, less data is available on the interaction between genetic variation, sodium status and the response to therapy. In hypertensive patients on high-sodium diet the C-allele of the A1166C polymorphism was associated with an increased sensitivity to angiotensin II, although the blood pressure response did not differ significantly between the genotype groups (36). Thus indicating there is gene–environment interaction between A1166CC with sodium status as well. Its implications for therapy response have not been explored so far.

MECHANISMS UNDERLYING THE INTERACTION BETWEEN SODIUM STATUS AND THE RESPONSE TO BLOCKADE OF THE RENIN-ANGIOTENSIN SYSTEM

Considering that the adverse effect of excess sodium on the response to ACE inhibition has been known for almost two decades now, it may be surprising that the mechanism of this blunting has not drawn more attention so far. This benign neglect may be due to the fact that the remedy seems to be obvious irrespective the underlying mechanism, namely, to correct the sodium excess by dietary sodium restriction and/or diuretics. However, the mechanisms of sodium-induced therapy resistance deserve more proper consideration for several reasons. First, despite the proven efficacy of RAAS blockade for target organ protection in chronic renal and cardiac failure, cardiac and renal disease still remain essentially progressive conditions, with a poor prognosis in many patients. Thus, it is important not to overlook any possibility to improve therapeutic efficacy. Next, correction of sodium status can be cumbersome, despite the availability of many diuretic agents. Renal sodium retention—inherent to renal and cardiac failure—and high sodium intake can both offset the effect of diuretics on sodium status. In the outpatient setting, especially during chronic treatment, such resistance to sodium-depleting measures is hard to detect, due to the lack of a simple, accurate and reproducible method to assess volume status. Whereas 24-hour sodium excretion is useful to monitor sodium intake, it does not provide information on the extracellular volume for that given sodium intake. Clinical symptoms of volume excess, such as edema, can be used to diagnose gross volume excess, but therapy resistance to ACE inhibitors is well-documented to occur already at a much milder degree of volume excess, without any clinical symptoms of volume overload. Third, as noted above, it should not a priori be assumed that sodium restriction is harmless. As mentioned above, this prompts for empirical evidence on hard end points. Moreover, this provides a strong rationale for analyzing the mechanisms of the interaction between sodium status and the responses to RAAS blockade, as this could help to design interventions that prevent or abolish possible unfavorable effects of sodium restriction during RAAS blockade, while leaving the favorable effects intact.

The most straightforward explanation would be that sodium repletion suppresses RAAS activity, and that blockade of a suppressed system, as opposed to blockade of a highly active system, is not likely to exert substantial biological responses. Whereas there is obviously truth in this, it also leaves important issues unaccounted for. That is, if pharmacological RAAS blockade is just the reciprocal of endogenous RAAS activation by sodium restriction, why does endogenous RAAS suppression by sodium loading not exert any therapeutic effect like those of pharmacological RAAS blockade? Other non-RAAS related associations have been put forward, such as the effect of ACE inhibition on bradykinin, but these fail to explain why sodium potentiates the effects of AT_1 receptor blocking as well.

The discovery of smaller angiotensins with vasodilator properties raised another possible explanation. RAAS blockade is associated with a clear-cut reactive rise in renin and angiotensin I that is enhanced during sodium depletion. During ACE inhibition, this was found to be associated with an enhanced rise in angiotensin (1-7) as well, whereas the drop in angiotensin II by ACE inhibition was similar during liberal and low sodium. Thus, during ACE inhibition, salt restriction may cause a shift in the balance between the vasoconstrictor angiotensin II and the vasodilator angiotensin (1-7), that could be postulated to be involved in the enhanced response to ACE inhibition (8,9). No such data are available for AT_1 receptor blockade, but if the rise in angiotensin (1-7) is related to the increased availability of angiotensin I, this mechanism could be relevant to AT_1 receptor blockade as well. However, it cannot be excluded that decreased breakdown of angiotensin (1-7) during ACE inhibition contributes to its rise as well, so separate studies during AT_1 receptor blockade are needed to substantiate the plausibility of this mechanism during AT_1 receptor blockade.

Experimental data provided several additional possibilities that are, however, difficult to substantiate in man. Sodium restriction can for instance alter the expression of angiotensin II subtype 1 and subtype 2 receptors. During high salt intake in rats the expression of AT_1 receptors (with vasoconstrictor and profibrotic properties) increases and the expression of AT_2 receptors, that have antihypertrophic and antifibrotic properties, decreases (37,38). Further studies would be needed to identify the possible role of these effects in the outcome of therapy with RAAS blockade.

An alternative explanation for the blunted effect of ACE inhibition during high sodium could be sodium-induced effects on tissue ACE. This is supported by a number of recent rat studies. First, high sodium intake was shown to induce renal ACE activity in rats, with, however, an unchanged plasma ACE level. The latter finding underlines the importance of specifically addressing tissue ACE. Moreover, when proteinuric rats treated with ACE inhibition were subjected to a shift in sodium intake, the responses of blood pressure and proteinuria were blunted by high sodium along with a rise in renal (but not plasma) ACE activity, with an opposite pattern upon institution of low-sodium diet (27). In additional studies, the effect of high sodium intake on the effects of ACE inhibition on tissue conversion of angiotensin I was addressed in isolated aortic rings, from the

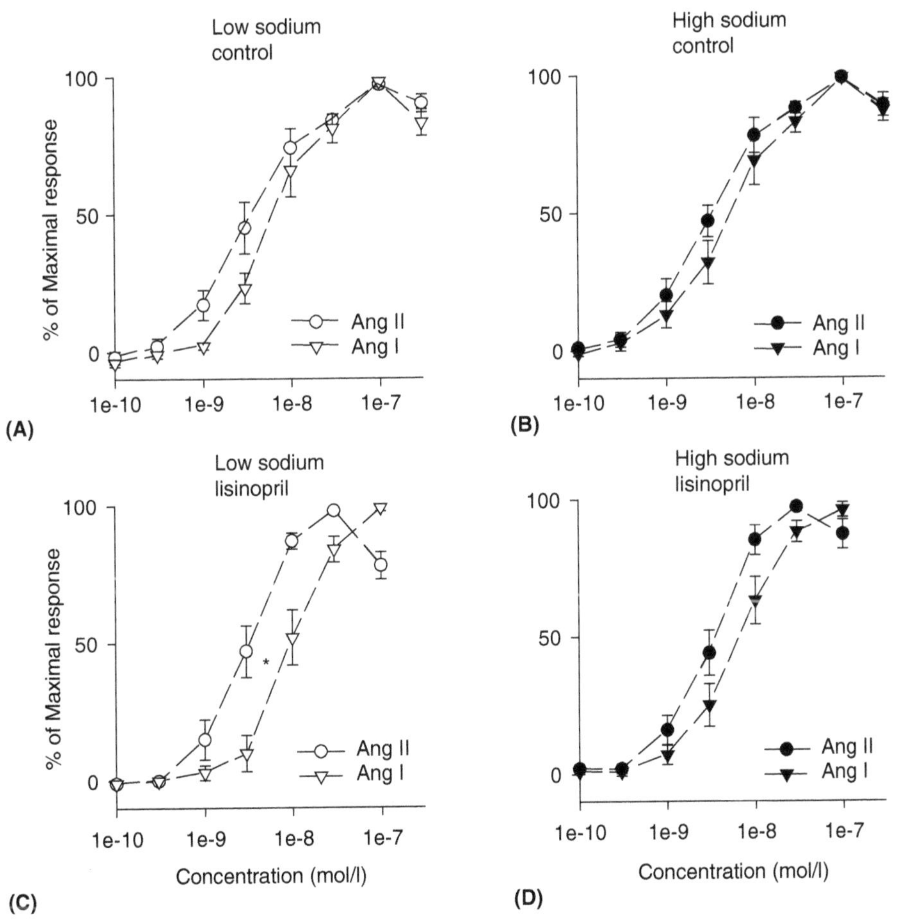

Figure 7 Concentration–response curves for angiotensin I and angiotensin II in isolated aortic rings of normal rats; (**A**) control group on low sodium, (**B**) control group on high sodium, (**C**) ACE inhibition-treated group on low sodium, and (**D**) ACE inhibition-treated group on high sodium. The area between the response curves for angiotensin I and angiotensin II reflects the efficacy of conversion of angiotensin I. During control, conversion is complete on both sodium intakes; during ACE inhibition conversion is significantly blunted during low sodium intake, but not during high sodium. *Abbreviation*: ACE, angiotensin-converting enzyme. *Source*: From Ref. 3.

vasoconstrictor responses to angiotensin I and angiotensin II. In this study the effect of ACE inhibition on vascular conversion of angiotensin I to angiotensin II was blunted by high sodium intake (Fig. 7) (3).

These animal studies support the hypothesis that sodium-associated effects on renal and vascular tissue ACE activity are involved in the potentiating effect of sodium restriction on the response to RAAS blockade. Such mechanisms at the tissue level are difficult to substantiate in man. Yet, the available human evidence supports an effect of sodium status on tissue ACE activity: Boddi found a larger vascular conversion of angiotensin I during high sodium (5). Effects of sodium on tissue ACE are also likely to be involved in the sodium-dependency of the genotype–phenotype relationship in the ACE (I/D) genotype described in the previous paragraph. However, obviously, further studies would be needed to explore the effects of sodium status on tissue ACE activity as a factor in therapy response, preferably also addressing these alleged mechanisms during AT_1 receptor blockade.

CLINICAL IMPLICATIONS AND CONCLUSIONS

Sodium status exerts a consistent effect on the response to RAAS blockade in different clinical conditions, with an increased response during sodium depletion by either dietary sodium restriction or a diuretic. This has been well-established for a quite sometime and, in fact, sodium depletion is an important clinical tool to improve the response to RAAS blockade, be it ACE inhibition or AT_1 receptor blockade. Overzealous volume depletion during RAAS blockade, however, is associated with hypotension and prerenal failure, but fortunately these adverse effects are reversible by volume repletion. In spite of the long-standing experience on RAAS blockade and sodium depletion, crucial questions remain to be answered. Most importantly, it has not been established whether the improved responses of intermediate parameters like blood pressure and proteinuria are also associated with improved long-term outcome with regard to cardiovascular and renal morbidity and mortality. In this regard, both long-term clinical outcome data and experimental studies exploring the direct effects on target organs are warranted.

REFERENCES

1. Ondetti MA, Rubin B, Cushman DW. Design of specific inhibitors of angiotensin converting enzyme: a new class of orally active antihypertensive agents. Science 1977; 196:441–4.
2. Dzau VJ, Bernstein K, Celermajer D, et al. The relevance of tissue angiotensin converting enzyme: manifestations in mechanistic and endpoint data. Am J Cardiol 2001; 88(9A):1L–20.
3. Kocks MJA, Buikema H, Gschwend S, et al. High dietary sodium blunts effects of angiotensin converting enzyme inhibition on vascular angiotensin I to II conversion in rats. J Cardiovasc Pharmacol 2003; 42(5):601–6.
4. van der Kleij FGH, de Jong PE, Henning RH, et al. Enhanced responses of blood pressure, renal function and aldosterone to angiotensin I in DD genotype are blunted by low sodium intake. J Am Soc Nephrol 2002; 13(4):1025–33.
5. Boddi M, Pogesi L, Coppo M, et al. Human vascular renin–angiotensin system and its functional changes in relation to different sodium intakes. Hypertension 1998; 31:836–42.
6. Hollenberg NK, Chenitz WR, Adams DF, et al. Reciprocal influence of salt intake on adrenal glomerulosa and renal vascular responses to angiotensin II in normal men. J Clin Invest 1974; 54(1):34–42.

7. Navis GJ, de Jong PE, Donker AJM, et al. Diuretic effects of ACE inhibition: comparison of low and liberal sodium diet in hypertensive patients. J Cardiovasc Pharmacol 1987; 9:743–8.
8. Kocks MJA, Lely T, Boomsma F, et al. High sodium status and ACE inhibition: effects on plasma angiotensin (1-7) in healthy man. J Hypertens 2005; 23(3):597–602.
9. Ferrario CM, Chappell MC, Tallant EA, et al. Counterregulatory actions of angiotensin (1-7). Hypertension 1997; 30(3872):535–41.
10. Navis GJ, de Jong PE, Donker AJM, et al. Moderate sodium restriction in hypertensive subjects: renal effects of ACE inhibition. Kidney Int 1987; 31:8159.
11. MacGregor GA, Markandu ND, Singer DR, et al. Moderate sodium restriction with angiotensin converting enzyme inhibitor in essential hypertension: a double blind study. Br Med J 1987; 294(6571):531–4.
12. Doig JK, MacFadyen RJ, Sweet CS, et al. Haemodynamic and renal responses to oral losartan potassium during salt depletion or salt repletion in normal human volunteers. J Cardiovasc Pharmacol 1995; 25(4):511–7.
13. Houlihan CA, Allen TJ, Baxter AL, et al. A low sodium diet potentiates the effects of losartan in type 2 diabetes. Diabetes Care 2002; 25(4):663–71.
14. Azizi M, Lamarre-Cliche M, Labatide-Alanore A, et al. Physiologic consequences of vasopeptidase inhibition in humans: effect of sodium intake. J Am Soc Nephrol 2002; 13(10):2454–63.
15. Heeg JE, de Jong PE, van der Hem GK, et al. Efficacy and variability of the antiproteinuric effect of ACE inhibition. Kidney Int 1989; 36:272–9.
16. Buter H, Hemmelder MH, Navis G, et al. The blunting of the antiproteinuric efficacy of ACE inhibition by high sodium intake can be restored by hydrochlorothiazide. Nephrol Dial Transplant 1998; 13(7):1682–5.
17. Esnault VLM, Ekhlas A, Delcroix C, et al. Diuretic and enhanced sodium restriction results in improved antiproteinuric response to RAS blocking agents. J Am Soc Nephrol 2005; 16(2):474–81.
18. Laverman GD, van Goor H, Henning RH, et al. Renoprotective effects of vasopeptidase inhibition versus ACE inhibition in normotensive nephrotic rats on different sodium intakes. Kidney Int 2003; 63(1):64–71.
19. Kober L, Torp-Pedersen C, Carlsen JE, et al. A clinical trial of the angiotensin converting enzyme inhibitor trandolapril in patients with left ventricular dysfunction after myocardial infarction. Trandolapril cardiac evaluation (TRACE) study group. N Engl J Med 1995; 333(25):1670–6.
20. Westendorp B, Schoemaker RG, Buikema H, et al. Dietary sodium restriction specifically potentiates left ventricular ACE inhibition by zofenopril and is associated with attenuated hypertrofic response in rats with experimental myocardial infarction. J Renin Angiotensin Aldosterone Syst 2004; 5(1):27–31.
21. Wapstra FH, van Goor H, Navis GJ, et al. Antiproteinuric effect predicts renal protection by angiotensin converting enzyme inhibition in rats with established adriamycin nephrosis. Clin Sci 1996; 90(5):393–401.
22. Vogt L, de Zeeuw D, Waanders F, et al. Independent and combined effects of low sodium diet and diuretic on the proteinuric efficacy of the AT1 antagonist Losartan in non-diabetic proteinuric patients. Provisionally accepted. J Am Soc Nephrol 2007.
23. Vogt L, Navis GJ, de Zeeuw D. Individual titration for maximal blockade of the renin–angiotensin system in proteinuric patients: a feasible strategy? J Am Soc Nephrol 2005; 16(Suppl.1):S53–7.
24. Luik PT, Hoogenberg K, Van der Kleij FG, et al. Short term moderate sodium restriction induces relative hyperfiltration in normotensive normoalbuminuric type 1 diabetes mellitus. Diabetologia 2002; 45(4):535–41.
25. Hamming I, Navis GJ, Kocks MJA, et al. ACE inhibition has adverse renal effects during dietary sodium restriction in proteinuric and healthy rats. J Pathol 2006; 209(1):129–39.
26. Westendorp B, Hamming I, Navis GJ, et al. Adverse renal effects of hydrochlorothiazide in rats with myocardial infarction treated with ACE inhibition. J Am Soc Nephrol 2005 (Abstract).

27. Kocks MJA, Gschwend S, de Zeeuw D, et al. Low sodium modifies the vascular effects of ACE inhibitor therapy in healthy rats. J Pharmacol Exp Ther 2004; 310(3):1183–9.
28. Kuivenhoven JA, Jukema JW, Zwinderman AH, et al. The role of a common variant of the cholesteryl ester transfer protein gene in the progression of coronary atherosclerosis. The regression growth evaluation statin study group. N Engl J Med 1998; 338(2):86–93.
29. Sciarrone MT, Stella P, Barlassina C, et al. ACE and alpha-adducin polymorphism as markers of individual response to diuretic therapy. Hypertension 2003; 41(3):398–403.
30. Kramer AB, Laverman GD, van Goor H, et al. Interindividual differences in antiproteinuric response to ACEi in established adriamycin nephrotic rats are predicted by pre-treatment renal damage. J Pathol 2003; 201:160–7.
31. Lufft V, Kliem V, Hamkes A, et al. Antiproteinuric efficacy of fosinopril after renal transplantation. Clin Transpl 1998; 12:409–15.
32. Ruggenenti P, Perna A, Zoccali C, et al. Outcomes and response to treatment in a prospective cohort of 352 patients: differences between women and men in relation to the ACE gene polymorphism. Gruppo Italiano di Studi Epidemologici in Nefrologia (Gisen). J Am Soc Nephrol 2000; 11(1):88–96.
33. Arnett DK, Davis BR, Ford CE, et al. Pharmacogenetic association of the angiotensin converting enzyme insertion/deletion polymorphism on blood pressure and cardiovascular risk in relation to antihypertensive treatment. Circulation 2005; 111(25):3374–83.
34. van der Kleij FGH, Schmidt A, Navis GJ, et al. ACE I/D polymorphism and short term renal response to ACE inhibition; role of sodium status. Kidney Int 1997; 63:S23–6.
35. Lely AT, Visser F, Kocks MJA, Zuurman MW, Navis GJ. Selective blunting of blood pressure response to ACE inhibition in ACE DD genotype in healthy men. J Am Soc Nephrol 2005 (Abstract).
36. Spiering W, Kroon AA, Fuss-Lejeune MMJJ, et al. Angiotensin II sensitivity is associated with the angiotensin II type 1 receptor A1166C polymorphism in essential hypertensives on a high sodium diet. Hypertension 2000; 36(3):411–6.
37. Gonzales M, Lobos L, Castillo F, et al. High salt diet inhibits expression of angiotensin type 2 receptor in resistance arteries. Hypertension 2005; 45:853–9.
38. Nickering G, Strehlow K, Roeling J, et al. Salt induces vascular AT1 receptor overexpression in vitro and in vivo. Hypertension 1998; 31:1272–7.

23
Mineralocorticoid Antagonists in Heart Failure and Chronic Renal Failure

Nancy J. Brown
Division of Clinical Pharmacology, Departments of Medicine and Pharmacology, Vanderbilt University Medical Center, Nashville, Tennessee, U.S.A.

RATIONALE FOR MINERALOCORTICOID RECEPTOR ANTAGONISM IN CONGESTIVE HEART FAILURE

In patients with congestive heart failure (CHF), activation of the sympathetic nervous system and decreased renal perfusion result in activation of the renin–angiotensin–aldosterone system (RAAS). Increased angiotensin (Ang) II and aldosterone concentrations, in turn, lead to increased afterload and sodium and water retention, and worsening congestion. In addition to these hemodynamic effects, Ang II and aldosterone cause vascular and renal injury and ventricular remodeling and fibrosis. Since the late 1980s many randomized clinical trials have demonstrated that treatment with angiotensin-converting enzyme (ACE) inhibitors or Ang II type 1 (AT_1) receptor antagonists reduces mortality in patients with CHF (1–4). However, during chronic interruption of the RAAS with ACE inhibition, aldosterone concentrations return toward baseline or "escape" (5,6), potentially attenuating the cardiac and renal protective effects of this class of drugs. Moreover, in patients with CHF, aldosterone concentrations correlate with mortality (7).

CLINICAL TRIALS OF MR ANTAGONISTS IN CHF

These observations provided the rationale for clinical trials examining the effect of combined ACE inhibition and mineralocorticoid receptor (MR) antagonism in patients with CHF. In the Randomized Aldactone Evaluation Study (RALES), the addition of the MR antagonist spironolactone (25 mg) in patients with New York Heart Association class 3 or 4 heart failure who were already treated with an ACE inhibitor, diuretics and digoxin reduced mortality by 30% (Fig. 1) (8). The Eplerenone Neurohormonal Efficacy and Survival Study (EPHESUS) trial studied the effect of the addition of the MR antagonist eplerenone (25–50 mg/day) to standard therapy with ACE inhibitors, AT_1 receptor antagonists, β-blockers, digoxin and diuretics on the primary end points of all-cause

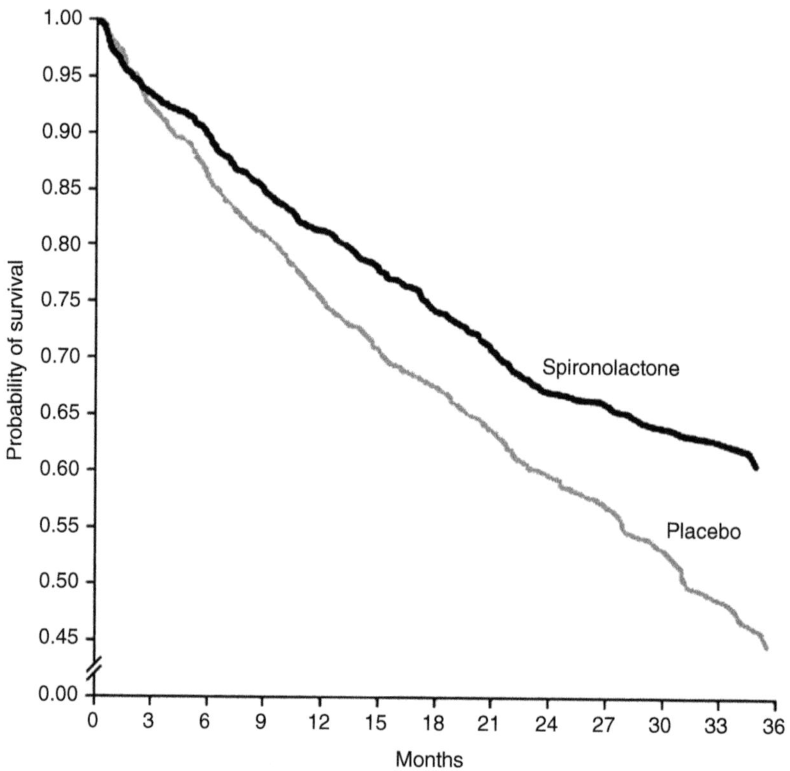

No. at risk

Placebo	841	775	723	678	628	592	565	483	379	280	179	92	36
Spironolactone	822	766	739	698	669	639	608	526	419	316	193	122	43

Figure 1 Effect of the addition of the mineralocorticoid receptor antagonist spironolactone on mortality in patients with New York Heart Association class 3 or 4 heart failure who were already treated with an angiotensin-converting enzyme inhibitor, diuretics and digoxin. *Source*: From Ref. 8.

mortality and the time to first occurrence of either cardiovascular mortality or morbidity leading to hospitalization in 6200 patients with left ventricular dysfunction (ejection fraction $<40\%$) following a recent (3–14 days) myocardial infarction (9). The addition of eplerenone resulted in reduced all-cause ($p=0.008$) and cardiovascular ($p=0.0002$) mortality (Fig. 2).

The RALES and EPHESUS trials were conducted in patients with systolic dysfunction. However, the most common cause of heart failure is diastolic dysfunction related to hypertension and left ventricular hypertrophy. The 4E-Left Ventricular Hypertrophy study compared the effects of the ACE inhibitor enalapril (40 mg/day), the MR antagonist eplerenone (200 mg/day), or combination enalapril (10 mg/day) and eplerenone (200 mg/day) (10). Both enalapril and eplerenone decreased left ventricular mass as measured by magnetic resonance imaging, but the combination ACE inhibitor/eplerenone decreased left ventricular mass to a greater degree than the MR antagonist alone. Although it is attractive to attribute this effect to increased interruption of the RAAS, systolic blood pressure was also reduced to a greater degree in the combination arm compared with the MR antagonist treatment arm.

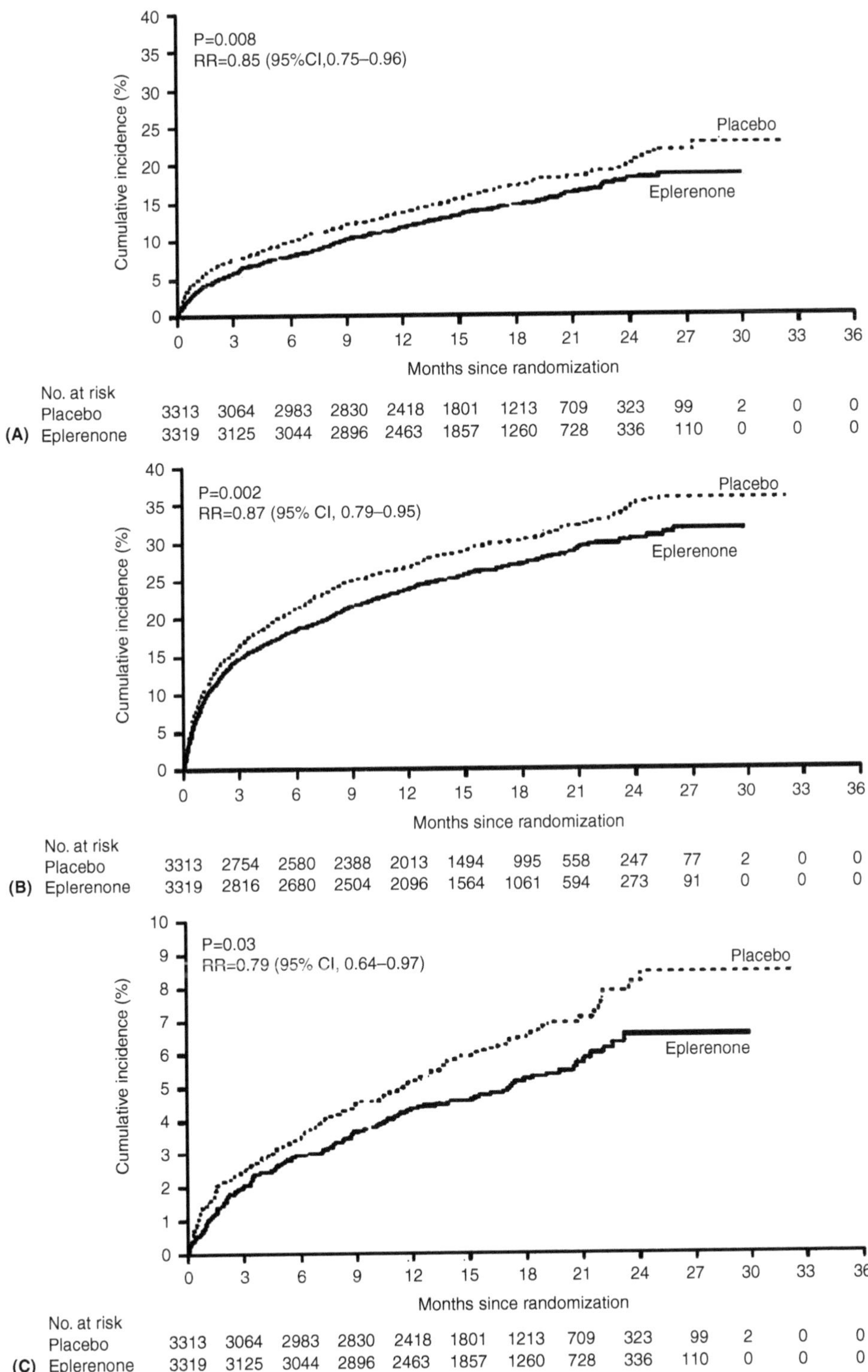

Figure 2 Effect of the addition of the mineralocorticoid receptor antagonist eplerenone on (**A**) total mortality, (**B**) cardiovascular mortality and hospitalization, and (**C**) sudden cardiac death in patients with left ventricular dysfunction following anterior myocardial infarction. *Source*: From Ref. 9.

MECHANISMS OF THE FAVORABLE EFFECT OF MR ANTAGONISTS IN CHF

Improvement in Endothelial Function

The mechanisms whereby MR antagonists reduce mortality in patients with systolic dysfunction and CHF have not been fully elucidated. Patients with CHF have impaired endothelial dysfunction as defined by vasodilation in response to sheer stress or pharmacological agonists that stimulate nitric oxide synthase (11). Impaired endothelial function is associated with decreased exercise capacity, but also with increased mortality (12). Increased aldosterone concentrations are associated with endothelial dysfunction in human hypertension (13,14) and acute aldosterone administration induces endothelial dysfunction in healthy individuals in some studies (15,16). In animal models, aldosterone infusion induces endothelial dysfunction via activation of cyclooxygenase-2 (COX-2) (17,18). Importantly, Struthers and coworkers have demonstrated that administration of an MR antagonist improves endothelial dysfunction in patients with CHF (19).

Effect on Ventricular Arrhythmias

Ventricular arrhythmias are a common cause of death in patients with CHF and may result from electrolyte imbalance in patients treated with loop diuretics. MR antagonists increase serum potassium and magnesium concentrations in patients with CHF and reduce the frequency of ventricular arrhythmias in this patient population (20). High circulating catecholamine concentrations may also contribute to the increased risk of ventricular arrhythmias and sudden death in CHF and MR antagonists increase extraneuronal norepinephrine uptake (21).

Decreased Ventricular Remodeling

In CHF, aldosterone-induced myocardial fibrosis may also promote left ventricular dysfunction and provide the substrate for arrhythmias. Chronic aldosterone infusion at doses that yield concentrations similar to those observed in CHF causes myocardial fibrosis in rat models in the setting of inappropriately high sodium (22). The development of fibrosis is preceded by coronary and myocardial inflammation characterized by monocyte and macrophage infiltration and by increased expression of inflammatory markers such as cyclooxygenase-2, osteopontin, monocyte chemoattractant protein-1 and intracellular adhesion molecule-1 (23,24). Both the inflammatory changes and subsequent fibrosis can be blocked by MR antagonism (22,25).

Aldosterone can induce the expression of several profibrotic molecules that may contribute to the pathogenesis of heart failure. For example, aldosterone induces transforming growth factor (TGF)-β_1 expression in cultured cardiomyocytes (26) and in vivo in the heart in some studies (24,27). TGF-β_1 could contribute to cardiac fibrosis both by increasing extracellular matrix (ECM) production and by blocking matrix degradation (28). In addition, TGF-β_1 can induce the expression of plasminogen activator inhibitor-1 (PAI-1) (29). PAI-1, a member of the serpin (serine protease inhibitor) superfamily and the major physiological inhibitor of tissue-type plasminogen activator and urokinase plasminogen activator in vivo, can in turn promote fibrosis by decreasing both direct and indirect effects of plasmin on ECM (30). Treatment of mice or rats with aldosterone increases cardiac PAI-1 expression, whereas MR antagonism reduces cardiac PAI-1 expression (24,31). MR antagonism reduces circulating PAI-1 concentrations in individuals with hypertension (Fig. 3) (32).

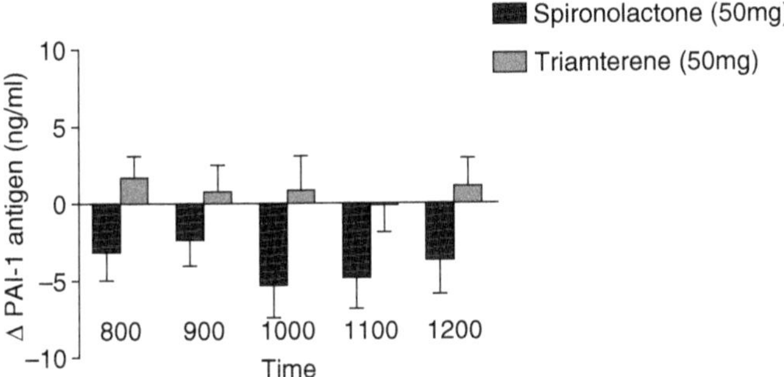

Figure 3 Effect of the mineralocorticoid receptor antagonist spironolactone versus the mineralocorticoid receptor-independent potassium-sparing diuretic triamterene on circulating PAI-1 concentrations in patients with hypertension. *Abbreviation*: PAI-1, plasminogen activator inhibitor-1.

Based on these findings, one might predict that PAI-1 deficiency would decrease aldosterone-induced cardiac fibrosis. Indeed, genetic PAI-1 deficiency protects against bleomycin-induced pulmonary fibrosis and treatment of PAI-1 knockout mice with tranexamic acid, an inhibitor of plasmin formation, reverses the protective effect of PAI-1 deficiency (33,34). As outlined below, PAI-1 deficiency also protects against renal injury in various animal models (35). PAI-1 knockout mice are protected against N-nitro-L-arginine (L-NAME)-induced perivascular fibrosis (36), as well as against the development of hypertension. In addition, several groups have reported that PAI-1 deficiency protects against perivascular cardiac fibrosis in rodent models of myocardial infarction (37). However, paradoxically, genetic PAI-1 deficiency increases Ang II- and aldosterone-induced cardiac fibrosis, as well as the expression of proinflammatory genes (38,39).

EVIDENCE THAT MR ANTAGONISM DECREASES CARDIOVASCULAR REMODELING IN CLINICAL TRIALS

Evidence for a favorable effect of MR antagonism on ventricular remodeling in patients with CHF derives from clinical trials that have investigated the effect of MR antagonism on serological markers of collagen turnover and mortality (40,41). For example, in RALES, elevated concentrations of procollagen type III amino-terminal peptide (PIIINP), a biochemical marker of myocardial fibrosis (42), were associated with an increased risk of death. Spironolactone significantly decreased procollagen type I amino-terminal peptide, procollagen type I carboxy-terminal peptide and PIIINP. Moreover, the effect of spironolactone on mortality was significant only in patients whose baseline markers of collagen turnover were above the median concentration. In a related study, patients with an acute anterior myocardial infarction treated with spironolactone had a significantly greater increase in left ventricular ejection fraction and significantly decreased circulating PIIINP concentrations compared with placebo-treated patients; PIIINP concentrations correlated significantly with left ventricular end-diastolic volume index (41). These studies support the hypothesis that aldosterone receptor antagonism affects ECM turnover in humans.

ROLE OF ALDOSTERONE IN THE PROGRESSION OF RENAL INJURY

The RAAS plays an important role in the progression to end-stage renal disease regardless of the inciting insult (43). Ang II causes endothelial and mesangial cell injury and fibrosis independent of hemodynamic effects (44). That interruption of the RAAS by ACE inhibition or AT_1 receptor antagonism slows the progression of renal damage in diabetic nephropathy has been well established in both animal models and clinical trials (45–48). Evidence for the contribution of aldosterone to renal injury during activation of the RAAS, stems from a seminal study of Hostetter and co-workers in the remnant kidney rat, a model associated with activation of the RAAS (49). In this study, treatment with an ACE inhibitor and an AT_1 receptor antagonist significantly decreased aldosterone concentrations, hypertension, proteinuria, and glomerular sclerosis. However, administration of aldosterone reversed the protective effects of ACE inhibition and AT_1 receptor antagonism. More recently, investigators have shown that MR antagonism decreases renal injury in animal models of hypertension such as the stroke-prone spontaneously hypertensive rat (50), nitric oxide synthase inhibitor-treated rats (51), and diabetic models such as streptozotocin-treated rats (52).

As in the heart, the mechanism through which aldosterone induces renal injury involves the generation of reactive oxygen species (53) and increased expression of inflammatory mediators (54). As in the heart too, the pathways involved in the progression from inflammation to glomerulosclerosis and tubulointerstitial fibrosis have not been fully delineated. Aldosterone induces mesangial cell proliferation in vitro and in vivo through a pathway that appears to involve reactive oxygen species and the activation of the mitogen-activated protein kinase 1/2, cyclin D1 and cyclin A pathway (53,55). Aldosterone induces the synthesis of type IV collagen, the principal component of glomerular basement membrane and matrix, in cultured glomerular cells (56). Aldosterone induces PAI-1 expression in the kidney (39). PAI-1 has been implicated in the pathogenesis of other forms of glomerulosclerosis and tubulointerstitial fibrosis (57–59). MR antagonism decreases PAI-1 expression and glomerular injury in parallel in a rat radiation injury model (60), as well as in streptozotocin-induced diabetic nephropathy (52). In addition, genetic PAI-1 deficiency protects against aldosterone-induced glomerular injury (39).

Increased expression of TGF-β_1 may also contribute to aldosterone-induced renal injury. Aldosterone has been reported to increase TGF-β_1 in a few studies (52). In addition, aldosterone may increase TGF-β_1 through a MR-dependent, potassium-independent posttranscriptional mechanism. TGF-β_1 had been implicated in the pathogenesis of renal injury in several animal models (61–63). TGF-β_1 may induce fibrosis in part by increasing PAI-1 expression; however, data obtained in β6 integrin-null mice treated with unilateral ureteral obstruction indicate that aldosterone can induce both PAI-1 expression and interstitial fibrosis through a TGF-β_1-independent pathway (64).

CLINICAL STUDIES ON THE EFFECT OF MR ANTAGONISM IN RENAL DISEASE

While ACE inhibitors and AT_1 receptor antagonists slow the progression of diabetic and nondiabetic nephropathy, albuminuria can return to baseline levels with chronic therapy (65). Interestingly, escape from the renoprotective effects of ACE inhibitors has also been associated with aldosterone escape in patients with type 2 mellitus (66).

Several studies have examined the effect of MR antagonism on microalbuminuria in individuals with essential hypertension. In addition to portending progression to renal insufficiency, urinary albumin excretion has been associated with an increased risk of cardiovascular events (67). In the aforementioned 4E study, combination treatment with the ACE inhibitor enalapril and the MR antagonist eplerenone reduced the urine albumin-to-creatinine ratio (UACR) to a significantly greater degree than did either eplerenone or enalapril alone (10). Again, it is not possible to conclude whether this renoprotective effect of combination ACE inhibition/MR antagonism resulted from interruption of the RAAS or superior blood pressure reduction. However, in a study of patients with mild-to-moderate hypertension, eplerenone (50–200 mg/day) reduced urine albumin excretion to a significantly greater extent than did enalapril (10–40 mg) despite equivalent effects of the two drugs on blood pressure (68). Similarly, in older patients with systolic hypertension, eplerenone reduced urine albumin to a greater extent than did amlodipine at comparable hypotensive doses (69).

Likewise, MR antagonism reduces microalbuminuria in patients with mild diabetic nephropathy. For example, Sato et al. reported that addition of the MR antagonist spironolactone (25 mg/day) in patients with type 2 diabetes with aldosterone escape reduced significantly urinary albumin excretion without affecting blood pressure (66). Rachmani et al. reported the effect of randomized treatment with either spironolactone (100 mg/day) or the ACE inhibitor cilazapril (5 mg/day) on a background of atenolol and hydrochlorothiazide in a group of hypertensive, postmenopausal female diabetic patients (70). Despite equivalent effects on blood pressure and hemoglobin A_1C, spironolactone reduced urinary albumin excretion to a greater extent than did cilazapril. Moreover, addition of spironolactone enhanced the effect of cilazapril on urine albumin excretion when both groups were crossed over to combination therapy with spironolactone and cilazapril at the end of the study. In patients with type 2 diabetes, eplerenone (50–200 mg/day), enalapril (10–40 mg/day), and eplerenone + enalapril (10 mg) reduced UACR 62% ($p=0.015$ vs. enalapril), 42%, and 74% ($p=0.018$ vs. eplerenone and $p<0.001$ vs. enalapril), respectively (71).

More recent studies have examined the effect of adjuvant MR antagonism on renal function in patients with more overt proteinuria or renal insufficiency. For example, in patients with residual proteinuria despite ACE inhibition and blood pressure control, the addition of spironolactone (25 mg/day) significantly reduced proteinuria and urinary excretion of type IV collagen, a potential marker of renal collagen turnover, without affecting blood pressure (Fig. 4) (72). In patients with depressed glomerular function, treated with ACE inhibitors and/or AT_1 receptor antagonists, the addition of spironolactone (25 mg/day) significantly reduced urinary protein excretion through a blood pressure–independent mechanism (73).

Taken together, these clinical studies suggest that MR antagonism reduces urine albumin excretion in hypertension, mild diabetic nephropathy, and mild-to-moderate chronic renal disease. However, whereas ACE inhibition and AT_1 receptor antagonism have been demonstrated to improve outcomes in patients with renal disease, the effect of MR antagonism on progression to end-stage renal disease and mortality has yet to be determined.

PHARMACOLOGY OF MR ANTAGONISTS IN HEART FAILURE AND CHRONIC RENAL FAILURE

Figure 5 illustrates the chemical structure of the MR antagonists, spironolactone and eplerenone. Eplerenone, pregn-4-ene-7,21-dicarboxylic acid, 9,11-epoxy-17-hydroxy-3-oxo, γ-lactone, methyl ester (7α,11α,17α), was derived from spironolactone by the

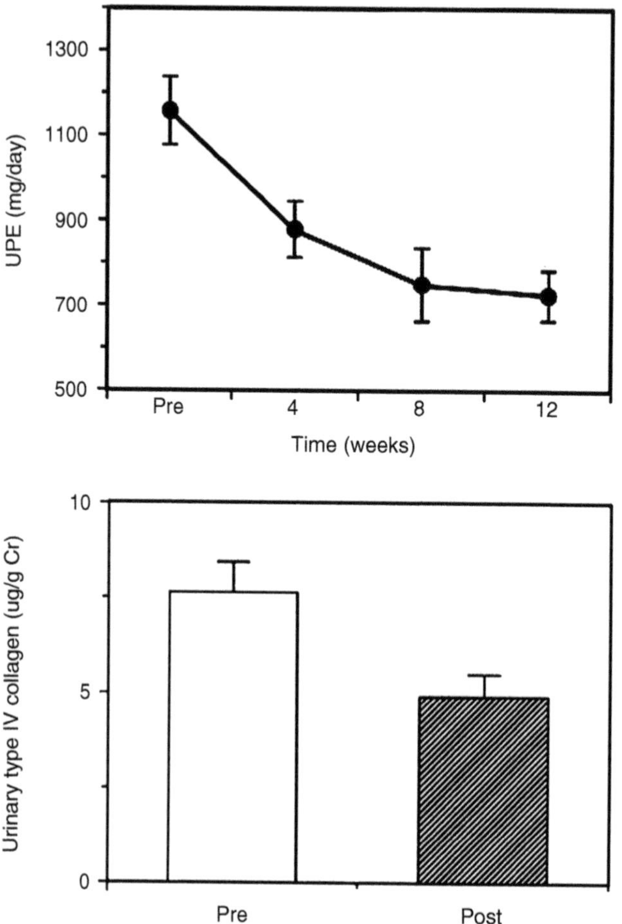

Figure 4 (*Top*) Effect of the addition of spironolactone on UPE in patients with chronic renal disease treated with angiotensin-converting enzyme inhibitor or AT_1 receptor antagonist. (*Bottom*) Effect of spironolactone on urinary collagen IV excretion in the same group of patients. *Abbreviation*: UPE, urinary protein excretion. *Source*: From Ref. 72.

introduction of a 9α,11α-epoxy bridge and by substitution of the 17α-thioacetyl group of spironolactone with a carbomethoxy group (74). The substitution of the 17α-thioacetyl group confers eplerenone with significantly increased selectivity for the aldosterone receptor over other steroid receptors. For example, in rats the IC_{50} of eplerenone for the aldosterone receptor was 360 nM, whereas the IC_{50}s half-maximal inhibitory concentration for the androgen, progesterone and estrogen receptors were >10,000 nM. In clinical trials, the increased specificity of eplerenone compared with spironolactone manifests in lower rates of progesterone-related side effects such as gynecomastia—e.g., 0.5% in EPHESUS (9) versus 10% in RALES (8).

While eplerenone exhibits 10- to 20-fold lower affinity for the aldosterone receptor in vitro compared with spironolactone (74), studies in humans suggest that eplerenone is 50% to 75% as potent as spironolactone (75). Mean peak concentrations are reached approximately 1.5 hours following oral administration of eplerenone in humans (data on file, GD Searle LLC, Pfizer Inc., New York, New York, U.S.A.). Eplerenone is cleared

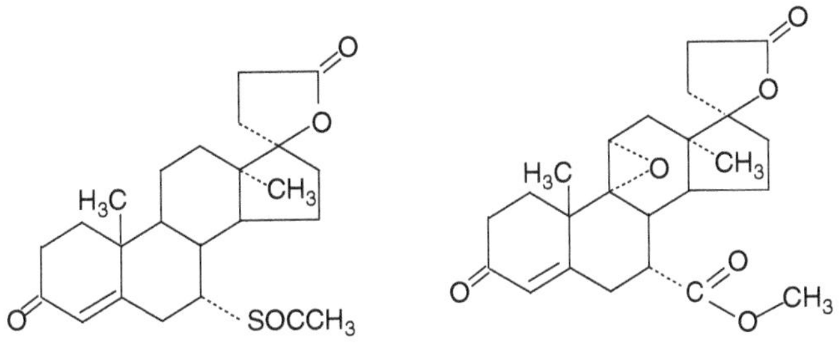

Figure 5 Chemical structures of spironolactone (*left*) and eplerenone (*right*).

primarily via metabolism by CYP4503A4 to inactive metabolites, with an elimination half-life of four to six hours (76). By comparison, spironolactone is converted to the active metabolites, canrenoate and canrenone, which have half-lives between 17 and 22 hours (77). Thus, while both spironolactone and eplerenone may be given once daily, twice-a-day dosing may provide better 24-hour MR antagonism with eplerenone.

SIDE EFFECTS RELATED TO THE USE OF MR ANTAGONISTS

An important side effect of both spironolactone and eplerenone, particularly in combination with ACE inhibition or AT_1 receptor antagonism, is hyperkalemia. The risk of hyperkalemia may be reduced by the concurrent use of loop diuretics, as in patients with CHF. On the other hand, the risk of hyperkalemia is increased in patients with renal insufficiency or diabetes, in which patients may also have a type IV renal tubular acidosis. In the study by Rachmani et al., 15% of hypertensive women with type 2 diabetes developed hyperkalemia during combined spironolactone/cilazapril therapy (70). Sato reported no effect on serum potassium and no hyperkalemia in type 2 diabetic patients with proteinuria but normal creatinine clearance treated with ACE inhibitor and spironolactone (72). On the other hand, Bianchi et al. reported a significant increase in serum potassium from patients with chronic renal disease treated with ACE inhibitor or AT_1 receptor antagonist.

Patients with renal insufficiency and diabetes were excluded from clinical trials of eplerenone in hypertension. However, rates of hyperkalemia, defined as a serum potassium >5.5 mmol/L, as a function of calculated creatinine clearance have been analyzed across all studies at the time of drug approval and were 2.6%, 5.6%, and 10.4% in patients with baseline creatinine clearances >100 mL/min, 70 to 100 mL/min, and <70 mL/min, respectively (data on file, GD Searle LLC). In a study of patients with type 2 diabetes and microalbuminuria, the frequency of hyperkalemia was 33% in patients receiving eplerenone 200 mg/day and 38% in patients receiving eplerenone and the ACE inhibitor enalapril.

SUMMARY

Increased aldosterone concentrations may cause cardiac dysfunction and glomerular injury by affecting electrolyte and volume homeostasis, by inducing endothelial dysfunction, and by causing inflammation and fibrosis. While ACE inhibitors and AT_1 receptor antagonists improve outcomes in patients with CHF and nephropathy, aldosterone concentrations escape with chronic treatment. The addition of MR antagonism reduces mortality in patients with CHF. MR antagonism reduces proteinuria, although the effect on mortality remains to be determined in chronic renal failure. MR antagonists must be used with caution in combination with ACE inhibitors and AT_1 receptor antagonists as they can cause serious hyperkalemia.

REFERENCES

1. Pfeffer MA, Braunwald EA, Moye LA, Basta L, Brown EJ, Jr., Cuddy TE, Davis BR, Geltman EM, Goldman S, Flaker GC, et al. Effect of captopril on mortality and morbidity in patients with left ventricular dysfunction after myocardial infarction. N Engl J Med 1992; 327:669–77.
2. Yusuf S, Pepine CJ, Garces C, et al. Effect of enalapril on myocardial infarction and unstable angina in patients with low ejection fractions. Lancet 1992; 340:1173–8.
3. Cohn JN, Tognoni G, Valsartan Heart Failure Trial Investigators. A randomized trial of the angiotensin-receptor blocker valsartan in chronic heart failure. N Engl J Med 2001; 345:1667–75.
4. Pfeffer MA, Swedberg K, Granger CB, et al. Effects of candesartan on mortality and morbidity in patients with chronic heart failure: the CHARM-Overall programme. Lancet 2003; 362:759–66.
5. Lijnen P, Staessen J, Fagard R, Amery A. Increase in plasma aldosterone during prolonged captopril treatment. Am J Cardiol 1982; 49:1561–3.
6. McKelvie RS, Yusuf S, Pericak D, Avezum A, Burns RJ, Probstfield J, Tsuyuki RT, White M, Rouleau J, Latini R, et al. Comparison of candesartan, enalapril, and their combination in congestive heart failure: randomized evaluation of strategies for left ventricular dysfunction (RESOLVD) pilot study. The RESOLVD Pilot Study Investigators. Circulation 1999; 100:1056–64.
7. Swedberg K, Eneroth P, Kjekshus J, Wilhelmsen L. Hormones regulating cardiovascular function in patients with severe congestive heart failure and their relation to mortality. CONSENSUS Trial Study Group. Circulation 1990; 82:1730–6.
8. Pitt B, Zannad F, Remme WJ, et al. The effect of spironolactone on morbidity and mortality in patients with severe heart failure. N Engl J Med 1999; 341:709–17.
9. Pitt B, Remme W, Zannad F, et al. Eplerenone, a selective aldosterone blocker, in patients with left ventricular dysfunction after myocardial infarction. N Engl J Med 2003; 348:1309.
10. Pitt B, Reichek N, Willenbrock R, et al. Effects of eplerenone, enalapril, and eplerenone/enalapril in patients with essential hypertension and left ventricular hypertrophy: the 4E-left ventricular hypertrophy study. Circulation 2003; 108:1831–8.
11. Drexler H, Hayoz D, Munzel T, Just H, Zelis R, Brunner HR. Endothelial dysfunction in chronic heart failure. Experimental and clinical studies. Arzneimittelforschung 1994; 44:455–8.
12. Bauersachs J, Schafer A. Endothelial dysfunction in heart failure: mechanisms and therapeutic approaches. Curr Vasc Pharmacol 2004; 2:115–24.
13. Taddei S, Virdis A, Mattei P, Salvetti A. Vasodilation to acetylcholine in primary and secondary forms of human hypertension. Hypertension 1993; 21:929–33.
14. Nishizaka MK, Zaman MA, Green SA, Renfroe KY, Calhoun DA. Impaired endothelium-dependent flow-mediated vasodilation in hypertensive subjects with hyperaldosteronism. Circulation 2004; 109:2857–61.
15. Farquharson CA, Struthers AD. Aldosterone induces acute endothelial dysfunction in vivo in humans: evidence for an aldosterone-induced vasculopathy. Clin Sci (Lond) 2002; 103:425–31.
16. Romagni P, Rossi F, Guerrini L, Quirini C, Santiemma V. Aldosterone induces contraction of the resistance arteries in man. Atherosclerosis 2003; 166:345–9.
17. Iglarz M, Touyz RM, Viel EC, Amiri F, Schiffrin EL. Involvement of oxidative stress in the profibrotic action of aldosterone. Interaction with the renin–angiotension system 6. Am J Hypertens 2004; 17:597–603.

18. Blanco-Rivero J, Cachofeiro V, Lahera V, et al. Participation of prostacyclin in endothelial dysfunction induced by aldosterone in normotensive and hypertensive rats. Hypertension 2005; 46:107–12.
19. Farquharson CA, Struthers AD. Spironolactone increases nitric oxide bioactivity, improves endothelial vasodilator dysfunction, and suppresses vascular angiotensin I/angiotensin II conversion in patients with chronic heart failure. Circulation 2000; 101:594–7.
20. Ramires FJ, Mansur A, Coelho O, et al. Effect of spironolactone on ventricular arrhythmias in congestive heart failure secondary to idiopathic dilated or to ischemic cardiomyopathy. Am J Cardiol 2000; 85:1207–11.
21. Barr CS, Lang CC, Hanson J, Arnott M, Kennedy N, Struthers AD. Effects of adding spironolactone to an angiotensin-converting enzyme inhibitor in chronic congestive heart failure secondary to coronary artery disease. Am J Cardiol 1995; 76:1259–65.
22. Brilla CG, Weber KT. Mineralocorticoid excess, dietary sodium, and myocardial fibrosis. J Lab Clin Med 1992; 120:893–901.
23. Rocha R, Stier CTJ, Kifor I, et al. Aldosterone: a mediator of myocardial necrosis and renal arteriopathy. Endocrinology 2000; 141:3871–8.
24. Sun Y, Zhang J, Lu L, Bedigian MP, Robinson AD, Weber KT. Tissue angiotensin II in the regulation of inflammatory and fibrogenic components of repair in the rat heart. J Lab Clin Med 2004; 143:41–51.
25. Rocha R, Martin-Berger CL, Yang P, Scherrer R, Delyani J, McMahon E. Selective aldosterone blockade prevents angiotensin II/salt-induced vascular inflammation in the rat heart. Endocrinology 2002; 143:4828–36.
26. Chun TY, Bloem LJ, Pratt JH. Aldosterone inhibits inducible nitric oxide synthase in neonatal rat cardiomyocytes. Endocrinology 2003; 144:1712–7.
27. Wahed MI, Watanabe K, Ma M, et al. Effects of eplerenone, a selective aldosterone blocker, on the progression of left ventricular dysfunction and remodeling in rats with dilated cardiomyopathy. Pharmacology 2005; 73:81–8.
28. Noble NA, Harper JR, Border WA. In vivo interactions of TGF-beta and extracellular matrix. Prog Growth Factor Res 1992; 4:369–82.
29. Dennler S, Itoh S, Vivien D, ten Dijke P, Huet S, Gauthier JM. Direct binding of Smad3 and Smad4 to critical TGF beta-inducible elements in the promoter of human plasminogen activator inhibitor-type 1 gene. EMBO J 1998; 17:3091–100.
30. Gils A, Declerck PJ. Plasminogen activator inhibitor-1. Curr Med Chem 2004; 11:2323–34.
31. Oestreicher EM, Martinez-Vasquez D, Stone JR, et al. Aldosterone and not plasminogen activator inhibitor-1 is a critical mediator of early angiotensin II/NG-nitro-L-arginine methyl ester-induced myocardial injury. Circulation 2003; 108:2517–23.
32. Ma J, Albornoz F, Yu C, Byrne DW, Vaughan DE, Brown NJ. Differing effects of mineralocorticoid receptor-dependent and -independent potassium-sparing diuretics on fibrinolytic balance. Hypertension 2005; 46:313–20.
33. Eitzman DT, McCoy RD, Zheng X, et al. Bleomycin-induced pulmonary fibrosis in transgenic mice that either lack or overexpress the murine plasminogen activator inhibitor-1 gene. J Clin Invest 1996; 97:232–7.
34. Hattori N, Degen JL, Sisson TH, et al. Bleomycin-induced pulmonary fibrosis in fibrinogen-null mice. J Clin Invest 2000; 106:1341–50.
35. Eddy AA. Plasminogen activator inhibitor-1 and the kidney. Am J Physiol Renal Physiol 2002; 283:F209–20.
36. Kaikita K, Fogo AB, Ma L, Schoenhard JA, Brown NJ, Vaughan DE. Plasminogen activator inhibitor-1 deficiency prevents hypertension and vascular fibrosis in response to long-term nitric oxide synthase inhibition. Circulation 2001; 104:839–44.
37. Takeshita K, Hayashi M, Iino S, et al. Increased expression of plasminogen activator inhibitor-1 in cardiomyocytes contributes to cardiac fibrosis after myocardial infarction. Am J Pathol 2004; 164:449–56.

38. Weisberg AD, Albornoz F, Griffin JP, et al. Pharmacological inhibition and genetic deficiency of plasminogen activator inhibitor-1 attenuates angiotensin II/salt-induced aortic remodeling. Arterioscler Thromb Vasc Biol 2005; 25:365–71.
39. Ma J, Weisberg A, Griffin JP, Vaughan DE, Fogo AB, Brown NJ. Plasminogen activator inhibitor-1 deficiency protects against aldosterone-induced renal injury. Hypertension 2004; 44:514.
40. Zannad F, Alla F, Dousset B, Perez A, Pitt B. Limitation of excessive extracellular matrix turnover may contribute to survival benefit of spironolactone therapy in patients with congestive heart failure: insights from the randomized aldactone evaluation study (RALES). Rales Investigators. Circulation 2000; 102:2700–6.
41. Hayashi M, Tsutamoto T, Wada A, et al. Immediate administration of mineralocorticoid receptor antagonist spironolactone prevents post-infarct left ventricular remodeling associated with suppression of a marker of myocardial collagen synthesis in patients with first anterior acute myocardial infarction. Circulation 2003; 107:2559–65.
42. Poulsen SH, Host NB, Jensen SE, Egstrup K. Relationship between serum amino-terminal propeptide of type III procollagen and changes of left ventricular function after acute myocardial infarction. Circulation 2000; 101:1527–32.
43. Ibrahim HN, Rosenberg ME, Hostetter TH. Role of the renin–angiotensin–aldosterone system in the progression of renal disease: a critical review. Semin Nephrol 1997; 17:431–40.
44. Ichikawa I, Brenner BM. Glomerular actions of angiotensin II. Am J Med 1984; 76:43–9.
45. Lewis EJ, Hunsicker LG, Bain RP, Rohde RD. The effect of angiotensin-converting-enzyme inhibition on diabetic nephropathy. The Collaborative Study Group. N Engl J Med 1993; 329:1456–62.
46. Agodoa LY, Appel L, Bakris GL, Beck G, Bourgoignie J, Briggs JP, Charleston J, Cheek D, Cleveland W, Douglas JG, et al. Effect of ramipril vs. amlodipine on renal outcomes in hypertensive nephrosclerosis: a randomized controlled trial. JAMA 2001; 285:2719–28.
47. Lewis EJ, Hunsicker LG, Clarke WR, et al. Renoprotective effect of the angiotensin-receptor antagonist irbesartan in patients with nephropathy due to type 2 diabetes. N Engl J Med 2001; 345:851–60 (see comments).
48. Brenner BM, Cooper ME, de ZD, et al. Effects of losartan on renal and cardiovascular outcomes in patients with type 2 diabetes and nephropathy. N Engl J Med 2001; 345:861–9.
49. Hostetter TH, Olson HG, Rennke MA, Venkatachalam MA, Brenner BM. Hyperfiltration in remnant nephrons: a potentially adverse response to renal ablation. Am J Physiol 1981; 241:F85–93.
50. Rocha R, Chander PN, Zuckerman A, Stier CT, Jr. Role of aldosterone in renal vascular injury in stroke-prone hypertensive rats. Hypertension 1999; 33:232–7.
51. Zhou X, Ono H, Ono Y, Frohlich ED. Aldosterone antagonism ameliorates proteinuria and nephrosclerosis independent of glomerular dynamics in L-NAME/SHR model. Am J Nephrol 2004; 24:242–9.
52. Fujisawa G, Okada K, Muto S, et al. Spironolactone prevents early renal injury in streptozotocin-induced diabetic rats. Kidney Int 2004; 66:1493–502.
53. Nishiyama A, Yao L, Nagai Y, et al. Possible contributions of reactive oxygen species and mitogen-activated protein kinase to renal injury in aldosterone/salt-induced hypertensive rats. Hypertension 2004; 43:841–8.
54. Blasi ER, Rocha R, Rudolph AE, Blomme EA, Polly ML, McMahon EG. Aldosterone/salt induces renal inflammation and fibrosis in hypertensive rats. Kidney Int 2003; 63:1791–800.
55. Terada Y, Kobayashi T, Kuwana H, et al. Aldosterone stimulates proliferation of mesangial cells by activating mitogen-activated protein kinase 1/2, cyclin d1, and cyclin a. J Am Soc Nephrol 2005; 16:2296–305.
56. Wakisaka M, Spiro MJ, Spiro RG. Synthesis of type VI collagen by cultured glomerular cells and comparison of its regulation by glucose and other factors with that of type IV collagen. Diabetes 1994; 43:95–103.

57. Oda T, Jung YO, Kim HS, et al. PAI-1 deficiency attenuates the fibrogenic response to ureteral obstruction. Kidney Int 2001; 60:587–96.
58. Matsuo S, Lopez-Guisa JM, Cai X, et al. Multifunctionality of PAI-1 in fibrogenesis: evidence from obstructive nephropathy in PAI-1-overexpressing mice. Kidney Int 2005; 67:2221–38.
59. Huang Y, Haraguchi M, Lawrence DA, Border WA, Yu L, Noble NA. A mutant, noninhibitory plasminogen activator inhibitor type 1 decreases matrix accumulation in experimental glomerulonephritis. J Clin Invest 2003; 112:379–88.
60. Brown NJ, Nakamura S, Ma L-J, et al. Aldosterone modulates plasminogen activator inhibitor-1 and glomerulosclerosis in vivo. Kidney Int 2000; 58:1219–27.
61. Yu L, Border WA, Anderson I, McCourt M, Huang Y, Noble NA. Combining TGF-beta inhibition and angiotensin II blockade results in enhanced antifibrotic effect. Kidney Int 2004; 66:1774–84.
62. Ma LJ, Jha S, Ling H, Pozzi A, Ledbetter S, Fogo AB. Divergent effects of low versus high dose anti-TGF-beta antibody in puromycin aminonucleoside nephropathy in rats 21. Kidney Int 2004; 65:106–15.
63. Grygielko ET, Martin WM, Tweed C, et al. Inhibition of gene markers of fibrosis with a novel inhibitor of transforming growth factor-beta type I receptor kinase in puromycin-induced nephritis. J Pharmacol Exp Ther 2005; 313:943–51.
64. Ma LJ, Yang H, Gaspert A, et al. Transforming growth factor-beta-dependent and -independent pathways of induction of tubulointerstitial fibrosis in beta6(−/−) mice. Am J Pathol 2003; 163:1261–73.
65. Shiigai T, Shichiri M. Late escape from the antiproteinuric effect of ace inhibitors in nondiabetic renal disease. Am J Kidney Dis 2001; 37:477–83.
66. Sato A, Hayashi K, Naruse M, Saruta T. Effectiveness of aldosterone blockade in patients with diabetic nephropathy. Hypertension 2003; 41:64–8.
67. Gerstein HC, Mann JF, Yi Q, et al. Albuminuria and risk of cardiovascular events, death, and heart failure in diabetic and nondiabetic individuals. JAMA 2001; 286:421–6.
68. Williams GH, Burgess E, Kolloch RE, et al. Efficacy of eplerenone versus enalapril as monotherapy in systemic hypertension. Am J Cardiol 2004; 93:990–6.
69. White WB, Duprez D, St Hillaire R, et al. Effects of the selective aldosterone blocker eplerenone versus the calcium antagonist amlodipine in systolic hypertension. Hypertension 2003; 41:1021–6.
70. Rachmani R, Slavachevsky I, Amit M, et al. The effect of spironolactone, cilazapril and their combination on albuminuria in patients with hypertension and diabetic nephropathy is independent of blood pressure reduction: a randomized controlled study. Diabet Med 2004; 21:471–5.
71. Coats AJ. Exciting new drugs on the horizon—eplerenone, a selective aldosterone receptor antagonist (SARA). Int J Cardiol 2001; 80:1–4.
72. Sato A, Hayashi K, Saruta T. Antiproteinuric effects of mineralocorticoid receptor blockade in patients with chronic renal disease. Am J Hypertens 2005; 18:44–9.
73. Bianchi S, Bigazzi R, Campese VM. Antagonists of aldosterone and proteinuria in patients with CKD: an uncontrolled pilot study. Am J Kidney Dis 2005; 46:45–51.
74. deGasparo M, Joss U, Ramjoue HP, et al. Three new epoxy-spirolactone derivatives: characterization in vivo and in vitro. J Pharmacol Exp Ther 1987; 240:650–6.
75. Weinberger MH, Roniker B, Krause SL, Weiss RJ. Eplerenone, a selective aldosterone blocker, in mild-to-moderate hypertension. Am J Hypertens 2002; 15:709–16.
76. Cook CS, Berry LM, Kim DH, Burton EG, Hribar JD, Zhang L. Involvement of CYP3A in the metabolism of eplerenone in humans and dogs: differential metabolism by CYP3A4 and CYP3A5. Drug Metab Dispos 2002; 30:1344–51.
77. Sadee W, Dagcioglu M, Schroder R. Pharmacokinetics of spironolactone, canrenone and canrenoate-K in humans. J Pharmacol Exp Ther 1973; 185:686–95.

Index

Milton Keynes UK
Ingram Content Group UK Ltd.
UKHW052023071024
449327UK00027B/2403